"Good Tuberculosis Men":
The Army Medical Department's Struggle with Tuberculosis

For sale by the Superintendent of Documents, U.S. Government Printing Office
Internet: bookstore.gpo.gov   Phone: toll free (866) 512-1800;   DC area (202) 512-1800
Fax: (202) 512-2104 Mail: Stop IDCC, Washington, DC 20402-0001

ISBN 978-0-16-092198-8

"Good Tuberculosis Men": The Army Medical Department's Struggle with Tuberculosis

Carol R. Byerly

Borden Institute
Daniel E. Banks, MD, MS, MACP
LTC MC USA
Director & Editor-in-Chief

Editorial Staff: Linette Sparacino
Volume Editor

Douglas Wise
Senior Layout Editor

Gayle Mueller
Layout Editor

Marcia Metzger
Technical Editor

The opinions or assertions contained herein are the personal views of the authors and are not to be construed as doctrine of the Department of the Army or the Department of Defense.

CERTAIN PARTS OF THIS PUBLICATION PERTAIN TO COPYRIGHT RESTRICTIONS. ALL RIGHTS RESERVED.

NO COPYRIGHTED PARTS OF THIS PUBLICATION MAY BE REPRODUCED OR TRANSMITTED IN ANY FORM OR BY ANY MEANS, ELECTRONIC OR MECHANICAL (INCLUDING PHOTOCOPY, RECORDING, OR ANY INFORMATION STORAGE AND RETRIEVAL SYSTEM), WITHOUT PERMISSION IN WRITING FROM THE PUBLISHER OR COPYRIGHT OWNER.

Published by the Office of The Surgeon General
Borden Institute
U.S. Army Medical Department Center and School
Fort Sam Houston, Texas 78234-6100

Library of Congress Cataloging-in-Publication Data
Byerly, Carol R.
  Good tuberculosis men : the Army Medical Department's struggle with tuberculosis / Carol R. Byerly.
     pages cm.
  Includes bibliographical references and index.
  1. Tuberculosis--United States--History. 2. Medicine, Military--United States--History. 3. World War, 1939-1945--Medical care. 4. World War, 1914-1918--Medical care. I. Title.
  RC313.A2B94 2013
  614.5'4209--dc23
                    2013033607

PRINTED IN THE UNITED STATES OF AMERICA
20, 19, 18, 17, 16, 15, 14, 13   5 4 3 2 1

Contents

Acknowledgments	vii
Foreword	xi
Introduction	xiii

Chapter One
    The Early Years: Fort Bayard, New Mexico   1

Chapter Two
    Life at Fort Bayard   39

Chapter Three
    The Congressman as Tuberculosis Patient   85

Chapter Four
    Tuberculosis in World War I   105

Chapter Five
    "A Gigantic Task": Treating and Paying for Tuberculosis in the Interwar Period   155

Chapter Six
    "Good Tuberculosis Women": Tuberculosis Nursing during the Interwar Period   205

Chapter Seven
    Surviving the Great Depression: Fitzsimons and the New Deal   233

Chapter Eight
    Camp Follower: Tuberculosis in World War II   273

Chapter Nine
    Miracle Drugs?   315

Selected Bibliography   xxix

Index   xli

Acknowledgments

This book began as a history of the Fitzsimons Army Medical Center in Denver, in operation from 1918 to 1996, but soon grew into a more expansive study of the Army Medical Department's experience with tuberculosis. John T. Greenwood, Ph.D., director, and Colonel (Col.) William T. (Tom) Gray, (ret.), of the Office of Medical History of the Office of The Surgeon General, US Army, supported this project financially and encouraged me at every step. They, along with the Office of Medical History staff, enabled me to explore a wide range of primary sources to tell the Army tuberculosis story from the point of view of individual patients and medical personnel as well as examine the broader impact of the disease on military operations and government policy at home and abroad. The Office of Medical History also supported travel to present my research findings at the annual conference of the Organization of American Historians in San Jose, California (2005), the annual conference of the Society of Military Historians in Ogden, Utah (2008), and enabled me to attend the nationally known "TB Course" taught by Michael Iseman, M.D., at the National Jewish Hospital Center (2006).

I relied on the expertise of many archivists and librarians to negotiate such a rich and varied historical record and thank the following navigators: Mitchell Yockelson, Rich Boylan, and Trevor Plant at the National Archives I and II in the Washington, DC, area; Eileen Bolger and Marene Baker at the National Archives and Records Administration (NARA) Regional Branch in Denver, Colorado; staff at the NARA regional branch in Fort Worth, Texas; Stephen Greenberg and Ginny Roth at the National Library of Medicine in Bethesda, Maryland; David Keogh and Richard Sommers at the U.S. Army Military History Institute at Carlisle, Pennsylvania; Tom McMasters at the Fort Sam Houston Medical Museum in San Antonio, Texas; editors of the Army Nurse Corps Association *Connection*; Jessy Randall at the Tutt Library, Colorado College, Colorado Springs; and archivists at the Central City Museum in Central City, New Mexico; the South Carolina

Historical Society in Charleston; the Oregon Health and Science University Historical Collections and Archives in Portland; the United States Holocaust Memorial Museum, Washington, DC; the Colorado Historical Society, Denver; and the Western Center for History and Genealogy at the Denver Public Library in Denver, Colorado. A number of people helped me work through the immense amount of material. Thanks goes to Crystal Avitia, A. J. Ballou, Kate Goodman, Kate Jankovsky, and Alma Moore for easing my research load and making the work more enjoyable with their company and conversation. I also heartily thank the Borden Institute, especially editor Linette Sparacino, for seeing the manuscript through to a book.

Not medically trained, I benefitted greatly from others who were. Mary Ann DeGroote, M.D., and Carolyn Bargman, R.N., generously and patiently responded to my queries about tuberculosis, and saved me from various errors and misconceptions. Two of today's "Good Tuberculosis Men," Col. Stephen Cersovsky, MC, and Lt. Col. Jamie Mancusco, MC, also helped me in numerous ways. Special thanks go to Col. Robert J. T. Joy, MC, retired, who, with his unparalleled knowledge, not only painstakingly read the entire manuscript but also cheerfully answered my questions and helped me think through problems whenever I called. I am nevertheless responsible for the medical and scientific discussions in this book and, of course, for any errors.

Many friends and colleagues took time out of their own busy lives to read all or part of my work and have made it immeasurably better. My appreciation goes to Jeanne Abrams, Carolyn Bargman, Lisa Budreau, Steve Cersovsky, Mary Ann DeGroote, Tina Gianquitto, John Greenwood, Mary Griffin, Jon Hoffman, Bob Joy, Thomas Krainz, Peggy Lamm, Jamie Mancusco, Anne Meyering, Hannah Nordhaus, Wendy Orent, Stephen Ortiz, Harry Reed, and Rosemary Stevens for their thoughtful comments and suggestions. To others I give thanks for answering the phone or email when I needed help. They include: Nancy Bristow, Michael D. Iseman, Susan D. Jones, Beth Linker, Sanders Marble, Howard Markel, Steve McGeary, and Mary Sarnecky. I am especially grateful to Margaret Gaule, R.N., and her family, for sharing her life story with me. As an Army nurse in a tuberculosis ward, a tuberculosis patient, and a tuberculosis veteran, she was all too familiar with the story that I tell in this book.

Research trips can be lonely affairs, but I often had wonderful company. Stephanie and Marty Maley helped my husband Rad and I explore Fort Bayard; Alma Moore was researcher and traveling buddy par excellence at the Military History Institute in Carlisle; Alice and John Goodman opened their home to me during visits to Washington, DC; and Pam Cicetti rescued me from the motels with friendship, food, and shelter during my weeks in the National Archives. Other friends patiently helped me develop my stories and deepen my understanding of tuberculosis in the military. They include Jeanne Christiansen, Tina Gianquitto, Julie Greene, Mary Griffin, Betty Hoye, Jim Hutchinson, Susan Kent, Tom Krainz, Peggy Lamm, Eric Love, Barb Miley, Scott Miller, David Paradis, Harry Reed, Dan Sarewitz, Mitch Stahl, Kathy Strand, and Nancy Vavra.

I am also grateful to my extended family of Byerlys, Rieses, Brandenburgs, Neuhausers, and Millses who accommodated family visits to my research and teaching schedule, listened to my disease stories, and helped me celebrate the various milestones on the path of book writing. And finally, my love and appreciation goes to Rad, for reading every word of this book at least once, helping me sort out myriad research, analysis, and writing problems, and supporting my work in so many ways. But most of all, for being the love of my life.

Foreword

During the past 239 years, our fighting forces have been stopped more often by diseases such as smallpox, cholera, and malaria than by enemy bullets. Our lessons learned in fighting these diseases have never been more important than they are today, because the health and resilience of our men and women in uniform have never been a greater matter of national security. Throughout history, the Army Medical Department has used our past experiences to strengthen our capacity and our resolve as a healthcare organization to support and sustain the Army, enhance the care experience, and innovate Army Medicine.

Tuberculosis is one of the diseases that have incapacitated our fighting forces in the past. "*Good Tuberculosis Men: The Army Medical Department's Struggle With Tuberculosis*" details the history of the Army's battle with this disease. Carol R. Byerly's extensively researched and insightful publication highlights the adaptability, tenacity, and resourcefulness of Army Medicine in overcoming challenging obstacles in the past.

Early Army tuberculosis programs proved to be effective; tuberculosis dropped from first place among reasons for federal disability discharges after World War I to 13th place after World War II. By the 1960s, tuberculosis became a curable and controllable disease. The US Army Medical Department—as with many infectious diseases—was a leader in the global efforts to contain, control, and cure this disease.

While the prevalence of tuberculosis has decreased dramatically in the Western world, it is still common in other parts of the world where nearly two million people die each year from tuberculosis, and one-third of the world's population is infected. As a result, tuberculosis is a serious threat to our fighting capabilities should American fighting men and women deploy to areas where this disease is still endemic.

Our military will continue to deploy, and by necessity our practitioners will have to treat our service members, the local populations, and enemy combatants infected with tuberculosis. Multidrug-resistant tuberculosis and extensively drug-resistant tuberculosis continue as serious concerns today in diabetic patients, immunocompromised patients, and those who have failed to complete previous courses of therapy.

The battle against tuberculosis is not over. We will continue the fight and be prepared to provide the best preventive and postinfection care against tuberculosis possible.

I thank Carol R. Byerly for this important contribution to the literature and for helping us to ensure our fighting forces are ready and resilient.

Serving to Heal…Honored to Serve!

Patricia D. Horoho
Lieutenant General, US Army
The Surgeon General and
Commanding General, US Army Medical Command

Introduction

In 1917, as the United States prepared for war in Europe, Army Surgeon General William C. Gorgas recognized the threat of *Mycobacterium tuberculosis* to American troops and recruited one of the nation's top tuberculosis specialists, Colonel George E. Bushnell, to help. Bushnell was a brilliant, skilled, compassionate medical officer, committed to public health and given ample government funding. He developed a nationwide program to keep tubercular men out of the U.S. Army and to identify and isolate active cases of tuberculosis in the ranks in a timely and effective manner. The disease was difficult to detect, especially in its early stages, so Bushnell was not surprised when trainees and soldiers began to appear in Army camp hospitals with signs of tuberculosis. He was, however, disturbed to learn in early 1918 that hundreds of American doughboys were coming home from Europe *erroneously* diagnosed with tuberculosis. False diagnoses wasted manpower and resources and needlessly alarmed soldiers and their families. What the Army needed, wrote Bushnell, were some "good tuberculosis men." Experts deployed with the American Expeditionary Forces in France could reduce the false-positive diagnosis rates "over there."[1] Bushnell stepped up his recruiting and training of tuberculosis specialists, designated several tuberculosis centers in France to evaluate soldiers with suspected disease, and established a system of tuberculosis hospitals in the United States to care for the sick. These steps dramatically reduced the false diagnoses. Still, despite the efforts of the nation's best "tuberculosis men," the disease would become a leading cause of World War I disability discharges and veterans benefits.

The problem was both biomedical and political. Tuberculosis was a wily foe, and medical scientists and physicians at the time lacked the knowledge to accurately diagnose or effectively treat it. Tuberculosis bacteria could lie latent in a person's body for years but then exploit a weakened immune system and break into active disease, spreading within the host's body and infecting others. Sir Arthur

S. McNalty, chief medical officer of the British Ministry of Health (1935–40), called tuberculosis "one of the camp followers of war." War abetted tuberculosis, he explained, because of the "lowering of bodily resistance and increased physical or mental strain or both,…combined with increased opportunities for contact infection from one person to another."[2] Active tuberculosis could also recede in many patients, succumbing to their immune systems once again, becoming undetectable, but then reactivating years later. This pattern made it difficult for government officials to keep infected men out of the Army, and if individuals developed tuberculosis later, it was often impossible to determine whether they had contracted it during military service or in civilian life. Moreover, the fact that tuberculosis patients often experienced cycles in which they recovered their health and then fell ill again over several months or years challenged government officials to judge the degree to which a person was disabled and required government care and support. Federal policies concerning tuberculosis would, therefore, confound the U.S. Army Medical Department during much of the twentieth century.

Tuberculosis in the Army

This book tracks the impact of tuberculosis on the U.S. Army from the late 1890s, when it was a ubiquitous presence in society, to the 1960s when it became a curable and controllable disease.[3] The Army experience with the disease is both similar to and different from the broader civilian story of tuberculosis, but the historical literature has paid little attention to it.[4] The evolution of tuberculosis treatments—from the nineteenth-century approach of fresh air and exercise, to rest therapy, to surgical intervention, and finally to antibiotics—was similar in both military and civilian institutions. Many of the important players were the same, too, as civilian physicians and nurses joined the military in wartime and then returned to civilian life afterward. Tuberculosis hospitals also shifted between civilian and military status, providing the military increased capacity during the war years, and then converting back to civilian management in peacetime. As tuberculosis rates slowly declined after 1900, medical strategies against the disease moved from defense to offense—from simply caring for the sick, to isolating and treating patients with tuberculosis, to surveilling military personnel and civilian populations to find, isolate, and treat active cases, and finally to curing the disease. This process was generally more rapid and thorough in military institutions than in civil society.

The military and civilian tuberculosis experience also differed, however, beginning with the fact that military populations were particularly vulnerable to tuberculosis because the disease favored young adults, the age group comprising the bulk of the Army. But as a relatively closed institution, the Army could more easily exclude the disease from its ranks than could civilian communities, screening its personnel for infections and treating them with greater and more uniform control. The federal government was also obliged to treat military patients, who therefore often—but not always—received some of the best tuberculosis treatment available in the country, if not the world.

The story of the Army Medical Department's struggle with tuberculosis describes the experiences of thousands of active duty personnel and veterans who spent years as patients in the Army's tuberculosis hospitals, and of the medical officers, nurses, and enlisted personnel who cared for them, often at the risk of their own health. It also brings to light individuals who have been largely obscured in more general histories of military medicine.[5] George E. Bushnell in the early 1900s and World War I, Earl H. Bruns in the 1920s and 1930s, Esmond R. Long in World War II and its aftermath, and Carl W. Tempel and James H. Forsee in the 1940s and 1950s all made important contributions to tuberculosis research, education, and treatment, as well as crafting and executing Army policies and practices. But just as many Americans have forgotten about the scourge of tuberculosis, historians, too, have forgotten these men's accomplishments.

This book examines the history of tuberculosis in the Army through four, interrelated themes regarding government policies and institutions, disease transmission, and the patient experience. The first follows the Army Medical Department's management of tuberculosis and the often uneven, sometimes ragged development of federal policies regarding military personnel and veterans with the disease. Once laboratories could identify tuberculosis in the 1880s, government officials began to devise targeted policies regarding the employment, treatment, and disposition of military personnel who were positively diagnosed. But just as the tools of detection and knowledge about tuberculosis evolved haltingly, so too did policies governing the treatment of tubercular soldiers, sailors, Marines, military nurses, and veterans.

The second theme tracks the Medical Department's efforts to establish and maintain tuberculosis hospitals and services to meet the needs of the military and the nation, and shows that its physicians and institutions were often leaders in tuberculosis research and treatment. The Army's program began with a small, insular community of tuberculars on a high plateau at Fort Bayard, New Mexico, serving the equally small and isolated Army of the early 1900s. Over the decades the program evolved into a nationwide network of government tuberculosis hospitals, which in the 1940s included a bustling military post of 10,000 in Denver, Colorado. During World War II, the Army tuberculosis program spanned the globe, as its hospitals and personnel cared for American prisoners of war (POW) and refugees in Europe and Asia, as well as for German, Italian, and Japanese POWs held in the United States. Tuberculosis hospitals also rode the national economy, booming in wartime, and almost "going bust" during the Great Depression. Questions of whether and when to terminate tuberculosis institutions and services involved both medical and political decisions, and engaged municipal, state, and federal governments, soldiers, veterans and their families, and, of course, the press.

This book's third theme explores the interaction between biology and society—how the evolution of scientific and patient understanding of tuberculosis transmission shaped patient and healthcare worker behavior, medical practice, and government policies. During much of the twentieth century, military and civilian medical personnel alike believed that contagious tubercular material was confined to patients' sputum and other excreta, and that careful disposal of that material and good patient hygiene could prevent transmission to other people. In fact, however, tuberculosis is largely spread by tiny airborne particles (droplet nuclei) expelled by a person with infectious tuberculosis while coughing, sneezing, talking, or even simply breathing. These droplet nuclei can remain suspended in the air for minutes or even hours, depending on the ambient ventilation, so an uninfected individual does not have to have direct contact with someone or their bodily fluids to become infected. Sources of tuberculosis contagion are also difficult to track because active tuberculosis does not demonstrate the dramatic, explosive contagion seen with diseases such as influenza or measles. Medical scientists and public health officials therefore did not fully understand and agree on the nature of airborne tuberculosis transmission until convincing scientific evidence emerged in the 1950s. As a result, they unwittingly exposed generations of caregivers, family members, and the general public to tuberculosis infection.

The fourth and final theme of this book examines the tuberculosis experience from the perspective of the military patients and the medical personnel who cared for them.[6] For several decades in this story, medical personnel were often both caregivers and patients. While this could increase their credibility as experts and healers, it also left some of them dead or disabled and vulnerable to disease recurrence. The evolution of tuberculosis treatment from fresh air and exercise to antibiotic therapy shaped and reshaped the tuberculosis experience, including the patients' interactions with medical institutions and staff and their discomfort, anxiety, hope, and fear. Rich archival sources including medical records and patient correspondence reveal the daily experience of tuberculosis and also underscore that tuberculosis often cruelly took young adults in the prime of life.

"Good Tuberculosis Men" explores these themes—tuberculosis policy, institutions, transmission, and the disease experience—over nine chapters in largely chronological order. The first third of the book examines the Army's first tuberculosis hospital established in 1899 at Fort Bayard in the mountains of New Mexico. Chapter 1, "The Early Years," describes the Medical Department's early efforts to find the right leadership and regime for the institution. In such an isolated community of active-duty soldiers, sailors, Marines, and veterans of the Indian and the Spanish-American wars, post commanders often struggled as much with poor patient and troop morale and discipline as with tuberculosis itself. The second chapter, "Life at Fort Bayard," explores the more stable and therapeutic world created by Colonel (Col.) Bushnell, who commanded the hospital from 1907 to 1917. Bushnell employed his authority both as a physician and as an Army officer to establish rigorous yet compassionate policies governing the benefits, rights, and responsibilities of tuberculosis patients and staff. His efforts transformed Fort Bayard into a model tuberculosis sanatorium that became a training school for both civilian and military tuberculosis specialists. For many patients the hospital also provided a seamless transition from active-duty to veteran status in the era before the nation had a separate hospital system for veterans. The third chapter, "The Congressman as Tuberculosis Patient," contributes to the scholarship on tuberculosis patients' struggles with the meaning of their disease by providing an intimate view of Fort Bayard life through the letters of Congressman George Legare of South Carolina.[7] His daily letters to his wife while he was a patient in 1908 and 1909 show a politician at the peak of his powers as an elected official and the *pater familias* of his extended clan, struggling with the consequences of his disabling disease.

World War I transformed the Army Medical Department's tuberculosis program, and the next two chapters examine that process. Chapter 4, "Tuberculosis in World War I," describes Bushnell's wartime efforts to contain tuberculosis cases and costs as thousands of tuberculosis patients flooded Army hospitals. The dramatic influx compromised care and put some hospitals and their patients at risk, but it also led to the establishment of the Army's largest and most important tuberculosis hospital, Fitzsimons General Hospital, in Denver, Colorado. Constructed in the final months of the war, Fitzsimons admitted patients before it was completed and fully prepared, which led to patient complaints, press exposés, and a congressional investigation before the hospital was a year old. Chapter 5, "'A Gigantic Task': Treating and Paying for Tuberculosis in the Interwar Period," examines the postwar impact of tuberculosis on government institutions and resources. As Congress extended benefits to more and more veterans in the 1920s, negotiations as to which veterans would get what benefits and for how long involved numerous federal agencies, medical specialists, interest groups, and military personnel and their families. The chapter also shows how and why the cost of tuberculosis treatment required longer hospital stays and became increasingly expensive after the war, examining Col. Earl H. Bruns' work at Fitzsimons on new tuberculosis therapies such as rehabilitation and surgery.

Invasive procedures that probed tuberculosis material also increased the risk of infection to medical personnel, especially nurses who cared for the sickest patients on a daily basis. Chapter 6, "Good Tuberculosis Women," examines tuberculosis nursing and the imperfect and evolving understanding of tuberculosis transmissibility during the interwar period. Despite evidence that tuberculosis nurses had higher rates of infection than other medical personnel, until a strong consensus on airborne transmission finally emerged in the late 1950s, many institutions were reluctant to impose time-consuming and costly protective measures. The result was that countless nurses and nursing students contracted the disease from their patients.

Chapter 7, "Surviving the Great Depression," shows how federal tuberculosis policy became the object of political controversy during the contraction of the Great Depression when Army Surgeon General Robert U. Patterson, required to make draconian budget cuts, tried to close down Fitzsimons Hospital in 1933. He ran into energetic and politically adept opposition from Congressman Lawrence Lewis, Denver's representative in Washington. With Lewis' detailed diary as a guide, the chapter traces his efforts to save the hospital using every political lever available, from medical opinion and patients' pleas to New Deal funds and intervention by President Franklin Roosevelt.

By the time the United States entered World War II, tuberculosis was but a minor threat to military operations, but the disease nevertheless continued to elude detection in the ranks; indeed, just one case could endanger an entire unit. Tuberculosis also exploited the most desperate conditions of the war—Nazi concentration camps, German and Japanese POW camps, and war-torn Europe. This time, the Army's tuberculosis expert was a civilian, Esmond Long of the Henry Phipps Institute of Philadelphia, Pennsylvania, who was commissioned as a colonel in the Medical Corps to fight tuberculosis in the Army. Chapter 8, "Camp Follower," tracks Long's various wartime activities and policies that successfully demoted tuberculosis from first place after World War I to thirteenth place as the cause of federal disability discharges. The ninth and final chapter, "Miracle Drugs?" describes how tuberculosis was finally brought under control with the development of antibiotic treatments in the 1940s and 1950s. The remedy did not involve a single "miracle drug," but rather a complicated antibiotic regime that still requires months to complete and contends with the continuous development of drug-resistant strains of bacteria. But years of research, trial, and error finally did produce a cure—and some of the important clinical trials were conducted at Army hospitals. Fitzsimons medical officers Cols. Carl Tempel and James Forsee were in the forefront of research on how to employ antibiotics to finally cure tuberculosis patients. Chapter 9 also tells the story of Margaret Gaule, an Army nurse and veteran of World War II, whose tuberculosis experience reveals how the struggle over fair and reasonable policies regarding tuberculosis in the military continues to this day.

Tuberculosis in Brief

An important character in this story is tuberculosis itself, which, in 1905, famed physician Sir William Osler labeled "the most universal scourge of the human race."[8] This book spans the often excruciating period in the history of tuberculosis (and in the history of medicine generally), from the 1890s to the 1950s, during which time physicians could *diagnose* tuberculosis but could neither *cure* it nor even *treat* it effectively.[9] Tuberculosis has plagued societies for millennia, and continues to thrive today. Archeological evidence of tuberculosis in humans dates back to prehistoric times, and in antiquity Hippocrates accurately described the disease then known as consumption. Though eclipsed by plague, leprosy, and other deadly diseases during the Middle Ages, tuberculosis steadily took its toll. When the early anatomists began to systematically study cadavers in the sixteenth and seventeenth centuries, they regularly found signs of tuberculosis in the bodies they opened. The development of the stethoscope and the art of percussion (tapping the chest and the upper back to learn the conditions of the lungs) in the late eighteenth century enabled physicians to better detect and describe tuberculosis in the living. Soon, there was more of it to describe: the disease surged in the poverty and crowded living conditions of the increasingly industrialized and urbanized societies to become the leading killer in Western Europe and the United States in the nineteenth century.

When the German scientist Robert Koch identified tuberculosis bacilli in 1882, he finally found the cause of all of the suffering. Reproducing tuberculosis by injecting the bacteria into guinea pigs, Koch also articulated germ theory—that a specific pathogen produced a specific disease—and accelerated the development of modern medicine. But unlike diseases such as diphtheria, typhoid, and tetanus, which quickly succumbed to vaccines and antitoxins, tuberculosis resisted control. Tuberculosis rates did decline in many industrialized nations throughout the twentieth century even before the antibiotic cures of the 1940s and 1950s due to improved standards of living and the isolation of many tuberculosis patients. Rates in the United States (Figure 1) fell from almost 200 deaths per 100,000 people in 1900 to around five deaths per 100,000 in 1955[10]. Similarly, in the Army tuberculosis declined from being the leading cause of disability discharges in the early 1900s to a rare occurrence by the latter half of the century. As one sign of increased control, in 1975, officials began to track *new cases* of tuberculosis rather than tuberculosis *deaths*. They found that new tuberculosis case rates in the country fell at a fairly steady rate of 5 to 6 percent annually during the second half of the twentieth century, from 52.6 per 100,000 per year in 1953 to 9.4 per 100,000 per year in 1984. Such dramatic decreases in the United States and other industrialized countries bred complacency on the part of many public health agencies. This complacency exploded in the 1980s when a mysterious new infection, the human immunodeficiency virus (HIV, the precursor to acquired immunodeficiency syndrome or AIDS), weakened people's immune systems enabling latent tuberculosis infections to become active and deadly, causing the first *increase* in tuberculosis rates in decades. New case rates increased from 9.2 per 100,000 in 1988 to 10.4 per 100,000 in 1991. Initially caught off guard, public

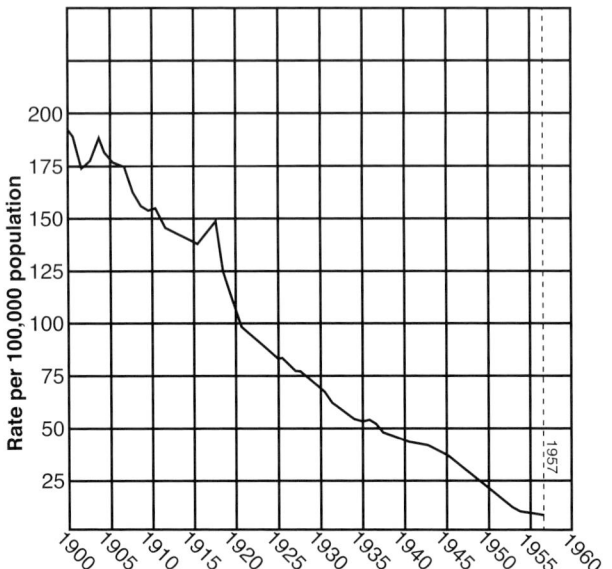

Figure 1. Chart showing the decrease in the tuberculosis death rates in the United States, 1900–57, in the civilian population.
Reproduced with permission from the *American Journal of Public Health* 48 (1958): 1440. Image available at: http://www.ncbi.nlm.nih.gov/pmc/articles/PMC1551815/pdf/amjphnation01081-0004.pdf.

health officials were able to reverse the trend. By 2008, the United States recorded 4.2 new cases of tuberculosis among 100,000.[11]

Tuberculosis has continued to flourish in other regions of the world, and today about one-third of the world's population—more than two billion people—is infected with the bacterium. Almost two million die every year.[12] The stresses of poverty, malnutrition, malaria, and HIV-AIDS suppress people's immune systems, allowing latent tuberculosis infections to flare across the world, including regions where Americans travel or the U.S. Army deploys. A deadly combination called TB-HIV (the co-infection of tuberculosis and HIV) is now ravaging a number of developing countries and threatens to become one of the biggest killers of the twenty-first century. Tuberculosis is a leading cause of sickness and death among people living with HIV because HIV compromises a person's immune system and can allow a latent tuberculosis infection to become active and fatal. Equally troubling, strains of *Mycobacterium tuberculosis* are developing resistance to life-saving antibiotic agents.[13] Multidrug-resistant tuberculosis (MDR-TB) bacteria are resistant to at least two of the best, first-line tuberculosis drugs. Extensively drug-resistant tuberculosis (XDR-TB) bacteria are resistant to the first line-drugs and at least two second-line drugs.[14] Treatment of MDR-TB and XDR-TB now involves long and expensive regimes of some 20 pills a day for two years. Some XDR-TB patients are virtually incurable, forcing physicians to return to tuberculosis medicine of the preantibiotic era resorting to bed rest and surgical removal of infected tissue.[15]

Tuberculosis defies definitive understanding to this day. Some cases continue to elude diagnosis and there is still no reliable, completely effective vaccine. Through the years the Army Medical Department has grasped all available tools to prevent and treat the disease, an effort that has challenged the intellectual and emotional resources of generations of medical personnel. Those challenges are particular to tuberculosis because of the unique etiology of tuberculosis, the human immune response to the bacteria, the difficulty diagnosing and treating the disease, and the politically sensitive and financially costly problem of treating military patients.

Etiology

Tuberculosis can develop in almost any part or organ of the body, but the great majority of cases are pulmonary, perhaps because the bacteria thrive in oxygen-rich environments. The other "extrapulmonary" cases include tuberculosis of the lymphatic system (once known as "scrofula"), tuberculosis of the spine (Pott's Disease), tuberculosis of the skin (including *lupus vulgaris*), and tuberculosis of the bones and joints or one or more vital organs. In most cases of initial infection, the body's general defenses can prevent active tuberculosis disease by walling off the invading bacteria and producing a calcified lesion in the lungs or elsewhere, so that a person may never know he or she has been infected. Only about 10 percent of people infected with *Mycobacterium tuberculosis* will go on to develop an active form of the disease. For that unfortunate minority, the immune response is inadequate or fails, and the bacteria multiply, destroying tissue and producing moist lesions or "spots" on the lungs. These areas can infiltrate lung tissues, causing "caseation," which gives a cheese-like texture to the lungs, and then progress to cavitation, or the erosion of the lung tissue that is coughed up in bloody or purulent sputum. Patients' symptoms can include a prolonged cough, fevers, night sweats, weight loss, fatigue, and lung hemorrhages (which can occur when tuberculosis bacteria rupture blood vessels in the lungs). Human lungs have three lobes on the right and two lobes on the left, and cavitation of a lobe can cause a displacement of the heart and coronary disease. Patients can also develop secondary tubercular infections in the larynx from coughing up bacteria, or gastrointestinal tuberculosis from swallowing tubercular matter. The progression of the disease is usually slow—over months and years—but can also be rapid, killing patients, especially children, in a matter of weeks. Some forms of tuberculosis are especially lethal, such as miliary tuberculosis, in which tuberculosis bacteria are released into the bloodstream, or meninginal tuberculosis, which infects the spinal fluid. Tuberculosis patients can die of blood loss, sepsis, pneumonia, lung or heart failure, or the failure of other organs. During the time frame covered in this book, 1899 to 1960, some Army Medical Department patients did recover completely and lived to die of other causes. The majority of soldiers, sailors, Marines, and veterans with tuberculosis, however, experienced years of impaired health, with cycles of recovery and relapse until they succumbed to the disease.

Transmission

The evolving contemporary understanding of tuberculosis transmission is key to this story because it informed tuberculosis policies ranging from patient admission and discharge rules, to medical and nursing protocols, and hospital architecture. That tuberculosis bacteria can be transmitted through the air did not become a consensus view until experiments with guinea pigs in the 1950s presented irrefutable evidence.[17] Only then did hospitals and medical personnel universally adopt precautionary procedures such as isolating patients in negative air pressure rooms to ensure that tuberculosis bacteria did not escape to the rest of the hospital; requiring healthcare workers to wear gowns, gloves, and masks or respirators when caring for patients; and monitoring staff with annual tuberculin tests and chest X-rays to catch new infections. Until this understanding, however, caregivers were repeatedly exposed to infection, and tuberculosis patients, including soldiers and veterans, often moved freely about the country, spreading disease to their families, friends, and communities.

Immunity

Some people who are repeatedly exposed to tuberculosis bacteria will never develop the disease and are presumably immune to it. Others, especially children, may succumb rapidly, their bodies' immune systems unable to wall off the bacteria. This is not the place for a discussion of the human immune response to tuberculosis—it is so technical and complex that even an article on the immune system in the *New England Journal of Medicine* for medical professionals had a glossary to assist readers.[19] But the unpredictability of immune responses and the bacteria's susceptibility to changes in the environment made it difficult for the Army Medical Department to develop clear and fair policies regarding benefits, treatment, eligibility, and even military assignments for tuberculosis patients. Military training, combat, or time spent as a POW could weaken soldiers' immune systems. In peacetime, service in the tropics could also be risky if military personnel or their families became ill with malaria, dysentery, sexually transmitted diseases, or anything else that could compromise their immune systems and give a latent tuberculosis infection the opportunity to become active.

Diagnosis

Tuberculosis diagnosis remains as much an art as a science, and an infection can still be mistaken for other diseases of the lungs or chest. As with most diseases, the earlier it is discovered the better the patient's chances of recovery. By the time tubercular people have physical symptoms such as a chronic cough, fever, weight loss, and the most telltale sign of all—lung hemorrhage or spitting up blood—they are seriously ill. Military physicians therefore eagerly adopted the microscope to identify tuberculosis bacteria and X-ray technology to detect lesions and cavities in the lungs or other organs. They also quickly learned to track the regression or progression of the disease over time. Despite diagnostic tools that today include blood tests and genetic analysis, tuberculosis detection is still imperfect and medical professionals continue to debate the usefulness of various diagnostic technologies.[20]

Treatment

Tuberculosis bacteria grow slowly and have a waxy coating on the cell surface, which enabled them to elude effective treatment or "magic bullets" until the development of antibiotic regimes in the 1940s and 1950s. The progression of tuberculosis therapies evolved from fresh air and exercise and various medicinal and chemical concoctions of the nineteenth century, to twentieth-century treatments including extended bed rest, a nutritious diet, exposure to the sun, lung collapse procedures, and surgery—all of which had debatable degrees of success. During the second half of the twentieth century antibiotics enabled many countries to cure thousands of patients and dramatically reduce their tuberculosis rates. But because tuberculosis rates were falling steadily decades before antibiotics, historians and scientists have debated the historical significance of various antituberculosis measures in reducing tuberculosis morbidity and mortality rates during the twentieth century, including:

- natural selection whereby tuberculosis survivors have produced more resistant progeny and/or tuberculosis bacteria have decreased in virulence;
- improved standards-of-living such as less crowded housing, better ventilation, and better diets, reducing chances of transmission and improving people's ability to resist disease;

- public health measures such as milk pasteurization, the isolation of tuberculosis patients in sanatoriums, and the surveillance of specific populations to identify and isolate disease carriers; and
- medical interventions such as rest therapy, lung collapse and the surgical removal of diseased tissue, vaccines, and antibiotics.[21]

The slow yet steady decline of tuberculosis in the United States suggests that the confluence of all of these factors was required to weaken this powerful adversary. It would be unwise, however, to declare victory. Physician and historian Barron Lerner points out that tuberculosis has remained a major health problem, particularly in poor urban communities, and another physician and historian, Howard Markel, states, "We must accept that we will never completely conquer tuberculosis.... The best we can hope for is to contain it enough to limit its influence."[22]

Disposition

The issue of "disposition," or what to do with both civilian and military tuberculosis patients once their treatment has been completed, has been one of the most vexing and politically sensitive issues the Army Medical Department has faced. Some patients recovered from the disease enough to return to duty, as many wanted to, especially officers and enlisted men who had planned on a military career. But some government officials questioned whether former tuberculosis patients would be able to perform their duties satisfactorily and whether they would infect others with the disease. Patients too disabled to return to duty also posed serious questions. Who should pay for their care? How long must the soldiers serve in the military before the government was responsible for their care? How long should treatment be provided? When were veterans and military patients well enough to go home? Did they pose a risk to themselves and to others? What about soldiers who wanted to go home to die? These issues would be heatedly debated in the War Department, Congress, and American society. Peoples' lives and livelihoods depended on the answers.

Throughout its history, the U.S. Army—like the rest of society—has had to contend with a complex, resilient, and deadly disease in its ranks. The emergence of germ theory in the late nineteenth century and successful identification of tuberculosis bacteria finally enabled public health officials to move against the disease, but it still defeated the brightest and most vigorous of its adversaries— "good tuberculosis men" like Col. George Bushnell and other medical officers who served with him and after him. In 1899, as the nineteenth century waned and the United States gained international power and responsibilities, the Army Medical Department took its first and perhaps most important step when it established its first tuberculosis hospital in the mountains of New Mexican Territory. Here, in the American wilderness, medical officers would enlist new scientific knowledge against an ancient foe.

Notes

1. G. E. Bushnell to G. B. Webb, 7 August 1918, Record Group [hereafter cited as RG] 112, Entry 29, Gen., 1917-27, Box 396, National Archives and Records Administration [hereafter cited as NARA].

2. Arthur S. McNalty, "Tuberculosis in Peace and War," *Tubercle* 23 (1942): 266.

3. Because the vast majority of people with tuberculosis in the Army and elsewhere—about 90 percent—had tuberculosis of the lungs, all references to "tuberculosis" will mean pulmonary tuberculosis unless otherwise stated.

4. Studies of tuberculosis in the United States include Barbara Bates, *Bargaining for Life: A Social History of Tuberculosis, 1876-1938* (Philadelphia, PA: University of Pennsylvania Press, 1992); Sheila Rothman, *Living in the Shadow of Death: Tuberculosis and the Social Experience of Illness in American History* (New York, NY: Basic Books, 1994); Georgina D. Feldberg, *Disease and Class: Tuberculosis and the Shaping of Modern North American Society* (New Brunswick, NJ: Rutgers University Press, 1995); Katherine Ott, *Fevered Lives: Tuberculosis in American Culture since 1870* (Cambridge, MA: Harvard University Press, 1996); Barron H. Lerner, *Contagion and Confinement: Controlling Tuberculosis Along Skid Row* (Baltimore, MD: Johns Hopkins University Press, 1998); Emily K. Abel, *Suffering in the Land of Sunshine: A Los Angeles Illness Narrative* (New Brunswick, NJ: Rutgers University Press, 2006); Emily K. Abel, *Tuberculosis and the Politics of Exclusion: A History of Public Health and Migration to Los Angeles* (New Brunswick, NJ: Rutgers University Press, 2007); and Cynthia A. Connolly, *Saving Sickly Children: The Tuberculosis Preventorium in American Life, 1908–1970* (New Brunswick, NJ: Rutgers University Press, 2008).

General histories include Thomas Dormandy, *The White Death: A History of Tuberculosis* (New York, NY: New York University Press, 1999); Flurin Condrau and Michael Worboys, *Tuberculosis Then and Now: Perspectives on the History of an Infectious Disease* (Montreal and Kingston: McGill-Queens University Press, 2010); and the classic Rene and Jean Dubos, *The White Plague: Tuberculosis, Man, and Society* (New Brunswick, NJ: Rutgers University Press, 1952, 1987).

5. Examples of works that give short shrift to tuberculosis and Army tuberculosis specialists include Mary C. Gillett, *The Army Medical Department, 1865–1917* (Washington, DC: Center of Military History, 1995); Percy M. Ashburn, *A History of the Medical Department of the U.S. Army* (Boston, MA and New York, NY: Houghton Mifflin, Co., 1929); Richard V. N. Ginn, *The History of the U.S. Army Medical Service Corps* (Washington, DC: Office of the Surgeon General and Center of Military History, 1997); and Clarence McKittrick Smith, *The Medical Department: Hospitalization and Evacuation, Zone of Interior*

(Washington, DC: Office of the Chief of Military History, Department of the Army, 1956).

6. Memoirs include Betty MacDonald, *The Plague and I* (Philadelphia, PA: J. B. Lippincott, 1948); Robert G. Lovell, *Taking the Cure: The Patient's Approach to Tuberculosis* (New York, NY: MacMillan 1948); Will Ross, *I Wanted to Live* (Milwaukee, WI: Wisconsin Anti-Tuberculosis Association, 1953); Elizabeth Mooney, *In the Shadow of the White Plague* (New York, NY: Thomas Y. Crowell, 1979); and Dorothy Simpson Beimer, *Hovels, Haciendas, and House Calls: The Life of Carl H. Gellenthien, M. D.* (Santa Fe, NM: Sunstone Press, 1986).

Novels about the tuberculosis experience include Thomas Mann's iconic *The Magic Mountain*, 1924, various editions; Julian Green, *The Closed Garden* (New York, NY: Harper and Brothers, 1928); A. E. Ellis, *The Rack* (London, UK: Penguin Books, 1958, 1961); Donald Stewart, *Sanatorium* (New York, NY: Harper and Brothers Publishers, 1930); and Eamonn McGrath, *The Charnel House* (Belfast, UK: Blackstaff Press, 1990).

7. See, for example, Rothman, *Living in the Shadow of Death;* Bates, *Bargaining for Life;* Ott, *Fevered Lives;* Abel, *Suffering in the Land of Sunshine;* and Carolyn June McQuien, "Tuberculosis as Chronic Illness in the United States: Understanding, Treating, and Living with the Disease," Ph.D. dissertation, University of Texas at Austin, 1993. Thomas Mann also explores these issues with Hans Castorp in *Magic Mountain*.

On the importance of examining the patient experience see Roy Porter, "A Patient's View: Doing Medical History from Below," *Theory and Society* (1985): 175–98. Also on the patient experience, see Arthur Kleinman, *The Illness Narratives: Suffering, Healing, and the Human Condition* (New York, NY: Basic Books, 1988); Chris Feudtner, *Bittersweet: Diabetes, Insulin, and the Transformation of Illness* (Chapel Hill, NC: University of North Carolina Press, 2003); Robert A. Aronowitz, *Making Sense of Illness: Science, Society, and Disease* (New York, NY: Cambridge University Press, 1998); Ray Fitzpatrick, John Hinton, Stanton Newman, Graham Scambler, and James Thompson, *The Experiences of Illness* (London, UK: Tavistock Publications, 1984); and Kathy Charmaz, *Good Days, Bad Days: The Self in Chronic Illness and Time* (New Brunswick, NJ: Rutgers University Press, 1991).

8. William Osler, *The Principles and Practice of Medicine,* 4th ed. (New York, NY: Appleton and Company, 1905), 284.

9. On the medical and scientific nature of tuberculosis, see Michael D. Iseman, *A Clinician's Guide to Tuberculosis* (Philadelphia, PA: Lippincott Williams & Wilkins, 2000); also Dormandy, *The White Death*; J. Arthur Myers, *Tuberculosis: A Half Century of Study and Conquest* (St. Louis, MO: Warren H. Green, Inc., 1970); and Lawrence Geiter, *Ending Neglect: The Elimination of Tuberculosis in the United States*, National Academy Press, Committee on the Elimination of Tuberculosis in the United States, Division of Health Promotion and Disease Prevention, Institute of Medicine (Washington, DC: Government Printing Office, 2000).

10. Geitner, *Ending Neglect,* 28.

11. Centers for Disease Control, "Morbidity Trend Tables, United States, at http://www.cdc.gov/TB/statistics/reports/2008/pdf/4_MorbTrend.pdf, accessed 26 October 2012.

12. Tuberculosis has been specifically targeted by the World Health Organization, see the Web site http://www.stoptb.org/, accessed 26 October 2012. See also the CDC Web site, http://www.cdc.gov/tb/topic/drtb/xdrtb.htm, accessed 26 October 2012; John D. H. Porter and John M. Grange, eds., *Tuberculosis: An Interdisciplinary Perspective* (London, UK: Imperial College Press, 1998); Charles W. Schmidt, "Linking TB in the Environment: An Overlooked Mitigation Strategy," *Environmental Health Perspectives* 11 (November 2008): A479–85; Kent A. Sepkowitz, "Tuberculosis and the Health-Care Worker: A Historical Perspective," *Annals of Internal Medicine* 120 (January 1994): 71–79; and "Some Ne-

glected Diseases Are More Neglected Than Others," *Science* 323 (6 February 2009): 700.

13. Matthew Gandy and Alimuddin Zumla, eds. *The Return of the White Plague: Global Poverty and the 'New' Tuberculosis* (London, UK: Verso, 2003).

14. WHO Web site, "Tuberculosis and HIV," http://www.who.int/hiv/topics/tb/en/, accessed 26 October 2012; and CDC Web site, http://www.cdc.gov/tb/topic/drtb/xdrtb.htm.

15. Just one example is Sohaila Mohsin Ali, Abdul Aziz Siddiqui, and Joseph S. McLaughlin, "Open Drainage of Massive Tuberculous Empyema with Progressive Re-Expansion of the Lung: An Old Concept Revisited," *Annals of Thoracic Surgery* 62 (1996): 218–24. See also Gwen Huitt, "MDR-TB," in the Denver TB Course, National Jewish Medical and Research Center," 26–29 April 2006; J. A. Caminero, "Treatment of Multidrug-Resistant Tuberculosis: Evidence and Controversies," *International Journal of Tuberculosis and Lung Disease* 10 (2006): 829–37; Benjamin J. Pomerantz, et al., "Pulmonary Resection for Multi-Drug Resistant Tuberculosis," *Journal of Thoracic and Cardiovascular Surgery* 121 (2001): 448–53; and Jose G. Somocurcio, et al., "Surgery for Patients with Drug-Resistant Tuberculosis: Report of 121 Cases Receiving Community-based Treatment in Lima, Peru," *Thorax* 62 (2007): 416–21.

16. For an example of the difficulty of diagnosing tuberculosis today, see Frederick O'Donnell, "A Tuberculosis Event on a Navy Assault Ship," *Military Medicine* 171 (December 2006): 1198–1200; James E. LaMar II and Mark A. Malakooti, "Tuberculosis Outbreak Investigation of the U.S. Navy Amphibious Ship Crew and the Marine Expeditionary Unit Aboard, 1998," *Military Medicine* 168 (July 2003): 523; and Remington L. Nevin, et al., "Suspected Pulmonary Tuberculosis Exposure at a Remote U.S. Army Camp in Northeastern Afghanistan, 2007," *Military Medicine* 173 (July 2008): 684–89. See also David G. Russell, Clifton E. Barry III, and JoAnne Flynn, "Tuberculosis: What We Don't Know Can, and Does Hurt Us," *Science* 328 (14 May 2010): 852–56.

17. R. L. Riley, et al., "Aerial Dissemination of Pulmonary Tuberculosis: A Two-Year Study of Contagion in a Tuberculosis Ward," *American Journal of Hygiene* 70 (1959): 185–196. Chapter 6 discusses this at length.

18. Sepkowitz, "Tuberculosis and the Health-Care Worker"; Dick Menzies, et al., "Tuberculosis Among Health-Care Workers," *New England Journal of Medicine* 332 (12 January 1995): 92–98; E. T. Curran, P. N. Hoffman, and R. J. Pratt, "Tuberculosis and Infection Control: A Review of the Evidence," 2006; and G. de Vries, et al., "Health-Care Workers with Tuberculosis Infected during Work," *European Respiratory Journal* 28 (2006): 1216–21.

19. Peter J. Delves and Ivan M. Roitt, "The Immune System," review article, *New England Journal of Medicine* 343 (6 July 2000): 38.

20. James D Mancuso, Steven K. Tobler, and Lisa W. Keep, "Pseudoepidemics of Tuberculin Skin Test Conversions in the U.S. Army after Recent Deployment," *American Journal of Respiratory and Critical Care Medicine* 177 (June 2008): 1285–89; Iseman, *A Clinician's Guide to Tuberculosis*, 21–49; and M. Rene Howell, "Screening for Mycobacterium Tuberculosis in the U.S. Military: Considerations for a Cost-Effectiveness Model," 16 May 2000, The Johns Hopkins University, Division of Infectious Diseases, Baltimore, MD.

21. For a good discussion of this debate, see Amy Fairchild and Gerald M. Oppenheimer, "Public Health Nihilism vs. Pragmatism: History, Politics and the Control of Tuberculosis," *American Journal of Public Health* 88, (1998): 1105–17; also Leonard Wilson, "The Historical Decline of Tuberculosis in Europe and America: Its Causes and Significance," *Journal of the History of Medicine and Allied Sciences* 45 (July 1990): 366–96.

22. Lerner, *Contagion and Confinement*, 4; and Howard Markel, *When Germs Travel: Six Major Epidemics That Have Invaded America and the Fears They Have Unleashed* (New York, NY: Vintage Books, 2005), 46.

Chapter One
The Early Years: Fort Bayard, New Mexico

On 16 November 1899, African American regulars of the 9th U.S. Cavalry, known as the Buffalo Soldiers, departed Fort Bayard, New Mexico, for Fort Duchesne, Utah.[1] They had been garrisoned at the fort since June, but now the War Department was transferring control of the fort from line command to the Army Medical Department. As the cavalry left, another group of men arrived. Some of them came on horseback, others by train and mule-driven ambulances, many so sick they had to be carried on stretchers. Arriving from Army hospitals and soldiers' homes for disabled veterans from the East and West coasts, these soldiers and veterans came to Fort Bayard to rest and heal. They came to be treated for tuberculosis.

This "changing of the guard" at Fort Bayard reveals a broader transition that was taking place in the Army as the United States strode onto the world stage as an economic and military power. Industrialization and the military conquest of Native Americans had helped the federal government lay claim to all corners of the country. Now the nation looked outward, and the War Department's mission and that of Fort Bayard changed. In addition to protecting American interests and people, the Army post's nineteenth-century mission had been to defend the nation's acquisition and control of land and resources in the West. The twentieth century would be dedicated to caring for the casualties of that effort. From fort to hospital, from cavalry barracks to patient wards, from combat officers to medical officers, Fort Bayard transformed from a multipurpose post in an army of the Indian wars to a specialized institution in an army of an empire.

Fort Bayard had a rocky start as a tuberculosis hospital. The first commander, Major (Maj.) Daniel M. Appel, successfully established a hospital in 1899 that provided state-of-the-art care for American soldiers and veterans. But Appel had difficulty maintaining order and discipline in this half-sanatorium, half-Army post, and two years later the Army Surgeon General relieved him of command. His successor, Lieutenant Colonel (Lt. Col.) Edward Comegys, encountered similar difficulties; the Surgeon General relieved him of command within eighteen months. This time the Surgeon General put one of his best medical officers, Maj. George E. Bushnell, in command. Bushnell would manage Fort Bayard from 1904 to 1917, becoming a leading authority on tuberculosis, and bringing not only order and discipline to the hospital, but national and international praise as well. He would also shape U.S. government tuberculosis policy for a generation.

Bushnell's success was due to his deep interest and knowledge of tuberculosis, his clear sense of Fort Bayard's mission, and his efforts to employ the modern American military management techniques emerging in the early decades of the twentieth century. His authority to run Fort Bayard lay not only in his rank and military command, but also in the scientific knowledge and medical expertise that he skillfully deployed within the Army's corporate, professional bureaucracy. The modernization of the U.S. Army would take place over several decades; the early years of the Army's tuberculosis hospital exemplified many of the elements of that complex process.

The Fort

In the last third of the nineteenth century the Army was small in proportion to the national population, with only 25,000 to 30,000 soldiers in a population of more than 76 million. Isolated from the greater society in far-flung posts, poorly funded, and held in low esteem by Americans traditionally hostile to the military, soldiers and officers knew each other well and often formed tight communities.[2] The Army's primary missions were domestic: fighting Indians and containing them on government reservations; protecting settlers, ranchers, and miners from outlaws and Indian attacks; policing industrial labor disputes; and building roads and stringing telegraph wire across the country—in short, bringing industrial society to the West.[3] That was the Army of the Buffalo Soldiers. The twentieth-century U.S. Army would adopt new, more corporate and bureaucratic methods of management, modern scientific knowledge and technology, and would also extend its mission and responsibilities to American economic interests in the Western Hemisphere and the Pacific. As this Army fought in other countries—especially in the tropics, where it encountered new, debilitating diseases—it generated a growing population of sick and disabled soldiers, some of whom who would come to Fort Bayard.

A tuberculosis sanatorium was a far cry from Fort Bayard's original purpose. It began as a military outpost, situated in a valley between the Sierra Madre and Santa Rita ranges of mountains, sixty miles north of the Mexican border at an altitude of 6,040 feet.[4] For centuries Mexican peasants, ranchers, and Indians competed for control of the region's land and mining resources. White settlers entered the fray after the 1848 Treaty of Guadalupe Hidalgo transferred much of the land claimed by the Chiricahua Apaches from Mexico to the United States.[5] The discovery of gold, silver, and copper in the nearby mountains soon brought more fortune seekers to the region. In August 1866, after the Civil War, the Secretary of War established a fort in the region to protect the mines, naming it for Brigadier General George D. Bayard of the First Pennsylvania Cavalry, who was mortally wounded in the 1862 Battle of Fredericksburg.[6]

Fort Bayard (Figure 1-1) was a classic western settlement: predominantly male, ethnically diverse, dependent on one industry, and vulnerable to its booms and busts. In 1870 the post housed about 185 soldiers—one infantry and two cavalry units. The medical officer on duty estimated the local population to be about 300 Mexicans, Irish, and German immigrants, and some Americans, most of whom were engaged in mining. A few men had their wives and children with them, and although Fort Bayard had no chapel or schoolhouse, it boasted a library with sixty-five books.[7] The cemetery already had twenty-one graves and the hospital had one twelve-bed ward "which is used alike by white and colored patients."[8] These "colored" patients were members of the Black Regulars—the four Army units that Congress had designated after the Civil War for African Americans: the 9th and 10th Cavalry Regiments and the 24th and 25th Infantry Regiments. Dubbed "Buffalo Soldiers" by the Indians, almost 20,000 African Americans served in the Army between the Civil War and the Spanish-American War, comprising about 10 percent of the enlisted men of the Army in a given year.[9] Seeking to avoid racial hostilities in the East and South the War Department posted most African Ameri-

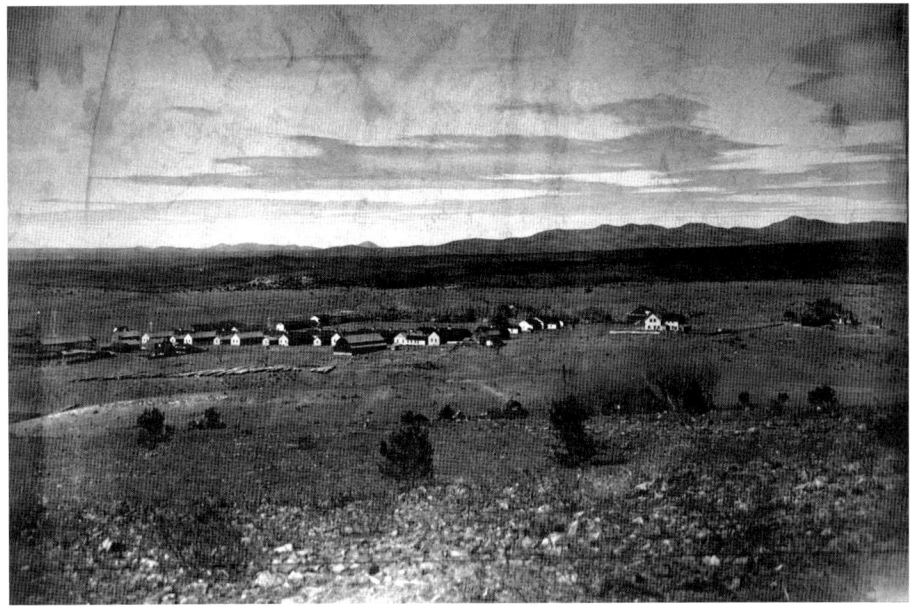

Figure 1-1. U.S. Army, General Hospital, Fort Bayard, New Mexico, General View, circa 1900, showing the isolation of the post on a high mesa in New Mexico Territory.
Photograph courtesy of the National Library of Medicine, Image #A02342.

can soldiers in the West during this period, many of them at Fort Bayard. Fort Bayard was a rung on the career ladder of other famous soldiers, including John Pershing, commander of the U.S. forces in Europe during World War I. Fresh out of West Point in 1886–87, Pershing commanded a troop of the 6th Cavalry at Fort Bayard.[10] Leonard Wood, who rode with Theodore Roosevelt and the Rough Riders during the Spanish-American War, served as Army chief of staff, and later ran for president. He also served as a medical officer at Fort Bayard early in his career.[11]

In the 1890s, however, with the West increasingly settled, there was less need for a military presence. Activity in the area further declined when local mines closed down after the 1893 economic crash. As the United States acquired new territories overseas, its military interests turned outward, and the War Department decommissioned forts across the West. As Fort Bayard soldiers dismantled Forts Selden and Stanton in New Mexico, they must have wondered if they would be doing the same to their own post. Rather than tear it down, however, the Army gave Fort Bayard a new mission.

From Climate Therapy to Sanatoriums

American medicine was in transition in the late nineteenth century, departing from the centuries-old practices of purging and bleeding, but not yet fully comprehending or embracing the power of germ theory—that specific pathogens caused specific diseases and could be passed from person to person.[12] With few effective medical remedies at their disposal, Americans resorted to a wide range of cures. Indians had long enjoyed the benefits of Rocky Mountains hot springs, and whites soon discovered that the warm waters and clear, dry mountain air offered relief from maladies such as arthritis, rheumatism, heart and skin ailments, and respiratory diseases.[13] As early as 1846 the Army erected a bath house and hospital at the hot springs at Las Vegas, New Mexico, for sick and wounded soldiers from the Mexican War, and during the nineteenth century many other people traveled west to visit similar springs, seeking health as well as land and riches.[14]

Tuberculosis is the disease that brought the most people to the West and Southwest. Eastern and midwestern physicians sent patients to Colorado, New Mexico, and California to regain their health, and medical journals such as the *Boston Medical and Surgical Journal* debated the merits of various resorts and locations.[15] Doctors traveled west for their own health, as well. Among them was John Henry "Doc" Holliday, a dentist who left Georgia in search of a cure for his tuberculosis and a chance to gamble. After gaining infamy at the gunfight at the O.K. Corral with the Earp brothers in 1881, he went to Colorado for his health and in 1887 died of tuberculosis in a hotel at Glenwood Springs, Colorado, at the age of 36.[16] At first health seekers had to be well enough to endure a journey on horseback or with wagons and mules, but the completion of the transcontinental railroad in 1869 opened the West to sicker and weaker patients. Some arrived at their destinations on stretchers and soon died. Many communities, with little appreciation of the contagious nature of tuberculosis, welcomed people with tuberculosis, especially if they brought adequate funds. In Denver more than 20 percent of the population was invalid in 1890.[17] By the early 1900s, New Mexico had forty-four tuberculosis sanatoriums, and as historian Jack Spidle put it, "tuberculosis dominated New Mexico medicine."[18]

Health seeking acquired a scientific aura during the 1880s and 1890s, as physicians and scientists developed the field of "climatology" to study the effect of climate on sickness and health. Men such as Charles Denison and Samuel Fisk of Colorado followed a European school that promoted the benefits of high altitude, fresh air, porous soil, and piney forests for recuperation from illness, especially tuberculosis. They believed that escaping dirty cities and getting rest, fresh air, hearty meals, and exercise would strengthen the body to fight disease and debated the relative merits of ocean breezes, mountain air, high altitude, and aridity on patients.[19] Denison, a physician who traveled west to cure his tuberculosis and indeed recovered his health, produced detailed tables and maps of the aridity and altitude of communities across the country to inform the debate.[20]

By the end of the century, however, climatology was losing its attraction. The lack of empirical evidence demonstrating the salubrious effect of certain climates fostered doubt. One Colorado physician was shocked and disappointed to learn that fewer than fifty of the one hundred tuberculosis patients he was studying were still alive after two years.[21] Others observed that recovery rates from tuberculosis were similar in New York, North Carolina, and Colorado—dampening any unique claims of high altitude therapy.[22] At the same time, and perhaps more importantly, people were coming to better understand the nature of infectious disease. By the early 1880s, germ theory had been developed by Louis Pasteur, Robert Koch, and other scientists, demonstrating that diseases like tuberculosis and typhoid were not inherited or caused by bad air (miasmas) but were transmitted by pathogenic organisms. After Koch identified tuberculosis bacteria in 1882, and other researchers began to find the pathogens causing various diseases, people began to view the sick with less sympathy and more fear. Some began associating tuberculosis with lower classes and treating those infected like lepers.[23] Health spas and resorts turned to soliciting healthy tourists rather than infectious invalids, and public health officials began to suggest that it would be safer to isolate sick people than to let them travel around the country infecting others.

New York City public health commissioner Hermann M. Biggs launched the first campaign against tuberculosis in 1889 by instituting routine bacteriological analysis of specimens from tuberculosis patients, and in 1893 required physicians to report all tuberculosis cases.[24] By the end of the century, at least twenty-four states had antituberculosis programs, as did many of the larger cities. Public health leaders formed the National Association for the Study and Prevention of Tuberculosis in 1904 to advance the view that tuberculosis was preventable and curable. Antituberculosis measures ranged in severity from outlawing spitting, to barring people with tuberculosis from food-handling or teaching jobs, to compulsory hospitalization for tuberculosis patients. Several states ruled that fraudulent concealment of tuberculosis was, like syphilis, sufficient grounds for marriage annulment, while a number of physicians opposed marriage for people with tuberculosis, especially women of childbearing age, and counseled patients to not kiss their husbands, wives, or children.[25] Some people called for the sterilization of the tuberculous. The *New Mexico Medical Journal* editorialized, "We cannot prevent the mating of the unfit, but we can prevent the procreation of the unfit." The journal also supported abortion for women with tuberculosis: "The command 'thou shalt not kill' is not violated when a fetus is taken from a tubercular woman and a life, problematic yet and probably a social unfit is sacrificed to prolong the existence of a social unit."[26] As historian Michael Worboys has written, "The campaign against consumption…ended in a war against the consumptive."[27]

As germ theory gained traction the federal government also took action against tuberculosis. The Public Health Service and Navy officials called for segregated train cars for people with tuberculosis traveling west and in 1907 immigration officials barred anyone with tuberculosis from entering the country.[28] Upon recommendation of the National Association for the Study and Prevention of Tuberculosis, President Theodore Roosevelt ordered an inspection of the sanitary conditions of all government buildings and issued regulations to prevent the spread of tuberculosis in government offices. These prohibited spitting on the floors, required ventilation and regular cleaning of all work spaces, and ordered that government employees with tuberculosis "be separated when possible from others while at work" and "provide their own drinking glasses, soap, and towels, and shall not use those provided for the general use." The federal government also began funding a program to eradicate tuberculosis from cattle and dairy herds and thereby prevent contagion by milk.[29]

Physicians and public health officials also increasingly turned to sanatoriums and tuberculosis hospitals to isolate and care for patients. Hospitals at the time were just emerging as a key element in American healthcare. The first national hospital survey in 1873 tallied 178 hospitals with about 50,000 beds, while one in 1909 counted 4,359 hospitals with more than 420,000 beds.[30] Nursing pioneer Florence Nightingale's admonitions and instructions on sanitation, fresh air, light, and good ventilation, along with professional, well-trained nursing care, helped reduce death rates in hospitals. New technologies such as aseptic surgery, X-rays, and laboratory diagnostics also increased the value of hospitals.[31] Massachusetts established the first state sanatorium for people with tuberculosis in 1895 and by 1916 there were more than 200 sanatoriums in the country, with 70 percent of the beds provided by local, state, or federal governments.[32] Religious and ethnic voluntary organizations established sanatoriums for special communities of tuberculosis sufferers. In Denver, groups established the National Jewish Hospital for Consumptives, the Jewish Consumptives' Relief Society, the Evangelical Lutheran Sanitarium, and the Swedish National Sanatorium for Consumptives.[33] Tuberculosis hospitals provided a threefold solution of isolating patients, treating the disease, and educating tuberculosis patients on how to care for themselves. The War Department's establishment of a tuberculosis hospital in New Mexico put the Army in the first wave of this movement.

Tuberculosis and the Army

Like the rest of society, the Army struggled with a range of diseases. Hospitalization rates for disease during the 1890s averaged more than one a year per soldier or 30,670 admissions for a mean strength of 29,308 men.[34] Although the War Department sought to screen sick men from the ranks—rejecting 64 percent of recruits in 1891 for poor health—soldiers still fell ill.[35] Malaria was the most common reason, accounting for 16 percent of hospital admissions, followed by diarrheal diseases at 12 percent. Respiratory diseases, influenza, tonsillitis, rheumatism, and sexually transmitted diseases each generated between 5 and 10 percent of admissions. Tuberculosis accounted for less than 1 percent of the hospital admissions but was responsible for 7 percent of the deaths from disease. After the Spanish-American War (1898–99), in which the United States supported Cuba's rebellion against Spanish control and challenged Spanish dominance of the Philippines, the Surgeon General noted with alarm a doubling in sickness rates over those of the previous decade, largely due to increases in malaria and dysentery among troops deployed overseas. In 1900 soldiers required hospitalization more than twice a year on average: the Army with a mean strength of 100,389 men had 212,377 annual admissions, with malaria still in the lead, followed by diarrhea, dysentery, and sexually transmitted diseases. Thirty percent of the Army's 2,283 deaths in 1900 were from wounds and injuries, the rest from disease. Dysentery caused one-third of the deaths from disease (565 of 1,585) and typhoid, malaria, and smallpox each killed more than 100 men. Another troubling development was that ninety-six men died of tuberculosis in 1900 compared to 140 during the entire previous decade.[36]

By 1900 tuberculosis caused about 20 percent of all American deaths. That was down from a horrifying 40 percent in the mid-nineteenth century, but tuberculosis still remained the single greatest killer in the country and a problem for the military.[37] During the Civil War more than 20,000 Union troops had been hospitalized with the disease and at least 6,000 died. Military surgeons conducting autopsies on soldiers killed in action or who had died of another disease noted that they often bore calcified lesions on the lung, signs of pulmonary tuberculosis, and concluded that "consumption was truly a development of the hardships and exposures of military life."[38] In peacetime, during the last two decades of the nineteenth century, Army hospital admissions for tuberculosis ranged from 1.5 to 4.7 per 1,000 annually.[39] Although these rates were lower than in the civilian population, any infection in the Army created a risk of contagion to healthy soldiers and could generate lifelong pension obligations to disabled soldiers.

In 1893 the War Department turned to Army Surgeon General George Sternberg (Figure 1-2) to solve its tuberculosis problem. A leader in American bacteriology, Sternberg was one of the first medical officers to acquire a microscope, one of the first American scientists to attempt to reproduce Robert Koch's famous experiments isolating tuberculosis bacteria, and author of the first American textbook on bacteriology in 1893.[40] As Surgeon General from 1893 to 1902, he would guide the Medical Department into the era of modern medicine, establishing the Army

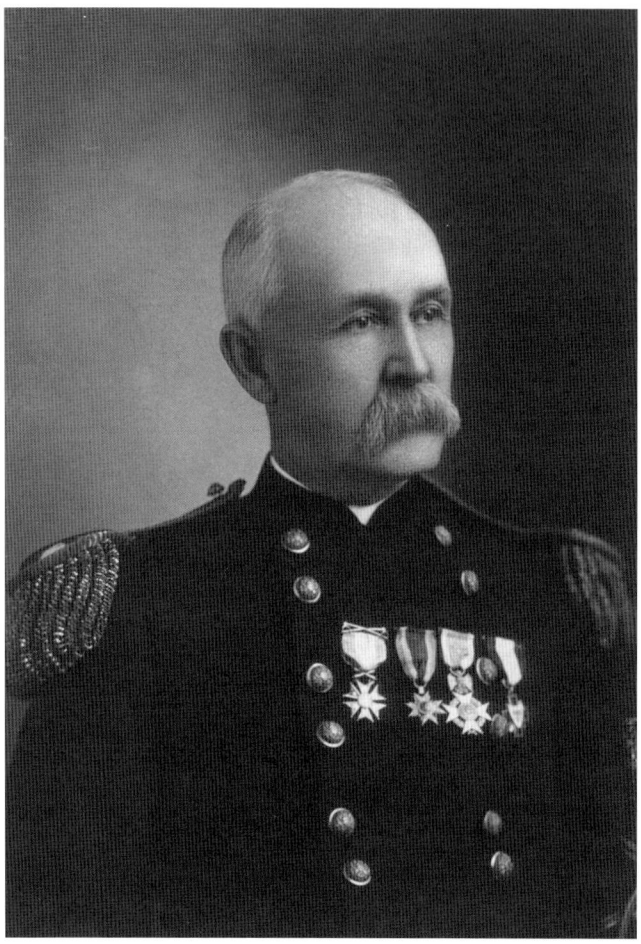

Figure 1-2. Brigadier General George Miller Sternberg, the Surgeon General who established the Army's first tuberculosis hospital in Fort Bayard, New Mexico.
Photograph courtesy of the National Library of Medicine, Image #B011438.

Medical School and the Army Nurse Corps, promoting professional dentistry and nursing, and creating a special surgical hospital in Washington, DC.

As Sternberg grappled with tuberculosis he faced four factors contributing to the problem: First, high rates of alcoholism and sexually transmitted diseases in the Army undermined soldiers' immune systems and rendered them susceptible to developing active tuberculosis; second, the War Department's expansion and increased activities in the tropics exposed soldiers to diseases such as malaria and dysentery, which also weakened their resistance to active tuberculosis; third, increasing numbers of aging Civil War and Indian wars' veterans crowded the

Soldiers' Homes in Washington, DC, and elsewhere, increasing the risk of contagion; and finally, rising expectations about the powers of new medical knowledge and technology to keep soldiers healthy reduced public tolerance for disease in the military.[41]

Alcoholism and venereal disease have long histories in the military, and physicians understood that these conditions could make people more susceptible to active tuberculosis. Before the Spanish-American War, hospital admission rates for syphilis averaged 7 percent, but in 1898 the rate nearly doubled to 13 percent, with almost one in five men in the American forces in Cuba hospitalized for sexually transmitted diseases.[42] The standard medical text of the time, William Osler's *Principles and Practice of Medicine,* noted that syphilis and other diseases could facilitate tuberculosis and that "chronic drinkers are much more liable to acute and pulmonary tuberculosis." Alcoholism, Osler suggested, "altered the tissue-soil, the alcohol lowering the vitality and enabling the bacilli more readily to develop and grow."[43] Hospital admissions for alcoholism in the Army averaged 6 percent to 7 percent in the 1890s, and virtually every Army post contended with drunkenness and the resulting fights, injuries, and desertions.[44] In 1896 the Soldiers' Home in Washington, DC, reported that 10 percent of residents suffered from alcoholism and 7.5 percent from tuberculosis.[45] Medical officers experimented with various methods of discouraging drunkenness. Lt. Edmund Munson injected patients with sulphate of strychnine, morphine, and other medicines that would make them very sick if they took a drink. Another medical officer pumped drunken soldiers' stomachs and then gave them beef broth with cayenne pepper. "The deterrent effect of this treatment is excellent," he reported.[46] The War Department also instituted post canteens in 1890 to sell beer and wine, but not spirits, and in 1899 concluded that the canteen reduced alcoholism admissions to Army hospitals from 6 percent to 3 percent of troops and was therefore "an aid to discipline as well as to the health and morals of the troops."[47]

The second factor framing the Army tuberculosis problem was the effect of tropical diseases such as malaria and dysentery on U.S. troops overseas. During the Spanish-American War the Army increased tenfold, from 25,000 to 275,000 men. So did the diseases that raged through the crowded camps. After the victory at San Juan in the summer of 1898, yellow fever and typhoid drove the Fifth Corps from Cuba in an ignominious retreat to Long Island. Dysentery and diarrhea rates in the Philippines were three times higher than among soldiers in the United States.[48] The 122,000 soldiers who served in the Philippines between 1898 and 1902 suffered at least 500,000 cases of illness, about four per capita.[49] Tuberculosis cases increased sixfold, from fewer than 100 annually to 547 cases in 1898, abetted by malaria, dysentery, and tropical fevers such as dengue, Malta, and yellow fever that could weaken or "break down" an individual's immune system and allow latent tuberculosis infections to flare.[50] So many Philippine Scouts (employed by the U.S. War Department) were developing tuberculosis that the Medical Department had to construct special hospitals in country to care for them.[51]

The case of one young officer is instructive. Lt. Watts C. Valentine was an infantry officer whose father had been a congressman from Nebraska. Young Valentine served in Puerto Rico (1898–99), but then went on sick leave for four months for an unspecified illness. Upon recovery, he was ordered to the Philippines where in a single year he experienced dysentery, Malta fever, dengue fever, and rheumatism. When he returned to the United States his weight had dropped from 155 to 83 pounds. Medical officers found malarial parasites in Valentine's blood and tuberculous infiltration of the upper and middle lobes of his right lung. Valentine spent three months at Fort Bayard in 1902 and the next year was forced to resign from the Army on disability.[52]

Alcoholism, malaria, dysentery, and tuberculosis not only damaged Army health and morale, but also generated increased federal costs when veterans had to retire on disability. Career Army enlisted men earned a pension after thirty years of service, and by the 1890s Congress had so expanded pension eligibility requirements that the vast majority of Union veterans of the Civil War received monthly stipends. Enlisted men and officers who were injured or became disabled due to illness during duty could also retire—or were compelled to retire—on disability and therefore received monthly pensions. Although lawmakers intended the pension system to obviate the need for government institutions to care for impoverished or disabled veterans, the nation cobbled together a system of domiciliary care for veterans in three parts: (1) the U.S. Soldiers' Home in Washington, DC, for poor and disabled career veterans of the Regular Army, established before the Civil War and administered by the War Department; (2) the National Home for Disabled Voluntary Soldiers, established after the Civil War to provide food, shelter, medical care, and companionship for lonely or destitute veterans, with a network of homes from Maine to California; and (3) various state-run homes. In 1899 the U.S. Soldiers' Home reported 1,296 "beneficiaries," the National Home for Disabled Volunteer Soldiers had 18,814 "members" in eight regional branches, and twenty-nine state homes served 9,140 more veterans.[53] As Civil War veterans aged and Spanish-American War veterans swelled the disabled rolls of these homes, government officials became concerned that tuberculosis was an increasing threat to the residents.[54]

Finally, the War Department and Surgeon General Sternberg faced rising public expectations regarding their abilities to keep soldiers healthy. A generation of improvements in public sanitation and medicine had largely banished water- and filth-borne diseases from American cities, and many people expected that soldiers would be as safe in the Army as at home. Such was not the case, however. Deaths by disease during the Spanish-American War outnumbered combat deaths sevenfold, 2,565 to 345.[55] Disease not only drove Americans from Cuba in 1898, but crippled the Army at home. In the summer of 1898, more than 20,000 soldiers contracted typhoid in Army training camps. At Camp Thomas, in Chickamauga, Georgia, almost 10 percent of the 80,000 men there came down with typhoid. These outbreaks outraged the public and infuriated Congress. Many people considered typhoid a disease of filth and poverty caused by poor sanitary conditions and personal hygiene; therefore, the epidemic signaled the War Department's failure to care properly for its men. A special commission established to investigate the scandal ultimately faulted the War Department leadership—not the Army Medical Department—for the failure of line officers to grasp the urgent need for sanitary efficiency and discipline, and criticized Congress for failing to provide sufficient funds to carry out the required measures. The episode, however, still humiliated the Medical Department and its officers.[56]

In 1899, with his Medical Department reeling from scandal, Surgeon General Sternberg surveyed the resources available to him to control the spread of tuberculosis in the Army. He had only three major hospitals: (1) the Army and Navy General Hospital located in Hot Springs, Arkansas, for the treatment of injuries and illnesses such as rheumatism; (2) the hospital in Washington, DC (later named for Walter Reed), where Sternberg had established a specialized surgical service; and (3) the new general hospital at the Presidio in San Francisco (later named for Jonathan Letterman), for care of the sick and wounded coming from the Philippines.[57] Sternberg commanded only 181 medical officers, 385 contract surgeons (civilian physicians hired on a contractual basis), several hundred contract nurses, and 3,300 enlisted men of the Hospital Corps, specially trained to carry out medical and hospital duties. In addition to supporting hospital ships, the Army Medical School, the Army Medical Museum, and the Surgeon General's Library, this staff had to care for a postwar Army of 99,000 officers and men located in more than 100 posts in the United States, Cuba, Puerto Rico, Hawaii, Alaska, and the Philippines.[58]

Sternberg's department was stretched thin, but the War Department's decommissioning of forts presented opportunities. In the 1890s Congress considered using government posts in the West as tuberculosis sanatoriums, and in April 1899, the Public Health and Marine Hospital Service established the first federal sanatorium at Fort Stanton, New Mexico.[59] The Army had been caring for some tuberculosis patients at the Army and Navy General Hospital in Arkansas and, since 1892, had transferred men in the early stages of tuberculosis to posts in Arizona, New Mexico, and southern California—"in order to give them the advantages of a more favorable climate."[60] In 1899 a medical officer at Whipple Barracks, Arizona, reported to Sternberg that several tuberculosis patients regained their health in the warm weather, and other Army physicians commented on the freedom from consumption of the New Mexico native population despite their poverty.[61] Anecdotal accounts of soldiers improving from tuberculosis also contributed to the belief that the environment did not "breed tuberculosis."[62] When a quartermaster officer inspected various southwestern forts as prospective hospitals, he reported favorably on Fort Bayard, estimating that $90,000 could make the buildings and barracks "suitable for occupation."[63] Given the crowding at the Soldiers' Home in Washington, DC, Sternberg proposed to the governing board that it send its tuberculous residents to a special Army hospital for tuberculosis. The Board agreed and the Secretary of War approved the proposal in 1899.[64]

Arrival of Daniel Appel and Early Optimism

When Sternberg sought a commander for the new tuberculosis hospital, he knew the medical officers from whom he could choose; small and spread thin, the Medical Corps was like a professional club. Most medical officers had worked together overseas or in training camps during the Spanish-American War and their business correspondence included inquiries about their families and one another's health. The Surgeon General's annual reports to the Secretary of War included information on individual officers' research and medical activities, the surgical procedures they had performed, and special reports on epidemics, scientific experiments, or case studies that might be of interest to their colleagues. Some reports even included medical charts, such as one tracking the temperature of a patient with appendicitis.[65]

Anticipating a favorable report for Fort Bayard's suitability, Sternberg had already chosen the medical officer to run the Army's first tuberculosis hospital. Maj. Daniel M. Appel (Figure 1-3), forty-five years old, was a respected officer with twenty-three years of experience, skilled in bacteriology, and had suffered from tuberculosis. His annual job evaluations, or "efficiency reports," deemed him "an excellent medical officer."[66] Born and raised in Pennsylvania, Appel graduated from Jefferson Medical College in Philadelphia in 1875 and received his commission as a medical officer the next year. He was married, with one child, Robert. Sternberg perhaps assumed that because Appel had had tuberculosis himself, he would have a keen interest in the disease and welcome a chance to live in the salubrious New Mexican climate. In assigning him to command at Fort Bayard, he explained, "The intention is to have a model sanitarium under the best climatic conditions, and where proper diet, an out-door life and approved methods of treatment we may expect a large proportion of recoveries." Given the urgency of the situation, Sternberg asked Appel to forgo the balance of his leave, and "report to duty at the earliest possible moment."[67] Appel's initial response to the assignment was not enthusiastic, however. He took more than two weeks to answer the Surgeon General and arrived at Fort Bayard five weeks later, 3 October, telegraphing Sternberg that he was "prepared for patients as soon as they can get here."[68]

The Soldiers' Home in Washington, DC, immediately began to send tubercular veterans west. The first patient to reach the hospital was an African American veteran of the 10th U.S. Cavalry, Private (Pvt.) Clifford Thornton. He arrived 12 October 1899, according to Appel, with "only the clothes he wore, an old civilian suit."[69] If the new patients were poorly provisioned, some were also virtually moribund. Pvt. Peter Murphy, of the 1st Artillery, died within weeks of his arrival and was buried at the Fort Bayard cemetery.[70] Appel complained to the governor of the Soldiers' Home that the disease was so advanced in some of the men they were sending that "there is no prospect for recovery."[71] But Fort Bayard became so useful that the Army also began transferring tubercular active-duty enlisted men and officers there, so that by January 1900, Fort Bayard had forty-seven patients, only one-third of them from the Soldiers' Home.[72]

As Appel took stock of Fort Bayard's resources he identified housing for him-

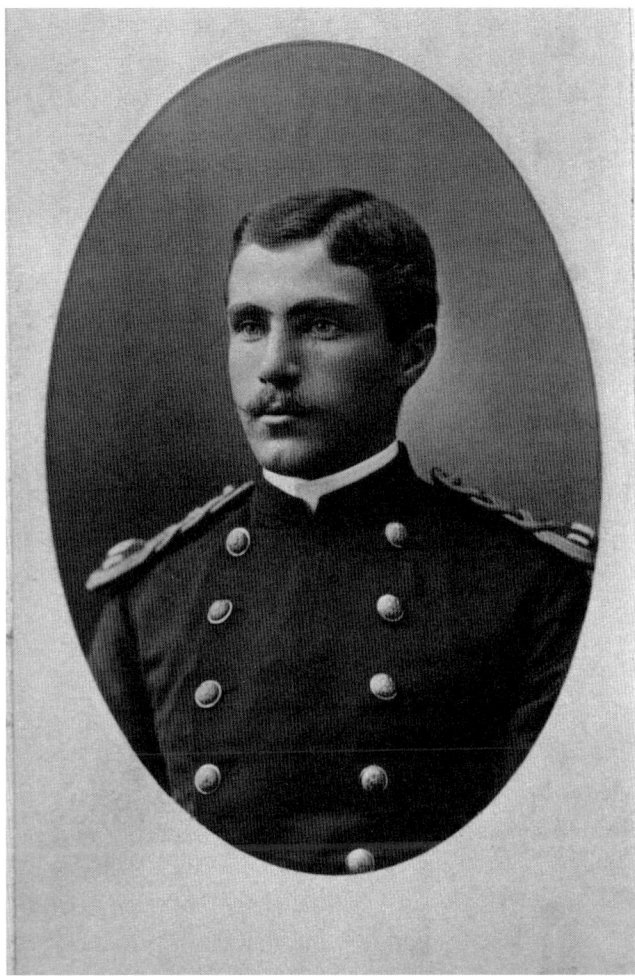

Figure 1-3. Daniel M. Appel, first commanding officer of the Army tuberculosis hospital at Fort Bayard, New Mexico.
Photograph courtesy of the National Library of Medicine, Image #B011271.

self and other officers but found most of the buildings dilapidated, with only one suitable for "a Model Sanitarium." He requested the assignment of a quartermaster officer to oversee the "necessary extensive repairs, alterations, and construction," and the authority to purchase four milk cows and employ laborers, a cook, and a baker. He also requested a garrison at the fort, "owing to the disreputable character of the inhabitants of the adjacent town," and "the extreme isolation of this post."[73] The War Department declined to send the garrison, but approved Appel's other requests, sending as quartermaster Lt. Robert Powers, who had recently been diagnosed with tuberculosis, to oversee the construction and refurbishment as he recovered his health.[74] Appel and his staff ordered medical and hospital supplies, stocked the library with medical journals and other periodicals, and acquired the requisite Army manuals. They hashed out myriad details and logistics such as arranging for the transportation of patients to the hospital. Fort Bayard was located three miles from the nearest rail line at Silver City, a spur from the Southern Pacific Railroad at Deming, New Mexico, and patients too ill to care for themselves could miss connections and languish for hours or days at the Deming station. The Army Medical Department therefore arranged to pay rail station employees to telegraph the hospital of the arrival of patients so they could ensure their safe travel on to Silver City.[75]

The local community watched events at Fort Bayard with interest. In November the *Silver City Enterprise* reported that nineteen carloads of furniture and supplies arrived along with fifteen nurses who were preparing the post to receive patients.[76] One of the most urgent tasks was to find personnel for the hospital. The Fort Bayard workforce included Chinese launderers and cooks, Mexican laborers, and African Americans, such as Pvt. Rice of the 9th Cavalry, recruited by Appel to serve in the Hospital Corps.[77] Appel also tried to build a medical staff. T. S. Bullock, a local civilian expert in tuberculosis, first ran the hospital laboratory, but Appel told the Surgeon General that "he has tubercle bacilli in his sputum and should not be closely confined to the laboratory."[78] Similarly, Margaret Drum was a nurse who was also a patient, doing light duty as a dietician while she recovered. Because the laboratory microscope showed that she had tuberculosis bacteria in her sputum, Appel wrote, "it is not advisable that she continue on duty as a dietist."[79]

Appel soon established a hospital regimen. A mule-drawn ambulance would pick up new patients from the train station in Silver City and upon arrival a medical officer, usually Appel, evaluated the patient, conducting a thorough medical history and physical examination. While Fort Bayard had X-ray machines, they broke down repeatedly and few medical officers knew how to operate them or read the X-ray images. They instead relied on a physical examination of the chest and laboratory studies of the blood, urine, and sputum.[80] Patients provided sputum samples, which laboratory staff concentrated by chemical or centrifugal preparation, placed on a glass slide, dyed to reveal the acid-fast tubercle bacilli, and then examined through a microscope. Once Appel had confirmed a tuberculosis diagnosis, he assigned the patient to a ward according to his rank—enlisted man or officer—and condition. Absent a national medical standard for tuberculosis classification, Appel divided patients into three classes according to the severity of their tuberculosis and then tracked their progress to evaluate the effectiveness of treatment. Class 1 patients had normal temperatures and no tuberculosis bacilli in their sputum, and included both patients with incipient cases and those who were recovering from serious illness. Class 2 patients had no temperature but did have tuberculosis bacilli in their sputum and were therefore infectious. Class 3 patients had a constant temperature above 100 degrees and bacteria in their sputum. Fort Bayard housed Class 1 and Class 2 patients in separate dormitories to prevent reinfection from the other patients, and confined to bed Class 3 patients in the enlisted men and officers' infirmaries.

Patients followed a routine, centering on rest, an abundant diet, outdoor living, and the regular monitoring of their bodily functions.[81] Nurses recorded temperatures three times a day, weighed patients every Friday, and recorded pulmonary hemorrhages, sputum production, and bowel regularity as needed. Medical officers conducted daily rounds of the patients, and gave them full physical examinations every two months. Patients had to bathe at least once a week and every morning Appel led ambulant patients in breathing exercises, such as one involving slow inspiration and rapid expiration to increase lung capacity. Patients received cod liver oil to strengthen their resistance and disinfectant sprays on laryngeal lesions to prevent secondary infections. Appel prescribed narcotics such as morphine and heroin for pain and to control coughing, explaining that coughing "is easily allayed by heroin, in the extensive use of which I have yet to see tolerance produced or a habit formed."[82] To combat the weight loss that accompanied consumption, Fort Bayard offered patients "abundant good nutritious food," dominated by milk and eggs provided by resident dairy cattle and chickens. Hospital rules instructed patients to eat slowly, "chew your food thoroughly," and refrain from coughing at meals. Appel noted that "to prevent eating too rapidly and bolting the food (so common among soldiers) it was found necessary to direct that ambulant patients must remain in the dining room for at least twenty minutes during each meal."[83] The patients needed to gain weight. Of 160 male patients weighed in April 1902, for example, 22 percent weighed less than 120 pounds; four patients weighed less than 100 pounds. Only twenty-eight patients, or 17 percent, weighed more than 142 pounds, the average weight of an American soldier during World War I.[84]

In addition to treating the disease, Fort Bayard (Figure 1-4) also educated patients on how to take care of themselves and practice proper hygiene.[85] Hospital staff instructed patients in the elaborate spit cup system intended to collect and

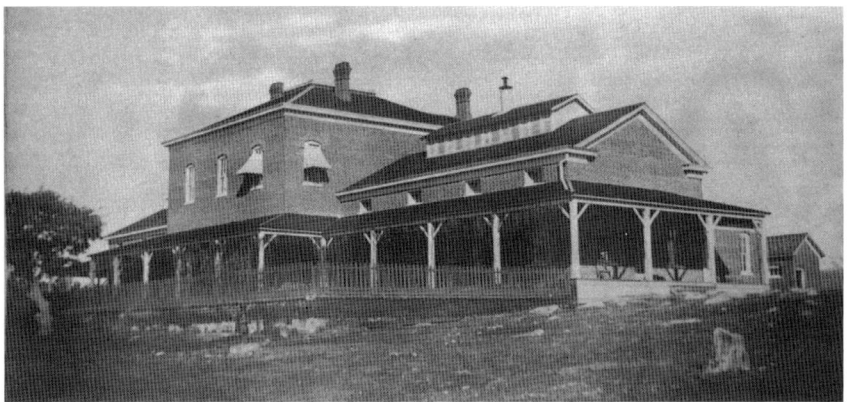

Figure 1-4. Post Hospital, Fort Bayard, New Mexico. It became one of several patient wards when the post became a tuberculosis hospital.
Photograph courtesy of the National Library of Medicine, Image #A01206.

destroy sputum infected with tuberculosis bacteria. General Order No. 2, "Instructions to Patients," explained that tuberculosis germs were found "in the spit," and "should it be allowed to dry and in the form of dust float around in the air, millions of these germs would be set free, and would not only endanger those who are well, but would often re-infect the sick."[86] The hospital gave patients tin cups with spring-loaded covers and paper inserts to carry with them at all times, placing them on shelves beneath the dining room chairs during meals. Patients had to spit into the cups carefully, never swallow the spit, and deposit the liners in large covered spittoons, also fitted with paper receptacles that were located throughout the facility. Four crematories burned the spit cups and other infected material daily.[87]

Ambulant patients were to make their beds every day and keep their belongings off the floor to avoid contamination. Fort Bayard prohibited the use of "stimulants," meaning whiskey, wine, or beer, and cigarettes, but cigars and chewing tobacco were allowed "in moderation." Above all, Fort Bayard required all patients to get as much fresh air and rest as possible by staying outside at least eight hours a day year-round, occupying their quarters only at night, and sleeping for at least ten hours a night with the windows wide open. Patients had to stay within the camp boundaries. An armed guard patrolled the area to ensure that these rules were enforced, especially the prohibitions against alcohol and leaving the post without permission.

Fort Bayard patients met one of several fates: some died, some were falsely diagnosed, and many others cycled in and out of the hospital as their health improved or deteriorated. The lucky ones recovered their health to leave Fort Bayard and live out the rest of their lives. Captain (Capt.) Charles L. Steele was one of the unfortunates. He arrived at Fort Bayard on 5 November 1899 very ill and was immediately put to bed.[88] A graduate of West Point and an officer in the 18th Infantry, Steele had enjoyed good health until 1881 when he contracted "mountain fever" in Montana, followed by malaria in 1883, from which he did not fully recover. His condition worsened on the long voyage to duty in the Philippines in 1899, and during just four months in the Philippines, Steele had two recurrences of malaria. His commanding officer recommended that he retire for his health, but Steele declined and applied for sick leave to return to the United States. After two months of rest, and then duty as a recruiting officer, Steele developed a sore throat and persistent cough. After a New York physician diagnosed him with tuberculosis of the larynx, the Army ordered him to Fort Bayard, and when he arrived Appel found that the disease had also "made giant strides in the lungs." Steele's condition deteriorated. He continued to lose weight and his medical record noted that the lungs were "universally involved," with "both upper lobes excavated." Appel put Steele on a liquid diet, and nurses monitored his temperature and tried to make him comfortable. Steele lived to see the turn of the century, but on the morning of 18 January 1900, he died at the age of forty-two. The immediate cause of death was listed as "exhaustion."[89]

Other Fort Bayard patients fought tuberculosis for years until they succumbed. Just weeks after a medical panel in the Philippines declared Albert B. Henderson fit for promotion, he fell ill with tuberculosis. The War Department promoted him to first lieutenant anyway, and ordered him back to the United States where he spent four days in the hospital at the Presidio in San Francisco, and then took the five-day trip by train and wagon to Fort Bayard. Arriving on 5 August 1901, Henderson was a sick man, with tuberculosis consuming most of his left lung and infiltrating his upper right one. Nurses described the twenty-two-year old as an "irritable and insubordinate" patient, and in 1904 he had to retire from the Army, disabled with tuberculosis. Henderson stayed in the West hoping the dry climate and altitude would cure him, but after five years, he died of tuberculosis in Denver.[90]

Pvt. Edward Long, an immigrant from Ireland, also struggled with tuberculosis for years, cycling in and out of Fort Bayard in his fight. He arrived at Fort Bayard in November 1901, having lost twenty-five pounds in five months and coughing constantly. Medical officers found active tuberculosis in the left lung and, after five months of treatment with little improvement, discharged him on disability. Long left Fort Bayard and went to New York, but returned in September 1902 with a fever and tuberculosis now in both lungs. He stayed five months, as a beneficiary of the Soldiers' Home, until he was "discharged at his own request." This time he stayed in the area, and over the next six years was in and out of Fort Bayard at least six times as his tuberculosis ebbed and flowed. On 25 June 1908, he disappeared from the historical record with his medical chart noting for the last time that he "left at his own request."[91]

Not all of Fort Bayard's patients would succumb. Two medical officers arrived at the hospital in 1904 with active tuberculosis but soon returned to duty at the hospital. In 1906 they went on a hunting trip in the mountains, and despite getting caught in a blizzard retained their health.[92] One of them, Lt. Paul Hutton, had developed tuberculosis in Beijing while on the China Relief Expedition to protect U.S. interests threatened by the Boxer Rebellion.[93] Ordered to Fort Bayard, after five months of sick leave as a patient there, he began light duty as a medical officer and two years later, once again feeling fit, requested foreign service and was assigned to Fort Seward, Alaska, where he continued his work on tuberculosis. Hutton served as a Medical Department inspector during World War I and became commander of a new Army tuberculosis hospital in Denver in 1923. He survived tuberculosis to die of a heart attack at the age of fifty-eight and was buried with honor in Arlington Cemetery. His hunting companion, Maj. Edward L. Munson, was already a bright star in the Medical Department when he came to Fort Bayard.[94] A graduate of Yale Medical School, Munson lectured at the Army Medical School, wrote one of its first textbooks, *The Theory and Practice of Military Hygiene* (1901), and was one of the medical officers present at the autopsy of President William McKinley after he was assassinated in 1901. Like Hutton, Munson fell ill during foreign deployment and was ordered to Fort Bayard. As he began to feel better, he went on part-time duty, caring for patients. With his health recovered, Munson continued his Army career in military medical education. During World War I Munson worked in the training division and headed the War Department's morale program. One of the few medical officers to be promoted to general before 1920, Munson continued his work in medical education and retired in 1932. He died in 1947, just short of his eightieth birthday.

Such successful recoveries fueled hopes for effective treatment or even a cure for tuberculosis. Surgeon General Sternberg required all Army hospitals to have a well-equipped laboratory and encouraged his medical officers at Fort Bayard and elsewhere to conduct research as time allowed. In 1900, with Appel's approval, contract surgeon Bullock gave thirty-three volunteer patients a series of injections of an experimental antituberculosis serum, but the results were discouraging. He had to stop the treatment on ten patients when they either left the hospital or refused more injections. Four patients had "extremely distressing" reactions, and twelve others' conditions appeared to worsen.[95] In a more benign experiment, Fort Bayard medical officers examined red and white cell counts in the blood of tuberculosis patients in 1900 and 1901 to learn if the blood tests "would furnish any diagnostic or prognostic value."[96]

In June 1902, Appel traveled to Saratoga, New York, to present the results of the first two years of Fort Bayard to the annual conference of the Association of the Military Surgeons of the United States.[97] He also participated in an American Medical Association (AMA) symposium on tuberculosis, along with Surgeon Paul M. Carrington, in charge of the Public Health Service sanatorium at Fort Stanton, Colorado. Appel told his colleagues that from October 1899 through March 1902, Fort Bayard admitted 623 patients, and discharged 449 after an average of five and one-half months in residence. Patients included officers, nurses, and civilians, but the vast majority were enlisted men and beneficiaries of the Soldiers' Home. Appel observed that about 80 percent of patients came from the tropics, "owing to enervating effects of the tropic climate," and that more than half of the patients had experienced pulmonary hemorrhaging. Of the "discharged patients," 21 percent had died and 7 percent were judged to be "clinically cured." Almost half, 46 percent, left the hospital with improved health but still bore signs of tuberculosis. Appel concluded that with regard to high-altitude therapy, "a larger variety of cases are amenable to its beneficial influence than is commonly believed."[98]

Surgeon General Sternberg seemed satisfied. The Medical Department's project at Fort Bayard had several goals—to prevent the spread of tuberculosis in the Army ranks and soldiers' homes, to provide healthcare to soldiers and veterans with tuberculosis, and to return to duty as many Army officers and enlisted men as possible to preserve the nation's investment in their training. In his last annual report in 1902, Sternberg told the Secretary of War that Fort Bayard had "proved to be of inestimable value for the treatment of victims of pulmonary tuberculosis," and that Appel had been "indefatigable in his effort to make this a model sanitarium and in his attention to the interests of the sick under his care."[99]

Bumps in the Road

Still, only two years after arriving at Fort Bayard, Appel departed for the Philippines with a clouded reputation. Although his superiors never questioned his work as a physician, they faulted his performance as an administrator. In 1904 he faced a court-martial for fraud and conspiracy in purchasing supplies for Fort Bayard.[100]

Although acquitted on all accounts, the War Department disciplined Appel several more times for rule infractions until his death of a heart attack in 1914.

Appel's first problem was his inability to handle the press. In the aftermath of the medical scandals during the Spanish-American War, Surgeon General Sternberg was sensitive to the Army Medical Department's public image. When a June 1900 *New York Tribune* story reported that twelve cases of "incipient consumption have been completely cured" at Fort Bayard and that Appel had characterized the results as "little short of marvelous," Sternberg may have worried that such pronouncements could lead to inflated public expectations about the Army's medical abilities.[101] Appel had to assure him that "no such statements…were ever made by me." He explained that "as far as I can ascertain, they originated in the brain of the newspaper canvasser who recently visited this hospital."[102] Several months later a similar wire story ran in newspapers across the country reporting the "remarkable success" in curing tuberculosis in government hospitals in New Mexico. The *Chicago Daily Tribune* reported that 30 of 121 patients had been discharged from Fort Bayard, "considered cured," and credited the Army hospital's treatment of outdoor living, abundant food, rest, and graduated exercise.[103] In March 1902 a *New York Times* front page story read: "You may quote me as saying that we can cure consumption in every stage." The speaker, Daniel Appel, also asked "that the statement be given the widest publicity."[104] On cue, a *New York Herald* reporter traveled to New Mexico to write a feature-length article. The story read like a travel article, describing the Fort Bayard grounds, its golf course, croquet field, and other amusements for recovering patients, and quoted Appel as saying "We have demonstrated at Fort Bayard Sanatorium for Soldiers that we can cure consumption at any stage."[105] The hospital, the reporter noted, had been "deluged by letters and telegrams" from physicians and tuberculosis sufferers eager for any new information on how to treat the disease. None of Appel's reports to the Surgeon General or the papers that he presented at scientific meetings in 1902 contained such boastful claims, but such stories suggest that Appel did not communicate well with the press, that he did brag about his record at Fort Bayard, or that they exaggerated his claims. The War Department, certainly not looking for new patients, did not need that kind of publicity, especially if it held out false hopes of a tuberculosis cure.

Appel also had difficulty managing the hospital staff. During his two years of command, Fort Bayard staff stole from the hospital, fought among themselves, and criticized his command. Trouble began within months. In June 1900 the local newspaper reported that two hospital employees had been stealing blankets and sheets and selling them to civilians in the area.[106] In 1902, Appel was again embarrassed when a hospital steward named Herbst deserted, taking with him more than $1,000 in patient funds. Slow on the uptake, Appel explained that, "I had no suspicion whatever that Steward Herbst was dishonest until several days after his desertion."[107] When Appel expelled patient Fred W. Wilkins from Fort Bayard for using profane language, and for refusing to clean out spittoons while on light duty, Wilkins protested to the Secretary of War. The Secretary referred the matter back to Appel, who was within his authority, but the fact that Wilkins went around the chain of command reflected Appel's lack of control.

Officers, too, questioned the commander's leadership. In 1902, a young cavalry officer, Lt. Robert L. Collins, filed two complaints against Appel, the first for insulting him. Appel, he charged, had broken up a card game Collins was playing with two other patients, saying that gambling was not good for their health and that the men could not afford to gamble because they had unpaid debts. Stung, Collins protested that he had money in the bank and resented Appel's accusation in front of another officer. An Army inspector came down from Chicago to investigate the charges and found that Appel's remarks were "unnecessary and showed a lack of consideration and tact, which justified the resentment on the part of Lt. Collins."[108] Collins also accused Appel of "irregularities" in the commander's practices of purchasing meat for the hospital's commissary; this charge led to Appel's trial by court-martial in 1904.[109] Other complaints included one by Pvt. Albert Henderson, who accused Appel of altering Henderson's medical record to force his retirement. Another medical officer and patient, Lt. H. D. Bloombergh, reported discourteous and unfair treatment. An investigating officer sided with Appel in these matters, but observed a lack of command: "I can see nothing in this case of importance beyond another outcropping of a spirit of insubordination among officers, both on duty and under treatment."[110] While the inspector recommended transferring several of the complainants out of Fort Bayard, in another case—that of a nurse who also challenged Appel's authority—it was Appel who had to leave.

Minnie H. Ruble entered Army service as a contract nurse during the Spanish-American War, serving in Cuba and the Philippines. Her supervisors rated her work "excellent" in those positions, but after being assigned to Fort Bayard in January 1902, she refused to carry out some duties and clashed with other staff members. By the summer Appel requested that Ruble be replaced "as early as practicable."[111] The Surgeon General declined, ordering instead that the Superintendent of Nurses give Ruble a warning, and then discharge her if there were further complaints. The superintendent, Dita H. Kinney, admonished Ruble for "insubordination" and "impertinence" in an August 1902 letter. "Your offensive manner under distasteful orders or toward those with whom you are not personally pleased is a thing that can not and will not be allowed," she warned. After Ruble refused to carry out duties in the officers' mess, which she considered outside her role as a nurse, Appel again requested her transfer. This time Ruble enlisted the support of her congressman, Rep. Frederick C. Stevens (R-MN), who asked for an investigation. An Army inspector gave Ruble a low evaluation score—6 of 10 points for efficiency—but with complaints piling up about Appel's leadership of Fort Bayard, the focus turned to him instead of her. The inspector concluded that Nurse Ruble could be continued at Fort Bayard on probation, in view of the "prospective change in the command."[112]

Appel's biggest problem was his failure to follow War Department rules and regulations. In March 1902, Army inspector Maj. James A. Irons deemed Appel "an exceedingly zealous and capable officer," noting the good condition of the post and restoration of the health of many of the patients. He was concerned, however, that the commander had not yet issued hospital rules, and instead was applying Army regulations by "changing them to suit existing conditions."[113] Another officer noted that Appel usually gave his orders verbally.[114] In September, the Army Medical Department ordered senior medical officer Col. John van R. Hoff to Fort Bayard to evaluate the hospital's progress and viability after two years in operation. He concluded that "it may be safely affirmed that the Army needs such an institution as the sanatorium at Fort Bayard, N. M.," but, he added, "the success or failure of this undertaking should not be permitted to rest upon the shoulders of any one man." Instead of verbal management, the hospital needed a comprehensive system of regulations to govern it, and recommended that the commanding officer "at once compile and forward for the consideration of the Surgeon General such a set of rules." He also questioned Appel's handling of patients' money, noting that a check for Fort Bayard was written out to Appel personally, rather than the "commander of Fort Bayard," and that the funds were held in a personal bank account in Silver City, not in a safe at the post.[115] The Surgeon General had already downgraded Appel's performance from the previous year's "excellent," to "good," but with van Hoff's report, relieved him of command in November 1902.[116]

Appel's career never fully recovered. Transferred to the Philippines, he was recalled to the United States for the court-martial. Ironically, it may have been Appel's lack of record keeping that prevented the court from convicting him of fraud. The Army charged him with buying beef on the open market for six to nine cents a pound and then reselling it to an Army commissary officer (also charged with conspiracy and fraud), at $0.10 a pound, accumulating a profit of more than $1,000 in two years. Appel said he did this to build up the hospital fund for patients, and without a paper trail proving fraud, the court acquitted both him and the commissary officer.[117] Secretary of War Elihu Root, however, found his conduct "highly reprehensible," and required him to repay the Army $1,238.86. In 1907 Appel's superiors again reprimanded him, this time for making "baseless accusations" of mismanagement against another officer, and in 1911 the Secretary of War sent him a letter of "emphatic censure" for failing to follow Army regulations in procuring diphtheria antitoxin during an epidemic. Appel's superior officer in 1913 rated him "good" but said he "would not choose him over other medical officers known to me."[118] On duty in Hawaii, Appel died in his sleep of a heart attack in April 1914.

As War Department officials wearied of the complaints and problems coming from the isolated hospital in New Mexican Territory, Fort Bayard was set to grow. The Navy had an especially serious tuberculosis problem due to the closed and crowded conditions aboard ships. Acutely aware that the formidable German and British navies had lower tuberculosis rates, Navy Surgeon General Presley M. Rixey chafed at not having his own sanatorium. He requested appropriations to enlarge Fort Bayard to accommodate sailors with tuberculosis, and in 1903 Congress approved $100,000 for improvements at Fort Bayard.[119] With the influx of funds, Washington officials wanted a trustworthy hand on the tiller—and in the till.[120]

Comegys in Charge

To replace Appel, Army Surgeon General Robert M. O'Reilly turned to a medical officer who had a mixed record in the Medical Corps. Lt. Col. Edward T. Comegys (Figure 1-5) arrived with his wife Grace and three children from Fort Meade, South Dakota, to take command in November 1902. He had served more than twenty-five years in the Army, receiving his commission in 1875 after his education at Harvard and Miami Medical College in Cincinnati, Ohio. He was also familiar with Fort Bayard, having served as post surgeon in the early 1890s. Most of his efficiency reports were positive, but in 1899 Surgeon General Sternberg had judged him "a medical officer of fair ability" and in 1901 stated, "I do not consider him a very active or efficient medical officer."[121] Comegys' poor health was perhaps hurting his performance. He had been hospitalized for malaria at least four times since 1894, and in 1901 suffered from "malarial cachexia"—physical wasting, including anemia and jaundice. Maj. John McDill, the examining physician in Manila, stated that "he is not fit for service in a tropical climate and should be sent back to the United States to prolong his life."[122] This condition may account for what his superiors perceived as a lack of energy. "He may be said to be rather an 'office man,'" observed another officer in 1903, "and lacks the energy in getting around which characterized the administration of Major Appel."[123]

Comegys did quickly promulgate rules for Fort Bayard, but his administration of these rules and regulations was not always satisfactory to the Office of The Surgeon General (OTSG).[124] OTSG staff considered Comegys' first requisition for surgical materials and drugs "excessive" and required an explanation before approving some items.[125] The office denied a requisition for carpeting because the Surgeon General considered it "undesirable furnishing for an institution for the treatment of contagious diseases," and scolded Comegys for "numerous uncorrected mistakes in spelling in this requisition," pointing out that articles were not arranged in alphabetical order and one item appeared in five places.[126] Other officials criticized Fort Bayard's administration. The Judge Advocate's Office in Denver thought that Comegys was quick to order general court-martial proceedings when less onerous and costly procedures were appropriate, and suggested that the commanding officer at Fort Bayard study the laws and regulations governing judicial proceedings.[127] Similarly, the Navy Secretary complained to the Secretary of War after Comegys asked him to convene a court-martial at Fort Bayard. The Navy, he said, did not have such authority and disciplinary problems at the hospital could be handled in other ways.[128]

In May 1903, the Secretary of War also received what was surely an unwelcome anonymous letter from a patient suggesting that all was not well at Fort Bayard. Written in a fine hand, but with poor spelling and grammar, the message was not subtle. "The commanding officer is drunk and smoking cigarettes all the time and letts the officers and lady nurses do as they please," the patient charged. "It seems as if he don't care [if] the officers sleep in the nurses quarters more than they sleep in their own quarters and when they are not doing that they

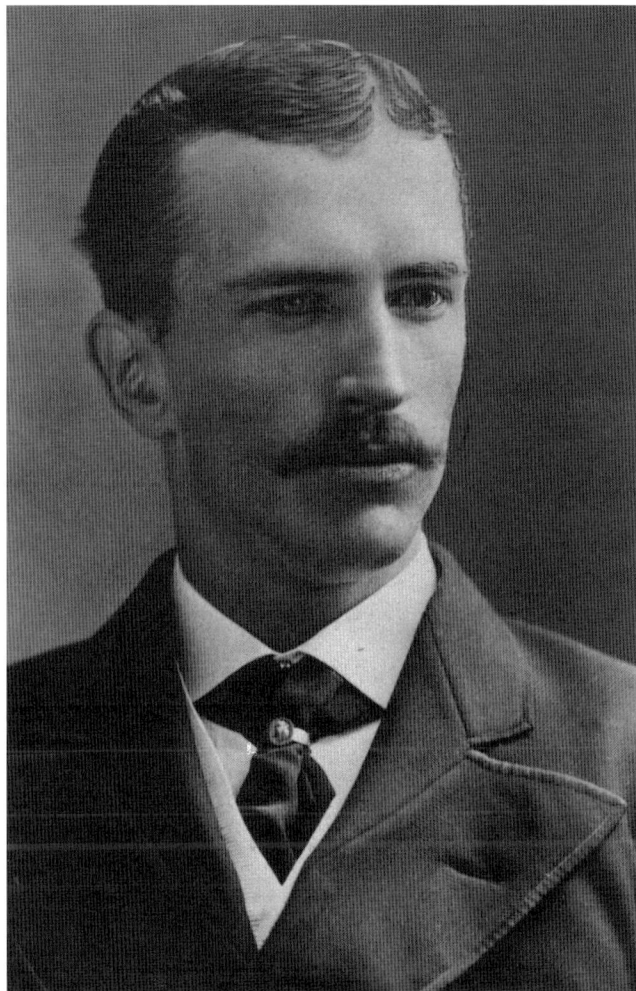

Figure 1-5. Edward T. Comegys, the second commanding officer of the tuberculosis hospital at Fort Bayard, New Mexico.
Photograph courtesy of the National Library of Medicine, Image #B011291.

are all out horse back ridding and laying around in bushes and hollows doing there dirt because patients here saw what they were doing." The writer identified them as "Lt. Patterson and Miss Rhubel, Miss Chamberlain and Liet. Collins and also the head nurse and Dr. Ohlinger and Miss Valentine. They carry on out here in the hills and bushes worse than dogs on the street." These distractions, the letter charged, caused the medical staff to neglect the patients, who were "dieing for the want of attention how can they help themselfs they are helpless and cant move without someone moves them." The solution was to bring back

Maj. Appel "so we can have some one to see to us so we can't starve and die." The correspondent closed with the threat that if the War Department did not investigate their complaints, "we turn it over to the newspapers so every body can see how the government let things go on," because, "you are not here [so] you don't know what is going on and we do."[129]

The Adjutant General's Office in Washington immediately sent Col. Charles H. Heyl to Fort Bayard. He arrived on 17 May 1903, and after a ten-day investigation determined that the charges against Comegys were "without foundation in fact and that on the contrary, Col. Comegys, while somewhat more lenient as compared with the former commanding officer, is nevertheless a competent officer and courteous gentleman." The real problem, he found, was a shortage of fully capable medical officers. Whereas Comegys had requested eight full-time officers, Heyl believed six would be sufficient if they were all well and able to work. A majority of the medical officers, however, were patients themselves and could not perform all of their tasks. "The practice of placing such officers on 'Light Duty,' requiring professional skill and mental as well as physical effort," he recommended, "should be discontinued." He added that while officers had generally disliked Appel, Comegys was popular with officers, "but not so much so with the enlisted class."[130]

Surgeon General O'Reilly's annual evaluation of Comegys was measured. He recognized that command of Fort Bayard was "a peculiarly difficult position" because the patient mix included officers, enlisted men, beneficiaries of the Soldiers' Home, and sailors. Comegys, he wrote, "is possibly deficient in energy and precision," but was discharging his duties "acceptably" and "must stand or fall on the record he is now making."[131] Signs that Fort Bayard was not being well managed continued to accumulate. When soldiers' families complained that Fort Bayard was losing patients' property, the Surgeon General observed that it indicated "a lack of system and adequate care in this respect."[132] At least one patient, medical officer Loren Ohlinger, who had pulmonary tuberculosis and developed tubercular appendicitis, was reviewing and signing his own medical chart.[133] Records during Comegys' tenure suggest that two officers, cavalry officer Lt. Robert L. Collins (who reported Appel's irregularities in procurement), and Maj. George Bushnell, who had arrived in August 1903, were assuming many of Comegys' duties. Bushnell represented the Army Medical Department at a tuberculosis conference in Baltimore in December 1903, for example, and made his report directly to the Surgeon General, and Collins signed numerous orders in Comegys' name.[134] The OTSG corresponded with Bushnell about the post construction program—something in which the hospital commander should have had an interest.

With such evidence of Comegys' carelessness and lethargy, on 21 April 1904 the Surgeon General relieved him of command of Fort Bayard, and put Bushnell in charge.[135] The War Department transferred Comegys to the Philippines, even though three years earlier a medical officer had judged him unfit to work in the tropics. Things did not go well for Comegys there. His 1905 efficiency report was so damning that the Army gave him the choice of retiring or being forced to do so. "The infirm condition of this officer is convincing to any one who has seen him that he is no longer qualified to discharge the duties of his position," reported his commanding officer, H. C. Corbin. And, he added, "It is beyond reasonable doubt that this condition is at least due to his inordinate use of drugs."[136] Comegys may have been using opium to treat chronic dysentery, which he had contracted in the Philippines, a common medical practice at the time. Within weeks of his negative efficiency report Comegys retired from the Army and died a year later in Los Angeles of heart disease and chronic dysentery.[137]

A New Hospital Commander for a New Army

When the Surgeon General named George Ensign Bushnell (Figure 1-6) to be the commander at Fort Bayard, he set the hospital on a steady course. Bushnell was one of the most esteemed members of the Medical Corps with uniformly

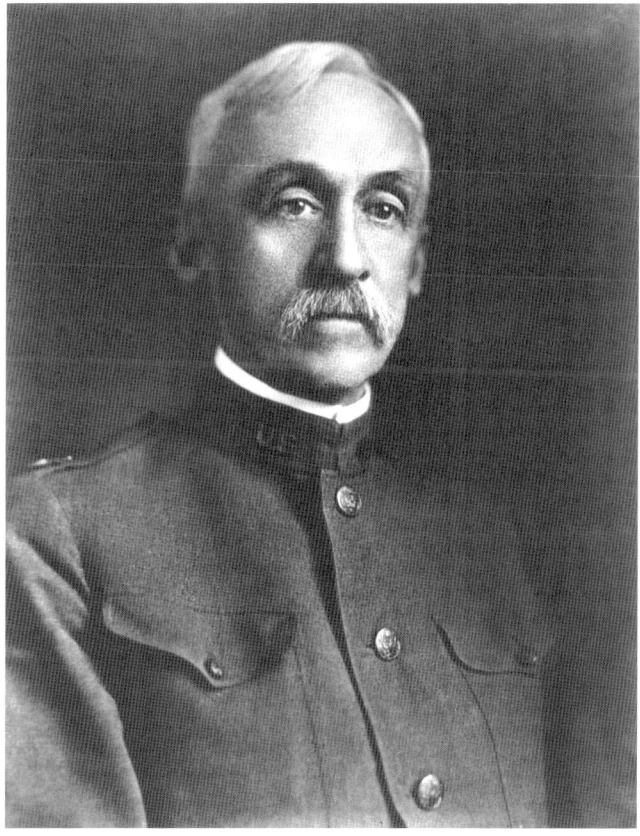

Figure 1-6. Colonel George E. Bushnell, commander of the tuberculosis hospital at Fort Bayard, 1907–1917.
Photograph courtesy of the National Library of Medicine, Image #B03218.

excellent efficiency reports and a strong record of medical scholarship that included the ability to translate medical articles in seven languages—a Renaissance man. Born in 1853, in Worcester, Massachusetts, he attended Yale University, receiving an A.B. in 1876, a Ph.D. in classical languages and literatures with a dissertation on the "the conditional sentences of Aeschylus," and an M.D. in 1880.[138] While working as an intern in a New York hospital, he developed tuberculosis, but soon regained his health and received his commission as an Army surgeon in 1881. Bushnell married twice, the first time in 1881 to Adra Holmes, with whom he had a daughter. After Adra died in 1896, Bushnell married Ethel M. Barnard in 1902, with whom he had no children. As a young officer Bushnell served at a number of frontier posts where his patients included Chinese laborers working on the railroads, and at Fort Yates, North Dakota, 3,000 Sioux prisoners of war, including Sitting Bull. During the long stretches of quiet common at frontier posts, he studied languages and botany. Called to Washington for the Spanish-American War, Bushnell worked in the medical supply depot until his health failed and his tuberculosis reactivated. He took a sick leave of absence in 1900 and spent six months in Asheville, North Carolina, in the care of tuberculosis specialist Charles L. Minor. Following the practice of sending tuberculous soldiers West, the Army transferred Bushnell to Fort Logan, Colorado. Ordered to Fort Bayard in August 1903, Bushnell took command the following May. One medical officer described him as "tall, thin, and rather ascetic in appearance, shy in manner, and very modest notwithstanding his learning and attainments, but," he added, "very positive in his opinions."[139]

Bushnell's deficiency as a medical officer was his physical condition, which his superiors believed precluded service in the field.[140] But tuberculosis also gave him a keen interest in the disease and he developed an expertise that impressed his superiors. In 1905, the Army inspector general concluded that Bushnell's leadership at Fort Bayard would "make a lasting success of the institution." The next year the inspector again stated, "the commanding officer, Major Bushnell, is an authority on tuberculosis and has acquired a reputation world-wide and second, perhaps, to none."[141] The War Department promoted him to lieutenant colonel in 1908 and colonel in 1911. In 1916, after Bushnell had been in command at Fort Bayard for twelve years, Surgeon General William Gorgas judged him "one of the most efficient officers ever developed in the Medical Corps."[142] Gorgas then called him to Washington, DC, in 1917 to take charge of the Medical Department's tuberculosis section during World War I.

Bushnell assumed command at Fort Bayard shortly after Elihu Root's tenure as Secretary of War, 1899 to 1904. President William McKinley had appointed Root, a lawyer and businessman, to shape up the War Department after the scandals of the Spanish-American War. The "Root Era" accelerated the modernization of the Army to better serve an urbanized, industrial society and the most powerful economy in the world.[143] In the 1890s, to professionalize the officer corps, Congress abolished promotion based only on seniority and the War Department established advanced training schools and increased standards for officers. It also improved living conditions for enlisted men and officers to make military service more attractive.

Secretary Root established the chief of staff and general staff system that would improve military policy development and planning, and convinced Congress to strengthen the nation's defense capability by creating a National Guard in 1903. Many of these reforms would not truly take hold until World War I, but Root set a new tone in the War Department, bringing its Army and Navy more in line with European powers as the United States assumed the world stage. In a similar vein, the Army Medical Department produced a manual in 1898 to standardize Army hospital and other medical unit supplies, equipment, and procedures, which it updated periodically. In addition to the Army Medical School and the Army Nurse Corps, the Army Medical Department developed a special curriculum for members of the Hospital Corps.[144] The Surgeon General's appointment of Bushnell reflected this new professionalism.

Tuberculosis had sidelined Bushnell during part of Root's tenure, but he clearly embraced the reforms. Although in the same generation as Appel and Comegys, Bushnell had perhaps a more modern, even corporate view of his military role than his predecessors and therefore less trouble enforcing Army regulations and standards. He wielded them as management tools.[145] In an article prescribing improvements in the recruitment, training, and promotion of the Hospital Corps, Bushnell sought to ensure that the force could be expanded in time of war, "yet contain only expert and well-disciplined men."[146]

Upon assuming command, Bushnell quickly issued new general orders for the hospital, and within months he began to shape Army tuberculosis policy, basing his arguments on science and professional knowledge as well as his military authority. Whereas Comegys' rules governed staff, including the guards, officers, nurses, and members of the Hospital Corps, Bushnell's also focused on patients' responsibilities and discipline. Instead of simply requiring ambulant patients to make their beds, Bushnell required them to be made by "nine o'clock A. M." Although Bushnell omitted detailed instructions on how patients should eat, he did require patients to pay for thermometers if they broke more than one.[147]

Bushnell's impact on Fort Bayard was both medical and military. Bushnell the physician proposed a change in the classification of patients at the hospital, objecting to Appel's system of three classes of patients because it "lays undue stress on the presence or absence of tubercle bacilli in the expectoration." He preferred a system that focused on "how far the lesions are advanced in the individual cases upon admission," and that, he added, "will make our reports more intelligible and interesting."[148] He also cut back on the amount of alcohol medical officers prescribed for their patients and cracked down on patient drunkenness.[149] Meanwhile, Bushnell the Army officer imposed strict discipline at the hospital. When superior officers questioned his frequent use of the court-martial against patients as well as staff, he stood his ground. In early 1905 the regional adjutant general objected to Bushnell's imposition of strict punishments for absence from roll call (which the commander no doubt implemented in part to discourage carousing). Bushnell responded that roll calls at the hospital were intended to prevent absences that would tire patients or "prove detrimental to their cure." He added, "These soldiers are in a status of privilege, being required to do no duty, absence on their part is therefore considered a more serious offense and should in my judgement in the interests of discipline of this Hospital be punished more severely than is permitted under the 32nd Article of War." He concluded by requesting that if the adjutant "does not approve of the views herein set forth, this paper be forwarded to higher authority for decision."[150]

A final example of Bushnell's change in command style reflects the transition from the "Old Army" to the new. In early 1904, the Medical Department circulated a memo describing a new system of medical forms for hospitalized patients, reflecting the increase in medical data now available and the Department's efforts to systematize data and patient care.[151] Instead of one single form, medical officers were to use a history sheet, a progress sheet, charts for temperature, weight, and pulse, and a treatment sheet, to be filled out by nurses. When Comegys departed, Lt. Robert Collins, the cavalry officer who had been working in the commander's office, asked to be transferred to his regiment in the Philippines. Bushnell gave Collins his final physical examination, noting that, "at the time of his departure he was considered clinically cured."[152] This entry was the first in Collin's medical record written with a typewriter instead of longhand.[153]

Bushnell's use of a typewriter reflects a departure from the nineteenth-century "Old Army" of the Indian Wars, cavalry raids, rifles, and documents written in fine hand. Bushnell's was more a technologically sophisticated, industrialized, and bureaucratic twentieth-century Army whose mission was not only to defend the homeland against its enemies, but also to protect American economic and political interests overseas. Surgeon General George Sternberg and his medical officers Daniel Appel and Edward Comegys had established the Army's first tuberculosis hospital in the West, putting the Army Medical Department in the vanguard of tuberculosis treatment and modern medicine. But George Bushnell would complete Fort Bayard's transition to the modern era. With his modern medical knowledge, firm military authority, and efficient typewriter, Bushnell would foster an oddly vibrant community of soldiers and patients living together in sickness and health, striving to rest or doing their duties, and united in common cause against a deadly disease.

Notes

1. "Fort Bayard Abandoned, to be Turned into Army Consumptives' Home," *Silver City Enterprise*, 17 November 1899.
2. Russell Weigley, *History of the United States Army* (New York, NY: The Macmillan Company, 1967), 292.
3. On the role of the federal government in the West see Richard White, *"It's Your Misfortune and None of My Own": A New History of the American West* (Norman, OK: University of Oklahoma Press, 1991); and Patricia Nelson Limerick, *The Legacy of Conquest: The Unbroken Past of the American West* (New York, NY: W. W. Norton, 1987).
4. On establishment of Fort Bayard see D. M. Appel, "United States General Hospital for Tuberculosis in Fort Bayard, N. M.," *Journal of the American Medical Association* 35 (1900): 1003–5; Daniel M. Appel, "The Army Hospital and Sanatorium for the Treatment of Pulmonary Tuberculosis at Fort Bayard, New Mexico," *Journal of the American Medical Association* 39 (1902): 1373–79; David Kammer, "National Register of Historic Places, Registration Form, Fort Bayard, United States General Hospital for Tuberculosis, Veterans Administration Hospital #55." 31 March 2001, New Mexico State Records and Archives, http://www.newmexicohistory.org/filedetails.php?fileID=9953, accessed 26 August 2012; and Eve E. Simmons, "It Took Blood, Bravery to Make Ft. Bayard History," *El Paso Times*, 20 January 1963.
5. On mining in New Mexico, see Christopher J. Juggard, "Copper Mining in Grant County, 1900–1945," in Judith Boyce DeMark, ed., *Essays in Twentieth-Century New Mexico History* (Albuquerque, NM: University of New Mexico Press, 1994).
6. War Department, Surgeon General's Office, *A Report on Barracks and Hospitals with Descriptions of Military Posts* (Washington, DC: GPO, 1870), 240.

In 2004 Congress designated Fort Bayard a National Historic District. See Public Law 108-209, "Fort Bayard National Historic Landmark Act," 108th Cong., 2nd sess.; and U.S. Congress, Senate, Report 108-8, "Fort Bayard National Historic Landmark Act," 108th Cong., 1st sess.

7. A. Judson Gray, "Notes on the History of Fort Bayard," 16 April 1870, Record Group [hereafter cited as RG] 112, Entry 386, Box 26, National Archives and Records Administration [hereafter cited as NARA].
8. War Department, Surgeon General's Office, Circular No. 4, *A Report on Barracks and Hospitals with Descriptions of Military Posts* (Washington, DC: Government Printing Office, 1870), 241.

9. On the Buffalo Soldiers see William A. Dobak, and Thomas D. Phillips, *The Black Regulars, 1866–1898* (Norman, OK: University of Oklahoma Press, 2001); Monroe Lee Billington, *New Mexico's Buffalo Soldiers, 1866–1900* (Boulder, CO: University Press of Colorado, 1991); Charles L. Kenner, *Buffalo Soldiers and Officers of the Ninth Cavalry, 1867–1898: Black and White Together* (Norman, OK: University of Oklahoma Press, 1999); and Frank N. Schubert, *Voices of the Buffalo Soldier: Records, Reports, and Recollections of Military Life and Service in the West* (Albuquerque, NM: University of New Mexico Press, 2003).

In 1992 a Buffalo Soldier Memorial Statue was dedicated at the Fort Bayard parade ground. See U.S. Congress, House of Representatives, "Fort Bayard National Historic Landmark Act," House Report 108-257, 108th Cong., 1st sess., 3 September 2003.

10. Pershing commanded white troops of the Sixth Cavalry at Fort Bayard, but earned his nickname as "Black Jack Pershing" when he commanded the African American soldiers of the 10th Cavalry at Fort Assiniboine, Montana, in the 1890s.

11. Jack Lane, *Armed Progressive: General Leonard Wood* (San Rafael, CA: Presidio Press, 1978).

12. Nancy J. Tomes, *The Gospel of Germs: Men, Women, and the Microbe in American Life* (Boston, MA: Harvard University Press, 1998).

13. On health seekers see Esmond R. Long, "Weak Lungs on the Santa Fe Trail," *Bulletin of the History of Medicine* 8 (1940): 1040–54; Billy Jones, *Health Seekers in the Southwest, 1817–1900* (Norman, OK: University of Oklahoma Press, 1967); Gregg Mitman, "Geographies of Hope: Mining the Frontiers of Health in Denver and Beyond, 1870–1965," *Osiris* 19 (2004): 93–111; Jake W. Spidle Jr., *Doctors of Medicine in New Mexico* (Albuquerque, NM: University of New Mexico Press, 1986); Jake W. Spidle Jr., "Coughing and Spitting and New Mexico History," in Judith Boyce DeMark, ed. *Essays in Twentieth Century New Mexico History* (Albuquerque, NM: University of New Mexico Press, 1994); Jeanne E. Abrams, *Blazing the Tuberculosis Trail: The Religio-Ethnic Role of Four Sanatoria in Early Denver* (Denver, CO: Colorado Historical Society, 1991); Jeanne E. Abrams, *Dr. Charles David Spivak: A Jewish Immigrant and the American Tuberculosis Movement* (Boulder, CO: University of Colorado Press, 2009); Judith L. DeMark, "Chasing the Cure—A History of Healthseekers to Albuquerque, 1902–1940," *Journal of the West* 21, no. 3 (July 1982): 49–58; and John Baur, "The Health Seeker in the Westward Movement, 1830–1900," *Journal of American History* 46 (1959): 91–110.

14. Jones, *Health Seekers in the Southwest*, 166.

15. See, for example, L. Huber, "The Climatic Treatment of Pulmonary Consumption in the Dry Elevated Regions of the Rocky Mountains," *Medical and Surgical Reporter* 55 (1887): 2227–29; J. Hilgard Tyndale, "New Mexico, Its Climatic Advantages for Consumptives," *Boston Medical and Surgical Journal* 108 (15 March 1888): 265–67; and Samuel A. Fisk, "The Effect of the Climate of Colorado upon Phthisis Pulmonalis, as Shown by the Analysis of One Hundred Recorded Cases," *Boston Medical and Surgical Journal* 121 (22 August 1889): 173–77.

16. Karen Holliday Tanner, *Doc Holliday: A Family Portrait* (Norman, OK: University of Oklahoma Press, 1998).

17. Jones, *Health Seekers in the Southwest*, viii and 97. See also Julius Lane Wilson, citing Edwin Solly in "Pikes Peak or Bust: An Historical Note on the Search for Health in the Rockies," *Rocky Mountain Medical Journal* 64 (1967): 59.

18. Spidle, *Doctors of Medicine in New Mexico*, 87.

Please note: I will use the spelling, "sanatoriums," in my discussion, but will retain the use of "sanatoria" and "sanitariums" in original quotes and publications.

19. For example, J. Hilgard Tyndale, "The Selection of a Suitable Climate for the Various Forms of Pulmonary Consumption," *Boston Medical and Surgical Journal* 112 (28 May 1885): 517–20; and Edward T. Bruen, "The Relative Importance of Different Climatic Elements in the Treatment of Phthisis," *Transactions of the American Climatological Association* 5 (1888): 36–45.

20. Charles Denison, *Rocky Mountain Health Resorts: An Analytical Study of High Altitudes in Relation to the Arrest of Chronic Pulmonary Disease* (Boston, MA: Houghton, Osgood, 1880); and "Dryness and Elevation, the Most Important Elements in the Climatic Treatment of Phthisis," *New York Medical Journal* 40 (1884): 283–89, and 309–15.

21. Jones, *Health Seekers in the Southwest*, 179. On the decline in popularity of the climate approach, see Frank B. Rogers, "The Rise and Decline of Altitude Therapy of Tuberculosis," *Bulletin of the History of Medicine* 43 (1969): 3.

22. Susan Jane Edwards, "Nature as Healer: Denver, Colorado's Social and Built Landscapes of Health, 1880–1930." Ph.D. dissertation, University of Colorado, 1994, 76.

23. Tomes, "The Making of a Germ Panic, Then and Now," *American Journal of Public Health* 90, no. 2 (2000): 191–98.

24. On the tuberculosis movement see Richard H. Shyrock, *The National Tuberculosis Association, 1904–1954: A Study of the Voluntary Health Movement in the United States* (New York, NY: The National Tuberculosis Association, 1957); Michael E. Teller, *The Tuberculosis Movement: A Public Health Campaign in the Progressive Era* (New York, NY: Greenwood Press, 1988); Ott, *Fevered Lives;* Rothman, *Living in the Shadow of Death;* Bates, *Bargaining for Life;* James A. Tobey, *Public Health Law*. 3rd ed. (New York, NY: Commonwealth Fund, 1947), 152–53; and James A. Tobey, *The National Government and Public Health* (Baltimore, MD: Johns Hopkins Press, 1926).

25. William Osler, *The Principles and Practice of Medicine*. 4th ed. (New York, NY: D. Appleton & Co., 1901); and Arnold C. Klebs, ed., *Tuberculosis: A Treatise by American Authors on Its Etiology, Pathology, Frequency, Semeiology, Diagnosis, Prognosis, Prevention, and Treatment* (New York, NY: D. Appleton & Co., 1909), 409.

26. Francis T. B. Fest, "Sociological Musings in Relation to Tuberculosis,"*New Mexico Medical Journal* 6 (January 1911): 68. See also Barron H. Lerner, "Constructing Medical Indications: The Sterilization of Women with Heart Disease or Tuberculosis, 1905–1935," *Journal of the History of Medicine and Allied Sciences* 49 (1994): 362–79.

27. M. Worboys, "The Sanatorium Treatment for Consumption in Britain, 1890–1914," in J. V. Pickstone, ed., *Medical Innovations in Historical Perspective* (London, UK: 1992), 58.

28. John William Trask, "The Dangers of Unrestricted Traveling of Consumptives," *Military Surgeon* 16 (1905): 322–33; L. W. Curtis, "Consumptives on Trains," letter to the editor, *New York Times*, 3 May 1905; and S. Adolphus Knopf, "Public Measures in the Prophylaxis of Tuberculosis," in Arnold C. Klebs, ed., *Tuberculosis: A Treatise by American Authors*, 418–20.

29. *Public Health Service Annual Report, 1906*, 207–214. On the bovine tuberculosis effort, see Susan D. Jones, "Mapping a Zoonotic Disease: Anglo-American Efforts to Control Bovine Tuberculosis Before World War I," *Osiris* 19 (2004): 133-48.

30. Charles E. Rosenberg, *The Care of Strangers: The Rise of America's Hospital System* (New York, NY: Basic Books, 1987), 5. See also Charles E. Rosenberg, "Inward Vision and Outward Glance: The Shaping of the American Hospital, 1880–1914," *Bulletin of the History of Medicine* 53 (1979): 346–91; David Rosner, "Social Control and Social Service: The Changing Use of Space in Charity Hospitals," *Radical History Review* 21 (1979): 183–97; Guenther Risse, *Mending Bodies, Saving Souls: A History of Hospitals* (New

York, NY: Oxford University Press, 1999); Rosemary Stevens, *In Sickness and in Wealth: American Hospitals in the Twentieth Century* (New York, NY: Basic Books, Inc., 1989); and Dianna E. Long and Janet Golden, eds., *The American General Hospital: Communities and Social Contexts* (Ithaca, NY: Cornell University Press, 1989).

31. Florence Nightingale, *Notes on Hospitals* (1859). See also Adrian Forty, "The Modern Hospital in England and France: The Social and Medical Uses of Architecture," in Anthony D. King and Paul Kegan, eds., *Buildings and Society: Essays on the Social Development of the Built Environment* (London, UK: Routledge, 1980), 61–93.

32. Michael E. Teller, *The Tuberculosis Movement: A Public Health Campaign in the Progressive Era* (New York, NY: Greenwood Press, 1988), 82.

33. Abrams, *Blazing the Tuberculosis Trail*; and Jeanne Abrams and Maryann Fitzharris, *A Place to Heal: The History of National Jewish Medical and Research Center* (Boulder, CO: Johnson Publishing, 1997). On segregating patients with different disease severity, see Edward O. Otis, "What is a Tuberculosis Sanatorium?" *American Climatological Association* (1911): 161–70.

34. *War Department Annual Report* [hereafter cited as *WDAR*], 1901, 866–71.

35. *WDAR*, 1892, 451–576.

36. *WDAR*, 1901, 855–68.

37. Twenty percent is an estimate because the United States was not yet compiling nationwide health statistics. Estimates on the percentage of deaths due to tuberculosis in the early nineteenth century range from 25 percent to 40 percent. See Bureau of the Census, *Tuberculosis in the United States* (Washington, DC: Department of Commerce and Labor, 1908), table 1.

38. United States Army, Office of The Surgeon General, *Medical and Surgical History of the War of Rebellion, 1861–1865* (Washington, DC: Government Printing Office, 1888), vol. 1, pt. III, 818.

39. "The Army Sanatorium for Tuberculosis at Fort Bayard, New Mexico," n.d., RG 112, Entry 26, Box 91, NARA. The rate in 1891, for example, was 2.97 percent, *Surgeon General Annual Report*, 1892 [hereafter cited as *SGAR*, year], 498.

40. George M. Sternberg, "Is Tuberculosis a Parasitic Disease?" *Medical News* 41 (July–December 1882): 6–7, 87–89, 311–14, 564–66, and 730–31; and George M. Sternberg, *A Manual of Bacteriology* (New York, NY: William Wood, 1892). For information on George Sternberg see Mary C. Gillett, *The Army Medical Department, 1865–1917*, Army Historical Series (Washington, DC: Center of Military History, 1995), 94–98; Martha L. Sternberg, *George Miller Sternberg: A Biography* (Chicago, IL: American Medical Association, 1920); John M. Gibson, *Soldier in White: The Life of General George Miller Sternberg* (Durham, NC: Duke University Press, 1958); Edgar Erskine Hume, "Sternberg's Centenary, 1838–1938," *Army Medical Bulletin* 46 (1938): 69–78; and Office of Medical History, Office of The Surgeon General, "The Surgeons General," http://history.amedd.army.mil/surgeongenerals/G_Sternberg.html, accessed 26 August 2012.

41. On rising expectations see Tomes, *The Gospel of Germs*.

42. *WDAR*, 1901, vol. 1, pt. 2, 709. See also Daniel Appel's observation at Fort Bayard, "A large majority of our patients have been addicted to the excessive use of alcohol, either occasionally or habitually," in Daniel Appel, *The General Hospital and Sanitorium for the Treatment of Pulmonary Tuberculosis at Fort Bayard* (Carlisle, PA: Association of Military Surgeons, 1902), 11.

43. William Osler, *The Principles and Practice of Medicine*. 4th ed. (New York, NY: D. Appleton & Co., 1901), 269, 382; and Thomas J. Mays, "Alcohol as a Factor in the Causation of Pulmonary Consumption," *Journal of the American Medical Association* 48 (2 February 1907): 398–99. On the relationship between alcoholism and tuberculosis see

Barron H. Lerner, *Contagion and Confinement: Controlling Tuberculosis along Skid Row* (Baltimore, MD: Johns Hopkins University Press, 1998).

Also on problems of alcoholism in the Army see Edward M. Coffman, *The Old Army: A Portrait of the American Army in Peacetime, 1784–1898* (New York, NY: Oxford University Press, 1986); James Marten, "Nomads in Blue: Disabled Veterans and Alcohol at the National Home," in David A. Gerber, ed., *Disabled Veterans in History* (Ann Arbor, MI: University of Michigan Press, 2000); Anton Paul Sohn, *A Saw, Pocket Instruments, and Two Ounces of Whiskey: Frontier Military Medicine in the Great Basin* (Spokane, WA: Arthur H. Clarke, 1998); 82, 102–4, and 354–56; Charles A. Byler, *Civil-Military Relations on the Frontier and Beyond, 1865–1917* (Westport, CT: Praeger Security International, 2006); and Earl F. Stover, *Up From Handyman: The United States Army Chaplaincy, 1865–1920,* vol. 3 (Washington, DC: Office of the Chief of Chaplains, Department of the Army, 1977).

On the history of alcoholism in the United States, see Sarah Tracy, *From Vice to Disease: Alcoholism in America, 1870–1920* (Tulsa, OK: University of Oklahoma Press, 2004); and David Courtwright, *Violent Land: Single Men and Social Disorder from the Frontier to the Inner City* (Cambridge, MA: Harvard University Press, 1996).

44. *WDAR*, 1899, vol. 1, pt. 1, 275.

45. *WDAR*, 1896, vol. 1.

46. W. H. Arthur to Surgeon General, 27 August 1894, RG 112, Entry 52, Box 2, NARA; and Gillett, *Army Medical Department, 1865–1917*, 103–4.

47. *WDAR*, 1899, vol. 1, pt. 1, Appendix C, "Report of the Adjutant General of the Army to the Secretary of War on the Canteen Section of the Post Exchange," 81–279.

48. Gillett, *Army Medical Department, 1865–1917*, 216; and Vincent J. Cirillo, *Bullets and Bacilli: The Spanish-American War and Military Medicine* (New Brunswick, NJ: Rutgers University Press, 2004).

49. Ken DeBevoise, *Agents of Apocalypse: Epidemic Disease in the Colonial Philippines* (Princeton, NJ: Princeton University Press, 1995), 41–42.

50. *WDAR*, 1900, 783. On tropical medicine and imperialism see DeBevoise, *Agents of Apocalypse*; Gillett, *Army Medical Department, 1865–1917*, 201–306; Warwick Anderson, "Immunities of Empire: Race, Disease, and the New Tropical Medicine, 1900–1920," *Bulletin of the History of Medicine* 70 (Spring 1996): 94–118; and Marcos Cueto, "Sanitation from Above: Yellow Fever and Foreign Intervention in Peru, 1919–1922," *Hispanic American Historical Review* 72 (1992): 1–22.

51. Isaac W. Brewer, "Tuberculosis Amongst the Philippine Scouts (native troops) of the United States Army," *Boston Medical and Surgical Journal* 163 (1910): 940–42.

52. "Clinical History, Valentine, Watts C.," RG 112, Entry 396, Box 82, NARA; and "Efficiency Report, Watts Crawford Valentine," RG 94, Adjutant General's Office [hereafter cited as AGO] 111610, Box 781, NARA.

53. Carol R. Byerly, "Army Sanctuary for Tuberculous Veterans: Fort Bayard, New Mexico, 1899–1919," in Stephen P. Ortiz, ed., *Veterans' Policy, Veterans' Politics: New Perspectives on Veterans in the Modern United States* (Gainesville, FL: University Press of Florida, 2012); Paul R. Goode, *The United States Soldiers' Home: A History of Its First Hundred Years* (Richmond, VA: n.p., 1957); Patrick J. Kelly. *Creating a National Home: Building the Veterans' Welfare State, 1860–1900* (Cambridge, MA: Harvard University Press, 1997); Patrick J. Kelly, "Establishing a Federal Entitlement," in Larry M. Logue and Michael Barton, eds., *The Civil War Veteran: A Historical Reader* (New York, NY: New York University Press, 2007); David A. Gerber, *Disabled Veterans in History* (Ann Arbor, MI: University of Michigan Press, 2000); William A. Dobak and Thomas D. Phillips, *The Black Regulars, 1866–1898* (Norman, OK: University of Oklahoma Press, 2001); and Trevor K. Plante, "Genealogy Notes: The National Home for Disabled Volunteer Soldiers," *Prologue* 36, no. 1 (Spring 2004): 56–61.

54. *WDAR*, 1899, vol. 1, pt. 1, 482. Also Eve E. Simmons, "It Took Blood, Bravery to Make Ft. Bayard History," *El Paso Times* 20 January 1963.

55. Cirillo, *Bullets and Bacilli*, 32; see also Mary Gillett, *Army Medical Department, 1865–1917;* Vincent J. Cirillo, "Fever and Reform: The Typhoid Epidemic in the Spanish-American War," *Journal of the History of Medicine and Allied Sciences* 55 (October 2000): 363–97; Percy M. Ashburn, *A History of the Medical Department of the U.S. Army* (Boston, MA and New York, NY: Houghton Mifflin, Co., 1929); and George M. Sternberg, *Sanitary Lessons of the War and Other Papers* (Washington, DC: Press of Byron S. Adams, 1912).

56. Walter Reed, Victor C. Vaughan, and E. O. Shakespeare, *Reports on the Origin and Spread of Typhoid Fever in the U.S. Military Camps During the Spanish War of 1898*, 2 vols. (Washington, DC: GPO, 1904); United States, Congress, Senate, *Report of the (Dodge) Commission Appointed by the President to Investigate the Conduct of the War Department in the War with Spain*, 56th Cong., 1st sess., Senate Doc. 221; Gillett, *Army Medical Department, 1865–1917*, chapter 7; and Stanhope Bayne-Jones, *The Evolution of Preventive Medicine in the United States Army, 1607–1939* (Washington, DC: Office of The Surgeon General of the Army, 1968), 123–46. On the impact on the Medical Department see Carol R. Byerly, *Fever of War: The Influenza Epidemic — The U.S. Army during WWI* (New York, NY: New York Univ Press, 2005).

57. The Medical Department was closing two hospitals it no longer considered useful— the Army General Hospital in Savannah, Georgia, and the Josiah Simpson Hospital at Fort Monroe, Virginia.

58. *WDAR*, 1899, vol. 1, pt. 1, 5, 371; and Gillett, *Army Medical Department, 1865–1917*, 319–25.

59. See, for example, Parker W. Thorton, "A National Sanatorium for Consumptives," *Journal of the American Medical Association* 26 (1896): 570–72; Jones, *Health Seekers in the Southwest*, 191–92; and "An Army Sanitarium for Tuberculosis," *Boston Medical and Surgical Journal* 141 (7 September 1899), 248–49. The federal government also established the Navajo Agency Sanatorium, with twenty beds, at Fort Defiance, Arizona, in 1915. See Robert A. Trennert, *White Man's Medicine: Government Doctors and the Navaho, 1863–1955* (Albuquerque, NM: University of New Mexico Press, 1998).

60. "An Army Sanitarium for Tuberculosis," *Boston Medical and Surgical Journal* 141 (7 September 1899): 248; and Gillett, *Army Medical Department, 1865–1917*, 339.

61. Porter, "Whipple Barracks," 328.

62. Esmond R. Long, "Weak Lungs on the Santa Fe Trail," *Bulletin of the History of Medicine* 8 (1940): 1046–47, 1045.

63. M. I. Ludington to Quartermaster General, 18 August 1899, RG 112, Entry 26, Box 359, NARA.

64. *WDAR*, 1899, vol. 1, pt. 1, 482.

65. *WDAR*, 1897, vol. 1, 502–44.

66. Efficiency Records of Daniel M. Appel, RG 94, Appointment, Commission and Personnel Branch, Office of the Adjutant General [hereafter cited as ACP], Box 631, NARA.

67. George Sternberg to D. M. Appel, 8 August 1899, RG 112, Entry 382, Box 1, NARA.

68. Appel to Office of The Surgeon General, telegram, 3 October 1899, RG 112, Entry 26, Box 359, NARA.

69. Appel to Board of Commissions, Soldiers' Home, 12 October 1899, RG 112, Entry 377, NARA.

70. Appel to Governor, Soldiers' Home, 12 December 1899, RG 112, Entry 377, NARA; and records of the Fort Bayard National Cemetery at http://www.interment.net/data/us/nm/grant/ftbaynat/index.htm, accessed 26 August 2012.

71. Appel to Governor, Soldiers' Home, 16 December 1899, RG 112, Entry 377, NARA.

72. *WDAR*, 1900, vol. 1, pt. 2, 784 and 538.

73. D. M. Appel to Office of the Surgeon General, 10 October 1899, RG 112, Entry 26, Box 359, NARA.

74. Sternberg to Appel, 17 October 1899, RG 112, Entry 26, Box 359, NARA.

75. D. W. Powell to Signal Officer, Department of Colorado, U.S. Army, 6 January 1900, RG 112, Entry 382, Box 1, NARA.

76. "The Bayard Sanitarium," *Silver City Enterprise*, 20 October 1899.

77. Appel to Adjutant General, Department of Colorado, 10 January 1900, RG 112, Entry 377, NARA.

78. Appel to Surgeon General, 17 December 1899, RG 112, Entry 377, NARA.

79. Appel to the Office of the Surgeon General, 15 August 1900, Entry 377, NARA.

80. This description of a sputum test is drawn from a tuberculosis manual that was listed as being in the Fort Bayard Library, Arnold C. Klebs, ed., *Tuberculosis: A Treatise by American Authors*, 327–30.

81. From *WDAR*, 1901.

82. Daniel M. Appel, "The Army Hospital and Sanatorium for the Treatment of Pulmonary Tuberculosis at Fort Bayard, New Mexico," *Journal of the American Medical Association* 39 (1902): 1378. See also Morris Manges, "Treatment of Coughs with Heroin," *New York Medical Journal* 69 (26 November 1898): 768–70; and Henry D. Fulton, "Heroin in Affections of the Respiratory Organs," *New York Medical Journal* 70 (1899): 760–61.

83. Appel, *The General Hospital and Sanatorium for the Treatment of Pulmonary Tuberculosis at Fort Bayard* 15.

84. Appel, "The Army Hospital and Sanatorium for the Treatment of Pulmonary Tuberculosis at Fort Bayard, New Mexico," *Journal of the American Medical Association* 39 (1902): 1378; and Appel, *The General Hospital and Sanatorium for the Treatment of Pulmonary Tuberculosis at Fort Bayard,* 13.

85. On education see also Evelyn Fisher Frisbee, "Education of the Consumptive in Home Care," *New York Medical Journal* 6 (January 1911): 86–89.

86. U.S. General Hospital, Fort Bayard, 26 October 1900, RG 112, Entry 26, Box 369, NARA.

87. *WDAR*, 1901, vol. 1, pt. 2, 552.

88. Charles Steele, "Efficiency Report," RG 94, Box 578, and RG 112, Entry 52, Box 3, NARA.

89. Daniel M. Appel, "Clinical History #4820," RG 112, Entry 53, Box 3, NARA.

90. Information on Albert B. Henderson can be found in RG 94, AGO 391621, Box 2727, NARA; and RG 112, Entry 26, #92255, Box 639, NARA.

91. Clinical History, Edward Long, RG 112, Entry 396, Box 50, NARA.

92. E. L. Munson, S. P. Vestal, and Paul Hutton to Adjutant, Fort Bayard, 20 November 1906, RG 112, Entry 386, Box 2, NARA.

93. Information on Paul Hutton from RG 94, AGO 229172, Box 1461, NARA.

94. Information on Edward L. Munson is from RG 94, AGO 2115, Box 1440, NARA; RG 112, Entry 396, Box 59, NARA; Edward L. Munson biography, from "U.S. Army Surgeon General's Office Biographical Sketches of Medical Officers," Manuscript Collection 44, History of Medicine Division, National Library of Medicine; and Dale C. Smith, "In Days Gone By: Edward Lyman Munson, M.D.: A Biographical Study in Military Medicine," *Military Medicine* 164 (January 1999): 1–5.

95. *WDAR*, 1901, vol. 1, pt. 2, 559.

96. Appel, "The Army Hospital and Sanatorium for the Treatment of Pulmonary Tuberculosis at Fort Bayard, New Mexico," *Journal of the American Medical Association* 39 (1902): 1379.

97. The following discussion is from Daniel M. Appel, "The Army Hospital and Sanatorium for the Treatment of Pulmonary Tuberculosis at Fort Bayard, New Mexico," *Journal of the American Medical Association* 39 (1902): 1373–79; and Daniel Mitchell Appel, "The General Hospital and Sanatorium for the Treatment of Pulmonary Tuberculosis at Fort Bayard, New Mexico," *Military Surgeon* 11 (1902): 203–21.

98. Appel, "Hospital and Sanatorium at Fort Bayard," *Military Surgeon*, 221.

99. *WDAR*, 1901, vol. 1, pt. 2, 849–50.

100. "General Court Martial of Major Daniel M. Appel," 1903, RG 153, Records of the Judge Advocate General, Box 3473, #35995, NARA; and RG 112, Entry 26, Box 40, NARA.

101. "Consumption Cured in New Mexico," *New York Tribune*, 14 June 1900, clipping attached to Appel to General Sternberg, RG 112, Entry 26, Box 359, NARA.

102. D. M. Appel to General Sternberg, date stamped 21 June 1900, RG 112, Entry 26, Box 359, NARA.

103. "Cured Thirty Consumptives," *Chicago Daily Tribune*, 30 September 1900. See also "Curing Consumption," *Fort Wayne Sentinel*, 6 October 1900.

104. "Can Cure Consumption," *New York Times*, 2 March 1902. See also "Benefits at Fort Bayard," *Chicago Tribune*, 6 March 1902.

105. "Consumption Conquered by United States Army," *New York Herald*, 30 March 1902.

106. "Employees Rob Uncle Sam," *The Enterprise*, 29 June 1900.

107. Appel to John G. McCartney, 20 September 1902, RG 112, Entry 377, vol. 3, NARA.

108. Surgeon General to D. M. Appel, 11 November 1902, RG 112, Entry 382, Box 1, NARA; and "Report of Investigation in the Case of 2d Lieut. R. L. Collins, 2d Cavy, U.S. Army General Hosp., Ft. Bayard, N. M." 14 October 1902, RG 112, Entry 26, Box 639, NARA.

109. "General Court Martial of Major Daniel M. Appel," 1903, RG 153, Box 3473, #35995, NARA.

110. See "The Case of Lieut. H. D. Bloombergh, Assistant Surgeon, U.S. Army," July 1902, RG 112, Entry 26, Box 639, NARA.

111. "The Case of Nurse M. H. Ruble, Nurse Corps," RG 112, Entry 26, Box 639, NARA.

112. "The Case of Nurse M. H. Ruble," 1902.

113. "Extracts from Annual Report Inspection of U.S. General Hospital, Fort Bayard, New Mexico, by Major James A. Irons, made March 5th, 6th, 7th, and 8th, 1902," RG 153, Box 3476, NARA.

114. "Synopsis of the Result of the Investigation of the General Hospital at Fort Bayard, New Mexico," 2 July 1903, RG 94, AGO 484491, Box 3393, NARA.

115. Hoff to Surgeon General's Office, 20 October 1902, Inspection Report, RG 112, Entry 26, Box 639, NARA.

116. Efficiency Record of Daniel M. Appel, RG 94, ACP, Box 631, NARA.

117. "General Court Martial of Major Daniel M. Appel," 1903, RG 153, Box 3473, #35995, NARA.

118. "Efficiency Report, Daniel M. Appel," RG 94, ACP, Box 631, NARA.

119. P. M. Rixey, "Hospital, Fort Bayard, For Tuberculosis Patients," U.S. Congress, House Committee on Naval Affairs, Committee Report 30-4, 1 December 1902, 57th Cong., 2nd sess., CIS-No H71-0.35. See also House Committee on Naval Affairs, "Hospital, Fort Bayard, N. Mex., for Tuberculosis Patients," 5 January 1903, Com. Serial Rpt. No.

28; and "Surgeon General Rixey's Recommendations on Personnel, Nurse Corps, Dental Corps, Fort Bayard Hospital, and Hospital Naval Academy," 7 January 1903, Com. Serial Rpt. No. 30, 57th Cong., 2nd sess., CIS-No H71 - 0.29 and 0.31.

120. "Appropriations for Ft. Bayard," *Silver City Independent,* 15 July 1902.

121. "Efficiency Reports, E. T. Comegys," RG 94, ACP, Box 311, NARA.

122. "Application for Leave of Absence," 26 March 1901, RG 94, Box 582, NARA.

123. "Synopsis of the Result of the Investigation of the General Hospital at Fort Bayard, New Mexico," 2 July 1903, RG 94, AGO 484491, Box 3393, NARA.

124. "General Orders No. 1," 12 January 1903, RG 112, Entry 389–91, Box 1, NARA. Please note: Fort Bayard, like all Army hospitals, communicated with a number of people within the Office of The Surgeon General. Unless it is important to the analysis, I will not introduce each staff person by name, but rather will use the designation OTSG to indicate surgeon general staff.

125. Surgeon General's Office to Commanding Officer, Fort Bayard, 3 December 1902, RG 112, Entry 382, Box 1, NARA.

126. Surgeon General's Office to Commanding Officer, Fort Bayard, 6 October 1903, RG 112, Entry 382, Box 1, NARA.

127. Judge Advocate to Adjutant General, Department of Colorado, U.S. Army, 19 August 1903, RG 112, Entry 382, Box 2, NARA.

128. Acting Secretary of the Navy to Secretary of War, 17 February 1904, RG 112, Entry 382, Box 3, NARA.

129. Anonymous to the War Department, 29 April 1903, RG 112, Entry 26, Box 639, NARA.

130. "Synopsis of the Result of the Investigation of the General Hospital at Fort Bayard, New Mexico, by Colonel Charles H. Heyl, Inspector General, U.S. Army," 2 July 1903, RG 94, AGO 484491, Box 3393, NARA.

131. Efficiency Report, Edward T. Comegys, RG 94, Box 311, ACP, NARA.

132. Surgeon General's Office to Commanding Officer, Fort Bayard, 18 August 1903, RG 112, Entry 381, Box 2, NARA.

133. Clinical History, L. B. Ohlinger, RG 112, Entry 396, Box 62, NARA.

134. G. E. Bushnell to the Surgeon General, 24 March 1904, RG 112, Entry 26, Box 91, NARA.

135. War Department, Special Orders, No. 94, 21 April 1904.

136. Efficiency Report, E. T. Comegys, RG 94, ACP, Box 311, NARA.

137. War Department, Special Orders No. 110, 19 May 1905; *Washington Post* 21 May 1905; and Grace Wilcox Comegys to General Ainsworth, n.d., and Chas. B. Nichols to "To whome it may concern," 21 October 1905, RG 94, ACP, Box 311, NARA.

138. Information on Bushnell's life is drawn from "Efficiency Report," George E. Bushnell, RG 94, ACP, Box 715, NARA; Earl H. Bruns, "Colonel Bushnell: An Estimate of His Character and Work," *American Review of Tuberculosis* 11 (June 1925): 275–91; James M. Phalen, "George Ensign Bushnell: Colonel, Medical Corps, U.S. Army," *Army Medical Bulletin* 50 (1939): 130–33; "Obituary: George Ensign Bushnell,"*Military Surgeon* 55 (September 1924): 423–24; and Yale University, *Obituary Record of Graduates Deceased During the Year Ending July 1, 1925* (New Haven, CT: Yale University, 1925), 1327–30.

139. "Obituary: George Ensign Bushnell," *Military Surgeon* 55 (September 1924): 424.

140. Surgeon General to Adjutant General, 21 November 1911, RG 94, AGO 1850340, Box 6734, NARA.

141. Efficiency Report, George E. Bushnell, RG 94, ACP, Box 715, NARA.

142. SGAR, 1916, vol 1, 469.

143. On the transition from the "Old Army" to the army of the twentieth century see Richard W. Stewart, ed. *American Military History*, vol. 1, *The United States Army and the Forging of a Nation, 1775–1917* (Washington, DC: Center of Military History, U.S. Army, 2005); Edward M. Coffman, *The Old Army: A Portrait of the American Army in Peacetime, 1784–1898* (New York, NY: Oxford University Press, 1986); Stephen Skowronek, *Building a New American State: The Expansion of National Administrative Capacities, 1877–1920* (New York, NY: Cambridge University Press, 1982); Paul A. C. Koistinen, *Mobilizing for Modern War: The Political Economy of American Warfare, 1865–1919* (Lawrence, KS: University Press of Kansas, 1997); and Ronald J. Barr, *The Progressive Army: US Army Command and Administration, 1870–1914* (New York, NY: St. Martin's Press, 1998).

144. *WDAR*, 1901, has a lengthy discussion of Hospital Corps training; and Gillett, *The Army Medical Department, 1865–1917*, 313–39.

145. Comegys was born in 1849, Appel in 1854, and Bushnell in 1853.

146. George E. Bushnell, "The Expansion of the Hospital Corps in War," *Military Surgeon* 14 (1904): 144.

147. See "General Orders No. 28, U.S. General Hospital, Fort Bayard, New Mexico," 17 October 1904, RG 112, Entry 26, Box 359, NARA, and "General Orders, No. 1," 12 January 1903, RG 112, Entry 389–91, Box 1, NARA.

148. G. E. Bushnell to Charles F. Mason, 14 February 1905, RG 112, Entry 380, NARA.

149. Earl H. Bruns, "Colonel Bushnell: An Estimate of His Character and Work," 277.

150. G. E. Bushnell to Adjutant General, Department of Colorado, U.S. Army, 5 January 1905, RG 112, Entry 380, NARA.

151. Charles Lynch, Office of the Surgeon General, memorandum, 15 April 1904, RG 112, Entry 381, Box 2, NARA.

152. "Clinical History," Robert L. Collins, RG 112, Entry 396, Box 17, NARA.

153. Christopher Crenner, "Diagnosis and Authority in the Early Twentieth-Century Medical Practice of Richard C. Cabot," *Bulletin of the History of Medicine* 76 (2002): 30–55; Christopher Crenner, "Professional Measurement: Quantification of Health and Disease in American Medical Practice, 1880–1920," Ph.D. dissertation, Harvard University, 1993; Stanley Joel Reiser, "Creating Form Out of Mass: The Development of the Medical Record," in Everett Mendelsohn, ed., *Transformation and Tradition in the Sciences: Essays in Honor of I. Bernard Cohen* (Cambridge, UK: Cambridge University Press, 1984); and Joel Howell, *Technology in the Hospital: Transforming Patient Care in the Early Twentieth Century* (Baltimore, MD: Johns Hopkins University Press, 1995).

Chapter Two
Life at Fort Bayard

On 5 September 1904 Private (Pvt.) Richard Johnson reported for duty—not hospitalization—at Fort Bayard, yet he arrived with a sense of dread. Traveling from his previous assignment in the Philippines he had steamed across the Pacific to San Francisco, and then ridden on the Southern Pacific and Santa Fe rail lines to Deming, New Mexico. It then took almost four hours to travel forty miles on a branch line up from Deming, and a bumpy wagon ride for the final three miles to his new assignment. To his despair Johnson "found the surrounds fully warranted the lugubrious description I had heard about the place." Although he ended up enjoying his Fort Bayard assignment, Johnson later wrote that most enlisted men of the Hospital Corps "found conditions quite forbidding because of its isolation, lack of social contact, limited recreational diversion and a distaste for association with tubercular disease."[1] Tuberculosis, he explained, was "regarded as a much dreaded disease that was easily contracted by association."[2] In fact, so many hospital corpsmen requested transfers out that the Surgeon General established a policy that no such requests would be considered until after two years of service.[3] Consequently, Johnson noted, "During my time there we had a high percentage of desertions." For example, all four of the men who arrived with Johnson deserted within a year—"two of them," he dryly observed, "owing me money."[4]

Four years later another young man arrived at Fort Bayard. He, too, remarked on the long journey by rail through the "desert waste of New Mexico," and then the wagon ride over "dry desolate foothills," to the post. But his reaction was different from Johnson's. Captain (Capt.) Earl Bruns and his wife, Caroline, both had tuberculosis and came to heal. They ended up staying for almost ten years, as Bruns moved from being a patient to a physician at the hospital. For Bruns Fort Bayard was "a veritable oasis in the desert, studded with shade trees, green lawns, shrubbery, and flowers." He credited the hospital commander, Colonel (Col.) George E. Bushnell, writing that, "[i]n this one spot one man had made the desert bloom like a rose."[5]

Johnson's and Bruns' different views from 1904 and 1908, respectively, may reflect the fact that Johnson was healthy and assigned grudgingly to work at the tuberculosis hospital, whereas Bruns had few other options and came in hopes of regaining his health—or it may reflect the improvements Bushnell made during his first years in command. But every week for the more than twenty years that Fort Bayard was an Army tuberculosis hospital, workers and patients arrived with dread and foreboding, or joy and relief—or a mix of them all. Fort Bayard would be a pivotal experience for many; some would arrive dying and find life, others would arrive healthy and die, and all would wonder at their fate.

The approach Fort Bayard and George Bushnell took to tuberculosis was similar to how physicians manage the disease today in that it involved isolating the patient, treating the disease, and educating the patient and his family on how to maintain their health. But without the antibiotic cures of today, success was elusive. The community that Bushnell fostered at Fort Bayard was therefore a place of contradictions and tensions in several ways. First, the Army hospital offered patients sanctuary from the demands, fears, and prejudices regarding tuberculosis in the outside world; while some men embraced that refuge, others felt imprisoned. Second, Fort Bayard treated tuberculosis patients with prolonged bed rest, fresh air, and a healthy diet, but undertaking this "rest treatment"—confining oneself to bed for months—proved difficult if not impossible for many patients, so some rebelled and others fled. The third tension at Fort Bayard involved patients' adaptation to new lifestyles as people with tuberculosis, or "lungers." As one tuberculosis sufferer put it, "Once a T. B....always a T.B."[6] For some this new identity simply required resting, using a spit cup, and guarding their health for the rest of their lives; for others, it meant the loss of their livelihoods and families. Some adjusted well to a new life of fragile health and circumscribed opportunities, but others despaired. Finally, Fort Bayard managed patients' transition back to the outside world. For the dead, it meant caring for their bodies and property and helping their loved ones come to terms with the loss. For the living, it meant providing shelter and medical care when their health broke down over the years. For the fortunate patients who recovered their health, Fort Bayard prepared them to reenter the outside world by educating their families about their disease, helping them get government disability benefits, or finding work suitable for a person with weak lungs. These aspects of the Fort Bayard experience—the hospital as a sanctuary or prison; the treatment as a *struggle* to *rest*; patient's acceptance and/or resistance to this new lifestyle; and finally, the departure from Fort Bayard—were all fraught with sorrow or joy, or both.

The World George Bushnell Made

When Johnson and Bruns arrived at Fort Bayard they entered a world apart from the desert around it. New Mexico did not become a state until 1912, and like most mining communities, the region experienced boom–bust economic cycles. But the local economy was generally thriving during much of Bushnell's command (1904–17) as open-pit mining operations extracted copper deposits to make wire to carry electricity throughout the country. In contrast to the rugged life of mining and ranching, however, Fort Bayard was a place of infirmity.

One of the most striking aspects of Fort Bayard was that many of the medical staff had tuberculosis themselves, including George Bushnell. Tuberculosis weakened Bushnell's lungs and shaped his life in numerous ways.[7] He tired easily, had to carefully monitor his health, and as Earl Bruns observed, "was never a well man."[8] Bushnell had active tuberculosis five times in his life: first, in 1881 during his medical training; then in 1900–01, while working in Washington, DC; and again in 1909–10, when he took a six-month sick leave of absence from Fort Bayard for bed rest in the California Sierra Madres; the fourth time in 1919 with a breakdown from the strain of wartime work; and the fifth and the final illness in 1924 that lead to his death at age 70.[9] Tuberculosis interfered with Bushnell's role as an Army officer in a particularly public and perhaps embarrassing way. In 1909 medical officer Charles N. Barney (who himself had tuberculosis) detected active disease in the middle lobe of Bushnell's right lung and found that tuberculosis had also caused swelling in the testicles, which made it difficult for him to ride horseback.[10] This was a serious matter because the War Department required all officers to take an annual horseback riding test to demonstrate their fitness. Bushnell at first requested permission to substitute the test with a long hike, but by 1911 advised his superiors that, "I did not consider myself strong enough to carry on the work of commanding this Hospital and keeping myself in condition for active duty."[11] The War Department generally required officers in poor physical condition to retire, but the Surgeon General secured a waiver for Bushnell, because "the interests of the service would suffer by his retirement."[12] After a leave of absence in 1909–10, Bushnell's annual reports on the competency of his officers included his own name on the list of those competent for hospital duty, but "unfit for active field service."[13] This must have been a bitter pill for a career Army officer.

Bushnell was not unique, however, because scores of tuberculosis specialists in the United States had the disease. "What would our sanatorium movement and our anti-tuberculosis crusade amount to," wrote tuberculosis expert Adolphus Knopf, "were it not for the labors of tuberculous physicians, or one-time tuberculous physicians, who, because of their infirmity, had become interested in tuberculosis?"[14] Well-known leaders in the antituberculosis movement such as Edward Trudeau and Lawrence Flick established their sanatoriums after they recovered from tuberculosis in order to offer others the treatment. Twenty-one of the first thirty recipients of the Trudeau Medal, established in 1926 for outstanding work in tuberculosis, had the disease.[15] James Waring, a Colorado tuberculosis physician who arrived at a Colorado Springs sanatorium on a stretcher in 1908, later wrote, "It has been my good fortune to serve three separate and extended 'hitches' as a 'bed patient,' the time so spent numbering in all about nine years."[16] He, like many physicians, saw his personal experience as an asset in his practice. Most Army tuberculosis experts knew the disease well. The three key figures in the Army tuberculosis program during World War I were Bushnell, Bruns, and Gerald Webb of Colorado Springs who started a tuberculosis sanatorium after his wife died of the disease.[17] During World War II, the man in charge of the Army's tuberculosis program, Esmond R. Long, also had the disease as a young man.

Bushnell turned tuberculosis into an asset for the Army Medical Department, making Fort Bayard a center of national expertise on the disease. His personal experience with chronic pulmonary tuberculosis gave him good rapport and credibility with many of his patients. Medical officer Earl Bruns wrote that, "[H]e went among the patients and talked to them individually" and thereby provided "a living example of a cure due to rational treatment." Bruns described how Bushnell spent his days attending to patients, carrying out administrative duties, and devoted hours to supervising the work in the gardens and grounds of Fort Bayard. Bushnell also had a scholarly side, said Bruns, so that "[a]ll spare moments were spent in improving his mind," as he continued to study languages at Fort Bayard and translate medical articles in German for the Army Medical Department. Bruns characterized Bushnell as "modest and sweet," but noted, "I have seen him angry in his office over official matters, but never at any other time."[18] Hospital corpsman Richard Johnson recalled that although Bushnell was in his early fifties, he had white hair, so "some of the witty guys occasionally referred to him as 'old cotton-top.'" But, he observed, Bushnell "was not the kind of person to whom a burlesque nickname would cling very tenaciously." He remembered him as "a wise old man peering over his glasses from behind his roll-top desk, or a somewhat ungainly, white-haired, figure plodding industriously across the parade ground in a short cut between the office and his quarters—with his ever-present pipe in his mouth." Bushnell, he concluded, was "mild mannered and dignified without ostentation, but could be stern on warranted occasions."[19]

Two incidents demonstrate this sternness. The first involved manure. While Bushnell was on sick leave in 1909, an Army inspector observed flies in the officers' mess room and blamed the proximity of a horse stable and a manure pile from the dairy herd, ordering their relocation.[20] When Bushnell returned to command in May 1910 he fired off a ten-page response to the inspection, refuting the notion that the "present location of the horses makes any difference whatever as to the number of flies in the officers' mess or elsewhere." Noting that he required the removal of manure from the stables every day to control flies, he launched into an exegesis on the *musca domestica*, pointing out that they lay their eggs in horse manure, not cow manure. The inspector, he argued, should have endeavored to "prove to himself that the manure pile was a nuisance before recommending its removal." Indeed, wrote Bushnell, "It is my opinion that the composting of cow manure is a praiseworthy act rather than an irregularity." That was apparently the last word on manure at Fort Bayard.

Fort Bayard Chaplain Cephas Bateman ran into a similar buzzsaw. In late 1912 he had questioned Bushnell's use of funds designated for the officers' stables to pay one of the guard post corporals, suggesting that it was "unmilitary" and "establishes a dangerous precedent."[21] When Bushnell took offense, Bateman apologized abjectly, stating he had been "crazy from grippe" when he complained, and "I have not found any rest in body or mind since I ran amuck like a juramentao in that letter to you."[22] The matter seemed closed until March 1913 when Chaplain

Bateman told the post teacher who had broken his collarbone that he was not well enough to teach and should cancel school for the day. Lieutenant (Lt.) Joseph Walkup, who had treated the teacher and cleared him to work, believed Bateman had undermined his authority and appealed to Bushnell who agreed with him. When Bateman characterized Bushnell's stance as "unwarranted and exasperating," the commander told the chaplain to request a transfer or face "official action" for insubordination. After more than seven years at Fort Bayard, Bateman and his family were gone within a few weeks.[23] Bushnell, while mild and white-haired, maintained command.

Bushnell presided over a community of more than 1,000 people, including patients, military personnel and their families, and civilian laborers and trades people. The hospital admitted 600 to 1,000 patients annually, many of whom stayed six months or more, and discharged almost as many.[24] Fort Bayard had about 400 hospital beds. The lowest patient population listed was 217, in October 1910, and the highest was 372, in December 1916. Hospital personnel generally included ten medical officers, an Army chaplain, ten to twenty nurses, and about 100 enlisted men of the Hospital Corps. Noncommissioned officers managed the post exchange, commissary, and any construction projects, and a quartermaster contingent was in charge of the guard house and patrol of the post reservation. Several dozen civilians served as laborers on the post. Although a creature of the federal government, Fort Bayard under Bushnell developed a degree of self-sufficiency in its isolated location, not unlike a ship at sea.

The Physical Plant

Upon assuming command in 1904, Bushnell, who had studied botany for years, immediately began to plant flowers, shrubs, and trees. When President Theodore Roosevelt created the Gila Forest Reserve in 1905, Bushnell ensured that Fort Bayard, which adjoined the Reserve, was part of a government reforestation project. The first year alone the Forest Service gave the hospital 250 seedlings of Himalayan cedar and yellow pine.[25] Bushnell also got approval to fence in land for pasturing dairy cattle and arranged to recultivate long-neglected garden plots. The first year he predicted that the garden would generate "about 1300 dollars worth of produce."[26] After the quartermaster located an underground water source, Bushnell redoubled his cultivation efforts, planting trees, flowers, and grass to mitigate the wind and dust, and "to beautify the Post."[27] In later years Bushnell successfully grew beans from ancient cave dwellers (Anasazi beans), and made a less successful effort to grow Giant Sequoia from California.[28] By 1910 Fort Bayard had four acres of vegetable gardens, a greenhouse, an orchard of 200 fruit trees, and alfalfa fields and hay fields for the dairy herd of 115 Holsteins, which the *Silver City Enterprise* proclaimed "one of the finest in the west."[29] The hospital also raised all of the beef consumed at the hospital (thereby avoiding Daniel Appel's purchasing problems) and consumed pork at small expense by feeding the pigs the waste food. The hospital laboratory raised its own Belgian hares and guinea pigs for experiments.[30]

Bushnell also oversaw years of construction at Fort Bayard. In the wake of Florence Nightingale's writings, nineteenth-century sanitation practices stressed cleanliness and ventilation, giving rise to pavilion style hospitals, narrow one- or two-story buildings lined with windows to provide patients with ample ventilation. In March 1904, Bushnell sent the Surgeon General plans for an "open court building" in modified pavilion style (Figure 2-1). The building consisted of a quadrangle of long, narrow dressing rooms around an open court with porches along both the exterior and interior of the building. The rooms could be used for sleeping in inclement weather and the porches allowed patients to seek sun or shade as they wished. Wide doors enabled the easy movement of beds between the rooms and the porches. "The object of this style of building is to facilitate sleeping out of doors, which is now considered so important in modern sanatoria for the treatment of tuberculosis," Bushnell explained. He added two-storied corner

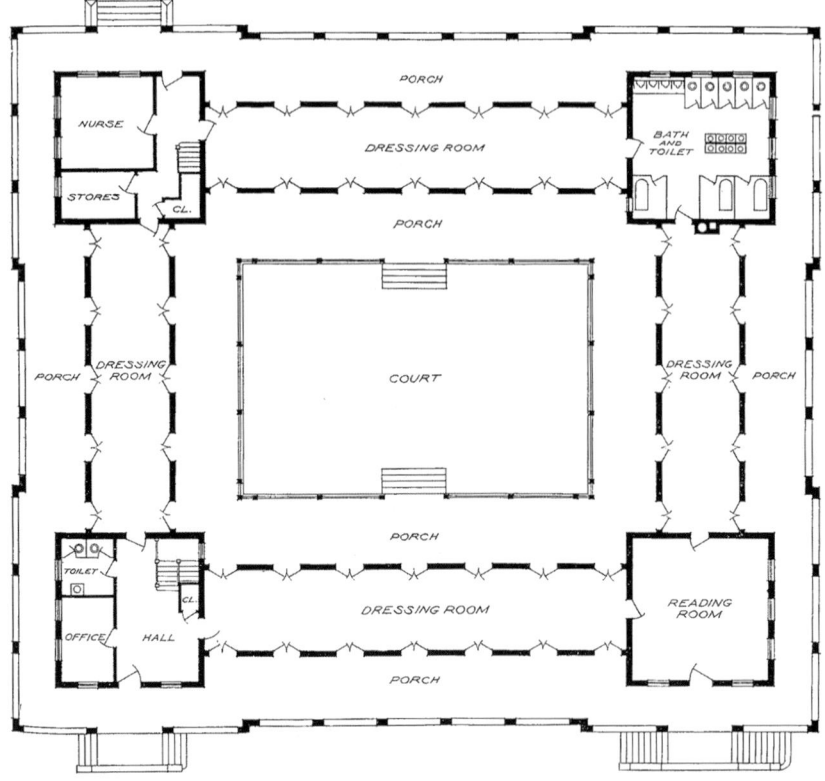

Figure 2-1. Plan for tuberculosis patient ward, as designed by George E. Bushnell, providing fresh air porches for each patient, in "United States Army Tuberculosis Hospital in New Mexico," *Modern Hospital* 3 (1914): 103.

towers to provide a reading room, storage, and bathroom facilities for the Hospital Corps, and to "add greatly to the architectural effect by relieving the monotony of the long and low sides."[31]

In his annual report for 1910 Bushnell provided a general overview of the hospital (Figure 2-2), noting that for the first time in years there was no construction underway.[32] His description would be familiar to a ship captain: an isolated, hierarchical

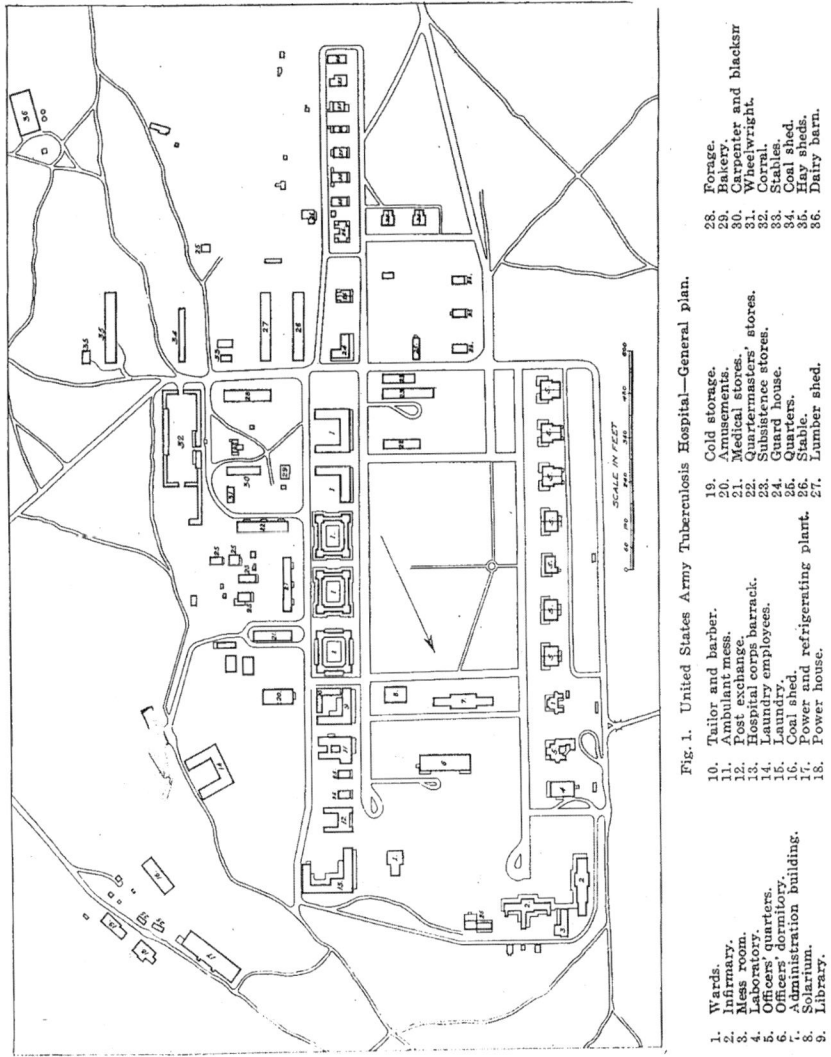

Figure 2-2. General plan of the Army tuberculosis hospital at Fort Bayard in 1914, from "United States Army Tuberculosis Hospital in New Mexico," *Modern Hospital* 3 (1914): 102.

46   "Good Tuberculosis Men"

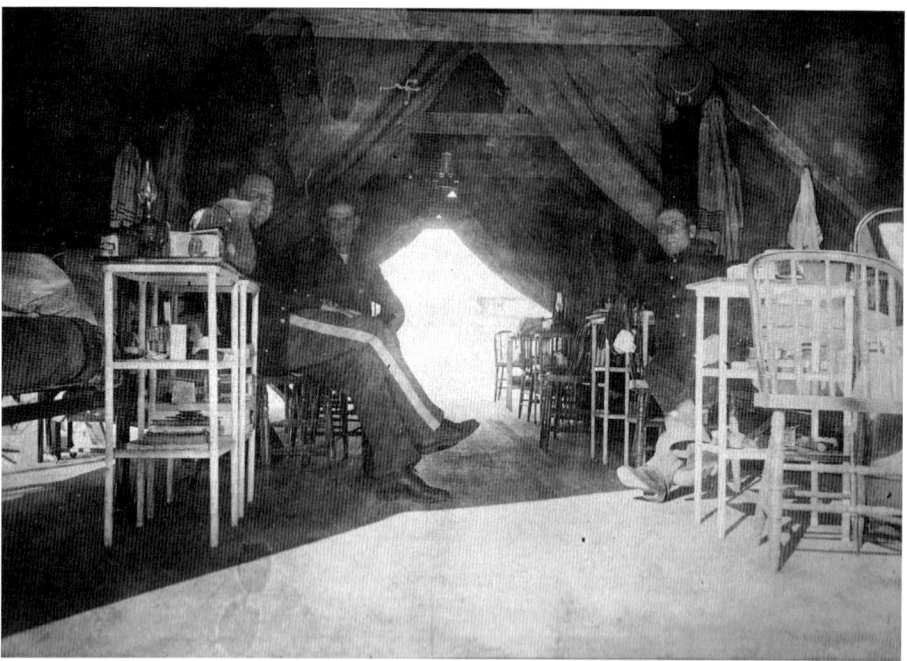

Figure 2-3. U.S. Army, General Hospital, Fort Bayard, New Mexico, Interior view of a tent ward, circa 1907.
Photograph courtesy of the National Library of Medicine, Image #A030247.

social compound on a desert, supplying much of its own food, supplies, entertainment, and, of course, healthcare.[33] The post was a collection of almost 100 buildings, some from the old fort, others new, and patient wards (that were designated for patients according to rank and severity of disease). The sickest enlisted men were housed in the former post hospital, which had a glass porch for those too ill for exposure to extreme weather. Ambulant patients lived in the three new quadrangle buildings, which accommodated about forty men each. Others lived in tent wards of twelve beds, with wood floors, electric lights, and wood stoves, and had an open flap design to allow fresh air throughout the day and night (Figure 2-3). Officer patients lived in two buildings with their own kitchens: one for the infirm, and the other one for ambulant patients. One of the former Army barracks served as the detention ward for the "punishment of patients too sick to endure other disciplinary measures." The complex also included a solarium, amusement hall, library, and a laboratory and surgical facility near the infirmaries. Bushnell noted that the nurses' residence occupied "a commanding position on the hill west of the post," with twenty bedrooms, kitchen, dining room, office, and parlor. The hospital administration building was equipped with a telephone, telegraph, and post office, and wings for the officers' club on one side, and a court-martial room on the other. To support both patients and the staff, the hospital had a range of resources and services such as shops for the carpenter, wheelwright, blacksmith, and plumber, as well as barns and granary for horses. Finally, Bushnell noted that, "pains have been taken to beautify the cemetery, installing underground irrigation to water the pine trees planted around it."[34]

The Patients

The majority of patients at Fort Bayard were, of course, military men. Unlike most civilian sanatoriums, which could limit admissions to members of a church or social organization, or patients whom physicians believed they could help, Fort Bayard had to admit all eligible individuals as space allowed. First priority was given to beneficiaries of the Soldiers' Home and military officers and enlisted men with tuberculosis, then family members of Army personnel, and finally civilians, with the Secretary of War's approval. Medical staff delivered several babies each year, and treated people at the post for a range of medical and surgical problems. In addition, from May 1904 to May 1905 Fort Bayard cared for 110 sailors and Marines. A hurricane destroyed a makeshift military tuberculosis camp at Pensacola, Florida, in 1906, and the War Department gave the Navy Fort Lyon, Colorado, for the care of tuberculosis sailors and officers, but Navy Surgeon General Preston Rixey still sent more than half of his tuberculosis patients to Fort Bayard. He told members of Congress, "There has been no question of the benefit resulting to many of the patients transferred for treatment at this institution."[35]

Fort Bayard periodically convened a board of three medical officers to determine which patients were so disabled by tuberculosis that they could not continue in active service. The War Department would then discharge them on a "certificate of disability," which made them eligible for military hospital care and the Soldiers' Home. A large percentage of patients did change from active duty status to beneficiaries of the Soldiers' Home during their treatment at Fort Bayard. Unlike soldiers and sailors, beneficiaries were generally free to enter and leave the hospital as they wished. Many chose to leave the hospital immediately, against doctors' orders. In 1905, for example, 33 percent of patients who were discharged from Fort Bayard with advanced tuberculosis were listed as "unimproved" when they returned to civilian life.[36]

Family members of military personnel gained admission to Fort Bayard only as beds were available. These patients included the children of Army officers, such as Daniel Appel's son, Robert, age nineteen, admitted by Bushnell in 1908, and Theodore Wilson, the stepson of a cavalry officer.[37] As Fort Bayard's good reputation spread, civilians also sought admission. Although the War Department referred many of them to private sanatoriums, people with political influence did get admitted. In 1908 Assistant Attorney General Alford W. Cooley came to Fort Bayard at the request of President Roosevelt, as did Congressman George Legare of South Carolina, at the advice of Secretary of War William Taft.[38] Some of the civilian patients developed tuberculosis while they were working on the construction and operation of the Panama Canal—of ninety-nine men sent home from Panama in 1915 due to debilitating illness, twenty-seven had tuberculosis.[39]

William C. Gorgas, who became Surgeon General in 1914 and had served in Panama for ten years, authorized the admission of several such patients. In one case, Harry C. Bradley, a United Fruit Company employee in Panama, came to Fort Bayard for treatment, and when he ran out of money to pay for his care, with Gorgas' approval, Bushnell arranged for the hospital to pay for his care.[40]

Fort Bayard had female patients from the start, most of them nurses who developed tuberculosis during service in the tropics or while caring for tuberculosis patients. The War Department also transferred Army officers whose wives had tuberculosis to the post so they could benefit from the climate and receive treatment. When medical officer Alexander Murray's wife was diagnosed, Bushnell offered him a position so she could be at Fort Bayard.[41] These arrangements were informal and unofficial; female patients stayed in the nurses' dormitory. In 1909, the Surgeon General told a member of Congress that women were not admitted to Fort Bayard.[42] But Bushnell sought permission to convert a dormitory into a ward for eight women, and beginning in 1910 the hospital formally admitted female patients.[43] Some of them had good connections like Helen Kress Gurley, the daughter of a retired brigadier general; Dena Watkins, daughter of a congressman from Louisiana; and Mrs. Edward C. Heasley, the wife of one of President Taft's office clerks. In the latter case, Secretary of War Henry Stimson also assigned Edward Heasely to duty at the Quartermasters Corps at Fort Bayard to facilitate his wife's admission and to maintain their income.[44]

Bushnell drew the line at young children, however. Army families had children at Fort Bayard, of course, but rules required them to stay away from hospital wards and messes, not only for the children's safety but also to avoid disturbing patients.[45] When the Secretary of War authorized the admission of Mrs. Donald P. Branson and her child, Bushnell noted that "noises made by one patient are very annoying to other patients," so that "the presence of a child in this institution would be in my judgement almost intolerable unless the child is extremely well trained and old enough to be left practically to its own resources." He strongly recommended, therefore, "that no authority be given in the future for the admission of children in this hospital."[46]

A variety of funding sources supported Fort Bayard patients. The War Department paid medical personnel salaries and operating costs of the hospital, and $1.00 per day for officers' and $0.50 per day for enlisted men's hospital subsistence. The Soldiers' Homes and the Navy paid $5.00 per week for patients under their jurisdiction, and civilian patients and family members of the military paid from $1.00 to $1.50 per day.[47] At all Army hospitals these monies went into the "Hospital Fund," which, after paying for patients' subsistence, hospital commanders could use to pay for special programs or patient services or for charity cases.[48] Patients used personal funds for laundry and postage, gambling, and drinking. Fort Bayard's costs compared favorably with those at other tuberculosis sanatoriums. The Saranac Lake sanatorium in the Adirondacks charged $8.00 per week in 1915.[49] When William Gorgas surveyed hospital costs in the United States, he found that in 1910 the costs per patient ranged between $1.00 and $2.00 per day.[50]

The different costs to support different classes of patients and military personnel reveal the military and social hierarchy. A 1910 inspection report listed the average cost per diem to feed enlisted Fort Bayard hospital corpsmen as $0.29; nurses, $0.46; ambulant patients, $0.47; infirmary patients, $0.51; and officers, $1.31. The latter figure included about $0.20 for the labor in the dining room because officers were served individually, on china, rather than barracks style. Although both enlisted men and officers each consumed an average of fifteen pounds of beef in March 1910, enlisted men were also offered ham, mackerel, and canned oysters, while officers ate fresh pork, veal, and fish. Enlisted men ate canned goods, including fruits, vegetables, and meats, while officers consumed fresh vegetables and fruits and few canned goods.[51] A congressman receiving treatment at Fort Bayard no doubt was on officers' rations when he told his wife in February: "Last night I had strawberries for supper, large saucer full. Now what about that! Temperature fifteen above zero and strawberries for supper!"[52] Another rule reflected Fort Bayard's hierarchy: "Enlisted men who are on duty at the Officers' Infirmary or who have business there (orderlies, etc.) will enter and leave the building by the rear."[53] Thus, while united by a common bond of living with tuberculosis either as patients or workers, and sometimes both, Fort Bayard remained a stratified military community.

Medical Officers

Bushnell gathered around him medical staff that shared his dedication to tuberculosis. He told the Surgeon General that "it would be much better if Medical Officers of this institution were to permanently settle here so that they could feel that their life work was to become experts in tuberculosis," and recommended that medical officers be assigned to Fort Bayard for at least four years. "There is no doubt in my mind that tuberculosis constitutes a specialty," he wrote. Men who are in charge of the patients "should have expert knowledge."[54] When the Office of The Surgeon General asked Bushnell to train civilian physicians under contract with the Army, thereby "giving them an opportunity of studying tuberculosis and spreading the knowledge gained for benefit of the community at large," Bushnell agreed as long as the men were "desirous of studying deeply internal medicine."[55]

Like Bushnell, many of these physicians had tuberculosis (Figure 2-4). In 1906, for example, six of the ten medical officers at Fort Bayard had the disease, one too ill to work, two on light duty, and the rest on full duty.[56] In 1910, five of ten medical officers had the disease, one on medical leave, one in bed, one on light duty, and two recovered enough for full duty.[57] The War Department supported Bushnell's approach, promoting him twice during his command of Fort Bayard, and advancing other medical officers even while under treatment for active tuberculosis. Edward Munson, for example, was promoted to major in 1906, while he was a patient at Fort Bayard, and Earl Bruns was promoted as well in 1908, with the War Department's comment that "[t]he precedent for promotion of this officer, though he is suffering from tuberculosis, has already been established....[and] his promotion to the rank of captain will not interfere with the promotion of any other officer."[58] The Public Health Service tuberculosis hospital at Fort Stanton

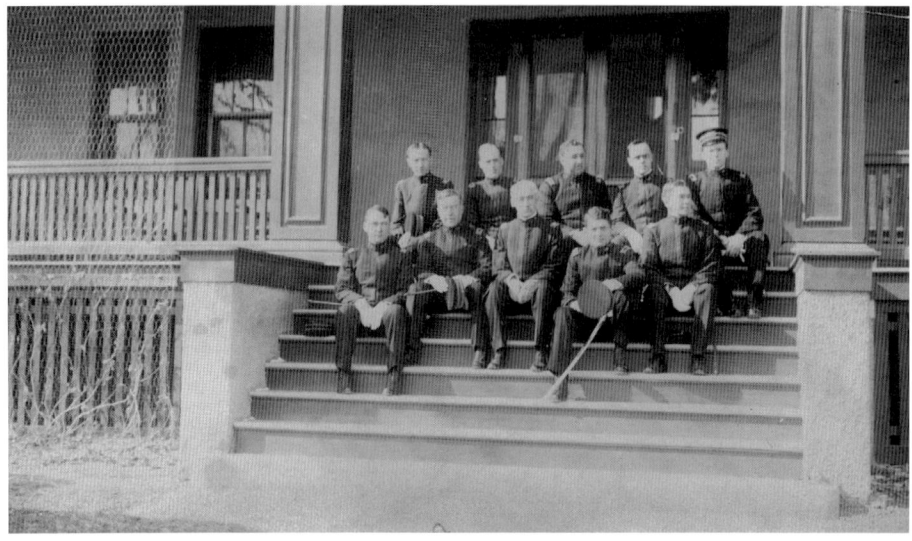

Figure 2-4. Colonel George E. Bushnell and medical staff, Fort Bayard. Photograph courtesy of Silver City Museum, Grant County, New Mexico, #01771.

had a similar practice. In 1908, five of the seven medical officers at Fort Stanton had tuberculosis, three were under treatment and two, including the commander, surgeon Paul Carrington, had recovered.[59] Carrington also reported that the Public Health Service sanatorium "was fortunate in having the free services of a dentist, who himself was suffering from pulmonary tuberculosis."[60]

When critics worried that some medical officers at Fort Bayard were too ill to perform their duties, they were less concerned about the transmission of disease than they were that the officers did not have the energy to do their jobs. In May 1906, Bushnell did ask for temporary duty medical officers because six of his officers were ill—four with tuberculosis, and two with other ailments.[61] But he was never apologetic or defensive about having people with tuberculosis on duty. Instead, he pointed out that practically all these medical officers "are here on account of lung trouble," and criticism that they were being worked hard is "only deserved in case men who are sent here perform duty which is beyond their strength. I have done my best to prevent this."[62] Not all medical officers at Fort Bayard were ill. Capt. W. H. Tefft (1910–14), 1st Lt. Roy C. Heflebower (1911–12), and Capt. George Scott (1911–13) all served at Fort Bayard without ever having the disease. In one sad irony, Capt. Joseph O. Walkup did not have tuberculosis but was struck by lightning and killed while driving an open automobile near Fort Bayard in 1914 just weeks after his promotion to captain.[63]

Fort Bayard physicians, regardless of whether they had the disease, became familiar with all aspects of tuberculosis. They examined hundreds of patients, tested thousands of laboratory specimens, surgically removed or repaired infected or damaged tissue, and conducted autopsies on the dead. The large number of cases provided an excellent opportunity to study the disease. Bushnell held weekly seminars on various aspects of tuberculosis and medical officers discussed cases and heard papers on one another's research.[64] According to Bruns, Bushnell at first scheduled such meetings after lunch, but after some men fell asleep, he "changed them to the evening and quizzed us over the previous lecture."[65] Medical officers also attended professional conferences; Bushnell was a charter member of the American Sanatorium Association and was made an honorary member of the New Mexico Medical Society.[66] Fort Bayard officers published a number of papers. In 1908 C. N. Barney published a paper on the use of tuberculin; in 1912 J. B. Van Horn reported on an experimental "modified flesh diet," which was heavy in meats, eggs, and prunes, for seriously ill patients; and in 1916 Thomas Johnson surveyed the various complications of tuberculosis at the hospital.[67] Bushnell and his staff also published a booklet in 1908, *Illustrations of Tuberculous Lesions*, containing case studies of patients who had died of tuberculosis with photographs of the damage to various organs found at autopsy.[68]

Other Staff

Fort Bayard also relied on a wide range of staff from hospital corpsmen, nurses, and post guards to gardeners, launderers, and cooks. And here Bushnell preferred to hire staff with a personal connection to tuberculosis because they were less inclined to be afraid of the patients. When the hospital chaplain left precipitously in 1905, Bushnell immediately requested the assignment of Chaplain Cephas Bateman to replace him, noting he "wishes to remain in the Southwest on account of the health of his wife."[69] Bateman's wife had tuberculosis and he would serve as Fort Bayard chaplain for seven years. Bushnell also recruited staff from among recovering patients. Cavalry officer Solomon Vestal arrived as a patient at Fort Bayard in 1903, and when he was well enough, served as quartermaster for construction.[70] Army engineer H. R. Robert, a patient in the hospital (1910–11), also served as Fort Bayard quartermaster, and artillery officer Stephen Abbot arrived as a patient, but later became the purchasing commissary officer.[71]

Bushnell's approach was not only practical, but also compassionate. He once told the Surgeon General, "It is better to admit some of the undeserving than to exclude any who has a right to admission."[72] In 1910, Walter Elliot, an infantry officer with fifteen years of service, came to Fort Bayard with his wife. They both had developed tuberculosis while in the Philippines, perhaps after bouts with malaria or dysentery. After examining Elliot, Bushnell determined that he would never recover his health, but instead of recommending retirement, which would have reduced Elliot's income and made his wife ineligible to stay at Fort Bayard, Bushnell asked that he be assigned as purchasing officer.[73] Elliot and his wife had both broken down with tuberculosis during military service, Bushnell pointed out, and "Captain Elliot's family affairs are in such a condition that they excite my sympathy and I believe should receive the consideration of the War Department." Elliot stayed at Fort Bayard and sat on several disability retirement boards, until the Army retired him on disability in 1913.[74]

In another example of compassion, when Congressman Nicholas Longworth of Ohio (Speaker of the House in the 1920s) requested admission to Fort Bayard for a constituent, a Mr. Barrett, Bushnell advised the congressman that admission of civilians was authorized only by the Secretary of War. Bushnell's current clerk was going to transfer to the U.S. Forest Service in Albuquerque, New Mexico, however, so Bushnell immediately arranged for Barrett, who had excellent clerical skills, to become his office clerk and take the Civil Service exam required for employment.[75] Bushnell thereby turned the problem of the loss of his clerk into an opportunity to get a new one, help a young man, and do a congressman a favor. Bushnell even built up the orchestra with tuberculosis patients when he arranged for the Hospital Fund to pay the costs of a destitute civilian patient, Julies Steyskal, noting "his services as director and musician much more than compensate for the extra expense involved."[76]

When Congress created the all-female Army Nurse Corps in 1901, Fort Bayard was one of the first assignments (Figure 2-5). Nurses generally cared for the sickest patients in the enlisted men's and officers' infirmary, feeding and bathing them, taking temperatures, giving medications, and assisting in surgeries. Like medical officers, some were patients as well. In 1910 four of ten nurses on duty had tuberculosis, two of them on "light duty" due to their illness.[77] Although most of these pioneer nurses welcomed the employment and the opportunity to serve in the military, some of them may have been dubious of their remote assignment. Jane Delano, Army Nurse Corps Superintendent, inspected the site in November 1909, and presented a positive report to the American Nurses Association. "One must expect to forego the pleasures of a city, but to any one who cares for the country, Fort Bayard offers many compensations." She explained, "Every provision for comfort has been made." Nurses lived in single rooms with balconies where they could sleep if they wanted to, and "electric lights, steam heat, and all the modern conveniences." Delano found that the hours of duty afforded time for outdoor recreation, and nurses could play tennis and have horses, "which are much cheaper than in the east, and can, as a rule, be sold without loss when the nurse is transferred."[78]

Created in 1886 to provide a cadre of soldiers trained in caring for the sick and wounded, the Hospital Corps, however, did the lion's share of the work. Richard Johnson, who had been so discouraged upon his arrival at Fort Bayard, wrote a memoir that provides a glimpse of life at the post. Johnson had three different jobs while at Fort Bayard—attendant in the ambulatory wards, worker in the hospital gardens, and orderly in Bushnell's office, doing errands, answering the telephone, and collecting and distributing the mail. He also served as bugler for the post, a job for which he considered himself "very fortunate."[79] He found his Hospital Corps colleagues were often better educated and from wealthier families than other enlisted men he encountered. "We had men who were medical students, law students, and at least one law graduate, pharmacist, one dentist, theatrical men and even one scion of British nobility." Most were in the Army because they had "back-slidden in some moment of weakness, and had resorted to the [A]rmy for solace, adventure or obscurity."[80] Johnson got to know some of these men by

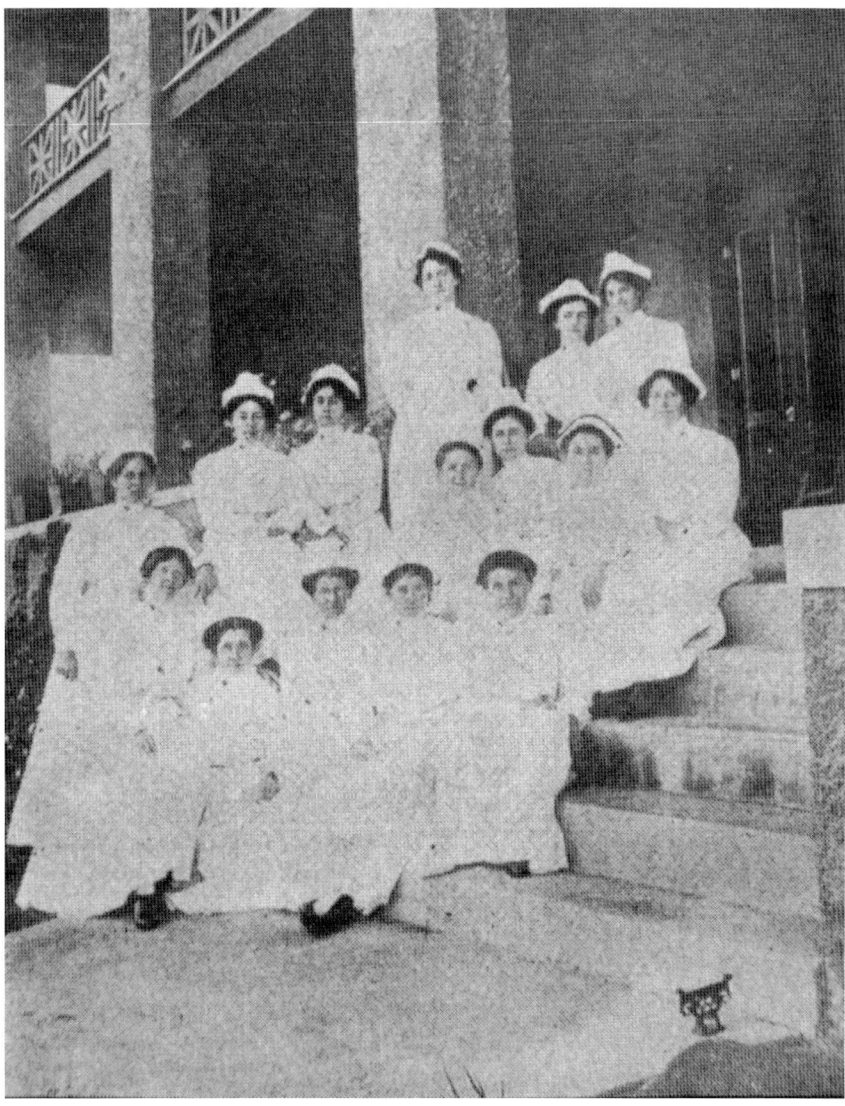

Figure 2-5. Group of trained nurses at Fort Bayard. Cephas C. Bateman, *The Army Hospital at Fort Bayard* (Lawrence: Kansas Collection, University of Kansas Libraries), circa 1911. Photograph courtesy of Spencer Research Library at the University of Kansas.

drinking with them or lending them money. Sedrick Dirks, the British scion, for example, was a former attorney, whose alcoholism drove him into poverty. When Johnson met him on his trip out to Fort Bayard, Dirks was broke, so he bought him drinks along the way. When they got to their new assignment, "To add to his humiliation this middle aged man of culture and refined background was assigned to the undignified job of mess attendant, which must have been the last straw in breaking his British pride."[81] Within a few months Dirks went absent without leave.

Hospital corpsmen could be an unwieldy bunch. During the first year of Bushnell's command, Fort Bayard had an average of 118 members of the Hospital Corps, and these men wracked up 123 disciplinary hearings and trials with 118 convictions.[82] Over the years Bushnell worked to reduce this rate and improve morale, and by 1910, he could report that he disciplined only 40 percent of the healthy soldiers who served in the Hospital Corps.[83] Most of the offenses involved minor rules violations for gambling, drinking, and fighting. Pvt. Charles Petersen, for example, was sentenced to confinement to his quarters for one month after being convicted of being drunk on the job and striking his sergeant.[84] Others, like Pvt. Clarence Miller in 1906, absconded to town without permission, and were tried by court-martial for going absent without leave.

The final category of Fort Bayard personnel was civilians from the local community who worked as laborers in and around the post. They included a Chinese laborer named Yee Hing, five members of another Chinese family named Fong, and workers with surnames such as Portillo, Delgado, and Villegas, mostly Mexicans and Mexican Americans, who worked in the kitchens, dairy, stables, and construction projects. Men working as teamsters and firemen with names such as Hill, Jones, Taylor, Harris, and Moore could have been black or white. These people left little trace of their experiences at Fort Bayard, though they do at times emerge in the historical record. African American Clara Blivins of the nearby town, Central, did laundry for some of the officers, and at one point complained to Bushnell that Chaplain Bateman owed her money.[85] Convalescent patients also worked in wards and the hospital gardens to earn a little money, test their health before returning to full duty, and, in Bushnell's view, "render men contented by giving them occupation."[86]

In this setting—an isolated place between mountain ranges, with trees, gardens, and flowers—lived a diverse community of medical officers, nurses, enlisted men, and civilian workers. Bushnell and his staff offered tuberculosis sufferers sanctuary from a busy and at times hostile world, providing rest and treatment for their disease, educating them on how to live with tuberculosis, and preparing them to rejoin the outside world.

Fort Bayard: Sanctuary or Prison?

Bushnell understood Fort Bayard as a sanctuary. "The primary object of the institution has not been to cure soldiers with a view to returning them to duty in the ranks," he wrote, but rather "to furnish asylum for all tuberculosis patients whose disease has been incident to the Military service as well."[87] Agnes Young, a nurse at Fort Bayard in 1906, compared this role to Fort Bayard's former one of fighting the Apaches. The post "now shelters those who fight a fiercer, more unrelenting and insidious foe than ever before stalked these wild plains, thirsting for victims."[88] Although many patients welcomed the protection and care of

Fort Bayard, others were ambivalent or outright resistant. "Consumptives as a rule are a sanguine, bright-eyed folk," observed Chaplain Bateman. "They are constantly over-rating their strength and the most intelligent appear frequently to be the poorest judges of their real condition." Consequently, he wrote, "[H]e who has led an active, efficient life may chafe under the confinement of a hospital and easily comes to regard an infirmary as a prison."[89]

Patients like Earl Bruns believed that Fort Bayard was their best chance to get well and welcomed the care they could not afford elsewhere. Some of these patients arrived begging. In 1905, civilian engineer L. C. Johnston arrived from the Philippines with advanced tuberculosis. As a civilian he was ineligible for admission, but he brought with him a letter from a medical officer he had met in Manila. Bushnell admitted him even though the hospital was full and requested authority to treat Johnson until he was well enough to travel to another sanatorium because "his condition is such that it is not considered humane to refuse him admission."[90] When Lt. Pedro A. Hernandez came to Fort Bayard in February 1915, he was well but his wife had tuberculosis and was pregnant. Bushnell requested permission for her to stay for several months to ensure a lesion on her lung cleared up and for Hernandez to be assigned to Fort Bayard. He noted that his wife did not speak English and "is quite helpless here since the personnel of the Hospital who come in direct contact with her are unable to speak Spanish. Under these circumstances her husband desires to stay here as long as she does."[91] At one point Bushnell detailed for the Surgeon General several cases of sick but ineligible patients, "in order to show the difficulties under which the Commanding Officer of this Hospital labors in his desire to avoid inhumanity on the one hand and on the other to reserve the funds of this Hospital for the class of patients for whom they are intended."[92] The Army Medical Department often supported Bushnell's practices, but occasionally resisted his charitable impulses. When he wanted to admit Joseph Fike, who had served two three-year periods of duty but was no longer in the Army, the Office of The Surgeon General gave permission with the caveat that it did "not view with favor the admission of discharged soldiers to the hospital under your command who are not beneficiaries of the Soldiers' Home."[93]

Fort Bayard served as home base or even a place to die for tubercular soldiers and veterans who had nowhere else to go for lack of funds, family, or both. One such man was 1st Lt. Olin R. Booth, a well-educated Army officer, born in Connecticut and graduated from Amherst College in 1895 with the ability to translate five languages. He enlisted in the Army shortly after graduation and served as an infantry officer during the Spanish-American War. After developing tuberculosis in the Philippines he arrived at Fort Bayard for treatment in March 1903 and stayed until he was retired on disability for tuberculosis in his entire left lung in 1906. Booth soon left Fort Bayard, but was in and out of the hospital four times, spending eight of a total of nine-and-one-half years at Fort Bayard until his death in September 1914. His records indicate that he never married and upon his death his body was shipped to his father in Brimfield, Massachusetts. Fort Bayard was the closest thing Booth had for a home during his adult life.[94]

Other men left Fort Bayard while they were sick but returned to die. Wilmot E. Brown, an Army contract surgeon, arrived in 1908 with advanced tuberculosis in both lungs. After two years, he left the hospital with a temperature of 100 degrees, and in "unfavorable" condition. He stayed in central New Mexico, but returned to Fort Bayard the following year so weak that Bushnell could not complete his physical examination. Medical staff kept Brown comfortable over the next months until he died in November 1911, at age thirty-eight.[95] In another example, William Gregg came to Fort Bayard with serious tuberculosis in April 1910, and six months later was granted a disability pension. He stayed on as a beneficiary of the Soldiers' Home only a few days. With a bad cough, pus in his sputum, and a low-grade temperature, his chart indicated that he "[l]eft the home at his own request." Gregg worked on a farm in Iowa and returned to Fort Bayard almost exactly four years later, in 1915, very ill. He stayed at the hospital for six months, recovered somewhat, and then left again. When Gregg returned three months later, he was dying. His last medical exam stated, "Patient is not doing well. Is a far advanced case with large involvement." On 24 January 1917 Gregg had a massive lung hemorrhage, died, and was buried at the Fort Bayard National Cemetery.[96]

Some patients wanted to leave but could not afford it. After receiving a grim prognosis, Pvt. Bernard Conroy wrote to his mother that he wanted to go home to die. She wanted him home, but asked Bushnell if her son would receive a pension if he were discharged from the Army. "I am a poor widow and am depending on his alottment [sic] of $10.00 a month which he made over to me and I still receive." Bushnell replied that it would be better for her son to stay at Fort Bayard because "your son is quite sick," and "he has every comfort here and his pay goes on, while if discharged he would probably have to wait some months before securing a pension."[97]

Not all patients had "every comfort" during their time at Fort Bayard, but they returned nonetheless. Pvt. Charles Tyler, an African American and member of the 9th Cavalry, had a long, sometimes painful relationship with Fort Bayard. He first arrived as a patient in late 1903 after he coughed up blood while on duty at Yosemite. During his stay at the hospital in 1904 he lost more than twenty pounds, going from 158 to 137, and requested a pension for disability.[98] Despite his weakened condition, a medical board denied his request and the Army returned him to duty at another post. Four months later, however, he was back at Fort Bayard, having lost ten more pounds, and finally received his discharge on disability in December 1905. Now at Fort Bayard as a beneficiary of the Soldiers' Home, Tyler gained back weight and began to work on the post for $30 a month and rations, the same as other laborers received.[99]

Although African American soldiers and veterans received similar pay and benefits as whites, and the Fort Bayard medical wards were not segregated by race, Bushnell and the War Department did impose the color line on social interactions. In 1907 Tyler complained to the Adjutant General that, "the CO [commanding officer] in command at Fort Bayard, N. M, has an Amusement Hall erected in that place and do[es] not want any of the colored patients to visit the Hall by no means." He continued in his letter, "There is no pleasure on earth for the Colored

Men at all in the BSH [Beneficiaries of the Soldiers' Home] in New Mexico they are barred from every thing there except the Guard House." Tyler was soon after suspended from Fort Bayard for three months, and while his medical chart does not give a reason for suspension, he told the governor of the Soldiers' Home that it was for writing a letter critical of Fort Bayard.[100] Diagnosed with tuberculosis, poor feet, and secondary syphilis, Tyler continued to cycle in and out of Fort Bayard six more times over the next eight years (1903–15). Tyler's medical record does not reveal his fate, but he was not buried in Fort Bayard's cemetery. The cemetery roster indicates, however, that many other "Buffalo Soldiers" did return to their old fort to die. The cemetery holds the graves of William Jones, a trumpeter in the 9th Cavalry (1903); Leon Ross, also of the 9th Cavalry (1907); and 10th Cavalry members George Cunningham (1905), Will Finney (1907), and William Ross (1914).[101] Unlike the amusement hall, the cemetery was not racially segregated. Men were buried in the order in which they fell.

Some patients did reject sanctuary entirely and left Fort Bayard at the first opportunity, usually the day after they received their disability pension. A patient who "left hospital at his own request" typically departed against medical advice. Pvt. Horace Smith, for example, was a twenty-year-old from North Carolina in the Hospital Corps, who had been in the Army only two years when in June 1910 he began to cough and lose weight. By the time he was admitted to Fort Bayard he had lost 25 pounds, down to 140 from 165. Medical officers found "very active lesions" in his lungs and tubercular laryngitis, and listed his condition as "unfavorable." Smith at first recovered some of the weight he lost, but was down to 130 pounds by the end of the year, with a persistent fever. In February, though he felt better, medical officers recommended that he be discharged on disability. Now a beneficiary of the Soldiers' Home, Smith was seriously ill with advanced tuberculosis in both lungs, a temperature of 101 to 102, and producing two cups of sputum daily. Smith chose not to stay at Fort Bayard, though, and as a very sick man he "[l]eft the home at his own request," most likely to die.[102]

Treatment: Rest and Effort

Fort Bayard became a tuberculosis hospital during a time of transition in tuberculosis treatment from a regime of exercise and fresh air intended to build up the body, to one of complete rest to allow the body to heal. George Bushnell made the transition complete stating, "upon taking command here I changed entirely the treatment and I believe with good results."[103] Under Daniel Appel and Edward Comegys patients had to rest two hours in the morning and two in the evening, but Bushnell established a more extensive rest regime, increasing both the daily time in bed and the length of time a patient would stay in treatment. Even before he took command, when he was only in charge of one of the wards in 1903, Bushnell began to implement the treatment regime and philosophy he had learned from civilian tuberculosis physicians Charles Minor in North Carolina and Carroll E. Edson in Denver. He asked volunteer patients to live in tents and spend longer periods in bed, and after several months reported to Comegys that patients were improving when they rested more and slept outside.[104] Bushnell then began to lobby the Surgeon General on his approach, telling him, "it is my opinion that many patients do badly here because they do not take sufficient rest."[105] When he attended a national tuberculosis conference, he told the Surgeon General of "a gratifying unanimity among the speakers...as to the treatment of tuberculosis," and that "rest, relative or absolute, as the activity of the disease may require, an abundance of nourishing food and outdoor life were the three essentials insisted upon in the treatment."[106]

The premise of the rest therapy was that although medicine could not control the disease, rest could help make the patient stronger to fight the "bug." "Repose in bed acts in two ways," explained Earl Bruns. "It affords a relative amount of rest to the damaged lungs and also conserves the energy of the weakened body."[107] Not all specialists subscribed to rest therapy, but Bushnell believed he had benefitted from rest, and his experiments with volunteers at Fort Bayard had further convinced him of its value.[108] He recognized, however, that "it is up-hill work to break the prejudice of the older patients in favor of exercise as well as their natural inclination to go and come at will," but added, "[i]t is my belief that we can cure almost any case if we get it early enough."[109] Once he convinced the Army Medical Department to adopt his method, the rest regime prevailed in the Army for the next five decades. The actual effectiveness of rest therapy was unclear at the time and is still debated. Some physicians reason today that bed rest must have helped some patients' immune systems fight off tuberculosis, and others point to the falling death rates from tuberculosis as evidence of the success of sanatoriums and the rest cure. Other scholars are more skeptical. Historian Barbara Bates suggested that late nineteenth-century microscopy and X-rays enabled physicians to identify tuberculosis bacteria and shadows on the lungs and thereby diagnosed tuberculosis earlier and "cured" patients who may have gotten better anyway.[110] Physician and historian Thomas Dormandy argues that the rest cure was largely futile, and "the credit almost always belonged to the patient's natural resistance, and the recuperative power of nature."[111]

Although Fort Bayard had an X-ray machine, it was not used routinely until the late 1910s. Responding to a survey on X-ray use, Bushnell replied that the X-ray laboratory was "a very valuable adjunct" to a tuberculosis sanatorium if the "apparatus is first-class and the operators skilled."[112] But, he said, "on account of the unsatisfactory character of the present instrument it has not been used as much as it would have been otherwise in the examination of patients." His hospital instead diagnosed the disease based on physical symptoms such as weight loss, coughing, persistent temperature, a physical examination of the lungs, and sputum samples that were chemically stained to reveal tuberculosis bacteria. An individual's sputum had to be free of tubercle bacilli at least ten times in a row before Bushnell's team deemed a patient's case cured or at least quiescent.[113] Bushnell's advocacy of physical examination for diagnosis followed the prescription of his mentor and personal physician, Charles Minor, who wrote the section on diagnosis in a leading textbook, *Tuberculosis*, edited by Arnold Klebs.[114] Minor recommended devoting at least an hour to examining the chest, and developed a chart (Figure

2-6) identifying eleven sounds in the lungs and heart detectable by percussion and thirty-eight sounds detectable by the stethoscope.

Bushnell and his medical officers used lung sounds to identify where the infection was and how far it had proceeded—from infiltration, to caseation, to consolidation, to cavitation—and to distinguish tuberculosis from other lung ailments, such as bronchitis or lung cancer. Bruns, a meticulous examiner, described the examination of one patient's left lung in the following manner:

> Dulness [sic] and tympany to 2nd rib. Slight dullness 2nd to 4th ribs. Impaired percussion resonance 4th rib to base. Increased vocal fremitus [vibration] apex to base. Increased vocal resonance to 3rd rib. Cavernous breathing to 4th rib. Area of whispered pectoriloquy, more marked bronchial breathing and cavity rales 2nd and 3rd intercostal spaces, parasternal line. Many medium moist rales apex to base, elicited by deep breather and hear both on inspiration and expiration.[115]

These findings told Bruns that the patient had tuberculosis infiltration in both lobes of the left lung and a cavity in the upper lobe. Fort Bayard medical officers thus became masters of the chest exam and conducted research on chest sounds as well. Several officers compared the chest sounds of healthy men to those of patients at Fort Bayard, and in 1912 Bushnell published a technical paper on those chest sounds that could lead to erroneous tuberculosis diagnoses.[116]

In 1905, the Army Medical Department adopted the National Association for the Study and Prevention of Tuberculosis classification system for disease severity. Class I was incipient tuberculosis, Class II was moderately advanced, Class III was far advanced, and Class IV was miliary or systemic tuberculosis, almost always fatal.[117] Fort Bayard medical records, however, also gauged the extent to which the lungs were infected, so a patient with incipient tuberculosis in part of one lung would be "Class I, Involvement I," while a patient with advanced tuberculosis in both lungs would be "Class III, Involvement III." Patients with similar classifications were segregated into wards and staff moved them around as their conditions improved or worsened.

Once a patient was assigned to a ward, he entered into the hospital's routine. A bugle call awoke patients every day. Nurses took infirmary patients' temperatures first thing in the morning, and hospital corpsmen took ambulatory patients' temperatures. Patients with high fevers or recent lung hemorrhages stayed in bed all day, even for meals. Those without fevers in the ambulant wards rested in bed at least two hours in the morning and two in the afternoon, ate together in their designated messes, and retired at eight o'clock at night. Most patients lived outside on porches or in tents to benefit from the fresh air, even in the cold winter months, with blankets and hot water bottles to keep them warm. Staff weighed patients once a week and Bushnell increased physical exams to monthly instead of every two months to monitor the extension or clearing up of lesions. When Richard Johnson was an attendant in an ambulatory ward, his duty "was to take and record temperatures twice daily, issue linen and spit-cups, keep water coolers filled and

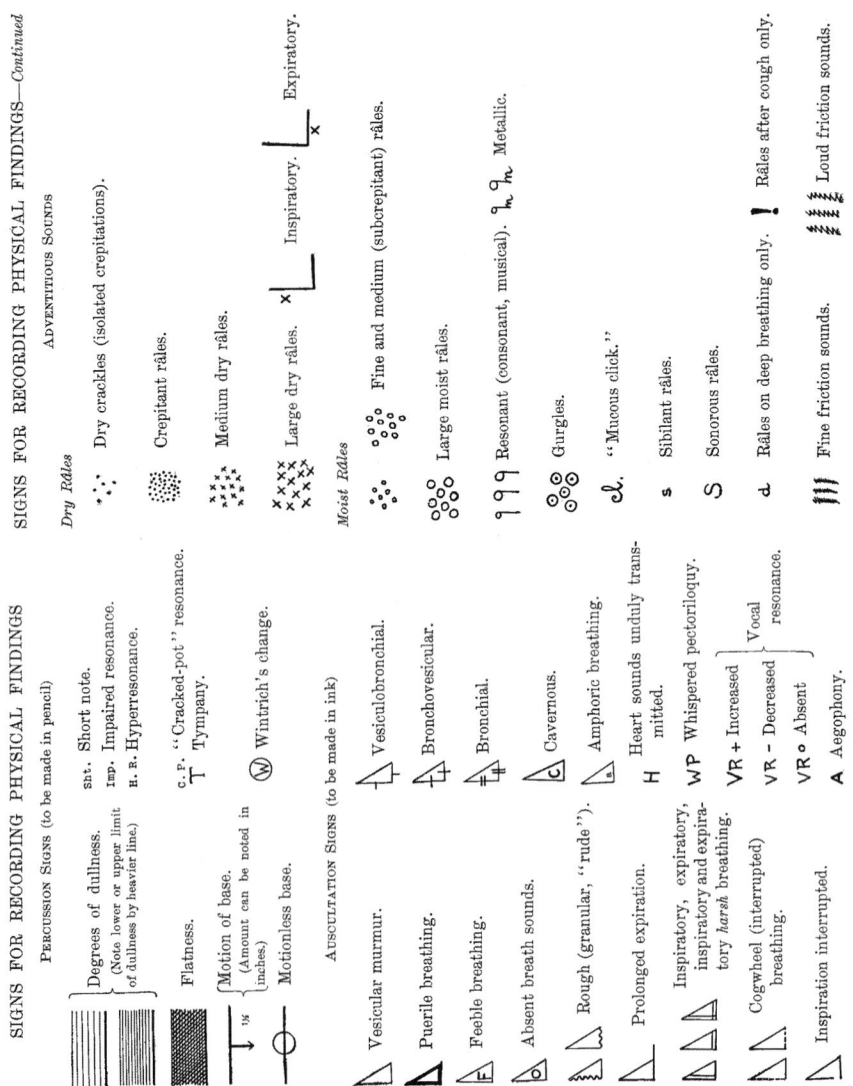

Figure 2-6. Auscultation chart. In Charles L. Minor, "Diagnosis," in Arnold C. Klebs, ed. *Tuberculosis: A Treatise by American Authors on its Etiology, Pathology, Frequency, Semeiology, Diagnosis, Prognosis, Prevention, and Treatment* (New York: D. Appleton and Co., 1909), 377–78.

to see that the tents and surrounding area was [sic] kept clean." He considered the work "a real soft job and I managed to hold on to it for six months."[118]

Bushnell discouraged strenuous exercise and stopped the practice of breathing exercises and hyperalimentation (overfeeding) found at many sanatoriums. He also did not use tuberculin therapy, which some tuberculosis physicians still used to treat tuberculosis. When Robert Koch discovered tuberculin, an antibody (antigen) to tuberculosis in 1890, he thought he had found the long sought-after cure. He was soon disappointed, but while it failed as a cure, scientists put tuberculin to other uses. In 1908 Clemens von Pirquet developed a tuberculin test that could detect if individuals had been infected by tuberculosis: if they had they were "tuberculin positive," if not, they were "tuberculin negative."[119] Once somebody received tuberculin as medicine, however, they would always test positive for tuberculosis infection. Bushnell believed that tuberculin therefore was both ineffective and interfered with the diagnostic process. He did not prescribe heroin, either, to calm coughing and recommended alcohol less often than his predecessors, explaining to one physician that, "[W]e do not use drugs in this institution with the idea of directly curing tuberculosis. Such drugs as are used are given on symptomatic indications."[120] During this period investigative journalists or "muckrakers" and some in the medical profession were warning the public about quackery, nostrums, and narcotics, and the American Medical Association cautioned that "[n]o other sick people are so easily influenced for better or worse [by patent drug venders] as those who suffer from pulmonary tuberculosis."[121] When a patient's condition worsened, however, medical officers prescribed morphine for pain, first orally and then by injection, at increasingly short intervals to a maximum of four times a day as the patient neared death.

Bushnell did believe that anything that was good for a person's health was bad for tuberculosis, and maintained orchards, gardens, and a dairy to provide a healthy diet for his patients. Medical officers adjusted the diet according to the patient's condition, prescribing a "soft diet" or "liquid diet," as well as laxative powders to relieve constipation that could accompany prolonged bed rest or the administration of narcotics. The few medical treatments they did prescribe included plasters on the chest to relieve pain and ease coughing, antiseptic gargles to soothe tubercular laryngitis, pain relievers such as aspirin, and straps around the chest to contract the chest walls to rest the lungs.[122] To stop lung hemorrhages, nurses placed ice bags over the chest for at least twenty-four hours, and used ice packs and caps or hot water bottles for pain. Some patients medicated themselves. Walter Robbins, for example, took mercury, which he claimed improved his appetite and digestion; another patient took olive oil before every meal.[123] The surgical treatment of tuberculous was not common at this time, but medical officers operated on patients for appendicitis and other infections or wounds, or to remove tumors and tuberculosis tissue from patients' limbs. In 1913, Fort Bayard medical officers performed 107 such operations.[124]

One patient's medical record reveals the roller coaster of recovery and decline many patients experienced at Fort Bayard. In March 1910, Sergeant (Sgt.) Homer McQueen, a Fort Bayard hospital corpsman, age 32, accompanied a convalescent patient from Fort Bayard to Jefferson Barracks, Missouri. Upon return, McQueen complained of "slight indisposition." Bruns admitted him to the hospital with diarrhea and a 100 degree temperature, but laboratory tests revealed no signs of malaria, typhoid, or tuberculosis. A "feeble breath sound" at the top of the left lung, however, did suggest pulmonary tuberculosis, and in late April his sputum revealed the telltale bacilli. By May Bruns found slight activity in the right lung and very active tuberculosis in the left, including a cavity that caused McQueen's heart to be displaced to the left. He received calomel and magnesium sulphur as purgatives, and a blister-producing plaster to his left side where the tuberculosis was the most severe, but little other medication. In June, Bruns classified McQueen's tuberculosis as Class III and Involvement II, but his patient recovered some weight, from 134 pounds to 141, and by the middle of June was well enough to eat in the mess hall.

After this rally, however, his condition worsened again. He was soon getting plasters on both sides and an antiseptic gargle, perhaps for tuberculous laryngitis. Nurses gave him quinine for his fever (which would have been ineffective unless he had malaria), but he continued to lose weight, and soon was spitting up blood. In September 1910 Bruns noted, "[g]eneral condition of patient at first improved has grown worse during last two months," and despite the fact that McQueen's left side had been strapped for four months, the "[l]eft lung seems to have broken down more with increased formation of fibrous tissue." He classified McQueen, "[a]bsolutely bed patient." Nurses gave him ice bags and phenacetin for fever and pain, and a soft diet, including eggs and brandy.[125] By his next examination, McQueen had lost seven pounds, had a "constant distressing cough," and was "losing ground rapidly." After a medical board found McQueen disabled on account of "far advanced" chronic pulmonary tuberculosis, the War Department discharged him on disability and immediately admitted him to the infirmary (Figure 2-7 and 2-8) as a beneficiary of the Soldiers' Home.[126] His condition stabilized.

In January, McQueen was improving. Medical officer Capt. Conrad Koerper noted that McQueen was sleeping better, had gained nine pounds in the last month, and "[a]ll lesions [in] both lungs show considerable decrease in activity." By mid-February he was able to return to the ward, but in less than a month was back in the infirmary with painful lung inflammation. Staff removed the straps from his chest, and for the first time gave McQueen morphine for pain. A nurse noted on March 30 that McQueen "appeared to sleep." Throughout April McQueen got morphine regularly, at first by mouth and then by injection. At this point medical personnel seemed to shift from combating tuberculosis to keeping McQueen comfortable. By late June he could not leave his bed for the physical examination and received four morphine injections daily, including one around midnight, as well as measures of whiskey. He also got a "cough mist" to ease the irritation of the constant coughing. On 2 July 1911, McQueen was too weak even to be examined, but staff observed that, "about twice daily he turns upon right side and empties cavity of large quantity of purulent foul smelling material." McQueen's nurses recorded the last days of his life:

> Cough medicine at 6 a.m.
> Whiskey, 15 cc
> Perspired profusely, considerable dyspnea [difficulty breathing] cough very severe at times, very restless from 9 P.M. to 1 A.M., slept about 1 hr.

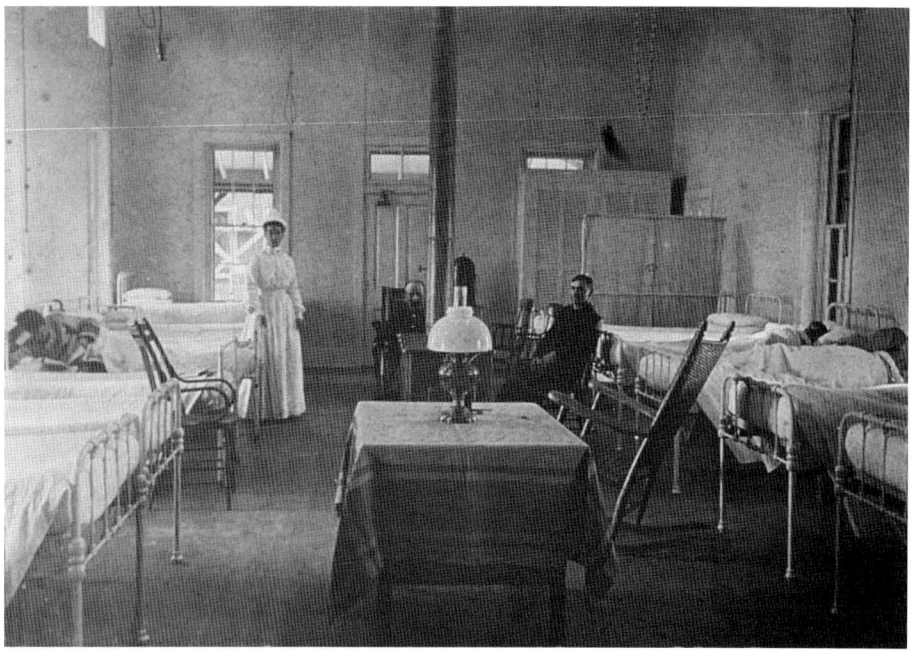

Figure 2-7. General Hospital, Fort Bayard, New Mexico, East Ward, Enlisted men's infirmary, circa 1907.
Photograph courtesy of the National Library of Medicine, Image #A030247.

> after 1 A.M. restless remainder of night.
> Hypo Morph and Atropine at 8:30 A.M., Had weak spell at 8 A.M.
> Whiskey 30 cc
> Morphine at 3:30 P. M.
> Did not take food
> Very restless from 11:45 P.M. to 12:30 A.M.
> Morphine and Atropine, 65 mg at 12:30 A.M.
> Respiration labored at 1:30 A.M., pulse imperceptible at 3:00 A.M.
> Appeared to be dead at 4:30 A.M.

Medical officer Roy Heflebower conducted an autopsy that afternoon, and found the internal organs distended and damaged, and the "thoracic cavity filled with 1,200 c.c. of foul smelling, greenish pus." He concluded the cause of death to be chronic pulmonary tuberculosis, with "associated conditions: empyema, [lung infection] unilateral, left. Addison's Disease. Chronic passive congestion all viscera." Only fifteen months had elapsed between his first diagnosis and his death due to tuberculosis. McQueen's father in River Sioux, Iowa, chose not to transport his son's body home, so Chaplain Bateman presided over McQueen's funeral and burial in the Fort Bayard cemetery on the hill behind the officers' quarters.[127]

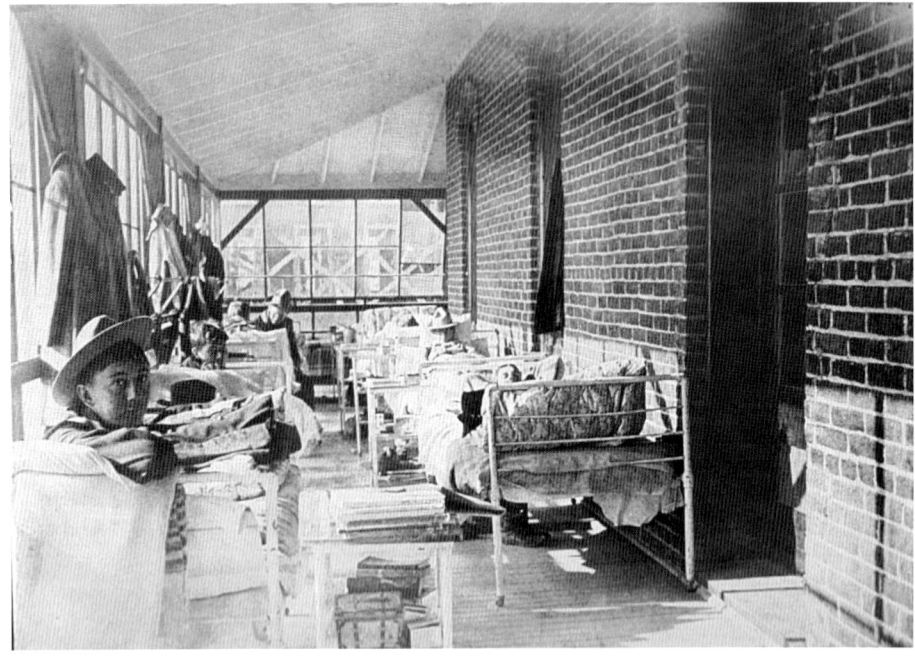

Figure 2-8. West Porch, enlisted men's infirmary, General Hospital, Fort Bayard, New Mexico, circa 1907.
Photograph courtesy of the National Library of Medicine, Image #A030248.

Homer McQueen's autopsy showed the destruction that tuberculosis could wreak on the body. In 1915–16, medical officer Capt. Thomas H. Johnson examined the records of 400 patients, 100 of whom died and were autopsied, to tabulate maladies that accompanied tuberculosis. He found that more than 20 percent of patients had syphilis, many at the secondary or tertiary stages that ravaged the body, and that 29 percent had tuberculosis complications, some more than one. Of these, 30 percent had pleurisy, an inflammation and collection of fluid around the lining of the lungs. Other common complications included tuberculous laryngitis (15 percent) and inner ear infections (11 percent). Some patients suffered inflammation of the gastrointestinal tract from swallowing tuberculous material, and Johnson also found that 90 percent of the autopsies showed kidney damage, a far greater percentage than had been diagnosed before death.[128] Another Fort Bayard study of cases showed a similar range of complications.[129]

Like all sanatoriums of the time, Fort Bayard's record in effectively treating tuberculosis was mixed. In the early 1900s many people believed that Fort Bayard and other sanatoriums could cure some cases of tuberculosis, especially those caught in the early stages. National tuberculosis rates were in decline in the early twentieth century, falling from 20 percent of deaths in 1900 to 15 percent in 1920.

By the time George Bushnell left Fort Bayard, tuberculosis had yielded first place to heart disease as the cause of death in the United States. During his tenure, the annual death rate at Fort Bayard dropped from around 21 percent in 1904 to less than 12 percent in 1917.[130] But if Bushnell was at first confident they could "cure almost any case if we get it early enough," a few years later he was more circumspect, telling one physician that "[i]t is dangerous to talk of absolute cure in tuberculosis."[131] In 1911 Chaplain Bateman observed, "the word 'cure' is sparingly used, when not evaded or omitted by the specialist in tuberculosis."[132] Death still resided in the hospital, claiming on average more than one patient every week. In 1908, 55 patients died; and in 1914, 66 patients died, 59 of tuberculosis.[133]

As the sanatorium movement expanded, people compared results among institutions across the country in hope of finding the best possible place for a cure. Admissions policies clearly affected sanatorium "success" rates. Some institutions, such as that run by Lawrence Flick in Pennsylvania, admitted only people with incipient or mild cases because they had the best chances for recovery, while others, such as the National Jewish Hospital in Denver, admitted only the very ill or indigent to provide them care and comfort as they died.[134] When people questioned Fort Bayard's record, Bushnell pointed out that comparisons with civilian hospitals were inappropriate because Fort Bayard admitted any eligible soldier or veteran, some of whom arrived moribund. It was not only a hospital, he explained, "it is also an asylum for discharged soldiers from the Regular Army who have tuberculosis, many of whom come and go for years and finally come back here to die."[135]

In 1908 Bushnell checked with the Army, Navy, and the Pension Office to determine how many former Fort Bayard patients from 1899 to 1904 had survived. He found that about 32 percent of Fort Bayard patients were still alive, 45 percent were dead, and 23 percent were unaccounted for.[136] A similar study by the Public Health Service tuberculosis hospital at Fort Stanton was "not gratifying in the number located or in the state of health of the individuals found." Of 1,924 patients who had been discharged for more than six months, only 149 were known living, 922 known to be dead, and 853 unaccounted for. Fort Stanton's director wrote, "The sanitary value of isolating a large number of open cases of tuberculosis can not be over-estimated," but "it must be admitted that the sanitarium for advanced cases plays no other part in the general campaign against the disease."[137] Given such evidence, many people began to consider tuberculosis sanatoriums more as places to isolate patients than as places to cure them.

Acceptance and Resistance of the Tuberculosis Lifestyle

The diagnosis of tuberculosis threatened a young man with disability, an uncertain future, and perhaps death, and could undermine his identity as warrior and wage earner, plunging him into depression.[138] The tuberculosis treatment itself was also a great trial for soldiers and sailors accustomed to a vigorous, masculine lifestyle. In addition to following the personal hygiene rules regarding coughing and sputum disposal, the patient's job was to accept total rest. Francis

Trudeau, who established one of the first and most popular sanatoriums at Lake Saranac, New York, said it required one to "[c]onquer fate by acquiescence"; another scholar called it "a draconian regimen of inactivity."[139] Bruns admitted, "[t]o me the news of the treatment came as a greater shock than had my tuberculosis diagnosis."[140] One had to rest for a long time. Thomas Johnson's 1916 study on tuberculosis complications revealed that the surviving patients in his sample population had been at Fort Bayard for an average of 3.3 years; those who had died had been there for an average of 1.9 years. The longest living patient had been at the hospital 15.9 years; thirty-eight had been "intermittently observed" for ten or more years; and sixty-nine for at least five years.[141]

As with any isolated Army post, boredom undermined morale. Many young, formerly active men on enforced bed rest, surrounded by sickness and death, forbidden to drink alcohol or to roam the hills, met their new life with despair and at times rebellion. Morale and discipline problems challenged Bushnell's medical and military authority.[142] Problems included promiscuous spitting, the scattering of spit cups, using foul language, disrespecting officers, engaging in sexual misconduct, possessing illicit firearms, going absent without leave, and smuggling whiskey into the hospital. Medical officer Paul Hutton even reported that one patient misbehaved by imitating the groans of others as they lay dying.[143] The use of opiates to control tuberculosis symptoms could also lead to drug addiction.[144] This was not a widespread problem for the Army Medical Department, but one Army study estimated that while fewer than 1 percent of enlisted men were drug users, they could tempt others into the habit, so that "a cocaine fiend is truly a loss as well as a danger to the Army."[145] Bushnell, therefore, refused to admit Soldiers' Home beneficiary Hugh T. Robbins, who California officials described as a "dope fiend," to protect his patients.[146]

One case involving sexual activity led to a dramatic arrest in Silver City. On a June night in 1909, Hospital Corps Pvts. Leslie Thomas and Charles F. Baker were found in bed together, against Army regulations. Thomas turned himself in the next morning, but Baker made a run for it. Medical officer Lt. Edgar Jones, also serving as the post constable, found Baker on a train departing from Silver City and confronted him with a revolver. Baker jumped off and reboarded the last car of the train with Jones in pursuit. Baker then climbed on a nearby freight train, only to be captured by Jones and taken to the Silver City jail. Fort Bayard officers wanted to dishonorably discharge both Thomas and Baker and thereby avoid publicly airing the incident, but the War Department insisted on a court-martial and both men were charged with sodomy—and Baker with resisting arrest—and tried within weeks.[147]

Illicit alcohol use and alcohol abuse were the biggest problems, leading to fights and unapproved absences. Patients snuck down "The Butterfield Trail" to a "gin mill" in the nearby village of Central, and once Bushnell caught a mail carrier smuggling whiskey in to a patient.[148] He cracked down especially hard on patient drunkenness. When a beneficiary of the Soldiers' Home, Thomas L. Kane, was convicted by court-martial of drunk and disorderly conduct, Bushnell suspended him from Fort Bayard for six months, a harsher punishment than the usual three-month confinement for members of the Hospital Corps.[149] In another case, when a court-martial dishonorably discharged two sailors for drunkenness, Bushnell made arrangements to purchase their train tickets and escort them to the train, because "[i]f this be not done it is anticipated that Sheppard [one of the men] will spend all his money on drink and return to this Hospital as a charity patient," he told the Navy. Sheppard had advanced syphilis and tuberculosis in both lungs, and was most likely contagious, but Bushnell the military officer would not have him in his hospital. "He is a thoroughly vicious man and his conduct in confinement has been bad."[150]

Bushnell had legal control over the active-duty Army officers and soldiers at Fort Bayard and exercised it vigorously. He believed that the soldier-patient's job was to get well. Excused from active duty he must therefore avoid "the acts which would tend to aggravate his disease."[151] In a report to his superior in Washington, Chaplain Bateman put it bluntly: "I am endeavoring to arouse and keep alive a profound sense of moral responsibility among the men who are under treatment here. Men who undo by evil habits and practices that which is done for them here, deserve and receive no sympathy, and are 'weeded out.'"[152] Fort Bayard officers often blamed—with some reason—recalcitrant patients when their health worsened. When Navy patient Luther F. Steward returned after being absent without leave, a medical officer found that his health had deteriorated "due in all probability to his own misconduct since on his return he showed unmistakable signs of debauchery."[153]

But if he had clear authority over Army personnel, Bushnell spent the early years of his command clarifying his authority over other patients.[154] He obtained approval from the Navy and the Soldiers' Home to discipline their patients under Fort Bayard rules and the court-martial system, and at times asked the Soldiers' Home to withhold a patient's pension money as a disciplinary measure.[155] He settled on suspension from Fort Bayard as punishment for patients not in the regular military, establishing a rule that patients expelled for bad behavior could not return until three months after the date of their discharge, and that "patients who are dishonorably dismissed from this Hospital need not expect to be readmitted under any circumstances."[156] Bushnell persuaded the War Department to support his efforts. In 1906 he suspended several beneficiaries of the Soldiers' Home for drunkenness with the proviso they could not reenter the post for three months. When they gained admission to the California branch of the National Home for Disabled Volunteer Soldiers (the domiciliary system for noncareer veterans of the Civil War and Spanish-American War), they complained to the War Department that Fort Bayard was not helping them. In response to the Department's inquiry, an unapologetic Bushnell fired back that many of the complainants had left Fort Bayard against medical advice or had been suspended for rules violations. James Duffey, he noted, had been in and out of the hospital eight times in five years, and "[t]his record will show how little responsibility the management here can have for his failure to improve." Joseph McGovern had been admitted and discharged from the hospital six times from 1902 to 1904, and had been punished four times. "He was the most troublesome and thankless patient I have known here," Bushnell stated. His staff often begged patients to stay because their health was not good enough to travel, so therefore "I wish to deny as emphatically as is in my power that patients with tuberculosis are ever sent away from here because they fail to improve." He closed his letter cautioning that, "[s]uspension from this hospital loses much of its force as a punitive measure if men suspended for misconduct are taken into volunteer homes without inquiry."[157] The War Department concurred, and the Soldiers' Home in Washington and the National Home for Disabled Volunteer Soldiers agreed thereafter to deny admission to patients expelled from Fort Bayard.[158]

Bushnell did negotiate with patients at times. Chaplain Bateman reported in 1909 that beneficiaries of the Soldiers' Home "created a mild sensation by a bill of grievances." The complaints, he said, "were heard and thrashed out by the Commanding Officer with marked tolerance and magnanimity and whatever could be done was done to restore contentment among the discontented." Putting the most positive face on it, the chaplain added that "discord will sometimes occur in the best regulated families."[159] Bushnell's discipline campaign seems to have made an impact because in February 1910 Bateman reported that "the guardhouse has been empty of prisoners for days at a time during this month."[160]

One of Chaplain Bateman's duties was to develop recreation programs and diversions to occupy staff and patients and improve morale at the isolated post. He relished the task, and opened a post exchange to sell items not available at the commissary, such as stationery and candy, and used the proceeds to fund entertainment. In 1906 he financed a Christmas party and bought a small printing press.[161] Over the years Fort Bayard acquired a moving picture projector, a camera and equipment to make lantern slides, a record player and "many excellent records," and a library, which subscribed to 82 periodicals and had 2,000 volumes of "light literature." Bushnell got funds to refurbish the amusement hall, which seated 400 for religious services, movies, dances, plays, and post orchestra performances. Medical officer Hutton loved the theater and one year wrote and directed a play, "The Tenderfoot Girl," that, according to the Silver City *Independent* "graphically depicted the cowboy life of Grant County, New Mexico."[162] Enthusiasm for the theater caused Bushnell to require that an officer preview plays or other entertainment to ensure "that the proposed production is free from vulgarity or indecency."[163] Fort Bayard also had a bowling alley and gymnastic equipment and fielded baseball and football teams.[164] Patients used a pool hall separate from that of regular duty soldiers and could not participate in all of these activities. As Bateman noted, "[a]ble-bodied men are forbidden to box with a patient, however good the latter's condition may be. No wise patient will play at ten pins, tennis or base ball."[165] Richard Johnson remembered "bronco-busting contests," with the local Mexican community, and hunting in the fall for quail, rabbit, or deer. "Thus life here was made tolerable for those of us who had the fortitude to make the best out of a bad situation."[166]

Reentry: Leaving Fort Bayard

Patients departed Fort Bayard in a number of ways. The majority entered as soldiers but left as beneficiaries of the Soldiers' Home, disabled by tuberculosis; others recovered their health and returned to duty and a long life; the unfortunate ones departed in a coffin. Due to their relative youth, active-duty enlisted men and officers had lower death rates than beneficiaries of the Soldiers' Home. In 1910, for example, the Regular Army death rate was less than half of the veteran death rate—4 percent versus 9.6 percent. Of the 496 officers and enlisted men discharged from the hospital, 260 were discharged on disability, 155 returned to duty, and 20 died. The same year, Fort Bayard discharged 383 beneficiaries of the Soldiers' Home, 37 of whom died, and 346 patients who simply "Left Hospital."[167] The War Department had different discharge policies regarding officers and enlisted men. Officers were kept on the active list "so long as there is a fair chance for cure," and the hospital sent the Office of The Surgeon General periodic reports on their progress.[168] Enlisted men disabled by disease, however, could be discharged from the Army rather quickly, sometimes within weeks. If the disability had been acquired during military service, a soldier could receive a pension—lower than duty pay—and be eligible for the Soldiers' Home and treatment at military hospitals. In 1907, however, Bushnell recommended that enlisted men be retained at the hospital at least six months before being discharged on disability. He argued that the longer period was required to determine a patient's prognosis, and would avoid "a possible injustice which may be committed if men of short service on admission here should be deprived of a pension and should not be admitted to the Soldiers' Home on the ground that the mode of their discharge showed them not to be disabled."[169] The Surgeon General agreed and approved the change.

The Army Medical Department did not provide systematic physical or vocational rehabilitation until World War I, but soldiers who recovered did a month of light labor before discharge to see if they were well enough to return to their units. The Army Medical Department advised against sending former tuberculosis patients to the tropics because it could be harmful to their health, but the War Department did not always oblige. Many disabled veterans stayed in the Southwest to take advantage of the climate; some stayed as close as Silver City, which had several private sanatoriums. Capt. Charles Barney was a patient and physician at Fort Bayard from 1906 until he was discharged on disability in 1910. He first went to Mexico, seeking a warm climate, but returned ill to Fort Bayard for a couple of months in 1911. After that he lived in Los Angeles and Tucson until his health deteriorated again in 1917, and he requested admission to Fort Bayard.[170] Hospital corpsman Charles Noyes was discharged on disability in 1910 and over the next five years was in and out of Fort Bayard at least four times, working at odd jobs in New Mexico, Texas, and Louisiana between his hospital stays.[171]

Many of these patients, like Noyes who had Class III, Involvement III tuberculosis, would have been highly infectious. Medical officers at the time, however, were more concerned that leaving treatment would jeopardize the patient's recovery than that they could be a danger to others. In the early twentieth century people understood that tuberculosis was contagious, but most hospitals and public health agencies did not impose strict anticontagion controls because of an incomplete understanding of the nature of tuberculosis transmission. Several factors may account for this. First of all, tuberculosis was so ubiquitous and usually developed so slowly that it was impossible to identify a single source of infection. It was also clearly not as contagious as other infectious diseases, such as measles, or typhoid, or influenza, which could sweep a town or Army post in days—and thus containment seemed less urgent. Secondly, the prevailing view held that some types of people were more likely to develop tuberculosis than others, and the nineteenth-century theory that tuberculosis was hereditary lingered. Tuberculosis physicians therefore focused on an individual's ability to resist tuberculosis, referring to a person who developed active disease as having "broken down." They considered an individual's internal resistance to be more important than external infection in the development of disease.

Perhaps the most important explanation for this lack of concern about disease transmission is that scientists and physicians of the time believed that bacteria existed only in droplets of sputum, blood, or other tubercular material and did not understand that tuberculosis could be transmitted through the air. A leading textbook in 1909 stated: "The germs from consumptives are carried by the sputum, not by the breath. The breath itself is harmless."[172] Medical personnel therefore believed that the daunting array of rules regarding coughing, the proper use and disposal of spit cups, and the avoidance of dried sputum could control the spread of tuberculosis. Hospital corpsman Richard Johnson gained confidence from these measures. He had worried about contagion from tuberculosis patients, but he later wrote that "essential measures of precaution were taught and enforced until they became a routine habit, ...and I do not recall a single case where an attendant contracted the disease during the time I was there."[173] Nonetheless, Fort Bayard active duty personnel had a tuberculosis rate almost double that of the next highest Army hospital, about 6 percent (seven cases among the hundred-plus active duty personnel) compared to 3 percent at the Presidio in San Francisco.[174] Although some of this was due to the transfer of military personnel with tuberculosis to Fort Bayard, staff may also have contracted the disease while caring for patients. But at the time, these differential rates prompted little official discussion about increased risk of infection at a tuberculosis hospital. The fact that Fort Bayard and other tuberculosis institutions allowed contagious patients to leave and reenter as they wished undoubtedly spread the disease to the larger population.

While some patients actively sought discharges from Fort Bayard for disability, others resisted it. Twelfth Cavalry Lt. Oscar Lusk's father, a judge in Los Angeles, wrote to U.S. Senator C. A. Culberson of California, in support of his son's retirement on disability. After the senator contacted the War Department, the Surgeon General supported the request, "if it can be done consistently with the public service."[175] Young Lusk soon got his pension and moved to Almagordo, New Mexico, where he survived five years until his death in 1908 at age thirty-seven.[176] Pvt. Charles Tyler, the former Buffalo Soldier, also sought retirement on disability, more on account of stomach ailments and painful feet due to corns than tuberculosis, but it took him a longer time (more than a year and three medical boards) before it was granted.[177] On the other hand, when Major (Maj.) Ogden Rafferty, a Medical Corps officer who had had a mountain peak in Yosemite National Park named after him, was ordered to go before a retirement board, he objected. He blamed his poor diagnosis and prognosis on "animus upon the part of Capt. Barney," the medical officer who had most recently examined him. The War Department rejected Rafferty's claims and retired him as "totally incapacitated" by pulmonary tuberculosis in 1909.[178] Similarly, Capt. Solomon P. Vestal, an officer with the 7th Cavalry, developed tuberculosis in 1903 and served light duty as quartermaster at Fort Bayard. Though he vigorously objected, he was forced to retire for disability in May 1910. With Bushnell's help he stayed on at the post to oversee construction on a contract basis.

Most patients who died at Fort Bayard succumbed to tuberculosis, but typhoid, appendicitis, peritonitis, and pneumonia claimed a few people every year, as did suicide. In 1909, two men (a patient and an active-duty private in the Hospital Corps) killed themselves. Unfortunate tuberculosis patients such as Homer McQueen (Figure 2-9) often died in a morphine-induced haze. Chaplain Bateman ministered to all of them in their last days. His monthly reports recorded the patient's name, status, military affiliation, date and cause of death, nearest relative or friend, and whether the person's remains were buried at the Fort Bayard cemetery or shipped home.[179] The commanding officer advised the next of kin on record, usually parents or a wife, and inquired as to how to dispose of his personal property. Loved ones often wanted to know the circumstances of the patient's death. John McCarty's wife, Medora, wrote to Bushnell: "Please give me some idea of how he died did he suffer? Was he many days confined to his bed? Did he say anything?" She explained, "Oh! I am most crazy. I would have liked so much to have seen him once before his death." She added, "I want every piece of paper that he has handled." Bushnell responded that her husband had expressed a desire to return home as soon as he was well enough to travel, but he "was unconscious for three days before his death. He died quietly and without pain."[180] Bushnell informed Samuel Hill's father, "Your son was a good patient and asked that the nurses be thanked for their kindness to him." He added that the son "left no messages, but a few days before he died he asked the Doctor to have his remains prepared so that they would look as well as possible for his folks to see."[181] Less sympathetic family inquiries asked for property or life insurance policies a deceased soldier or veteran might have left behind.[182] In a long-established tradition, hospital staff auctioned off unclaimed property and put the proceeds into the hospital fund. Many active-duty patients had wives or parents willing and able to pay for the body to be shipped home for burial, but Bateman's reports for 1909 and 1910 show that the majority of deceased—almost two to one—were buried at the post cemetery. Many of them, especially beneficiaries of the Soldiers' Home, Bateman noted as having "no relatives." The Fort Bayard cemetery not only received soldiers, but also sailors, civilians, and children of men on duty at the post, including a few infants who died at birth.

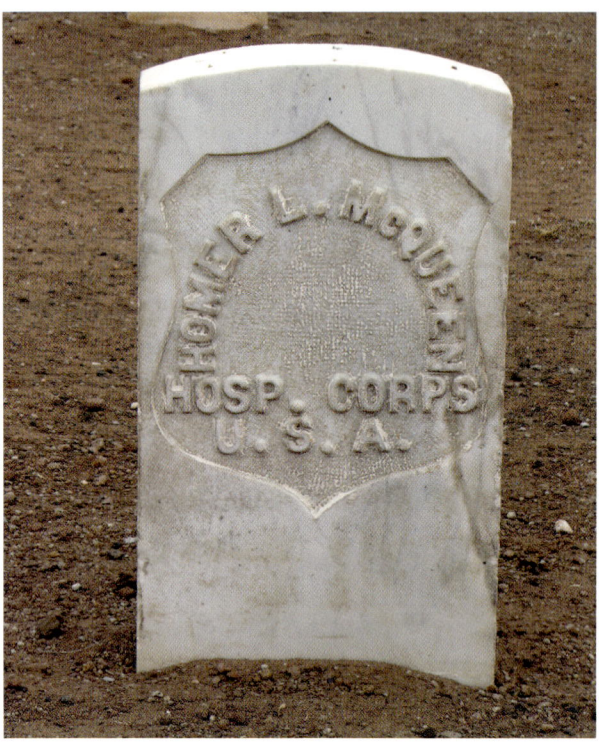

Figure 2-9. Grave marker of Homer L. McQueen, Fort Bayard National Cemetery, Fort Bayard, New Mexico (author's possession).

A number of patients were able to recover and live long lives, some returning to military service. In 1912, for example, Bushnell sent the Surgeon General a list of fifty-six Army officers who had been treated for tuberculosis at Fort Bayard over the years and returned to duty.[183] Nurse Agnes Young described what must have been a spectacular recovery. One of her patients arrived at Fort Bayard a nervous, "almost hysterical man," enduring nineteen hemorrhages in a month, totaling more than 4.7 liters of bloody sputum. Five months later, however, he was "able to hunt arrowheads on the old battlefields among the hills surrounding our post."[184] Another patient, Corporal (Corp.) Howard O. Watson, struggled with tuberculosis for more than fifteen years, in and out of Fort Bayard four times from 1905 to 1920. Although the Army discharged him for disability in 1911, he became well enough to return to active duty in the Army in 1920.[185] Some Fort Bayard patients went on to serve with distinction in World War I. Army cavalry officer Capt. Walter C. Babcock mapped the trans-Alaskan trail in 1899 before he developed tuberculosis while serving in the Philippines. He had two stints of treatment in 1906 and 1907, but recovered enough to earn the Distinguished Service Medal for his command of the 310th Infantry in the Meuse Argonne, 1918.[186]

And Earl Bruns, who had arrived at Fort Bayard in a state of such desperation and hope, would become a key figure in the War Department's tuberculosis program, writing a definitive report on tuberculosis in the American Expeditionary Forces in Europe during the war.

Some patients thus welcomed their treatment at Fort Bayard, while others resented it; some recovered their health, but most did not. Under George Bushnell's command (1904–17) the post remained isolated and self-sufficient, but still very much connected to the outside world through scientific research and medical correspondence and the cycling in and out of patients. As patients and medical staff struggled against tuberculosis on the high New Mexican plateau, they encountered the contradictions of the human condition: hope and despair, acceptance and resistance, and life and death. A close look at one patient's experience at Fort Bayard reveals those complexities.

Notes

1. Richard Johnson, "My Life in the US Army, 1899 to 1922," unpublished typescript, Richard Johnson Papers, Military History Institute, Carlisle, PA, 83.
2. Johnson, "My Life in the US Army," 82.
3. Correspondence between G. E. Bushnell and Adjutant General, June 1909, Record Group [hereafter cited as RG] 112, Entry 386, National Archives and Records Administration [hereafter cited as NARA].
4. Johnson, "My Life in the US Army," 83.
5. Earl A. Bruns, "Colonel Bushnell: An Estimate of His Character and Work," *American Review of Tuberculosis* 11 (1925): 277.
6. William Garrott Brown, "Some Confessions of a T.B.," *The Atlantic Monthly* 113 (June 1914): 747.
7. Patricia Paton, *A Medical Gentleman: James J. Waring, M.D.* (Denver, CO: Colorado Historical Society, 1993), provides a revealing view of how tuberculosis shaped the life of another tuberculosis patient and expert, James Waring. For more on the role of personal experience in a physician's work, see Stanley W. Jackson, "The Wounded Healer," *Bulletin of the History of Medicine* 75 (Spring 2001): 1–36; Chris Feudtner, "Patients' Stories and Clinical Care: Uniting the Unique and the Universal?" *Journal of General Internal Medicine* 13 (1998): 846–49; and Lawrence K. Altman, "At the Helm: Oncologists with Cancer," *New York Times* (24 May 2005).
8. Bruns, "Colonel Bushnell," 282.
9. Bushnell later disputed that he had a tuberculosis relapse in 1909–10, believing instead that he had been misdiagnosed. He wrote in 1918, "I myself have spent six months in physically harmful idleness under the diagnosis of active tuberculosis resting on the erroneous interpretation of normal physical signs." See George E. Bushnell, "Lessons from the War as to Tuberculosis," *Journal of the American Medical Association* 70 (9 March 1918): 665.
10. "Application for Medical Leave of Absence," C. N. Barney, Record Group 94, Records of the Adjutant General, (hereafter RG 94), Appointment, Commission and Personnel Branch, Office of the Adjutant General [hereafter cited as ACP], Box 715, NARA. The report reads, in part, "left epididymis is distinctly enlarged, nodular and quite tender and is associated with hydrocele [accumulation of water]. The right epididymis appears to be somewhat thickened. The condition of the epididymis was not noted last year, but the hydrocele at least is of long standing."

11. G. E. Bushnell to Adjutant General, 26 August 1911, RG 112, Entry 386, Box 40, NARA.

12. Efficiency Record, George E. Bushnell, 1910, RG 94, ACP, Box 715, NARA. See also Surgeon General to Adjutant General, 21 November 1911, RG 94, Adjutant General's Office [hereafter cited as AGO] 1850340, Box 6734, NARA.

13. G. E. Bushnell to Adjutant General, 26 November 1911, RG 112, Entry 386, NARA; and George E. Bushnell's efficiency reports, RG 94, Box 715, NARA.

14. S. Adolphus Knopf, "Is There Any Relation between Tuberculosis, Mental Disease, and Mental Deficiency?" *Medical Record* 91 (6 January 1917): 7.

15. This is for the years 1926–56; Fred L. Ayvazian, "The 55 Trudeau Medalists," *American Review of Tuberculosis* (April 1980): 757; and Julius L. Wilson, "Five Great Teachers in the Field of Tuberculosis," *American Review of Tuberculosis* (May 1981). For discussion of physicians who had tuberculosis see Julius Lane Wilson, "Pikes Peak or Bust: An Historical Note on the Search for Health in the Rockies," *Rocky Mountain Medical Journal* 64 (1967): 59; Jake W. Spidle Jr., *Doctors of Medicine in New Mexico* (Albuquerque, NM: University of New Mexico Press, 1986); Jake W. Spidle, "Coughing and Spitting and New Mexico History," in Judith Boyce DeMark, ed., *Essays in Twentieth-Century New Mexico History* (Albuquerque, NM: University of New Mexico Press, 1994).

16. James J. Waring, "The Patient and the Physician," *American Review of Tuberculosis* 62 (1950): 68.

17. Helen Clapesattle, *Dr. Webb of Colorado Springs* (Boulder, CO: Colorado Associated University Press, 1994).

18. Bruns, "Colonel Bushnell: An Estimate of his Character and Work," 277 and 282.

19. Richard Johnson, "My Life in the U.S. Army, 1899 to 1922."

20. Correspondence regarding inspection of Fort Bayard, 29 September to 3 October 1909, RG 112, Entry 386, Box 27, NARA.

21. Cephas Bateman to G. E. Bushnell, 4 December 1912, RG 94, Box 1283, NARA. Bateman's letter opened, "No one will ever know, apart from ourselves, of the contents of this letter unless you disclose the same."

22. Cephas Bateman to G. E. Bushnell, 11 December 1912, RG 94, Box 1283, NARA.

23. Memoranda relative to the conduct of Chaplain Bateman, March 1913, RG 94, Box 1283, NARA. The conflict flared again during Bateman's efficiency evaluation in May 1913. When asked about the matter, Bateman wrote that he believed he was the "aggrieved party in this matter," but "soon charged the whole matter to the disease from which Colonel Bushnell is said to suffer." For his part, Bushnell wrote that, "[T]he question may be fairly raised whether the usefulness of this officer as a chaplain in the Army service has not ceased." Correspondence regarding the Bateman efficiency report, May 1913 and June 1913, RG 94, Box 1283, NARA.

24. Information in this paragraph is drawn from Fort Bayard's annual reports to the Office of The Surgeon General, and the War Department Annual Reports, 1904 to 1917.

25. G. E. Bushnell, "Report for the Calendar Year 1905. U.S. General Hospital, Fort Bayard, N.M.," RG 112, Entry 380, NARA. Presidential Proclamation, Theodore Roosevelt, 21 July 1905, regarding Gila River Forest Reserve. In 1905 the forest reserves were transferred from the Department of the Interior to the Department of Agriculture, and the Bureau of Forestry was reorganized as the Forest Service. In 1907, the forest reserves were renamed national forests.

26. G. E. Bushnell to Surgeon General, 8 August 1905, RG 112, Entry 380, NARA.

27. G. E. Bushnell to M. W. Ireland, 20 November 1905, RG 112, Entry 380, NARA. See also, "Improvements at Fort Bayard," *Silver City Enterprise,* 3 August 1906.

28. "Giant Sequoias Set Out at Fort Bayard," *The Independent*, 20 April 1915.

29. "Improvements at Fort Bayard," *Silver City Enterprise*, 3 August 1906.
30. Earl Bruns to G. E. Bushnell, 4 July 1917, RG 112, Entry 31-K, Box 16, NARA.
31. G. E. Bushnell to Surgeon General, 3 March 1904, RG 112, Entry 381, Box 2, NARA; and "United States Tuberculosis Hospital in New Mexico," *Modern Hospital* 3 (1914): 102–4.
32. The following description is drawn from Bushnell to Surgeon General, 18 February 1912, RG 112, Entry 26, Box 919, NARA; and "U.S. Army General Hospital, Fort Bayard, N.M., 1908," RG 112, Entry 31-K, Box 15, NARA.
33. Sanatorium designer Thomas Carrington "suggested that the sanatorium landscape should be a microcosm of the world, self-contained and self-supporting with forest, orchard, cultivation, and light industry." Susan Jane Edwards, "Nature as Healer: Denver, Colorado's Social and Built Landscapes of Health, 1880–1930," Ph.D. dissertation, University of Colorado, 1994, 86.
34. E. L. Munson to E. A. Pierce, 12 February 1906, RG 112, Entry 380, NARA.
35. Presley Marion Rixey, *The Study of Tuberculosis in the United States Navy* (Carlisle, PA: Association of Military Surgeons, 1908), 9–10; and U.S. Congress, House of Representatives, "Fort Bayard Hospital for Tuberculosis Patients; Army Hospital Enlargement to Accommodate Navy Tuberculosis Patients," 1902, CIS H71-0.35, 1. See also, George H. Kress, "Antituberculosis Work in the United States Army, Navy and Marine-Hospital Services," *American Medicine* 10 (19 August 1905): 319–22.
36. "Record of Complete Cases of Tuberculosis, 1899–1907, United States Army General Hospital, Fort Bayard, New Mexico," RG 112, Old Entry 399, NARA. Only six cases of 120 patients discharged unimproved were listed as "incipient."
37. G. E. Bushnell to D. M. Appel, 2 January 1908, RG 112, Entry 386, Box 10, NARA.
38. Correspondence regarding Alford W. Cooley, RG 112, Entry 383, Box 1, and RG 112, Entry 386, Box 15, NARA. See also George M. Torney to J. A. Jaqua, 2 December 1912, RG 112, Entry 26, Box 92, NARA. Paul M. Carrington, "Further Observations on the Treatment of Tuberculosis at Fort Stanton, New Mexico," *Military Surgeon* 14 (1904): 207. RG 112, Entry 26, File #140768, Boxes 1000 and 1001, contains correspondence regarding the admission of civilian patients.
39. *War Department Annual Report*, 1916 [hereafter cited as *WDAR*, year], vol. 1.
40. Information on this case can be found in RG 112, Entry 26, Box 1000, NARA.
41. Correspondence between George E. Bushnell and William C. Gorgas, April–May 1906, Philip S. Hench Walter Reed Yellow Fever Collection, Historical Collections and Services of the Health Sciences Library, University of Virginia.
42. Surgeon General to W. H. Andrews, February 1909, RG 112, Entry 26, Box 892, NARA.
43. *WDAR*, 1910, 155; and George Bushnell to the Surgeon General, 18 February 1912, RG 112, Entry 26, Box 919, NARA.
44. John Kress to George Torney, 16 June 1913, RG 112, Entry 26, Box 892; Bushnell memo, 28 June 1913, RG 112, Entry 26, Box 892; and Henry L. Stimson to Charles D. Hilles, 14 January 1913, RG 112, Entry 26, Box 892, NARA.
45. "General Orders No. 18," U.S. General Hospital, Fort Bayard, NM, 1 August 1905, RG 112, Entries 389–91, Box 1, NARA.
46. G. E. Bushnell to Surgeon General, "Admission of women to the hospital at Fort Bayard," 17 April 1915, RG 112, Entry 26, Box 892, NARA.
47. Correspondence between Inspector General and U.S. General Hospital, Fort Bayard, NM, October 1910, RG 112, Entry 386, Box 24, NARA.
48. Hospital Fund ledger sheet, 1901 and 1902, RG 112, Entry 382, Box 1, NARA;

"Statement of the Hospital Fund," May 1912, RG 112, Entry 399, Box 1, NARA and "U.S. Army General Hospital, Fort Bayard, N.M., 1908" report, RG 112, Entry 31-K, Box 15, NARA, 16.

49. Christine R. Whittaker, "Chasing the Cure: Irving Fisher's Experience as a Tuberculosis Patient," *Bulletin of the History of Medicine* 48 (1974): 404.

50. E. Chaves-Carballo, "The Cost of Running American City Hospitals: The Gorgas 1910 Survey," *Southern Medical Journal* 93, no. 2 (February 2000): 191–4.

51. Correspondence between Inspector General and U.S. General Hospital, Fort Bayard, NM, October 1910, RG 112, Entry 386, Box 24, NARA.

52. George S. Legare to Frances Izlar Legare, 18 February 1909, Legare Family Papers, South Carolina Historical Society, Charleston, South Carolina.

53. "General Orders, No. 18," U.S. General Hospital, Fort Bayard, New Mexico.

54. G. E. Bushnell to Surgeon General, 28 November 1905, RG 112, Entry 380, NARA.

55. P. F. Straub to G. E. Bushnell, 26 November 1906, RG 112, Entry 386, Box 2, NARA, and G. E. Bushnell to P. F. Straub, 3 December 1906, RG 112, Entry 386, Box 2, NARA.

56. These were George E. Bushnell, Charles N. Barney, Edward L. Munson, Paul C. Hutton, Fred W. Palmer, and Clarence Treuholtz, as recorded by J. L. Chamberlain, Inspection Report, 22 October 1906, RG 112, Entry 386, NARA.

57. "List of Officers Treated at GH, Fort Bayard," 19 March 1912, RG 112, Entry 26, #134220, NARA.

58. Efficiency Report, Earl Bruns, 17 September 1908, RG 94, ACP, NARA.

59. P. M. Carrington, "The U.S. Marine Hospital Sanatorium for Tuberculosis at Fort Stanton, N.M.," *New York Medical Journal* (27 February 1909): 420; and Paul M. Carrington, "Further Observations on the Treatment of Tuberculosis at Fort Stanton, New Mexico," *Military Surgeon* 14 (1904): 234.

60. *Public Health Reports* 27 (30 August 1912): 1418.

61. G. E. Bushnell to Surgeon General, 4 May 1906, RG 112, Entry 380, NARA.

62. G. E. Bushnell to Surgeon General, 28 November 1905, RG 112, Entry 380, NARA.

63. "Lightning Kills Army Man," *New York Times*, 2 June 1914.

64. See "Lectures on Tuberculosis, Fort Bayard, 1910–1914, United States Army, Fort Bayard, New Mexico," Manuscript Collection [hereafter cited as MS C] 12, National Library of Medicine.

65. Earl H. Bruns, "Colonel Bushnell: An Estimate of his Character and Work," 278; Efficiency Report, George H. Scott, RG 94, AGO 458840, Box 3230; Efficiency Report, C. E. Holmberg, RG 94, AGO 1737980, Box 6381; and Efficiency Report, W. H. Tefft, RG 94, AGO 506387, Box 3534, NARA.

66. Lewis J. Moorman, *The American Sanatorium Association: A Brief Historical Sketch* (New York, NY: National Tuberculosis Association, 1947); and *New Mexico Medical Journal* 6 (September 1911): 305. Bushnell and Paul Carrington also appear in an advertisement titled, "Climate of New Mexico, Nature's Sanatorium for Consumptives," *New Mexico Medical Journal* 5 (December 1909).

67. C. N. Barney, "Ophthalmo-Reaction to Tuberculin," *Medical Record* (1908): 96–101; J. B. VanHorn, "Preliminary Report on Experience with Modified Flesh Diet," Fort Bayard, New Mexico lectures, MS C 12, National Library of Medicine; and Thomas H. Johnson, "Diseases Complicating Chronic Pulmonary Tuberculosis," unpublished paper, 1916, RG 112, Entry 26, Box 466, NARA.

68. *Illustrations of Tuberculous Lesions* (Fort Bayard, NM: U.S. Army General Hospital, 1908), National Library of Medicine.

69. G. E. Bushnell to Military Secretary, 19 July 1905, RG 94, ACP, Box 1283, NARA.

70. Efficiency Reports, Solomon P. Vestal, RG 94, ACP, NARA.

71. C. N. Barney to Office of The Surgeon General, 6 December 1909, RG 112, Entry 386, Box 27, NARA.

72. G. E. Bushnell to the Surgeon General, 10 April 1914, RG 112, Entry 26, Box 10610, NARA.

73. Bushnell seems to have done exams on officers (Munson, Lusk, Van Horn) and those where Washington, D.C. made an inquiry, such as Oscar Lusk, the son of a judge in California who contacted a U.S. senator from Texas to intervene. See RG 112, Entry 396, NARA.

74. Efficiency Reports, Walter B. Elliot, RG 94, NARA.

75. G. E. Bushnell to M. W. Ireland, 21 January 1909, RG 112, Entry 386, NARA.

76. Bushnell to Office of The Surgeon General, 24 August 1907, RG 112, Entry 386, Box 8, NARA.

77. Howard Priest to the Adjutant, 25 February 1910, RG 112, Entry 386, Box 29, NARA.

78. Jane Delano, "The Army Nurse Corps, Changes During November and December, 1909," *American Journal of Nursing* 10 (1910): 278–79.

79. Johnson, "My Life in the U.S. Army," 88.

80. Johnson, "My Life in the U.S. Army," 84.

81. Johnson, "My Life in the U.S. Army," 85.

82. J. L. Chamberlain, Inspection Report, 22 October 1906, RG 112, Entry 386, NARA.

83. Inspection report of General Hospital Fort Bayard, 15 October 1910, RG 112, Entry 386, NARA.

84. "Charges and specifications preferred against Private Clarence Miller, Hospital Corps, U.S. Army," RG 112, Entry 382, Box 5, NARA; and General Orders No. 36, 1908, U.S. Army General Hospital, Fort Bayard, New Mexico, RG 112, Entries 389–91, NARA.

85. Card on C. C. Bateman, #15860, RG 112, Entry 381, NARA.

86. G. E. Bushnell to M. W. Ireland, 20 November 1905, RG 112, Entry 380, NARA.

87. United States Army General Hospital, Fort Bayard, New Mexico, "Record of Completed Cases of Tuberculosis, 1899–1907." Fort Bayard, New Mexico, 1908.

88. Agnes G. Young, "Notes from Fort Bayard, New Mexico," *American Journal of Nursing* 6 (1906): 370.

89. Cephas C. Bateman, "The Army Hospital at Fort Bayard: Fort Bayard, New Mexico," Lawrence, KS: Kansas Collection, University of Kansas Libraries, c. 1911, p. 9.

90. G. E. Bushnell to Surgeon General, 5 January 1905, RG 112, Entry 380, NARA. In another case he admitted a former soldier who came to the hospital without permission because "his physical condition was such that his medical officer did not think that he should be sent away." See G. E. Bushnell to Surgeon General, 25 April 1907, RG 112, Entry 386, NARA.

91. G. E. Bushnell to Surgeon General, 1 March 1915, RG 112, Entry 26, Box 1089, NARA.

92. G. E. Bushnell to Surgeon General, 26 January 1907, RG 112, Entry 386, Box 3, NARA.

93. Correspondence regarding Joseph F. Fike, May 1909, RG 112, Entry 386, Box 22, NARA.

94. Efficiency Record, Olin R. Booth, RG 94, AGO 224422, Box 1417, NARA.

95. Medical Record, Wilmot Brown, RG 112, Entry 396, Boxes 10 and 11, NARA; and correspondence regarding Wilmot Brown, RG 112, Entry 383 and Entry 386, Box 41, NARA.

96. Medical Record, William H. Gregg, RG 112, Entry 396, Box 33, NARA. Bushnell may have invoked the three-month suspension rule for misconduct by beneficiaries of the Soldiers' Home, because Gregg sought readmission exactly three months after his departure.

97. G. E. Bushnell and Ellen A. Conroy correspondence, RG 112, Entry 386, Box 3, NARA.

98. Charles Tyler to Adjutant, Fort Bayard, 24 January 1905, RG 112, Entry 381, Box 3, NARA.

99. Correspondence between Inspector General and U.S. General Hospital, Fort Bayard, NM, October 1910, RG 112, Entry 386, Box 24, NARA.

100. Medical Record, Charles Tyler, RG 112, Entry 396, NARA; and Charles Tyler to Governor of the Home, Washington, DC, 20 March 1907, RG 112, Entry 386, Box 5, NARA.

101. See Interment.net, Cemetery Transcription Library, Fort Bayard National Cemetery, http://www.interment.net/data/us/nm/grant/ftbaynat/index.htm, accessed 26 August 2012.

102. Horace E. Smith, Medical Record, RG 112, Entry 396, Box 77, NARA.

103. G. E. Bushnell to Surgeon General, 4 April 1908, RG 112, Entry 386, Box 12, NARA.

104. See Cephas C. Bateman, "The Army Hospital at Fort Bayard: Fort Bayard, New Mexico." Lawrence, KS: Kansas Collection, University of Kansas Libraries, n.d., c. 1911–12; and Earl H. Bruns, "Colonel Bushnell: An Estimate of His Character and Work," 277.

For another physician's explanation of how he adopted the rest treatment after visiting Minor's sanatorium see Joseph H. Pratt, "The Development of the Rest Treatment in Pulmonary Tuberculosis," *New England Journal of Medicine* 206 (1932): 64–69.

105. G. E. Bushnell to Surgeon General, 3 March 1904, RG 112, Entry 381, Box 2, NARA.

106. G. E. Bushnell to Surgeon General, 24 March 1904, RG 112, Entry 26, Box 91, NARA.

107. Bruns quoted in Bateman, "The Army Hospital at Fort Bayard," 13.

108. For example, in 1908 the Navy Medical Department circulated an article advocating mercury to treat tuberculosis, declaring "the only question remaining to be decided is: how long will it [mercury] take to effect a cure?" and in 1914 a Navy medical officer downplayed the importance of rest and advocated graduated exercise in the treatment of tuberculosis. Barton Lisle Wright, "The Treatment of Tuberculosis by the Administration of Mercury," *U.S. Naval Medical Bulletin* 2 (1908): 25; and G. B. Crow, "Some Prevailing Ideas Regarding the Treatment of Tuberculosis," *U.S. Naval Medical Bulletin* 8 (1914): 541–54.

109. George E. Bushnell to Charles F. Mason, 22 November 1904, RG 112, Entry 26, NARA.

110. Bates, *Bargaining for Life*, 265, and 318–21.

111. Dormandy, *The White Death*, 149. See also Carolyn June McQuien, "Tuberculosis as Chronic Illness in the United States: Understanding, Treating, and Living with the Disease, 1884–1954," Ph.D. dissertation, University of Texas at Austin, 1993, who calls it "a draconian regimen of inactivity," 145.

112. G. E. Bushnell to C. C. Slemons, Board of Health and Poor Commissioners of Grand Rapids, Michigan, 5 January 1911, RG 112, Entry 386, Box 37, NARA.

113. Earl Bruns, cited in Bateman, "The Army Hospital at Fort Bayard," 11.

114. Charles L. Minor, "Diagnosis," in Arnold C. Klebs, ed., *Tuberculosis: A Treatise by American Authors on its Etiology, Pathology, Frequency, Semeiology, Diagnosis, Prognosis, Prevention, and Treatment* (New York, NY: D. Appleton & Co., 1909), 297–324 and 377–78. This book was included in a list of medical books at the Fort Bayard library in a 1910 inspection report. See correspondence between Inspector General and U.S. General Hospital, Fort Bayard, NM, October 1910, RG 112, Entry 386, Box 24, NARA.

115. William H. Gregg, Medical Record, entry for 16 September 1915, RG 112, Entry 396, Box 33, NARA.

116. George E. Bushnell, "Some Extrapulmonary Sounds Which Simulate Rales," *Medical Record* 82 (20 January 1912): 1–24.

117. G. E. Bushnell, "Report for the Calendar Year 1905, U.S. General Hospital, Fort Bayard, N. M.," RG 112, Entry 380, NARA. For a description of the classification system, see Klebs, *Tuberculosis,* 361–74.

118. Johnson, "My Life in the U.S. Army," 83.

119. Thomas D. Brock, *Robert Koch: A Life in Medicine and Bacteriology* (Madison, WI: Science Tech Publishers, 1988), chapter 18. On the more recent use of tuberculin testing see "Targeted Tuberculin Testing and Treatment of Latent Tuberculosis Infection," *Morbidity and Mortality Weekly Report* 49 (9 June 2000).

120. G. E. Bushnell to Millard Knowlton, 20 June 1906, RG 112, Entry 380, NARA. Also on treatment of tuberculosis, see Klebs, ed. *Tuberculosis*; and Paul M. Carrington, "Further Observations on the Treatment of Tuberculosis at Fort Stanton, New Mexico," *Military Surgeon* 14 (1904): 201–34.

121. *Nostrums and Quackery: Articles on the Nostrum Evil and Quackery Reprinted, with Additions and Modifications, from the Journal of the American Medical Association,* 2d ed. (Chicago, IL: Press of the American Medical Association, 1912), 76. For example, Oscar C. Young, "On the Use of the Opiates, Especially Morphine," *Medical News* (25 January 1902): 154–57, told of his own addiction and warned others to use morphine judiciously.

122. This discussion is based on examination of a number of medical charts in RG 112, Entry 396, NARA. Medical personnel kept charts only for medications given to patients while they were in the infirmary, and under the closest supervision and care. I am grateful to Mary Ann DeGroote, M.D., for helping me read the medical charts and diagnostics used at Fort Bayard.

123. Walter Robbins, Medical Record, RG 112, Entry 396, Box 70, NARA; and Charles S. Legare to Frances Izlar Legare, 4 December 1908, Legare Family Papers, South Carolina Historical Society, Charleston, SC.

124. Commanding officer to Surgeon General, "Annual Report for 1913," RG 112, Entry 26, Box 919, NARA.

125. According to Medline Dictionary, phenacetin is: "a compound [C_2H_5O–C_6H_4–$NHCOCH_3$] formerly used to ease pain or fever but now withdrawn from use because of its link to high blood pressure, heart attacks, cancer, and kidney disease."

126. A medical board had recommended disability discharge several months earlier, but the War Department did not approve it.

127. Details on Homer McQueen's case come from Medical Record, Homer L. McQueen, RG 112, Entry 396, Box 54, NARA; and Cephas Bateman, Monthly Reports, RG 94, ACP, Box 1283, NARA.

128. Correspondence regarding manuscript by Thomas H. Johnson, "Diseases Complicating Chronic Pulmonary Tuberculosis," unpublished paper, 1916, RG 112, Entry 26, Box 466, NARA.

129. *Record of Completed Cases of Tuberculosis at the United States Army General Hospital, Fort Bayard, New Mexico* (Washington, DC: GPO, 1917).

130. Fort Bayard annual reports, 1900 to 1917; and "Record of Complete Cases of Tuberculosis, 1899–1907, United States Army Hospital, Fort Bayard, New Mexico," RG 112, Old Entry 399, NARA.

131. George E. Bushnell to Charles F. Mason, 22 November 1904, RG 112, Entry 26, NARA; and G. E. Bushnell to Millard Knowlton, 20 June 1906, RG 112, Entry 380, NARA.

132. Cephas C. Bateman, "The Army Hospital at Fort Bayard: Fort Bayard, New Mexico." Lawrence, KS: Kansas Collection, University of Kansas Libraries, c. 1911, 9.

133. "The U.S. Army General Hospital, Fort Bayard, New Mexico, 1908," report, RG 112, Entry 31K, Box 16, NARA; and G. E. Bushnell to Surgeon General, "Annual Report for 1914," 15 February 1915, RG 112, Entry 26, Box 919, NARA.

134. Bates, *Bargaining for Life*, 135–38; and Jeanne Abrams and Maryann Fitzharris, *A Place to Heal: The History of National Jewish Medical and Research Center* (Boulder, CO: Johnson Publishing, 1997).

135. George E. Bushnell to Guy Hinsdale, 26 May 1908, RG 112, Entry 386, NARA.

136. United States Army General Hospital, Fort Bayard, NM, "Record of Completed Cases of Tuberculosis, 1899–1907," Fort Bayard, NM, 1908, Appendix, RG 112, Old Entry 399, NARA; and J. L. Chamberlain, Inspection Report, 22 October 1906, RG 112, Entry 386, NARA.

137. Public Health Service, *Annual Report*, 1913, 265.

138. Sheila Rothman makes this point especially well in *Living in the Shadow of Death*.

139. Quoted in Bruns, "Colonel Bushnell," 275; and McQuien, "Tuberculosis as Chronic Illness in the United States," 145.

140. Bruns, "Colonel Bushnell," 275. The boredom and difficulty of the rest cure are vividly described in tuberculosis memoirs such as Betty MacDonald, *The Plague and I* (Philadelphia, PA: J. B. Lippincott, 1948); and novels such as Thomas Mann, *The Magic Mountain*, 1924, various editions; and Eamon McGrath, *The Charnel House* (Belfast, UK: Blackstaff Press, 1990).

141. Thomas H. Johnson, "Diseases Complicating Chronic Pulmonary Tuberculosis," unpublished paper, 1916, RG 112, Entry 26, Box 466, NARA.

142. On the problem of patients who were absent without leave (AWOL), see Charles A. Byler, *Civil-Military Relations on the Frontier and Beyond, 1865–1917* (Westport, CT: Praeger Security International, 2006); on alcoholism among young men during this period, see David Courtwright, *Violent Land: Single Men and Social Disorder from the Frontier to the Inner City* (Cambridge, MA: Harvard University Press, 1996); and on discipline and the coercion of tuberculosis patients see Lerner, *Contagion and Confinement*; Barron H. Lerner, "New York City's Tuberculosis Control Efforts: The Historical Limitations of the 'War on Consumption,'" *American Journal of Public Health* 83 (1993): 758–66; and Richard Coker, *From Chaos to Coercion: Detention and the Control of Tuberculosis* (New York, NY: St. Martin's Press, 2000).

143. Paul Hutton to commanding officer, 20 January 1905, RG 112, Entry 381, NARA. Numerous records of discipline problems can be found in RG 112, Entry 380, NARA.

144. On drug addiction, see David Courtwright, "Opiate Addiction in the American West, 1850–1920," *Journal of the West* 21, no. 3 (1982): 23–31; David Courtwright, *Dark Paradise: A History of Opiate Addiction in America* (Cambridge, MA: Harvard University Press, 2001); and David F. Musto, *The American Disease: Origins of Narcotic Control*, 3d ed. (New York, NY: Oxford University Press, 1999).

145. Edgar King, "The Use of Habit-Forming Drugs (Cocaine, Opium and Its Derivatives) by Enlisted Men. A Report Based on the Work Done at the United States Disciplinary Barracks," *Military Surgeon* 39 (1916): 383.

146. Correspondence regarding Hugh T. Robbins, August 1909, RG 112, Entry 386, Box 24, NARA.

147. Correspondence regarding the court-martials of Leslie Thomas and Charles F. Baker, 1909, RG 112, Entry 386, Box 26, NARA. The records do not state the outcome of the trials.

148. Eve E. Simmons, "It Took Blood, Bravery to Make Ft. Bayard History," *El Paso Times* 20 January 1963; and G. E. Bushnell to Walter M. Murphy, 26 December 1905, RG 112, Entry 380, NARA.

149. General Orders No. 36, U.S. Army General Hospital, Fort Bayard, NM, RG 112, Entries 389–91, Box 1, NARA.
150. Correspondence regarding F. G. Sheppard, 1907, RG 112, Entry 386, Box 9, NARA.
151. G. E. Bushnell to Military Secretary, 27 December 1905, RG 112, Entry 380, NARA.
152. Cephas C. Bateman, Monthly Reports, RG 94, Box 1283, NARA.
153. E. L. Munson to Chief of Bureau of Navigation, 20 February 1906, RG 112, Entry 380, NARA.
154. See RG 112, Entry 26, Box 639, File #94449, NARA.
155. See documents in RG 112, Entry 26, Box 1000, File #149083, NARA.
156. G. E. Bushnell to Military Secretary, 27 December 1905, RG 112, Entry 380, NARA.
157. G. E. Bushnell to Chamberlain, 16 October 1906, RG 112, Entry 386, Box 1, NARA.
158. Military Secretary to the President, Board of Managers, National Home for Disabled Volunteer Soldiers, 1 December 1906, RG 112, Entry 386, Box 1, NARA.
159. C. C. Bateman, Monthly Reports, March 1909, RG 94, Box 1283, NARA.
160. C. C. Bateman, Monthly Reports, February 1910, RG 94, Box 1283, NARA.
161. G. E. Bushnell to Military Secretary, 5 January 1907, RG 94, Box 1283, NARA.
162. *The Independent*, 18 January 1907.
163. General Orders No. 32, U.S. Army General Hospital, Fort Bayard, NM, 30 June 1909, RG 112, Entries 389–91, Box 1, NARA.
164. J. L. Chamberlain, Inspection Report of General Hospital at Fort Bayard, New Mexico, 22 October 1906, RG 112, Entry 386, Box 1, NARA.
165. Bateman, "The Army Hospital at Fort Bayard," 8.
166. Johnson, "My Life in the U.S. Army," 86.
167. *Surgeon General Annual Report,* 1910, 153. In addition, two were discharged at the end of their term of service, two transferred to other hospitals, and fifty-seven were "otherwise disposed of."
168. RG 112, Entry 23, File #62565, NARA.
169. G. E. Bushnell to Surgeon General, 16 September 1907, RG 112, Entry 386, Box 3, NARA; and G. E. Bushnell to Charles M. Mason, 22 November 1904, RG 112, Entry 26, NARA.
170. Medical Record, Charles Barney, RG 112, Entry 390, NARA.
171. Medical Record, Charles H. Noyes, RG 112, Entry 390, Box 62, NARA.
172. Klebs, ed. *Tuberculosis,* 805.
173. Johnson, "My Life in the U.S. Army," 82.
174. *WDAR*, 1911, 70.
175. General R. M. O'Reilly, buck slip endorsement of U.S. Senate request, 30 November 1907, RG 112, Entry 386, Box 11, NARA.
176. Medical Record, O. S. Lusk, RG 112, Entry 396, Box 50, NARA; and Efficiency Reports, Oscar S. Lusk, RG 94, AGO, Box 1106, NARA.
177. Medical Record, Charles Tyler, RG 112, Entry 396, Box 41, NARA; and Charles Tyler to the Adjutant General, 24 January 1905, RG 112, Entry 381, Box 3, NARA.
178. Efficiency Reports, Ogden Rafferty, RG 94, Box 1142, NARA. Rafferty continued to pursue his military career, and was assigned to active duty at Fort Douglas, Utah, after the United States entered World War I.
179. Cephas C. Bateman, Monthly Reports, RG 94, Box 1283, NARA.
180. G. E. Bushnell and Medora H. McCarty, correspondence, March 1907, RG 112, Entry 386, Box 5, NARA.

181. G. E. Bushnell to S. H. Hill, 8 January 1909, RG 112, Entry 386, NARA.

182. See, for example, G. E. Bushnell to Richard Hepple, 9 May 1906, RG 112, Entry 380, and G. E. Bushnell and Henry K. Rymill correspondence, 27 March 1910 and 3 April 1910, RG 112, Entry 386, Box 30, NARA.

183. "List of Officers of the Army who have been under treatment for tuberculosis at the General Hospital, Fort Bayard, N.M.," RG 112, Entry 26, Box 938, NARA.

184. Agnes G. Young, "Notes from Fort Bayard, New Mexico," *American Journal of Nursing* 6 (1906): 372.

185. "Howard Watson," Medical Record, RG 112, Entry 396, Box 84, NARA.

186. Medical Record, Walter C. Babcock, RG 112, Entry 386, NARA; RG 95, Box 1451, NARA; and http://www.distantcousin.com/Military/wwi/units/usa/310infantry78division/, accessed 26 August 2012.

Chapter Three
The Congressman as Tuberculosis Patient

Congressman George Legare arrived at Fort Bayard in late November 1908 exhausted and frightened. He had just turned thirty-nine, had a wife and family, a thriving law practice, a busy life commuting between Charleston and Washington, DC, and had recently won a fourth term as a U.S. Representative from South Carolina.[1] But he was also facing death. He had struggled with tuberculosis for six years, visiting several specialists and sanatoriums in the Carolinas for help, and generally held the disease at bay. But the stress of the 1908 campaign brought him to a crisis, and he became so ill that Secretary of War William Howard Taft, who had just been elected president, arranged for the congressman's admission to Fort Bayard. So after celebrating his reelection, and bearing a grim prognosis from his doctors, Legare said goodbye to his family and took the train west.

After a five-day journey he arrived at Fort Bayard on 25 November. He would stay at the hospital for more than seven months, until July 1909, during which time he wrote to his wife, Mary Frances Izlar Legare ("Frances") every day, sometimes twice a day [hereafter references to these letters will be by date]. As for many patients, correspondence with family back home became an essential focus of his life. "I think I live from letter to letter rather than from day to day," he told Frances.[2] These intimate letters between a couple who had been married sixteen years and had six children, five surviving at the time, provide an extraordinary opportunity to scrutinize a tuberculosis patient's experience at Fort Bayard as he wrestled with the disease and he and his physician negotiated the terms of sanctuary, treatment, lifestyle, and departure from Fort Bayard. Few soldiers have left such a record, so the letters provide a rare glimpse inside an Army tuberculosis hospital.[3] They also present a portrait of an early twentieth-century marriage in a time of crisis.

Legare (Figure 3-1) seemed to sit and converse with Frances (Figure 3-2) as he wrote his letters. He usually began with the weather and responses to letters he had received from her and from other family and friends. He then discussed how he was feeling that day; often reporting on his weight, temperature, appetite and digestion, and sleeping; and providing at times detailed descriptions of his cough-

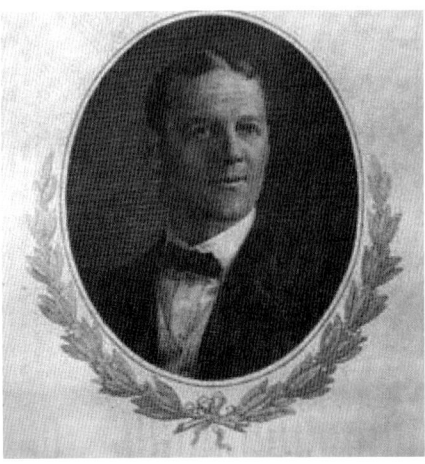
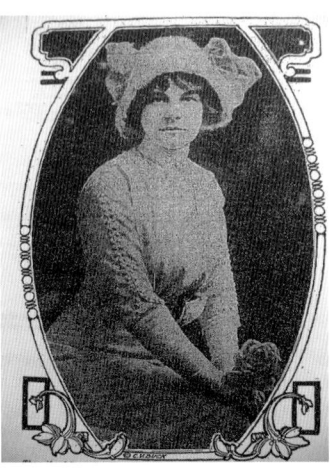

Figure 3-1. Hon. George S. Legare. Photograph courtesy of the South Carolina Historical Society.

Figure 3-2. Frances Izlar Legare. *The Washington Post*, 24 March 1912.

ing. On 6 February 1909 he wrote, "Just as Col. Bushnel[l] said the blood specks Thursday morning were nothing and evidently from the throat—possibly strained coughing." The letters inquired about Frances' health, the health and education of their children, the management of their home, problems with friends and family, and local and national politics and events. Legare's letters were also humorous, sprinkled with jokes, puns, and teases. "Why don't you tell me these little home news," he wrote the next day, "Why if the old gander lays an egg or one of the mules has a colt tell me, for all these little things are about home and so interesting to me." Two months later (8 April 1909), when Frances wrote that she could hardly wait for him to come home, he replied, "The only thing I see left for us to do is to swallow a small watch and then take a whole bottle of castor oil to pass the time away."

These were also love letters. He addressed Frances as "Darling Girl," "My Sweetheart," "My Own Sweet One," and "My Precious One," and said in every letter how much he missed her and the children. He flirted, as in the 7 February letter: "Tell me about yourself, if you have gotten rid of all the freckles yet and is your nose still inclined upwards at the end and, in fact, any old news about your dear self." He made sexy comments. On a cold winter day (28 January 1909), he wrote, "So I'm going out to the porch now and snuggle up in bed and think of you and wish I had you along side of me and under the same covering with me and well, you know." Several months later (2 June 1909) he wrote, "Sweet I do want to see you and love you in person. I'm so tired of doing it with a pen." Each letter ended with professions of love and a special signature, all in one word, "yourowndevotedgeo." Although Frances' letters to Legare have not survived, she probably responded in kind. Thanking her for some photographs she sent, he wrote on 7 March that he liked them, "Especially that mouth picture. I just felt how I would love to kiss you right in the middle of it while it was open that way." Another time (25 March 1909) he wrote, "Sometimes you write such good things that I actually blush."

Tuberculosis, however, was an undercurrent in Legare's letters and on that topic George Bushnell loomed large. Bushnell took charge of his very important patient, and Legare's letters contain at least sixty references to him, an average of more than two a week. They show how the patient and physician worked together, or, as historian Barbara Bates has written, how they "bargained" to determine the terms and conditions under which they would fight Legare's illness.[4] This struggle may again be seen as a fourfold experience. Fort Bayard offered Legare a sanctuary from the demands of the outside world and a chance to heal, but life there could also be depressing and boring. He had to learn to submit to the rest therapy, and with Bushnell's coaching, came to believe it was his best chance at life, though *fighting* a disease by doing *nothing* was both difficult to comprehend and endure for even the most compliant patient. Bushnell and his staff educated the congressman on how to live with tuberculosis without spreading it to his family, friends, or the public, and the difficult task of adjusting to his new life as a "lunger," or a person with tuberculosis, when this new identity could alienate him from his family and friends. Finally, Bushnell and his staff helped Legare prepare to reenter the world of South Carolina and Washington, DC, but the congressman's life as a tuberculosis sufferer would be forever changed. Unlike some Fort Bayard patients, Legare was a "good soldier" and embraced his treatment. "I'm here to be cured and propose to carry out everything in the line of instructions to the very letter no matter what it is," he told his wife on 4 December 1908. "With me, it is a matter of duty."

The Patient and His Physician

The decision to enter Fort Bayard was not easy for Legare. When in 1902 a physician recommended that he take a two-year rest cure, he told Frances, "I'd sooner die any time than do that." A social person, he had a "horror" of living in an isolated tuberculosis sanatorium under virtual quarantine, and he admitted: "I do hate to be 'bossed.' I think you know that if anyone does, don't you darling?"(23 October 1902). That year Legare recovered his health and won election to his first term in Congress. A child of privilege, Legare was a graduate of Georgetown University Law School, a member of a prestigious family in Charleston, South Carolina, and enjoyed a circle of friends that reached to the presidency. He was a popular member of Congress, and made friends among Democrats and Republicans alike, even catching the attention of Republican president Theodore Roosevelt, who supported Legare's efforts to secure federal funding for the Port of Charleston. Legare was also the *paterfamilias* of an extended household of wife and children, at least two foster children, and two generations of African American servants. He looked after his parents' affairs, advised his wife's siblings and their families, and served the constituents of Charleston.

Legare was a complex man. Although a southern aristocrat from a family with deep South Carolina roots, he was not wealthy, and in addition to practicing law, he ran a dairy operation for income. A proud South Carolina Democrat, he was part of a group of politicians who sought to breach the gap between the North and the South.[5] Legare befriended Republicans such as William Howard Taft and several members of Congress from the North. Rep. Charles Townsend (R-MI), for example, was in Legare's 1902 freshman class of Congress and later invited Legare to his district to deliver a Lincoln's Day speech. Legare in turn invited Townsend to Charleston to speak. They developed such a strong friendship that in 1906, when Legare and Frances thought they might have twins (they did not), Legare told Frances, "I'll feel like naming that new boy Charlie Townsend—the other you can name after me" (5 February 1906).

Legare's views on human rights were seemingly inconsistent. In 1912 he spoke in Congress against a United States treaty with Russia because of the regime's oppression of Jews, yet he remained committed to white supremacy in the South.[6] He spoke with affection about the black servants in his household, and wrote letters to several of them while at Fort Bayard, yet he also at times spoke of them as if they were property. On 4 January 1909 he wrote to Frances, "I am so thankful to God that despite my diseased condition I can still give you a carriage and pair of horses and darkey to go to the city and meet your friends on the street and money to shop with while you are meeting them." The next month (20 February 1909) he told Frances, "We have such a good gang of darkies and I only wish I could see them all right now."

Power and influence, however, meant little in the face of tuberculosis. The disease would become George Legare's master and shape the rest of his life in many ways. It made him weak, wracked his body with coughs, and caused him to spit up pus and blood. Bushnell did not minimize the extent of Legare's tuberculosis to his patient. As Legare told Frances on 10 January 1909, "Every now and then Col. Bushnell says something like 'fellow with such a big lesion as yours,' or 'fellow with a long standing case like yours,' etc. And that makes me fear he thinks it is going to take a long time to cure it."

The only surviving letters written by Frances are those she wrote to George Bushnell, preserved among the records of the U.S. Army Office of The Surgeon General in the National Archives. Perhaps concerned that her husband was protecting her from the truth of his condition, she corresponded directly with Bushnell several times to learn her husband's condition and prospects for coming home. Bushnell responded promptly and considerately, with a mixture of candor and optimism. "I would say that [he] has a considerably damaged lung and as you are aware the condition has proceeded for some time." He explained that "such cases are always slow in recovery, partly on account of the amount of the diseased tissue and partly because it seems to be the case that the longer a disease has lasted the longer it takes to cure it." He did believe, however, that Legare could recover. "So long as he can continue to be as well as he is now." He told Frances, "I have no doubt that he will ultimately arrest the disease." He added, however, "Just how long it will take, it is impossible for me to say." It is not clear whether Legare knew of this correspondence because his letters do not mention it. The patient–physician relationship was infused with goodwill, however. As Bushnell told Frances, "I thank you for the kind things which you say in your letter. We are all very fond of Mr. Legare."[7] She responded, "He should have been under your skilful[l] treatment a year ago." She told the commander, "My heart is full of thanks to you and yours for the interest and kindness in his behalf."[8]

With their politicians' instincts, Legare and Frances came to trust and respect both Bushnell's medical and military authority. After a few weeks at Fort Bayard, Legare weighed Bushnell's assessment of his case with that of a physician at another sanatorium and, on 11 December 1908, told Frances, "Of the two men I would of course take Dr. Bushnell's opinion." He said that "while they are both specialists and experts, Dr. B—has so many hundreds more to deal with and gather his experience from." Legare concluded, "I think if there is a man in the United States who ought to know and have a chance to find out about this disease it is Dr. Bushnell." After first referring to him as "Dr. Bushnell," Legare soon got in sync with his military surroundings and called him "Col. Bushnell." When Frances urged Legare to approach Bushnell about moving up Legare's departure date a few days, he would not, explaining on 21 June 1909 that Bushnell "is one of these military men who when he gives an order, considers it given and to be carried out and never thinks of it again." Legare and his wife yielded to Bushnell full control over Legare's disease—his treatment, how he should manage his life with tuberculosis, and when he could see his family again. Legare watched his physician closely and was deferential, at times even timid. When Frances encouraged him to ask Bushnell about when he would get out of bed, he wrote (3 May 1909), "No dear I'm not moving around in my clothes yet and it may be some little while before he (Col.) tells me to dress. He never hurries these matters and I'm not going to hurry him."

In the grip of tuberculosis, the man who hated to "be bossed" put himself under the complete control of George Bushnell. He did so in part because he was vulnerable and scared, but also because Bushnell's expertise and the rest therapy were Legare's only chance at a cure. In the same way, Bushnell had to believe in his approach because he had little else to offer and because he had to inspire the hope and optimism in his patient that he considered essential to his recovery.

Sanctuary

Legare slept for days after his arrival at Fort Bayard. After the first week, he wrote to Frances on 1 December 1908, "Oh love I'm so happy here!... A few months ago I began to feel the end was soon and there was no chance for me, but I'd soon have to leave you and the babies for all time." It was hard for him to make the decision to come to Fort Bayard, but now he was "happy to think that I will be able to get well and strong and live with and for my sweetheart and our dear babies and my dear old Dad and Mother." At Fort Bayard his appetite returned, and he soon believed his health was improving. On 14 December he wrote, "I can safely say I don't feel like the same man and I have only been at it three weeks."

Although Legare was deeply grateful for his care at Fort Bayard, he missed his family terribly, had long days of boredom, depression—even self-pity at times—and counted the days until he could leave.

Legare established a virtual office in his private room in the officers' infirmary, with subscriptions to local newspapers, the *Congressional Record*, and congressional stationery on which to correspond with colleagues, constituents, and government officials. The Agriculture Department sent a box of plants, which made his room look like a "Palm Garden" (18 January 1909). He continued some official duties, helping soldiers at Fort Bayard get promotions or transfers, and sought to keep in the public view with what he called a "little xmas Editorial" (2 January 1909) in the local paper, the Charleston *News and Courier*. He also set up what he called "my little household" with photographs of his family at which he gazed while he wrote his long, loving letters to Frances (15 May 1909). Once he became stronger, Legare became part of the community of tuberculosis patients. He enjoyed visits from other patients, reporting to his wife about them and their family situations, their tuberculosis symptoms, methods of cure, and prognoses.

In January, however, Bushnell began to circumscribe Legare's world. "Col. Bushnell says I'm doing entirely too much writing. And that I must confine it to one or two short letters each day," Legare wrote on the 17th. The day before, in fact, Legare had received fourteen letters. Bushnell suggested he "'write a short slip to each one of your friends and tell them I forbid your writing any more.'" Legare told Frances, "Here I obey orders and after this I'm going to follow this plan. One short letter to you every day. I can say a lot in one page, and one or two still shorter ones to my friends." Bushnell also stopped the visits from other patients and told Legare to rest completely.

When most patients got through their initial crises, medical staff moved them into an officers' or enlisted men's dormitory. Legare started worrying about this, though, concerned he might not be able to rest well in the dormitory among other patients (11 December 1908); Bushnell must have picked this up. "I think Col. Bushnell is going to keep me in this building all the time," he told Frances on 9 February 1909. The congressman could have gotten a "promotion" to the dormitory, but Bushnell "[t]old me he was mighty glad I was willing to lay quiet and not want to get up and move around like the rest...and that a man with the bug was better off in bed...and as long as I was willing to remain quiet where I was it was better for me." He concluded, "I am very comfortable in every way here and away from the crowd." He later reported that day, "...I don't have visitors any more. Col. Bushnell saw it was annoying me and stopped it.... It was too much of it." But solitude had its own challenges. "So all I can do now is to lay quiet and think all day long and day after day and week after week. So you don't blame me for getting homesick do you dear?" This letter, his second to Frances that day, was just one page, but in smaller handwriting than previously. Although Legare's letters did consume fewer pages, he managed to squeeze more words on each page. He probably cut back on his correspondence with others, but letters to Frances provided a lifeline on which he depended.

Frances considered joining Legare at Fort Bayard, but Legare told her that no other patients had their families with them. When she asked Bushnell about it he responded, "I know that it is hard for you to be separated from him, but feel that you do wisely in not coming here, especially with young children." He explained that, "Mr. Legare should be free from all family cares at the present time, if he is to make the most rapid progress possible."[9] Bushnell sought to protect all of his patients from cares that he believed distracted them from their treatment. One of his medical officers, Capt. Charles Barney, explained, "A patient who is to make the struggle against tuberculosis, if he is ill enough to require hospital treatment, should not be worried with domestic cares such as inability to secure servants, illnesses of wife and children, etc."[10] In 1908 a physician at a Rhode Island sanatorium asked Bushnell if he had found his patients unusually exhausted after sexual activity. Bushnell said he had no clear evidence of this, but had noticed that, "men are much better when their wives are away," but "whether the explanation of this is sexual rest, I do not know."[11]

Legare marked time by observing the holidays at Fort Bayard and home. At Christmas he said, "Everybody here is all agog about xmas, sending and receiving presents and getting mistletoes and fixing boxes and getting xmas trees for the soldiers." Despite his absence, he attempted to choreograph the family's holiday dinner table, instructing that his father should sit at the head of the table and carve the turkey (2 December 1908). He discussed New Year's resolutions with his nurses, but letters from 10 February to 14 February have not survived in the collection, so there is no record of Legare's thoughts on Valentine's Day (or Lincoln's Birthday, for that matter). He did jokingly observe another presidential birthday, though. "Yesterday (Birthington's Wash day) was a corker sure," he wrote on 23 February, "I never saw such weather in all my born days before. Snowed for over forty-eight hours." In March he imagined the excitement surrounding the inauguration of President Taft, a Republican, and asked Frances, "How'd you like to be there today?" (4 March 1909). Although a southern Democrat, he wrote, "We're going to have a great president I'm sure," but perhaps feeling his infirmity, admitted "I'm glad I'm not in that rush and turmoil." He regretted missing the Hibernian supper in Charleston, but told Frances on 17 March, "there'll come another St. Patrick's day I'll be home to enjoy it." And on Easter, one of the medical officers' wives made Easter baskets for the patients. "Mine is a pretty little green basket with a little bunny and some Easter eggs in it," he noted (11 April 1909). "How I would love to send it home to you all for the kids, its so pretty but would be all smashed before it got there."

If Legare never let go of his family and life back East, he also tried to run his household from his Fort Bayard sanctuary across the country. Legare continued to control the family finances, paying bills and sending Frances a check each month, and every letter contained instructions. When their youngest child fell ill, he told Frances to hire a "trained nurse," and "not one of the young husband-hunters" (31 December 1908). He advised Frances on which servants to take to their summer home, "Pickens," in the Carolina mountains (23 January 1909), and devoted pages and pages (e.g., 25 January and 23 February 1909) to plans and instructions for the gardens in Charleston and Pickens. When he sent silver bracelets to his daughters ("made by the wild Apache Indians with rude tools"), he advised, "Now they can own them together if they prefer and take turns wearing the bracelet, or if they can choose and each be satisfied, then let them choose and if they can't then let them draw straws for a choice." He asked Frances (19 February 1909) to represent him in the political world. When President-elect Taft and a congressional delegation made plans to pass through Charleston on the way to inspect the Panama Canal construction project, Legare encouraged Frances to meet them (16 January 1909): "I see that Mr. Taft is to be in Charleston two days, Saturday and Sunday. So you'll have no trouble to see him for a few minutes. How I would love to be there well and strong and help to entertain him." The visit remained on his mind and he repeatedly encouraged Frances to attend the festivities. Frances did meet the Taft delegation, and when she stayed up late that evening to write a letter describing the day's events for him, Legare was delighted.

Such letters suggest that Frances generally followed Legare's wishes and instructions; there is evidence of little debate or argument in the correspondence. But sometimes a request or suggestion on her part received a heated response. "You asked [a]bout getting a gun for Bill. By no means do so," he wrote. "In the first place he knows nothing about using it and will shoot himself, or someone else before he has it two weeks." Guns, he implied (14 December 1908), were a matter to be left to a man. "You don't know what kind of gun to get him and some cussed cheap gun would blow up with him or be too heavy or too long and not fit him. Tell him to wait until I get home and I will get him a gun that will fit him and at the same time I will be there to show him how to use it and how to shoot." When Bill and his cousin killed a cougar apparently just beating it with sticks, Legare arranged to send the cat to a taxidermist, and reiterated to Frances on 1 March, "Tell them they certainly are entitled to guns and I will sure give them each a gun when I get back home." He ached to be there. "I sure would love to have seen their excitement and pleasure when they reached home with the cat," he wrote (7 March 1909). Legare also bridled when his wife spoke of buying a car. "Dear, you frighten me when you talk of wanting an automobile and electric lights, etc.," he replied on 17 March. "Really you must think that I'm a millionaire instead of a lunger. No, cut the automobile idea right out of your head at once before it grows too large there." It would cost too much, and "I want to give you any pleasure within reason my pet but I can't indulge in automobiles until I have laid aside enough to take care of you and the babies in case of the rainy day." It was almost a plea.

Treatment

Despite his longing for home, Legare embraced what he called the "treatment and training" at Fort Bayard with the zeal of a convert (22 February 1909).[12] Living outside in the cold may have alarmed some southerners but Legare approved immediately. On 4 December 1908 he wrote, "I'm already catching the fresh air fever and by the time I get home think I'll be putting you *all* to sleep out of doors at night." A week later (12 December 1908) he reported, "I was put outside to sleep in the open air on the porch for the first time last night and it was fine." He had "covering enough on to do my whole family. I had a sheet, six blankets and a very thick eider-down comforter... Beside this I had on a thick suit of pajamas, my white sweater over that and a turkish bath robe over all this. Also had a large hot water bag at my feet and this was changed once during the night. So," he assured Frances, "I slept as snug as a bug in a rug." On 28 April 1909 he wrote, "I do think we would all be so much healthier, I mean mankind generally, if we lived almost entirely in the fresh air."

Legare's letters reveal some of the techniques Bushnell employed to get his patients to follow the prescribed treatment. Bushnell educated patients about tuberculosis and their particular case, explained the purposes of various measures, and also used advice rather than absolute injunctions to change behaviors. With the congressman he was more of a teacher than a disciplinarian, and Legare passed on what he learned to Frances. After one of his first meetings with Bushnell, for example, he drew a picture of his lung for Frances, to illustrate where the lesion was, and relayed Bushnell's analysis of his infection (4 December 1908). After another examination (15 January 1909), Legare reported that he was improving and that Bushnell "went into long detail which I understood but cannot explain." He tried nonetheless to explain to Frances that while his lungs were still diseased, his body was putting up a fight. "So to sum up his talk I would say I'm getting better because I'm not worse." Legare adopted Bushnell's explanation of immunity and the need to strengthen the body to fight the "bug," and on numerous occasions advised Frances to get more fresh air and rest. For example, on 30 December he told her Bushnell "makes all of the patients here, whether on the sick list or not, take an hours' rest before each meal." She should do the same, he wrote, locking her bedroom door so the children would not disturb her. Legare also convinced several people, including a friend, Duncan, to go to a sanatorium, and passed on Bushnell's advice. "Heard from Dunc that he had a small hemorrhage," he wrote, "but Col. Bushnell says hemorrhage often is the best thing that could happen to certain patients. That in the majority of cases all the poison goes out with the blood and the patient gets well, heals up, twice as quick." Legare conveyed this to Duncan (17 March 1909) and "also told him to stick to his couch and quit exercising."

Bushnell also used encouragement to change behavior. A pipe-smoker himself, he did not tell Legare to stop smoking outright, but instead, according to a 23 December 1908 letter, "Col. Bushnell said my pulse was a little too fast and he thought it was from smoking too strong tobacco. He would suggest I try a lighter brand and see if it wouldn't make a change." Legare quit smoking. As he reported to Frances (31 December 1908), when a nurse asked him if he had any New Year's resolution, he told her, "I had quit cussin' because there's nothing here to cuss about, I've quit chewing first, then cigar smoking, and lastly the pipe, and I've quit drinking so all my bad habits are gone and I have nothing to resolve about." A number of patients hunted game, Legare observed (4 December 1908), but "Col. Bushnell objects to it and while he does not say they positively must not hunt, they do it against his advice and wishes. So hunting is out of the question with me." Bushnell might also have confided in Legare regarding other patients. Of the rest treatment, he wrote on 17 December, "Col. Bushnell says that it is the hardest matter in the world to get them to look at it in the right light and not become restless and weary of it."[13] On 15 March 1909, Bushnell told Legare that "if he had all patients who would be as content [and] earnest to take the cure as I am, he'd have a wonderful record for cures." Comments such as these could help reinforce a patient's resolve to adhere to the treatment. They could also suggest that patients who did not follow doctor's orders had themselves to blame if they did not improve.

Legare heard from another patient, not Bushnell, that the colonel was hoping Legare would be "Exhibit B," or a second example of Fort Bayard's success in treating tuberculosis. "There is a General Edwards in the War Department in Washington who was very ill (had it in throat and lungs) and was cured here," he told Frances on 25 March.[14] "When Mr. Taft was Sect. of War he would introduce General Edwards to friends as a result of Col. Bushnell's rest cure." Legare liked the comparison because it meant Bushnell "wants to have me thoroughly cured as an advertisement."

A letter on 21 December 1908 provides an intimate view of both life in a sanatorium and the Legares' marriage. Frances apparently was concerned about female nurses' contact with her husband, and inquired about his bath. "So you are worried about the bathing process are you?" Legare almost crowed, "Old girl, I know you too well and you're just too cute for anything!" But he added, "Well don't 'wonder' any more it's all right and nothing for you to worry about." He proceeded to explain the process. The nurses, he began, "place two blankets on the bed and tell you when ready for your bath to ring for nurse (2 rings) and [then the nurses] leave the room. Then the patient slips off clothes and gets between two blankets and touches bell." The nurse then comes in, he continued, and washes each arm and leg out from under the covers, replacing it afterwards. Then she "slips hand under cover and washes as far down as possible and tells you to turn over when she washes back down as far as possible." After that, "the bed is pushed up close to basin and she says 'when you have finished your bath ring for me' and leaves you to wash your own possible." It is not known whether this relieved Frances, but the issue came up again as Legare prepared to go home. "This is bath day," he wrote on 24 June 1909, "Wonder if you will give me my baths when I get home?" If she did, he would not "make you do like the nurses here but will stand up in the tub and let you wash possible and all. Will you do it dear?"

Lifestyle

"In tuberculosis we prescribe not medicine, but a mode of life," wrote Bushnell. The challenge, he explained, was "to work upon the patient's mind so effectively that he will be willing to change entirely his mode of living and to persevere in the new way for months, perhaps for years, often through his whole life."[15] Tuberculosis patients at Fort Bayard, then, had to adjust to and adopt a new lifestyle, and even a new identity as individuals who had a deadly, contagious disease. George

Legare at first resisted the implications of tuberculosis. "I'm no consumptive," he wrote to Frances when he was in a South Carolina sanatorium on 23 October 1902. "They may think so, but I'm not." But by February 1909, his letters began to refer to himself as a "lunger" (6 February 1909). While at Fort Bayard Legare rarely used the word "tuberculosis," referring instead to "the bug," and to those with the disease as "lungers." In contrast, the physician Bushnell never used the term "lunger" or "bug" in his correspondence.

Legare's growing acceptance of himself as a "lunger" raised daunting concerns about his ability to earn a living and maintain his identity as the *paterfamilias*. Legare also clearly worried about infecting his family, especially Frances, with his coughing and the deadly sputum that Fort Bayard personnel treated like hazardous waste. "You have been so much with me that you may have the bug," he wrote on 30 January. When Frances became ill, his concern heightened. (She ended up undergoing a surgical procedure, probably gynecological, in March). "I am certainly glad to know your lungs are O.K. This is the thing that has been worrying me and yet I was afraid to even write about it," Legare later admitted (28 February 1909). On 7 March, however, he wrote about kissing her, noting, "Of course it would be dangerous but I'd be willing to take my chances."

Legare became insecure about social relationships. When some friends had not replied to his letters, he asked Frances on 27 January, "So let me know if your social standing is still good there." His feelings were hurt when his congressional secretary, Jerry, who was handling routine congressional matters and responding to constituents in Legare's absence, did not reply to his letters. "I couldn't have done more for him if he had been my own child," he complained on 12 April. "I have clung to him since he was a little fellow and can't help but feel deeply hurt at the way he has treated me with neglect." In June (9 June 1909) he was almost bitter: "How is my ex-secretary, the Congressman? He is sick too I suppose for he never writes." With repeated nudging by Frances, Jerry became more responsive in time for Legare's return home, but his boss had felt keenly the shift in power relations during his illness.

The tuberculosis that so weakened the body was not considered to be a "manly" disease, but Legare viewed his own struggle in masculine terms. In addition to framing his fight with tuberculosis as a "duty," he also vowed (30 December 1908) "to take whatever came like a man." When Frances complained about the separation, he told her on 22 January 1909, "I'm standing it like a man and you must do your share too." After a few weeks of separation and perhaps apprehensive that their marriage would falter, Frances suggested that Legare loved his mother more than her. Whether or not she was teasing, Legare took her seriously. "The love I have for you is different from that I have for anybody on earth," he assured her. "And it isn't any foolish mad kind of love but a strong manly love that nothing not even death could efface," he wrote on 6 January. But the disease did trouble his sense of his masculinity. At first he teased his wife about having another baby. When she told him she did not want another "papoose," he responded on 10 January, "I am satisfied that what you really want is to try. And dear I shall certainly let you try to your heart's content. Would you like to? *Very* much? I believe you would. How about right now?" But two months later (9 March 1909) he was of a different mind. "Idea of your talking another baby! Haven't you got troubles enough now old girl?" he wrote. "No more for me. I can hardly take care of those I have now and if we do this properly we will have done our share."

Legare's letters track a roller coaster of emotion. In February the usually cheerful congressman became depressed. There were plenty of reasons to be sad at Fort Bayard. In addition to being lonely, having a lethal disease, and living among scores of sick men, Chaplain Bateman's records show that seventeen patients had died since Legare had entered the hospital, including a nurse, Mrs. Halliday, who suffered a fatal cerebral hemorrhage in January.[16] Legare told Frances about Halliday's death, but on another day (15 March 1909) wrote, "Darling there are so many things to depress a man in a place like this and I don't write about them because it is only sad news and would tend to depress you even at a distance." Legare apologized on several occasions for writing "wretched letters," during his blue moods, which he called "indigo," but these letters do not appear in the collection. (Frances or Legare himself may have considered them unmanly or too intimate for public view and destroyed them at a later date.) On 4 January, he reminded Frances how very lucky they were, but remarked, "I am really the fellow who gets the worst of it, here in this wild, distant land all alone and sick and every habit taken from me and kept in bed day and night." When they decided to send money to Frances' sister Anne, whose husband also had tuberculosis, he wrote on 6 February, "It does seem hard tho that one lunger with so much load to carry should have to spend his substance on another when I ought to be saving it." Other letters reveal similar self-pity, such as the time he referred to his stay at Fort Bayard as a "hideous dream" (20 April 1909). Bushnell tried to dispel these fits of depression, believing that optimism was key to recovery. Legare reported on 9 April that one day Bushnell "told me that when I got homesick I must try to think of something pleasant to take my mind off of it," and suggested that he think of flowers to cheer him up. A few days later, on 22 April, Legare sent Frances a poem about the importance of being cheerful.

Leaving Fort Bayard

Although Legare counted the days until he could go home, he was apprehensive. His worries were multiple: he wondered about when he could go home and about how he would manage the travel across the country; he worried about being overworked into a relapse when he returned to Charleston and Washington; he agonized about changes in his relationship with Frances; and finally, he worried that he had not completely recovered his health. Legare was one of the lucky Fort Bayard patients who would depart the hospital in relatively good health, but his departure required weeks of planning and caused much anxiety. Legare and Frances began to contemplate when he could go home almost as soon as he arrived at Fort Bayard. They expected he would stay for six months and became almost obsessed with 1 June 1909 as the date when he could return home. (Richard Johnson observed that this was a common topic among patients, and noted that patients' "mental problems and discussions were mostly about the progress of their case, the probability of being discharged, and how soon, how much pension they would get."[17])

Legare needed Bushnell's approval for departure, and the medical officer was noncommittal for quite a while, perhaps wanting Legare to stay as long as required to become "Exhibit B," his second triumphal cure to show Washington officials. He also may have wanted to keep Legare calm as long as possible, worried that the excitement of returning home would retard his recovery. Bushnell ultimately decided Legare should stay until 1 July. Letters suggest that Bushnell told Frances of Legare's departure date at least a week before he told his patient, perhaps to avoid exciting his patient and to forestall Frances' entreaties (19 and 27 May 1909). With the 1 July date set, the couple debated whether this meant that Legare would be home by the first of July, or depart Fort Bayard that day. When Frances asked her husband to leave before the first to ensure that he would be home on the Fourth of July, Legare resisted. "I would like to be home on the Fourth but wouldn't care to ask the Colonel," he responded on 5 June. The next week (11 June 1909) he allowed, "I feel as if I simply must get away from here first of July and I'm so worried all the time something might happen and prevent it I am almost tempted to take off a little sooner." But, he wrote on the 13th of June, "I was so glad when [Bushnell] said first of July I wouldn't dare appear childish. No, let's be patient as we can. If you are impatient how do you suppose I must feel?"

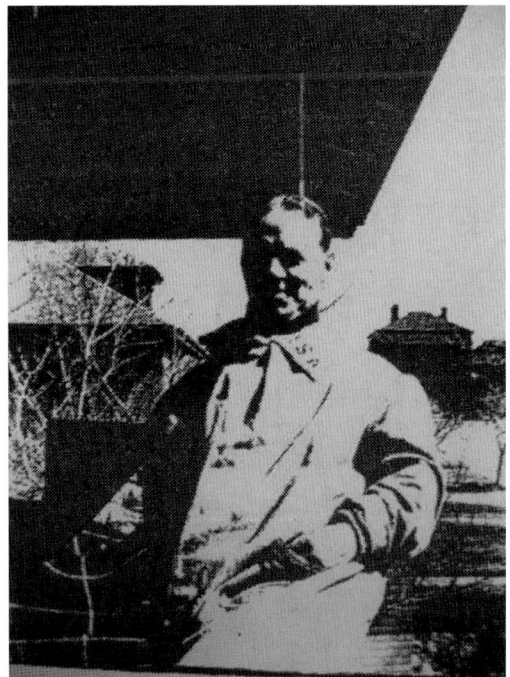

Figure 3-3. Photograph of Congressman George S. Legare that he sent to his wife, Frances, from Fort Bayard, writing, "I am looking east toward home." George S. Legare and Frances Islar Legare correspondence, Legare Family Papers.
Photograph courtesy of the South Carolina Historical Society.

As part of the reentry process, Bushnell prescribed graduated exercise for his patients in their last month to see how they would fare in the outside world. Legare got out of bed in mid-April and proudly sent Frances a photograph of himself in his clothes instead of pajamas (Figure 3-3), with the caption: "Sitting on the rail and looking homeward." The first day of June, physician and patient took a short walk together to look at some peonies. Bushnell also drove Legare in a wagon to see Fort Bayard's dairy operation, and on 21 June invited the congressman to visit him and his wife, Ethel, in their home, not far from the officers' infirmary. As Legare moved about Fort Bayard, he felt better, but he knew he was not strong.

Contemplating the four-to-five day trip home, Legare worried about how he would manage his considerable luggage and the transfers required en route. Fort Bayard often had men accompany patients to and from the hospital, as Corpsman Homer McQueen had done before he fell ill with tuberculosis. Legare worked out his own arrangements, helping a young soldier at Fort Bayard get a transfer to a post near his home in North Carolina so they could travel east together. Bushnell assisted this process, forwarding the transfer request to the Surgeon General with his own letter of endorsement (27 May 1909). This reassured Legare (8 June 1909): "Will get my soldier to accompany me home (as far as Easly) O.K. So while the trip will be long and hot and tiresome I'll have nothing to worry me and some one to do my packing and look after everything for me." His correspondence during the last two months discussed the trip in detail, going over his route; whether Frances would meet him in Atlanta or, near their summer home at Easly, South Carolina; who would come to the train station; and how they would communicate while he was traveling. Legare also worried about the actual homecoming. "[Legare's congressional assistant] Jerry says there's going to be so much hugging and kissing and screaming at Easly he's afraid I'll be knocked out," he wrote (22 June 1909) in only a partial tease. "But I'll have my soldier along so you'd better be careful or I'll have you arrested for abusing me." The next day he wrote, "The minute you pull me to pieces in Easly, I'm going to say to my soldier man, 'here arrest this woman at once,'" but he added (23 June 1909), "Darling I can almost taste those dear sweet lips of yours right now."

Worried that his constituents and legal clients would overwhelm him with work and reactivate his tuberculosis, Legare asked Frances to keep his homecoming plans a secret. He reminded her that he was not as strong as he used to be, explaining, "I get so many letters telling me how anxious they are for my complete recovery and how they hate to bother me but 'it is an important matter, etc.' and asking me to do thus and so." He asserted on 28 March, "I simply cannot do any work until Fall. Col. Bushnell would not hear of it." He laid out his plans in detail (2 May 1909):

> My plans are about as follows: Stay in Pickens until about Oct. 15th then go to Charleston to remain quietly at home in the country until first Monday in December when I have to be in Washington and then remain about ten days in Washington and then come home for the holidays which will give me about one more month at home so that I really will not begin work in earnest until the New Year. Now that is my plan but of course it's a long ways off so don't mention it.

Bushnell supported this caution, writing to Frances that although her husband could come home in July, "Of course he will need a thorough rest after his arrival and will have to be quite careful of himself for some time to come." He explained on 19 May, "It is as you know important that patients take no chances even after the activity of the disease should appear to be entirely arrested." Regarding their summer plans, Legare told Frances on 4 June he would like to have friends come to visit. "But of course I'm in no condition to entertain anyone this summer and will expect to be entertained, see?" Of the Pickens County Fair, he wrote two days later (6 June 1909), "Of course I can not have a thing to do with it this year." At Legare's request, Chaplain Cephas Bateman sent a letter to the Charleston *News and Courier* asking people to permit Legare "to remain in comparative quiet for some months after his return," so that he could complete his recovery.[18]

In addition to being "abused" by his family and friends, Legare worried that during his months at Fort Bayard he had changed. He joked that he had been away from "civilization" so long that the fashions were probably different (1 June 1909). On 27 June he told Frances, "I'm afraid I'll look strange to you. Think you'll know me?" He prepared her for his homecoming, as early as May: "Darling you 'all time speak about my gainin' so much weight and how I won't be able to button my clothes, etc. I don't think I weigh a pound more sweet than when I came. If anything I may be off a little." He hoped to be dancing with her soon (5 May 1909), "But the fox hunts you and I will have to cut out for awhile possibly a year or two to be on the safe side absolutely." He explained, "Colonel Bushnell thinks horseback riding very severe on a lunger." Another time (25 June 1909) he reported, "I still have some bronchial moisture caused by bronchitis. That is phlegm forming in the bronchial tubes like a fellow after a cold and it makes me cough a little at times." Both to himself and to her, he added, "But Colonel says this is to be expected and nearly always accompanies 'the bug.'" Furthermore, "'the bug' is walled in and fenced off and that's the fellow we're after so I'm O.K."

Legare's trepidations about his health were warranted. Bushnell's assessment was both heartening and sobering. In May he told Frances that her husband "has always been in a very satisfactory condition considering the amount of his disease and the length of time he has been sick. A change in his condition is more apparent in his general health than in the state of his lung disease." Legare's disquiet might have been due to problems with his digestion. Although at first he enjoyed the Fort Bayard fare, after a few months he began to complain of the food and his digestion, mentioning, for example, a "bum appetite" on 12 June. On the 15th he apologized, "That was a real bum letter I wrote yesterday, wasn't it? Well my stomach had me on the grouch and I couldn't help it—just did the best I could. Am feeling better in those regions today."[19] Later (20 June 1909) he explained, "When my indigestion gets a hold of me the days seem so long—feel as if they will never go by but when I'm feeling fine in my lower story it doesn't seem so long." A few days later (25 June 1909) he was more cheerful, writing, "If I can get my stomach straight, and I'm sure I will, I'll be all right."

Legare's last letter (30 June 1909) to Frances from Fort Bayard was short. It read in full:

This is my last letter to you from here and I will be only a few hours behind, thank God. You have been so good and true and faithful my sweet girl and I shall be so happy when I clasp you in my arms once more. Tomorrow I begin my journey and when I know you are at the other end of it, the train can't go fast enough. God bless and keep you safe and all my loved ones my dear little wife. Until we meet Monday afternoon or morning I'll be thinking of and longing for you. Love and kisses and prayers for you and all my dear ones. Yourowndevotedgeo.

A week later, Legare's assistant, Jerry, advised Bushnell of the congressman's safe arrival, and Legare followed up with letters of his own.[20] Bushnell replied, "I was pleased to learn from your two letters that you have reached home in safety and good physical condition and hope that the latter will continue indefinitely."[21] Correspondence then ceased as Legare continued his recovery.

Tuberculosis is a fickle disease that allows some patients to get well and others not. Legare never mentioned in his letters to Frances that Bushnell also suffered from tuberculosis, but less than four months after Legare departed, Bushnell himself left Fort Bayard for the mountains of California to treat a recurrence of active tuberculosis in his left lung.[22] He had to leave his own hospital to assume the role of the patient. Bushnell returned to duty after six months and lived for another fourteen years. George Legare, however, was not so fortunate. His digestive problems on the eve of his departure from Fort Bayard suggest that Legare's tuberculosis had not been arrested, but had spread to his gastrointestinal system (tuberculous enteritis), a common complication, often a result of a patient swallowing tubercular material. His disease was so advanced that he and Frances grappled with it for several more years.

During his tenure in Congress, Legare compiled a rather sparse record, no doubt due to his illness. Legare never spoke about tuberculosis on the floor of the House. His main achievement was procuring funding for improving the Charleston Harbor. He made only two major speeches on the floor of the House, one, opposing the recognition of Russia because of the oppression of the Jews, and the other opposing provisions in the proposed state constitution of New Mexico that would prohibit non-English speaking people from holding state office and allow popular recall of members of the judiciary.[23] Due to his frequent absences from Washington, he attracted a primary opponent in 1912, unusual in the Democratic South. The challenger, H. L. Larisey, charged that Legare missed too many votes in Washington and was becoming "too close to the Republicans."[24] Legare defeated Larisey, but after winning a fifth term in Congress he fell seriously ill and died in January 1913 at the age of forty-three. George Legare had every advantage a tuberculosis patient could have, but his disease killed him less than four years after his departure from Fort Bayard.

People in Charleston, Pickens, Washington, and Fort Bayard mourned his death. The Charleston *News and Courier* estimated that 2,000 people attended the funeral, inside the church and standing outside. Those who attended, according to the paper, "were from every order and class of people, and the fact that George Legare was loved by rich and poor, high and low alike was forcibly brought out."

Attendees included members of Congress and Charleston civic leaders as well as fifty African Americans, "men and women who had worked for the Legare family or had known the Congressman in one way or another." Some people blamed the Democratic primary race for ruining Legare's health, and the *News and Courier* noted that, "If anyone in Charleston should offer just now to run against George Legare for Congress there would probably be a lynching."[25]

A few weeks later in Washington, members of Congress gathered in the House and the Senate to eulogize Legare. Although remarks during such occasions always overflow with compliments about the departed colleague, those regarding Legare had a powerful unifying thread. Almost to a man, they described him as "lovable."[26] Rep. Joseph Johnson (D-SC) said that his colleague was "the most loving and lovable man I have ever known," and was laid to rest "in the presence of the largest crowd that I have ever seen at a funeral."[27] Rep. Asbury Lever (D-SC) explained, "No one ever liked George Legare, each loved him. He was the type to whom you go when the heart is harrowed with sorrow and the mind is afire with doubt."[28] Charles Townsend (R-MI), just elected to the Senate, echoed that sentiment: "Thus, went out from this Congress, one of the brightest and most lovable men I have ever known."[29]

George Legare was survived by three daughters and one son, as well as Frances, and the Legare family treasured his Fort Bayard letters for decades. Frances married again to Walter B. Logan and lived until 1948. She passed the letters along to her oldest daughter, Ferdinanda Legare Waring, who kept them until 1983, when, at the age of 87, she gave them to the South Carolina Historical Society.[30] Although she and her mother would survive much of the turbulent twentieth century, witnessing two world wars and the rise of the United States as a world power, tuberculosis prevented George Legare from knowing just how much war would change the world.

Notes

1. For information on George S. Legare, see Legare Family Papers, South Carolina Historical Society, Charleston, SC [hereafter, LFP]; *Transactions of the Huguenot Society of South Carolina*, No. 86, (Columbia, SC: R. L. Bryant, 1981), 69–70; and http://bioguide.con-gress.gov/biosearch/biosearch.asp, accessed 1 November 2012.

2. George S. Legare to Frances Izlar Legare, 1 January 1909, LFP. Hereafter references to these letters will be by date. Correct spelling and punctuation have been added where necessary to clarify the meaning.

3. On the tuberculosis patient experience, see Sheila Rothman, *Living in the Shadow of Death: Tuberculosis and the Social Experience of Illness in American History* (New York, NY: Basic Books, 1994); Barbara Bates, *Bargaining for Life: A Social History of Tuberculosis, 1876–1938* (Philadelphia, PA: University of Pennsylvania Press, 1992); Katherine Ott, *Fevered Lives: Tuberculosis in American Culture since 1870* (Cambridge, MA: Harvard University Press, 1996); Beth O'Donnell Linker, "In the Center of the Plague: Tuberculosis and the Experience of Space, Time and Teleology, 1910–1940," Master's thesis, Michigan State University, East Lansing, 1999; and Carolyn June McQuien, "Tuberculosis as Chronic Illness in the United States: Understanding, Treating, and Living with the Disease, 1884–1954," Ph.D. dissertation, University of Texas at Austin, 1993.

On the importance of examining the patient experience see Roy Porter, "A Patient's View: Doing Medical History from Below," *Theory and Society* (1985): 175–98. Also on the patient experience see Arthur Kleinman, *The Illness Narratives: Suffering, Healing, and the Human Condition* (New York, NY: Basic Books, 1988); Chris Feudtner, *Bittersweet: Diabetes, Insulin, and the Transformation of Illness* (Chapel Hill, NC: University of North Carolina Press, 2003); Kathy Charmaz, *Good Days, Bad Days: The Self in Chronic Illness and Time* (New Brunswick, NJ: Rutgers University Press, 1991); Robert A. Aronowitz, *Making Sense of Illness: Science, Society, and Disease* (New York, NY: Cambridge University Press, 1998); and Ray Fitzpatrick, John Hinton, Stanton Newman, Graham Scambler, and James Thompson, *The Experiences of Illness* (London, UK: Tavistock Publications, 1984).

Memoirs include Betty MacDonald, *The Plague and I* (Philadelphia, PA: J. B. Lippincott, 1948); Robert G. Lovell, *Taking the Cure: The Patient's Approach to Tuberculosis* (New York, NY: MacMillan, 1948); Julius A. Roth, *Timetables: Structuring the Passage of Time in Hospital Treatment and Other Careers* (Indianapolis, IN: Bobbs-Merrill, 1963);

Charmaz, *Good Days, Bad Days*; Will Ross, *I Wanted to Live* (Milwaukee, WI: Wisconsin Anti-Tuberculosis Association, 1953); Elizabeth Mooney, *In the Shadow of the White Plague* (New York, NY: Thomas Y. Crowell, 1979); and Dorothy Simpson Beimer, *Hovels, Haciendas, and House Calls: The Life of Carl H. Gellenthien, M.D.* (Santa Fe, NM: Sunstone Press, 1986).

Novels about the tuberculosis experience include Thomas Mann's iconic *The Magic Mountain* (several publishers) 1924; Julian Green, *The Closed Garden* (New York, NY: Harper and Brothers, 1928); A. E. Ellis, *The Rack* (London, UK: Penguin Books, 1958, 1961); Donald Stewart, *Sanatorium* (New York, NY: Harper and Brothers Publishers, 1930); and Eamonn McGrath, *The Charnel House* (Belfast, Ireland: Blackstaff Press, 1990).

4. Bates, *Bargaining for Life*.

5. On the reapproachment of the North and South around the turn of the twentieth century, see Nancy Silber, *The Romance of Reunion: Northerners and the South, 1865–1900* (Chapel Hill, NC: University of North Carolina Press, 1993); and Cecilia Elizabeth O'Leary, *To Die For: The Paradox of American Patriotism* (Princeton, NJ: Princeton University Press, 1999).

6. Rep. George S. Legare remarks on "Treaty with Russia," 13 December 1911, *Congressional Record*, 62nd Cong., 2nd sess., 317–18.

7. G. E. Bushnell to Frances Izlar Legare, 1 February 1909, RG 112, Entry 386, NARA.

8. Frances Izlar Legare to G. E. Bushnell, 8 February 1909, RG 112, Entry 386, NARA.

9. G. E. Bushnell to Frances Izlar Legare, 1 February 1909, RG 112, Entry 386, NARA.

10. Charles Barney to Surgeon General, 24 November 1909, RG 112, Entry 386, NARA.

11. G. E. Bushnell to W. H. Peters, 8 April 1908, RG 112, Entry 386, Box 12, NARA.

12. Christine Whittaker writes of Irving Fisher, a tuberculosis patient who adopted the open air sleeping for the rest of his life: "The convert became a zealot like many other former tuberculosis patients," in "Chasing the Cure: Irving Fisher's Experience as a Tuberculosis Patient," *Bulletin of the History of Medicine* 48 (1974): 415.

On tuberculosis education see also Evelyn Fisher Frisbee, "Education of the Consumptive in Home Care," *The New York Medical Journal* 6 (January 1911): 86–89; David R. Lyman, "The Control of the Careless Consumptive," *American Review of Tuberculosis/ American Review of Pulmonary Diseases* 2 (1918–1919): 36–42; Nancy J. Tomes, *The Gospel of Germs: Men, Women, and the Microbe in American Life* (Boston, MA: Harvard University Press, 1998); and Michael E. Teller, *The Tuberculosis Movement: A Public Health Campaign in the Progressive Era* (New York, NY: Greenwood Press, 1988).

13. Medical historian Christopher Feudtner has described how much work it takes patients and their families to manage diabetes, constantly monitoring one's diet and blood sugar, and keeping up with the latest therapies and technologies in *Bittersweet*.

14. This was Brigadier General Clarence Ranson Edwards who was a patient at Fort Bayard in 1906. See "List of Officers of the Army who have been under treatment for tuberculosis at the General Hospital, Fort Bayard, N.M.," RG 112, Entry 26, Box 938, NARA. Richard Johnson's memoir also mentions Edwards at Fort Bayard, in "My Life in the U.S. Army," 91. Edwards was a graduate of the U.S. Military Academy at West Point, served in the Philippines (1898–1901), was chief of the War Department Bureau of Insular Affairs (1906–13), and commanded the 26th Division in the United States and France during World War I. He retired as a major general in 1922 and died in 1931 at the age of seventy-two. War Department, *Army Register* (Washington, DC: Government Printing Office, 1916), 7.

15. George E. Bushnell, "The Treatment of Tuberculosis," *American Review of Tuberculosis* 2 (1918–19): 261.

16. Fort Bayard reported sixty-four deaths in 1909, including one by suicide. See United States Army General Hospital, Fort Bayard, NM, "Annual Report for 1909," RG 112, Entry 26, NARA.

17. Richard Johnson, "My Life in the U.S. Army," 87.

18. G. E. Bushnell to Frances Izlar Legare, 19 May 1909, RG 112, Entry 386, NARA. Newspaper clipping, *News and Courier*, Charleston, SC, June 1909, LFP.

19. G. E. Bushnell to Frances Legare, 19 May 1909, RG 112, Entry 386, NARA. No letters survived from 14 June 1909.

20. J. B. McMahon to G. E. Bushnell, 8 July 1909, RG 112, Entry 386, Box 24, NARA.

21. G. E. Bushnell to George S. Legare, 9 August 1909, RG 112, Entry 386, Box 24, NARA.

22. "Form of Medical Certificate," 23 October 1909, RG 94, Box 715, NARA.

23. George S. Legare remarks on "Treaty with Russia," 13 December 1911, *Congressional Record*, 62nd Cong., 2nd sess., 317–18; and George S. Legare remarks on "New Mexico and Arizona," 16 May 1911, *Congressional Record*, 62nd Cong., 2nd sess., 1250–53.

24. "Legare-Larisey Debate Features," *News and Courier*, 20 July 1912, Charleston, SC, LFP.

25. "George S. Legare Laid to Rest," *News and Courier*, 3 February 1913, Charleston, SC, LFP.

26. See "The Late Representative George S. Legare, of South Carolina," U.S. House, *Congressional Record*, 23 February 1913, 62nd Cong., 3rd sess., 3753–59; and "Memorial Addresses on the Late Representative Legare," U.S. Senate, *Congressional Record*, 1 March 1913, 62nd Cong., 3rd sess., 4395–99.

27. Rep. Joseph H. Johnson, "The Late George S. Legare, Memorial Address," *Appendix to the Congressional Record*, 63th Cong., 1st sess., 475.

28. Rep. Asbury Francis Lever, "The Late Representative George S. Legare, of South Carolina," U.S. House, *Congressional Record*, 23 February 1913, 62nd Cong., 3rd sess., 3754.

29. Sen. Charles Townsend remarks on "Memorial Addresses on the Late Representative Legare," U.S. Senate, *Congressional Record*, 1 March 1913, 62nd Cong., 3rd sess., 4396.

30. Legare Family Papers, 1886–1930 and Ferdinanda Legare Waring Papers, 1910–1984, South Carolina Historical Society, Charleston, SC.

Chapter Four
Tuberculosis in World War I

Although Europe went to war in the summer of 1914, the United States escaped the cauldron until April 1917. But after years of trying to maintain neutrality, President Woodrow Wilson's administration mobilized the nation to fight in the most deadly enterprise the world had ever seen. Modern industrialized warfare would kill millions of soldiers, sailors, and civilians and unleash disease and famine across the globe. Typhus flourished in Eastern Europe and a lethal strain of influenza exploded out of the Western Front in 1918, producing one of the worst pandemics in history. Although eclipsed by such fierce epidemics, tuberculosis also fed on the war.

As the United States entered the war, it rushed to build a mass industrial army. In eighteen months the Selective Service registered twenty-five million men for the draft, examined ten million for military service, and enlisted more than four million soldiers, sailors, and Marines.[1] To the dismay of many people, medical screening boards across the nation soon discovered that American men were not as strong and healthy as they had assumed. Of those eligible for military service, 30 percent were physically unfit; a number of them deemed ineligible to serve had tuberculosis.[2] Therefore, in 1917 Surgeon General William Gorgas called George Bushnell to Washington, DC, to establish the Office of Tuberculosis in the Division of Internal Medicine, leaving Bushnell's protégé, Earl Bruns, in charge of Fort Bayard. Given the Medical Department's mission to maintain a strong and healthy fighting force, Bushnell's new job was to minimize the incidence of tuberculosis among active-duty soldiers and avoid the high cost of disability pensions for men who incurred the disease during military service. It was a tall order.

Wartime tuberculosis had already received attention in 1916, when reports circulated that the French army had sent home 86,000 men with the disease, raising the specter that life in the trenches would generate hundreds of thousands of cases. One investigator found that tuberculosis rates in the British army were double those in peacetime, reversing the prewar downward trend. The head of the New York City Public Health Department, Hermann Biggs, declared that "tuberculosis offers a problem of stupendous magnitude in France."³ Subsequent studies revealed that only 20 percent or less of the French soldiers sent home with tuberculosis actually had the disease; others were either misdiagnosed or had had tuberculosis prior to entering the military and therefore had not contracted it in the trenches.⁴ The reports nevertheless galvanized public health officials to address the tuberculosis problem. The Rockefeller Foundation, for example, in cooperation with the American Red Cross, established a Commission for the Prevention of Tuberculosis in France to help the French and protect any Americans from contracting tuberculosis "over there."⁵

Bushnell established four "tuberculosis screens" by (1) examining all volunteers and draftees before enlistment, (2) checking recruits again in the training camps, (3) examining soldiers already in the Army for tuberculosis, and (4) screening military personnel at discharge to ensure they returned to civil life in sound condition. To implement these activities, Bushnell developed a protocol under which physicians could quickly examine men for tuberculosis as part of the larger physical examination process. He standardized the procedures for examinations throughout the Army, and crafted a narrow definition of what constituted a tuberculosis diagnosis to enable the Army to enlist as many young men as possible. Despite these efforts, soldiers developed active cases of tuberculosis throughout the war.

Like the rest of the Army, the Medical Department had to play catch up to meet the demands of a ballooning army. It coordinated with the American Medical Association and the American Red Cross to recruit thousands of civilian physicians and nurses for military service, many of whom were unfamiliar with the military, tuberculosis, or both. Bushnell's office also created eight more tuberculosis hospitals in the United States and designated three hospitals with the American Expeditionary Forces (AEF) in France to care for soldiers who developed active tuberculosis in the camps and trenches. Short of resources and knowledge, however, the Army Medical Department at times struggled just to provide beds for tuberculosis patients, let alone deliver the individual care Bushnell and his staff had provided at Fort Bayard before the war.

This chapter examines the power of disease in wartime—specifically tuberculosis—to challenge the American medical establishment. Patients at one tuberculosis hospital even conflated disease and war, depicting the fight against tuberculosis as going "over the top" in the trenches on the Western Front, braving bureaucratic red tape and intransigent doctors (Figure 4-1). Wartime stretched the limits of competent personnel and adequate supplies. Untrained medical officers incorrectly diagnosed soldiers with tuberculosis who actually had some other chest ailment, shuffling them from one Army hospital to another, increasing expenses, generating paperwork, and distressing the soldiers and their families. Overburdened medical personnel worked long hours, in often poor conditions. Thousands of tuberculosis patients resented the diagnosis and protested the conditions in which at times they were virtually warehoused. The draft, which brought millions of young men into government control and responsibility, also exposed the Army Medical Department to public scrutiny. Some wartime tuberculosis hospitals met the crisis well, but others were so widely criticized that the U.S.

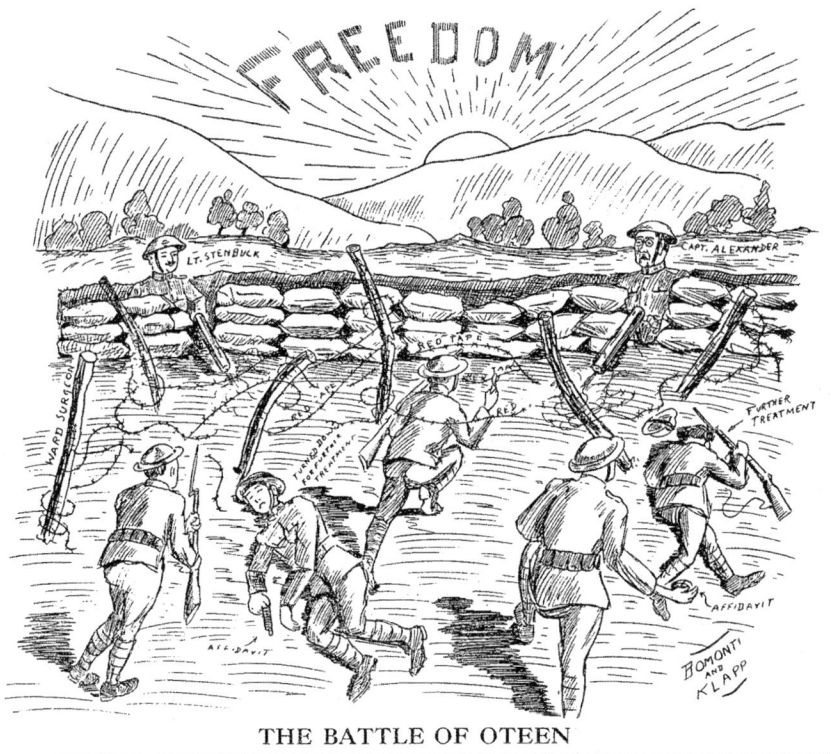

Figure 4-1. The Battle of Oteen," cartoon in *The Oteen*, patient newspaper at General Hospital, No. 19, Oteen, North Carolina, portraying the struggle men with tuberculosis faced getting discharged from the hospital.
Photograph courtesy of the National Library of Medicine, Bethesda, Maryland.

Congress launched an investigation in 1919. World War I, which so dramatically changed the world, profoundly altered the Army's tuberculosis program as well. It also challenged George Bushnell's expertise. The Army's tuberculosis expert had founded his policies on assumptions that, although widely held at the time, proved to be inaccurate and costly in lives and treasure. Wartime tuberculosis, therefore, shows the power of disease to overwhelm both knowledge and institutions.

Keeping Tuberculosis out of the Army

Bushnell based the Army Medical Department's tuberculosis program on four assumptions. The first was that most adults in the United States were already infected with tuberculosis and that this "tubercularization" provided them with a certain degree of immunity from the disease. "According to recent teachings," he wrote, "we all have a little tuberculosis."[6] Bushnell and his contemporaries were familiar with the concept of immunity and the power of vaccination, and the Army Medical Department vaccinated soldiers for smallpox and typhoid. Extending this concept of immunity to tuberculosis, medical officers differentiated between primary infection in childhood and secondary infection later in life. Observing that tuberculosis was often fatal for infants and young children, they reasoned that for survivors, an early infection of tuberculosis bacilli immunized a person against the disease later in life.[7] (This was accurate to some degree because children who did not develop or die of tuberculosis were more resistant than those who sucumbed.) A "primary infection," wrote Bushnell, gave a person some immunity, which "while not sufficient in many cases to prevent extension of disease [within the body]…is sufficient to counteract new infections from without."[8] In an article on "The Tuberculous Soldier," the revered physician William Osler agreed. For years autopsies had uncovered healed tuberculosis lesions in people who had died in accidents or of other diseases. Although it was not known how many men between the ages of eighteen and forty harbored the tubercle bacillus, Osler wrote, "We do know that it is exceptional not to find a few [lesions] in the bodies of men between these ages dead of other diseases." Thus, he argued, "In a majority of cases the germ enlists with the soldier. A few, very few, catch the disease in infected billets or barracks."[9] Bushnell reasoned if adults developed tuberculosis, "they do it on account of failure of their resistance."[10] Accordingly, the Medical Department often noted the cause of tuberculosis as "failure of immunity." If a primary tuberculosis infection could render one immune to the disease, soldiers with "a little tuberculosis" might even benefit the Army.

Bushnell's second assumption was that tuberculosis was not very contagious, and that a person already infected could be reinfected, "only by large amounts of tuberculosis virus [sic]."[11] At one point Bushnell told the chief surgeon of the AEF, "Personally I have no fear of the contagion of tuberculosis between adults and see no reason why patients of this kind should not be treated in the ordinary hospital."[12] He asserted that the "really cruel persecution of the consumptive… through the fear that he will infect others, is based on what I must characterize as highly exaggerated notions of the danger of such infection."[13] This, too, was the prevailing view. Boston bacteriologist Edward O. Otis, who served as a medical officer during the war, wrote that "Undue fear of the communicability of pulmonary tuberculosis from one adult to another is unwarranted in the present state of our knowledge."[14] A civilian nurse similarly wrote, "It is a popular belief that a tuberculous person is a constant source of infection to his associates. This is not true." If a person followed the hygienic rules of covering the mouth and nose while coughing and sneezing, she explained, "an advanced case whose sputum is full of bacilli, need not be isolated from the family except to have a separate bed."[15]

The third assumption informing Bushnell's tuberculosis program was that military life would not increase tuberculosis incidence. He recognized that epidemics of measles or influenza in Army camps and barracks could reactivate latent tuberculosis, but argued that, in general, military life made men stronger, increasing the body's immunity. He reasoned that if men infected with tuberculosis could indeed easily spread it to others, there would be much more tuberculosis in the Army than there was.[16] After the scare concerning the 86,000 French soldiers with the disease, tuberculosis specialists debated the increased risks and benefits of military service. British physician Leslie Murry, for example, reasoned that although the crowded and damp conditions of trench warfare would have unfavorable effects on soldiers' health, living outside with plenty of fresh air and good food and hygienic practices would improve their resistance to tuberculosis.[17] New York physician Maurice Fishberg suggested in a *Journal of the American Medical Association* editorial that although some people experienced the reactivation of dormant tuberculosis lesions in civil life, "it is doubtful whether it is more likely to occur in military life."[18] Not everyone agreed. Public health specialist George Thomas Palmer countered that although reactivation may not be higher in the military than in civil life, the United States had enough men without tuberculosis to bar anyone suspected of it from the military and thereby avoid an "added financial burden to the nation."[19]

Bushnell's final assumption was that what are now called "false positives" were harmful to the war effort, the Army, and the individual. "There is no reason why the possibly tuberculous alone should be excluded from the risks," he wrote. "He who in time of war excuses men for trifling or doubtful deviation from the normal does not properly conceive his duty toward his country."[20] The challenge, therefore, was to keep tuberculosis out of the Army and tuberculars off the disability rolls, but not to exclude so many men as to impair the nation's ability to amass an army.

Bushnell's views of tuberculosis immunity, contagion, interaction with military life, and the risk of overdiagnosis shaped the Army Medical Department programs for screening recruits. He knew he could not guarantee that all tuberculosis could be eliminated from the Army, but asserted that, "a sufficiently rigid selection of promising material in itself practically excludes tuberculosis."[21] In addition to enlisting the strongest men, Bushnell believed that a massive screening program would pay for itself by eliminating those who would later cost the government in medical services and disability benefits. He calculated that tuberculous soldiers in the United States cost an average $1,000, and that each patient returned from Europe would cost the government about $5,000.[22]

But the nation at war did not have the time or resources for the meticulous one-hour examination practiced at Fort Bayard, so Bushnell developed a protocol for civilian and military physicians to examine volunteers, draftees, trainees, and soldiers for tuberculosis in a matter of minutes. *Circular No. 20* detailed how physicians should examine recruits, and became the single most important Army tuberculosis document during the war.[23] The six-page circular began by cautioning examiners not to base a tuberculosis diagnosis on a man's word because he might be motivated to mislead. Some men may be anxious to enlist despite having tuberculosis so they could fight in the war or become eligible for treatment in Army hospitals; others might feign tuberculosis symptoms to avoid service or to get a discharge on disability. Examiners, therefore, must base their diagnosis on physical signs. The circular explained that the apices, or the tops of lungs, were the most common location for tuberculosis lesions, and that "the only trustworthy sign of activity in apical tuberculosis is the presence of persistent moist rales." It also outlined ten lung sounds that were *not* signs of tuberculosis but rather indications of bronchitis, pneumonia, or other lung ailments.

The next section described the various kinds of tuberculosis lesions examiners might encounter—acute, arrested chronic, active chronic, and disseminated—noting that arrested chronic tuberculosis was the most common. *Circular No. 20* directed that "the presence of tubercle bacilli in the sputum is a cause for rejection," and that "no examination for tuberculosis is complete without auscultation following a cough." It recommended that a sputum sample "be coughed up in [the examiner's] presence," to ensure that it was actually from the examinee.[24] The last one-third of the document detailed X-ray examinations, summarizing eight different kinds of conditions that may appear and that would be grounds for rejection, and which conditions would not. *Circular No. 20* ultimately counseled examiners to reject anyone with a lesion of considerable size. But as Bushnell told a gathering of tuberculosis specialists, "'Considerable' is not a good term, but we couldn't think of anything better."[25] The circular prescribed no time frames for the examination, but the Medical Department imposed speed by requiring examiners to see at least fifty men a day. Some physicians objected to this pace, while others got into the spirit. One team of three reported seeing 1,763, 1,854, and 1,944 men in three successive days, which raises the question of how thoroughly they conducted their examinations.[26]

The X-ray provisions of *Circular No. 20* generated controversy. Bushnell later wrote that, "considerable pressure was exercised…by a number of prominent physicians and radiologists to induce the Surgeon General to make the radiograph the decisive factor in the diagnosis of pulmonary tuberculosis."[27] The Medical Department had acquired X-ray equipment soon after it was developed in 1895 and immediately found it useful for locating bone fractures and bullets in wounds.[28] By 1915, a Fort Bayard medical officer stated that X-ray technology "has become one of the most valued procedures in the diagnosis of pulmonary tuberculosis," but stressed that it had to be employed by a skilled physician in conjunction with a careful physical examination.[29] During the war mobilization, some physicians wanted to rely primarily on X-rays, claiming that they could be made rapidly and accurately, and that the stored X-ray plates provided a medical record and an excellent resource for research. Medical officers F. E. Diemer and R. D. MacRae at Camp Lewis, Washington, carried this issue to the pages of the *Journal of the American Medical Association,* arguing that X-rays should be the primary diagnostic tool, not an "adjunct." A few months later one of their senior colleagues, Ralph C. Matson, countered that X-rays should be only one of several tools, because Diemer and MacRae "claim more for roentgenology [radiology] than it should be expected to yield."[30]

Bushnell took the Matson view and the Medical Department's tuberculosis program employed X-ray technology only in the quarter or third of cases where the physical examination was ambiguous. Bushnell believed that X-rays were unreliable because they could not catch early lesions or distinguish between active and healed lesions. He was also concerned that the nation's X-ray schools did not have the technical expertise to train the numbers of skilled radiologists the Army required. Nor did the Army have the equipment to X-ray all recruits, "not to mention the enormous costs of photographing the entire new Army and the impossibility of obtaining a sufficient number of plates within a reasonable time."[31] World War I ultimately, however, did encourage X-ray technology by revealing its power to thousands of physicians, stimulating the search for technical advances, and demonstrating the importance of specialization in reading X-rays. By the end of the war, the Army Medical Department had shipped to France hundreds of X-ray machines for use in Army hospitals and at the bedside, and developed various modes of X-ray equipment, including X-ray ambulances.[32]

The most sensitive tuberculosis controversy was whether to enlist men who had previously been diagnosed with the disease. Medical officers such as Clarence L. Wheaton at Camp Grant, Illinois, believed that soldiers with tuberculosis infection were a "liability" in the training camps.[33] Physicians in other armies agreed. For example, Thomas McCrae, Canadian medical officer and poet ("In Flanders fields the poppies blow"), argued that, "If you accept men who have had tuberculosis you are harming them and adding to the burden after the war."[34] Bushnell took a different view. When an American physician suggested rejecting all men who had any sign of tuberculosis, even old, apparently healed cases, Bushnell replied, "That is impossible," because "if we should say that all signs of tuberculosis should lead to rejection we would have no army at all."[35] Others would have gone further. Army officer J. F. Hammond wrote to Bushnell that he was dismayed that a disability board at his post recommended only five of fifty-three men for duty. Given the wartime emergency, he suggested that men with very slight tuberculosis or no symptoms be given special or light duty. Bushnell may have agreed with him, but responded diplomatically that employing such men "was not deemed advisable" because they were not fit for battlefield work. "In all events," he told Hammond, "this is the view of the War Department."[36]

The War Department took a more lenient position regarding tubercular medical officers than enlisted men. As Bushnell pointed out, "The men especially interested in tuberculosis work had themselves the disease, a fact which under ordinary conditions would debar them from admission into the Army."[37] The War Department assented, but did not issue a general waiver, rather allowing physicians with tuberculosis to serve on a case-by-case basis. Some of these were Fort Bayard "alumni" from the ranks of patients as well as medical officers. In addition to Bushnell, Earl Bruns joined the Office of The Surgeon General and traveled to Europe to evaluate the AEF program after the war. Former patients/medical officers such as Paul Hutton served as a Medical Department inspector; Conrad E. Koerper examined trainees at Camp Gordon, Georgia; Carl Holmberg commanded a tuberculosis hospital at Whipple Barracks in Arizona; and W. H. Tefft and Carl Bloombergh commanded evacuation hospitals in France.

Not everyone favored employing tubercular medical officers. In a letter marked "Personal," one officer touring the hospitals in the West to encourage reconstruction programs—education and rehabilitation programs for tuberculosis patients—wrote to a colleague that at Fort Bayard and Whipple Barracks, Arizona, he found, "the entire staff, commissioned and enlisted…are ex or active T.B.'s." He did not think such men had the energy or enthusiasm to administer reconstruction programs. "Everyone knows that the T.B. man is subject to mental and nervous crises and depressions and [that] unfits him much of the time for such functions as reconstruction which require inexhaustible energy, enthusiasm and 'Pep.'" He believed that "the Commanding Officer [C.O.] should always be a perfectly sound man physically," and then "the rest of the staff might be all ex-T.B.'s if necessary but it would be far better were all of the same physical class of the C.O." Taking direct aim at Bushnell, he wrote, "I fear for your program under the present administrative conditions in these hospitals which seems to be run more for the T.B. medical officers than for the good of the service."[38]

Throughout the war, however, Bushnell's views, correct or incorrect, prevailed. After testing the *Circular No. 20* protocol at Camp Dodge, Kansas, in October 1917, the Medical Department decided to proceed.[39] Calculating that it would require 600 examiners for the screening process, the Medical Department turned to training general practitioners from civil life who knew little about tuberculosis. Bushnell's office established a six-week tuberculosis course to prepare physicians. The first course at the Army Medical School in Washington, DC, was so popular that instructors offered it at several other training camps in the country. General Hospital No. 16, operating in conjunction with Yale Medical School, also offered a course on hospital administration to train medical officers to run tuberculosis hospitals.

Once prepared, these new medical officers participated in the massive physical examination of the nation's young men, taking part in a modern bureaucracy of impersonal queues and myriad forms.[40] Enlistees passed through a series of exam rooms (Figure 4-2) to undergo their physicals, including the "TB (tuberculosis) room." At Camp Lewis, Washington, X-ray specialists viewed 200 to 250 men daily, and reported chest examination findings for each man on "Form 1." If the examiner had concerns, "Form 2" summoned the recruit back for another examination. "Form 3" instructed men how to expectorate sputum and "Form 4" requested yet another X-ray exam. "Silence is maintained in the tuberculosis examining room," reported one medical officer—punctuated, no doubt, by the sounds of supervised expectoration.[41] The physicians filled out more forms if they suspected a man had other physical problems, referring him to various specialists, each with his own forms and procedures. The Army Medical Department also referred those with sexually transmitted diseases to treatment, but sent home men with other diseases such as trachoma, a potentially blinding eye infection, or carriers of the typhoid bacillus.

Despite *Circular No. 20* and Bushnell's efforts, tuberculosis inevitably slipped through the Army's screen. Warning his wife to not tell a soul, a tuberculosis specialist at Camp Russell, Wyoming, confided that "Everyone is very kind but

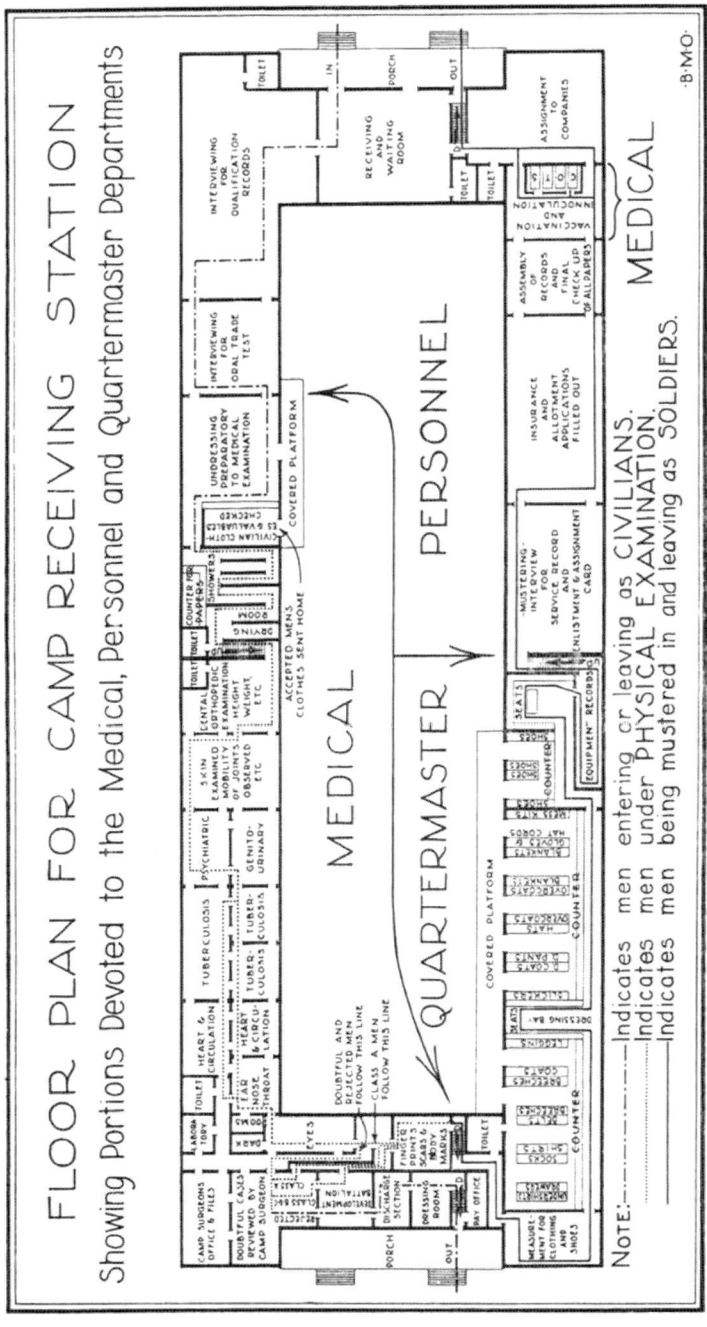

Figure 4-2. Diagram of medical screening facility plan for training camps. Source: The Medical Department in the World War, U.S. Army, Office of the Army Surgeon General, Washington, DC, vol 6, p. 458.

efficiency is not supreme here."[42] Another physician noted that, "There is a gross misconception on the part of men here as elsewhere as to what shall constitute tuberculosis sufficient for rejection."[43] Earl Bruns noted that examiners seeing more than one hundred recruits in a day became fatigued, and "very often the examiner was not to blame[,] for at times examinations were conducted amid noisy surroundings and without sufficient time to make an examination even according to the rapid Bushnell method."[44]

If examiners diagnosed a recruit or soldier with tuberculosis, the question became whether he should be immediately discharged or kept on the military rolls and treated, and whether he was eligible for disability benefits. The War Department initially ordered that a diagnosis of tuberculosis within the first three months of service *not* be considered in line of duty, unless it was an acute case or the product of extraordinary exposure to the elements.[45] This policy, issued in September 1917, was an attempt to achieve a balance between building up the disability roles at great cost to the government and taxpayers, or sending men back home sick to be cared for by their families.[46] In the following months medical officers determined that although 349 trainees diagnosed with tuberculosis had contracted it in the line of duty, 3,327 had not.[47] When the Army discharged sick draftees or trainees without treatment or benefits, however, people began to protest. Public health officials and the National Tuberculosis Association asked to be informed of any tuberculous individuals being sent to their communities, including the name and address of the "party assuming responsibility for such continued treatment and care."[48] The journal *American Medicine* published an article by British tuberculosis specialist Halliday Sutherland, who expressed concern that if men declined treatment and returned home they could spread tuberculosis to their families. He suggested that the U.S. Army retain men diagnosed with tuberculosis so that the government could provide treatment and discipline them if they resisted.[49]

Members of Congress also opposed simply discharging men with tuberculosis. Representative Carl Hayden of Arizona argued that such men had given up their civilian lives upon induction into the Army, only to discover "that they were afflicted with a dread disease which prevents them from earning a livelihood." He suggested that "some provision should be made for the care of such men until they are able to provide for themselves."[50] In response to such criticism, the Medical Department changed the policy in May 1918 so that "any soldier who shall have been accepted on his first physical examination…shall be considered to have contracted any subsequently determined physical disability in the line of duty."[51] Men therefore found to have tuberculosis were sent to hospitals until "maximum cure" had been achieved.[52] This policy further increased the pressure on Bushnell to keep tuberculosis out of the rank and file.

Medical officers in the training camps lectured soldiers on how to avoid tuberculosis. For example, George Brewer at Camp Ethan Allen, Vermont, spoke on "What the American Soldier can do to lessen his chances of becoming infected with Tuberculosis (Consumption)," noting that "a sick soldier is a double burden because of the extra men who must care for him." To avoid infection, he said, a soldier should maintain good physical condition; spend time in the fresh air and live in well-ventilated places; avoid sneezing and spitting on others; keep his tent or dugout clean; breathe deeply and hold the pure air in his lungs; and if "any of your comrades" violate these regulations, report him, "so he will not endanger your health by his carelessness."[53]

While Bushnell's policies succeeded in suppressing tuberculosis rates in the Army, the narrow definition of a tuberculosis diagnosis explicitly allowed men with healed lesions in their lungs to serve, and the rapid screening system caused some examiners to miss cases of active disease. For example, George W. Troutman, a brick mason from North Carolina, twenty-two years of age, enlisted with the 118th Infantry in July 1917, but not until the following February did medical officers at Camp Sevier, South Carolina, learn that he had been spitting up blood about twice a week for several months.[54] New York City public health officials also advised the Medical Department that Edward Waring, a soldier with the Signal Corps, had been diagnosed with tuberculosis, but "is reported to be in France." Surgeons at the AEF Base Hospital (BH) No. 20 had to amputate the right leg of Private (Pvt.) Walter P. Keating, 102nd Infantry, for tuberculosis of the bone.[55]

Bushnell recognized that "a standard, though imperfect, is believed to be an indispensable adjunct in Army tuberculosis work not only to support the examiner but also to secure the necessary uniformity of practice in the matter of discharge for tuberculosis."[56] Nationwide, local draft boards and training camps rejected more than 88,000 men for tuberculosis, about 2.3 percent of the 3.8 million men examined. Essentially all soldiers who traveled to France were examined two or three times for tuberculosis before crossing the Atlantic. Postwar assessments calculated that of the more than two million soldiers who went to France to serve in the AEF, only 8,717 were evacuated with a diagnosis of tuberculosis, an incidence of only 0.4 percent; Army-wide only 1,607 American soldiers died of the disease during the war.[57]

Tuberculosis in the American Expeditionary Forces

Bushnell recognized that some men with tuberculosis would emerge among the troops, but he was less tolerant of medical officers who generated "false positive" tuberculosis diagnoses. He became alarmed in early 1918 when a strep infection in the training camps in the United States caused medical officers to send hundreds of trainees to Army hospitals misdiagnosed with tuberculosis, crowding hospitals and generating paperwork and confusion. For a time, therefore, the Office of The Surgeon General ordered that no one should be discharged for tuberculosis from the training camps unless he had bacilli in his sputum—meaning the very severe cases.[58] Bushnell was even more disturbed to learn that more than 50 percent of the patients being sent back to the United States from France with a diagnosis of tuberculosis did not actually have the disease.[59] He viewed such overdiagnoses as "evil," because it took men out of the AEF and overburdened tuberculosis hospitals and naval transports, which had to segregate suspected tuberculosis cases in isolation rooms or on open decks.[60]

Faced with what he called "leaking" of soldiers from the AEF due to erroneous tuberculosis diagnoses, Bushnell turned to a specialist for assistance, Gerald B. Webb (Figure 4-3), from Colorado Springs.[61] An Englishman by birth, Webb had married an American, and when she developed tuberculosis the couple traveled to Colorado Springs, Colorado, for treatment. His wife struggled with the disease for ten years until her death in 1903, and afterward Webb stayed on in Colorado Springs, remarrying and building a medical practice specializing in tuberculosis.[62] In addition to his medical practice, Webb pioneered research into the body's

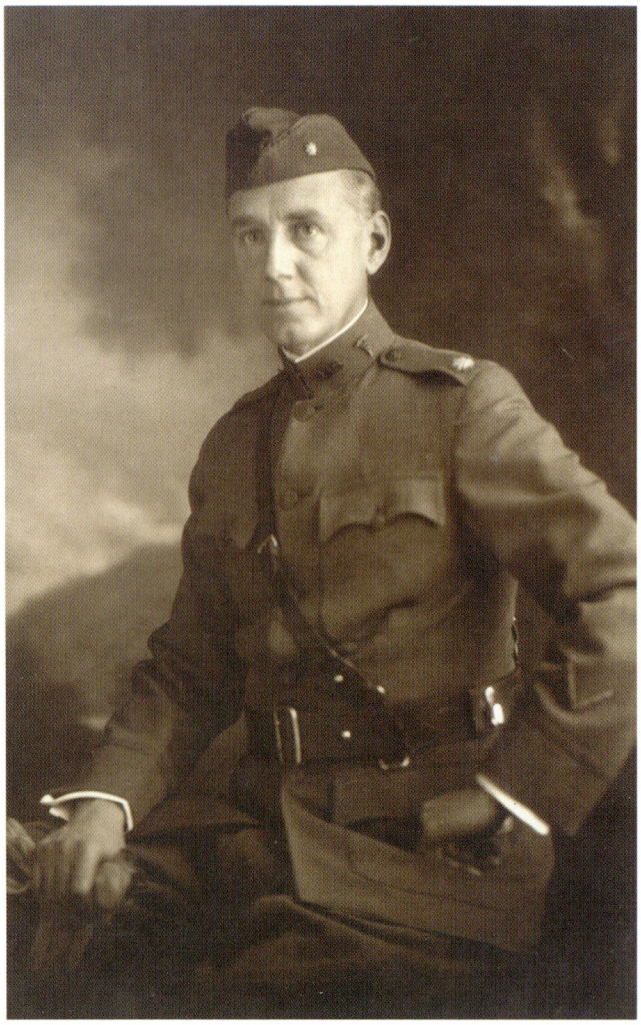

Figure 4-3. Gerald B. Webb, World War I, Gerald B. Webb Papers.
Photograph courtesy of Special Collections, Tutt Library, Colorado College, Colorado Springs, Colorado.

immune function, searched for a tuberculosis vaccine, and was a founder of the American Association of Immunologists (1913). Still somewhat bored in Colorado Springs, Webb volunteered for the Medical Corps soon after the United States declared war and helped organize and run tuberculosis screening boards at Camp Russell, Wyoming, and Camp Bowie, Texas. While in Wyoming, he published a research paper on the incidence of tuberculosis among draftees who smoked cigarettes, and wrote an editorial supporting Bushnell's tuberculosis program.[63] Bushnell noticed these articles, and after Webb brought order to a chaotic tuberculosis screening program at Camp Custer, Michigan, appointed him senior tuberculosis consultant for the AEF. After meeting with Bushnell in Washington and attending the Army War Course for senior officers at Columbia University, Webb sailed to France in March 1918.

Webb was one of a number of medical consultants who provided expertise to the AEF medical services in fields such as cardiology, urology, skin diseases, and neurological disorders. Johns Hopkins physician William Thayer commanded the medical consultants, who met once a month in Paris. One of Webb's colleagues suggested the importance of his job when he said Webb had to be "the Col. Bushnell on this side of the tuberculosis work."[64] Webb instituted a screening process similar to that in the United States, distributing *Circular No. 20*, and preparing an illustrated version for medical officers in the field.[65] He established a policy similar to that of the training camps, directing that only patients with sputum positive for tuberculosis should be sent back to the United States. Others would be tagged "tuberculosis observation" and sent to one of three hospitals designated as tuberculosis observation centers. There, specialists—Bushnell's "good tuberculosis men"—would distinguish tuberculosis signs from other lung problems such as bronchitis and pneumonia, test a patient's sputum ten to fifteen times before determining that he was free of disease, and thereby send only patients who were indeed positive for tuberculosis back to the homeland. In one of his daily letters to his wife, Varina, Webb described his work as "tactfully putting a cork into the bottle from which so much T.B. leaked."[66]

Headquartered in Neufchateau in the Vosges, Webb traveled to field and base hospitals throughout France. He would typically spend three days at a hospital, examining patients, leading conferences, giving lectures, and, according to his biographer, Helen Clapesattle, "preaching his gospel of fresh air and absolute rest."[67] He recruited a radiologist to teach the proper reading of X-ray plates, and advocated the early detection of tuberculosis, explaining, "Just as the wounded do better if they are got to the surgeons quickly, so the tuberculosis-wounded are more likely to recover if they are spotted and sent to the doctors early."[68] After the Armistice in November 1918, Webb based himself at port hospitals, where he worked to ensure that only properly diagnosed demobilizing soldiers were sent to tuberculosis hospitals in the United States.

Webb designated three large AEF hospitals as tuberculosis centers. BH No. 3, at Vauclaire (Figure 4-4), organized by Mount Sinai Hospital in New York City, operated in an old Trappist monastery, and during its service from May 1918 to January 1919, cared for 9,127 patients, 222 of whom were suspected of having

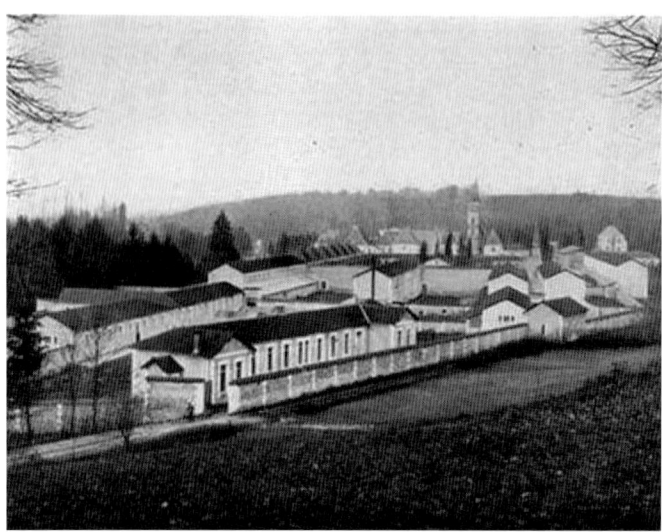

Figure 4-4. Base Hospital No. 3, Vauclaire, one of the hospitals designated to receive patients suspected of having tuberculosis.
Source: The Medical Department in the World War, in U.S. Army, Office of the Army Surgeon General, Washington, DC, vol. 2. Available at http://history.amedd.army.mil/booksdocs/wwi/adminamerexp/ch24fig125.jpg.

tuberculosis.[69] BH No. 8, organized at the Post-Graduate Hospital in New York City, got off to a slow start when its transport ship *Saratoga* was accidentally rammed by another ship, dumping hospital equipment into the New York Harbor. After finally arriving in France, BH No. 8 set up in Savenay and ultimately saw more than 35,000 sick and wounded during its war service, taking 12,000 X-rays, a large percentage of them for suspected tuberculosis.[70] BH No. 20, organized by the University of Pennsylvania in Philadelphia, was located at a French health resort at Chatel Guyon and operated from May 1918 to January 1919. At first it cared for only a few suspected cases, but as the AEF grew, so did its tuberculosis load, averaging seventy-five tuberculosis patients in its care by the end of the war.[71]

Webb loved the work. He wrote enthusiastic letters to Thayer and Bushnell, detailing his activities and observations, and asking for "any criticisms or suggestions you will have." Webb told Bushnell that he was widely distributing Bushnell's *Military Surgeon* article on tuberculosis screening, and that "it gave me great pleasure to introduce your name to my audiences and to tell of the Army's preparedness for the situation thanks to your years of work and research at Fort Bayard."[72] But when he said he admired many of the physicians he was encountering in the AEF, Bushnell cautioned, "I am well aware that many very excellent internists were sent over with the early base hospitals.… That is not, however, exactly equivalent to having a lot of tuberculosis men." They had not been trained in "our methods," he pointed out, so that Webb would have to work with them. Bushnell added, however, that given the shortage in the United States, he was "glad that you have not made a call for a considerable number of tuberculosis specialists."[73] Webb also told Thayer, "This work has been one of the greatest pleasures of my life, and I am daily thankful that I can do my small share." His superiors responded with praise. Webb was delighted to report to Varina, "Col Bushnell wrote me I had cut the 60% leak home to 15%!"[74]

The war, therefore, provided once-in-a-lifetime experiences for participants behind the lines as well as in the trenches. The carnage of World War I, like most wars, offered physicians opportunities for medical and surgical research unimagineable in peacetime. The advent of poison gas in 1915, for example, raised the question of chemical weapons' effects on tuberculosis incidence. Physicians speculated that exposure to poison gas could cause tuberculosis or reactivate quiescent cases. Some conducted animal experiments to test their hypotheses and found that gassed rabbits did not develop tuberculosis more easily than those not gassed, and that gassing rabbits with tuberculosis did not accelerate the tuberculous process in their bodies.[75] After the war, the Surgeon General's Office surveyed tuberculosis hospitals to determine the number of tuberculosis patients who had been gassed, and whether, in the medical officers' judgment, the disease had been caused by gas. Although a few medical officers saw a correlation, the majority responded that chemical weapons had little impact on tuberculosis.[76] The Medical Department concluded that "gassing, even in fairly high concentration, cannot initiate a tuberculosis process, the extent to which it may be operative in relighting a quiescent lesion has not been determined."[77] Research continued on the effect of war gases on tuberculosis until 1927, when the *Journal of the American Medical Association* concluded that after a decade of clinical observations, "A man is no more liable to tuberculosis as a result of gassing than is a man who has never been gassed."[78]

An issue of greater consequence was the impact of military life on tuberculosis, and this question would test Bushnell's assumption that most soldiers had gained some immunity against the disease by being previously exposed, or "tubercularized." Although most medical scientists understood that immunity to tuberculosis was not binary—as it was with smallpox, or yellow fever, where survivors, or those who had been vaccinated, acquired immunity for life—they did theorize that childhood tuberculosis infections increased one's immunity to the disease and would to some degree protect soldiers from developing active tuberculosis in the barracks or trenches. One way to test this theory would be through postmortem examinations of soldiers killed in combat or by other diseases to see if they had healed tuberculosis lesions. The Medical Department had the legal authority to perform autopsies on its soldier-patients; Fort Bayard medical officers conducted autopsies on most patients who died there (cattle, too), often holding seminars on the findings. But the lack of Army pathologists and the wartime conditions in France made such a systematic autopsy program difficult in the early months of the AEF. By the fall of 1918, however, AEF pathologists were performing autopsies on 95 percent of all patients who died in a hospital, and the Office of The

Surgeon General had requested special autopsy studies for deaths from gunshot injuries, chemical weapons, and influenza and pneumonia.[79]

To pursue the question of tubercularization, Gerald Webb persuaded several Army pathologists to search specifically at autopsy for healed tubercular lesions, indicated by walled-up tubercles. Having devoted years of research to tuberculosis immunology, Webb had written as late as December 1917 that "practically every post-mortem examination of those who had escaped [tuberculosis] shows such a spot [healed tuberculosis lesion], and it is now known that through having this spot their bodies have been protected against tuberculosis."[80] He therefore did not question the theory that childhood infection gave a person some immunity to tuberculosis, but was seeking data on the actual rate of infection. After gathering approximately 2,000 autopsy reports of soldiers who had died of something other than tuberculosis, though, Webb was surprised to find that only 25 percent of the bodies examined had healed tubercular lesions. This suggested that three-fourths of American soldiers had never been infected with tuberculosis bacilli and therefore lacked the theorized immunity.[81] The fact that some 300 AEF soldiers died of miliary tuberculosis, an acute and lethal form of the disease that most often struck children who had never been exposed to the disease, also ran counter to the immunity theory.

Such results challenged Bushnell's assumption of infection and immunity because they suggested that 75 percent of U.S. soldiers had not been "tuberculized" and could develop active disease if they were exposed to the bacteria in the Army. Troubled by the criticism, Bushnell and Bruns responded vigorously. When Bruns arrived in France after the Armistice to evaluate the Army's tuberculosis program, his May 1919 report generally praised Webb's work, but took sharp exception to the autopsy findings. These and the miliary tuberculosis cases, wrote Bruns, had been "interpreted as meaning that a large percentage of our soldiers have not been 'vaccinated to tubercule,'" and that this "establishes a heresy which should be corrected."[82] Bruns requested a retroactive study of all AEF autopsies to get a larger sample, and contended, with some reason, that Webb's sample was incomplete, even faulty. He noted that it took great care to detect small lesions deep within the lungs, and cited a British study that found calcified tubercle deposits in 70 percent of British soldiers autopsied. He also argued that the tuberculosis rate was twice as high for noncombatant troops as those at the front because troops on the front lines "lived an out-of-door life, were free from dissipation and had plenty of good nourishing food which more than offset the fatigue and exposure." He concluded that "the suggestion that deaths from tuberculosis among the American Expeditionary Forces...[were] due to infections acquired in [F]rance [i.e., from other soldiers] is contrary to the modern theory of tuberculosis and has not been borne out by facts."[83]

This issue erupted during the 1919 National Tuberculosis Association conference when Webb summarized the AEF pathology data. He reported that although H. E. Robertson found that 70 percent of the German soldiers he autopsied had lesions, D. J. Glomsett had found tuberculosis lesions in only 14 percent (44 of 308) of the autopsies he performed on Americans, and Webb himself had "been unable to detect deposits of tubercle in even as much as 25 percent of the [American] cases."[84] Bushnell rose to respond that, "I do not believe that the situation is as bad as Colonel Webb thinks." Deaths from miliary tuberculosis were "not a proof that the case is one of primary tuberculosis," that is, the results of a soldier's first exposure to tuberculosis bacteria. Following Bruns' line of argument, Bushnell cited other armies' studies of high infection rates among soldiers, and pointed out that some of the pathologists had not used microscopes and were therefore unlikely to find the small, deep lesions other researchers had.[85] The issue remained unresolved and Bushnell pursued it after the war, writing a book on his theory of the tubercularization of the "civilized" races.[86] At an international conference in London in 1921, he asserted that, "It has been established beyond the shadow of a doubt that the large majority of civilized mankind are infected with tuberculosis." Therefore, he could conclude, "That they do not die of it is the best of proofs that tuberculosis is not necessarily evil."[87] Bushnell must have felt compelled to reject the implication that his wartime tuberculosis policies could have exposed soldiers to fatal tuberculosis infections. He may also have been resisting the implication that soldiers and officers who had ever had tuberculosis—such as himself—did not belong in the Army.

But Webb was on to something. The issue would see resolution only in the 1930s, when scientists came to recognize that early tuberculosis infections did not provide protection and that adults could be reinfected with tuberculosis and develop active disease.[88] In the meantime, with his AEF work done, in January 1919 Webb returned to his family and medical practice in Colorado Springs. The National Tuberculosis Association recognized Webb's war work by electing him president in 1920, and Webb set the Association on a course of tuberculosis research on the immunity question and the standardization of X-ray diagnostics. He did not return to military service, but was a mentor for young physicians Esmond Long and James Waring, who would be leaders in the Army Medical Department's tuberculosis program during the next war. Unlike so many of his colleagues, Webb never developed tuberculosis. He died of a heart attack in 1948.

Overwhelmed

As Gerald Webb worked to standardize and strengthen the AEF tuberculosis program in Europe, conditions deteriorated in the United States. When Medical Department inspector Col. Jere B. Clayton visited Fort Bayard in late February 1919, several months after the end of World War I, he did not like what he found. The wartime emergency had exploded admissions but stripped the facility of its best personnel and equipment.The patient population had increased fivefold from some 300 patients in February 1917 to 1,533 in December 1918, and despite the recent transfer of 500 to another hospital, Fort Bayard still had twenty more patients than beds. The physical plant was crowded and rundown. Fifty-five officers lived in thirteen sets of quarters, and most of the motor pool had been shipped to France for the war, leaving one mule ambulance and three motor ambulances, one of which was "unserviceable."[89] Clayton also found the medical staff wanting.

The commander, Lieutenant Colonel (Lt. Col.) Edward P. Rockhill, had been called out of retirement to run the post, and although he had been a patient at Fort Bayard and was therefore knowledgeable in the treatment of tuberculosis, he was "not familiar with the best base hospital procedure" as established by the wartime Medical Department. Clayton judged the chief of medical service to be an "unknown quantity" and the dental service so understaffed it "could do little more than emergency work." He rated ward conditions as "fair only" because some areas of the post were dirty or in ill repair. Clayton reported that the nurses were generally efficient, but that the chief nurse, Samantha C. Plummer, was a "poor executive for a large hospital," and could not provide proper supervision because she was cooking meals for the ninety-six nurses in her charge. He was particularly critical of the Fort Bayard kitchens: "This is probably the richest hospital fund in the country and the patients are not being well fed." The food was too heavy for bed patients, served cold on cracked dishes, and more patients had complained to him about the food than at any other hospital around the country. Patients even had to *purchase* extra milk from the hospital.

Clayton concluded that "as a whole the patients were not receiving the care and consideration that they get in a first class base hospital." He fired off thirty-eight recommendations, including the relief of the Fort Bayard commander, the chief of medical service, the chief nurse, and the head of the Hospital Corps, and a reduction in the number of patients to the authorized capacity of 1,046.[90] The Army Surgeon General, Merritte Ireland, adopted many of the inspector's recommendations, but did not relieve Rockhill—he had no one to replace him. Instead he sent Rockhill a stern memo outlining twenty-three steps he should take to remedy the deficiencies at Fort Bayard. Ireland was particularly disturbed by the sale of milk to patients, stating that "milk should not be sold to a patient in a hospital by the hospital or an agency of it."[91]

This inspection revealed a hospital in crisis. Fort Bayard was one of several Army hospitals that, overwhelmed by patients and bereft of competent staff, struggled to meets its responsibilities during and after World War I. Before the war, Fort Bayard's 300 beds were sufficient to care for an army of 175,000. But what of an army that had grown to four million by late 1918? There was no way Fort Bayard could carry the load.

The Medical Department ultimately faced more than 22,000 cases of tuberculosis, about 18,500 from training camps in the United States and 3,500 from Europe.[92] Tuberculosis patients required treatment for longer periods than many other sick and wounded, thus they consumed a disproportionate amount of Medical Department resources. The Department calculated that during 1918 alone, tuberculosis stood third in loss of days for officers (50,341 days) and seventh for enlisted men (1,255,009 days).[93] Fort Bayard scrambled to meet these needs (Figure 4-5). Although the local economy was booming as the Burro Mountain Copper Company in Grant County increased its copper production tenfold in 1918, Fort Bayard's boom was less profitable.[94] In eighteen months the patient population increased fivefold, but medical officers only tripled, from fourteen to thirty-nine, and nurses and enlisted staff quadrupled, from twenty-three to eighty-six, and from 145 to

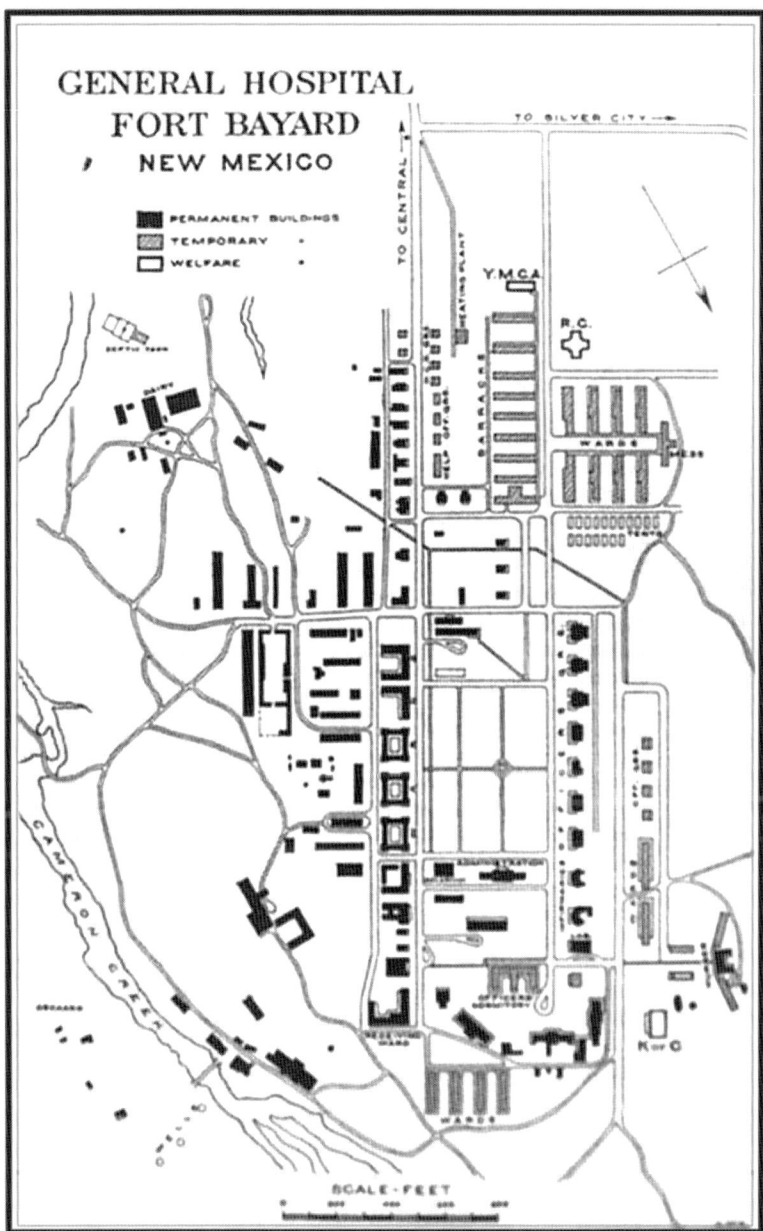

Figure 4-5. Map of Fort Bayard, New Mexico, during World War I, showing the extensive temporary structures (shaded gray) erected to accommodate patients and staff during the wartime emergency.
Source: The Medical Department in the World War, in U.S. Army, Office of the Army Surgeon General, Washington, DC, vol. 5. Available at http://history.amedd.army.mil/booksdocs/wwi/MilitaryHospitalsintheUS/chapter25figure166.jpg.

604, respectively. Patients and staff lived in tents and once-condemned buildings.[95] Food stocks and budgets were stretched to the point that the hospital laboratory, which raised Belgian hares for experiments, handed them over to the kitchen for food.[96] And as the AEF claimed able-bodied medical officers, the Medical Department turned to retirees and disabled medical officers to operate its hospitals.

When Bushnell called Bruns to Washington to assist him in the fall of 1917, he appointed Rockhill to command the Army's tuberculosis hospital. Rockhill, forty-five years old, had been invalided out of the Philippines and sent to Fort Bayard in 1907 for tuberculosis of the bladder. Retired for disability in 1909, he returned to active duty in 1916 first as a medical officer at Fort Bayard before he assumed command.[97] As crowded conditions and staff shortages generated myriad problems, Rockhill kept up a prodigious correspondence with Bushnell and Bruns, seeking guidance, support, and an opportunity to complain. "You and Colonel Bushnell are the only two men in Washington," he told Bruns, "who have any connection with and any interest in Fort Bayard."[98] Discipline deteriorated, and while Rockhill issued orders prescribing proper uniform attire and prohibiting the use of "profane or vulgar language," he was at his "wits' end" because many of the men in the hospital had no sense of military order—they were going "hog-wild," Rockhill wrote.[99] Compounding his problems, Rockhill did not always display good judgment. Despite a shortage of thirty medical officers, he advised the Office of The Surgeon General that "the services of a woman anesthetist are not desired at this Hospital."[100] And when a congressman sought admission for his son to the crowded hospital, Rockhill suggested that if the congressman could get an appropriation for a new wing, there might be enough room. To this idea, Bushnell responded curtly that the War Department did not ask for special appropriations during wartime.[101] By mid-1918, recognizing his own limitations and under tremendous stress, Rockhill asked to be replaced, explaining that "the relief of responsibility would be more than a compensation for the loss of prestige."[102]

The nursing staff at Fort Bayard was also in an uproar. When nursing inspector Anna C. Jamme came to Fort Bayard in early 1919, nurses complained about their living conditions, and some of them signed a letter alleging that several coworkers were entertaining men in their quarters.[103] Jamme told Annie Goodrich, the head of the Army School of Nursing, "I cannot begin to tell you how very deeply I was disturbed by the serious and undignified conditions which I found at Ft. Bayard." Although the patients appeared to be well-cared for, she observed a laxness of discipline throughout the hospital, and the chaplain was "filled with anxiety" about the "absence of supervision of the nurses in their social relations." She added that "every one smokes at Ft. Bayard." Jamme blamed the chief nurse. "I believe the whole difficulty lies with Miss Plummer." Samantha C. Plummer had been in the Army Nurse Corps since its inception in 1901, and had spent ten years at Fort Bayard. In peacetime, Jamme explained, the unit "maintained more of a family than a military life," but Plummer could not cope with the wartime expansion.[104] She was not aware of the problems in nurses' quarters because she went to bed early. Jamme did the rounds, though, and at 1:30 a.m. found lights on. Within days of receiving Jamme's report, the Army Nurse Corps dismissed the women accused of misbehavior, relocated Plummer to a small Army hospital in California, and transferred the nurses who signed the letter of complaint.[105] At about the same time, Jere Clayton issued his disastrous inspection report. With Fort Bayard's leadership in disarray, the Office of The Surgeon General began to ponder the future of its first tuberculosis hospital, now twenty years old and struggling.

To relieve pressure on Fort Bayard and as part of the nationwide effort to increase military hospitalization capacity, Bushnell surveyed the Medical Department's needs and options for expansion. When he asked Canadian officials how many tuberculosis beds he would need, they told him that 3,500 to 4,000 beds per million soldiers should be sufficient. That translated into 14,000 to 16,000 beds for an army that by the fall of 1918 numbered four million.[106] The Secretary of War ultimately approved eight additional tuberculosis hospitals, providing a peak capacity of 8,000 patients in January 1919. Some of these facilities were new construction, and others were conversions of existing facilities. These were General Hospital (GH) No. 8, at Otisville, New York; GH No. 16, in association with Yale University, in New Haven, Connecticut; GH No. 17, in Markelton, Pennsylvania; GH No. 18, in a converted hotel in Waynesville, North Carolina; GH No. 19, newly constructed in Oteen, North Carolina, and later named O'Reilly General Hospital; GH No. 20, at the former Army fort at Whipple Barracks, Arizona; GH No. 21, also newly constructed near Denver, Colorado; and, after the war had ended, GH No. 42 in Spartansburg, South Carolina, taking over the hospital of a former training camp.[107]

In the rush to accommodate thousands of patients, it was difficult, if not impossible, to reproduce the cloistered environment of Fort Bayard. New hospitals faced construction delays and shortages of competent and experienced medical officers and often received patients before they could care for them properly. The Surgeon General had to advise the new tuberculosis hospitals on such rudimentary matters as keeping tuberculosis patients in bed and ordered that "moribund or extremely advanced cases of tuberculosis should not be evacuated to other hospitals or sanatoria."[108] The new medical officers, or "emergency men," most of them civilian physicians, had little knowledge of tuberculosis or the military, and lacked the time to develop relationships such as those that medical officers had with many patients at Fort Bayard. For some hospitals, just providing good, nourishing food was a challenge. This was not a trivial problem because many people considered weight gain a key measurement of recovery, and tuberculosis patients often had tricky appetites due to their feverishness, or because the disease had spread to their gastrointestinal tract. Meals were even less palatable because the AEF had claimed most trained mess personnel, and many hospital kitchens lacked steam tables and carts, which meant they served hot food cold.

Two Troubled Hospitals

An examination of two wartime tuberculosis hospitals—GH No. 8 and GH No. 18—illustrates how the Medical Department struggled to meet the needs of tuberculosis patients. One of the first new hospitals was GH No. 8, in Otisville, New York. Although this facility was well funded and constructed to order, it suffered from poor management. In the fall of 1917, the Medical Department leased land owned by New York City and began construction in February 1918 on a 1,000-bed hospital (500 of the beds in tent wards), with a final cost of $1.5 million, or $1,500 per bed.[109] Patients began to arrive in June, several weeks before construction was completed. One of the first Medical Department inspectors to tour GH No. 8 declared it "an excellently constructed hospital." But there were warning signs that it would not be well administered, because the commanding officer, William J. Hammer, a civilian tuberculosis specialist who had joined the Medical Corps for the war, was absent. The inspector deemed him "a comparatively new officer, but should prove to be efficient," but by the fall, patients were complaining of poor treatment and bad food in insufficient quantities.[110]

When Bushnell visited the hospital in December, he gave Hammer the benefit of the doubt because of his extensive professional experience in tuberculosis hospitals, and because he was "more of a medical man than military executive and has had a difficult proposition organizing and equipping this hospital." Hammer also had to work with "officers of mediocre ability on his staff not of his own choosing but who were the best obtainable under the exigencies of war time service."[111] Soon, however, thirty patients signed a petition charging that they were not getting enough food, and a Medical Department inspector confirmed that the mess "did not meet the nutritional requirements of tuberculosis patients."[112] Inquiries by members of the U.S. Congress spurred the Army Inspector General to investigate and his inspectors were less sympathetic than Bushnell. They found conditions at GH No. 8 "unsatisfactory" due to the "lack of administrative ability of Major William J. Hammer," and recommended replacing him with a "field officer of the Medical Corps of suitable service, ability and experience."[113] Bushnell and the Surgeon General, perhaps preferring a poor administrator who knew tuberculosis to a good administrator who did not, initially rejected this recommendation.[114] But by late spring of 1919, with more medical officers returning from Europe, the Medical Department replaced Hammer with another "emergency man" from the civilian sector, Allen M. Smith, who proved to be an equally poor administrator. Food complaints persisted and inspectors declared that although the kitchen at GH No. 8 was well constructed and equipped, the "mess officer is manifestly unable to properly feed the patients at this hospital."[115] Surgeon General Ireland had to admit as much to a congressman and promised that he would take action.[116]

In late July 1919, the Army Inspector General, still on the case, took the unusual step of calling for the relief of Smith as commander, for "inefficiency and neglect of duty," and recommended disciplinary action against him for violating Army regulations regarding the purchase of meat and the use of Army transportation.[117] The Surgeon General's own inspector, Paul C. Hutton, who had been a patient and medical officer at Fort Bayard, was also appalled by conditions there. He called for disciplinary action against one of the hospital's medical officers, Edward W. Granger, "who failed to render adequate professional treatment to patients in #9 ward Sunday, August 17th."[118] The short-staffed Surgeon General still did not relieve the commander until the Army Adjutant General ordered him to do so.[119]

After eighteen difficult months, the Department finally closed the shiny new hospital and transferred the patients from GH No. 8 to other facilities.

Other hospitals contended with more competent staff, but problem facilities. The Medical Department established two hospitals near Asheville, North Carolina, home to some twenty private sanatoria and Charles Minor, Bushnell's mentor and a leading tuberculosis physician. The hospital at Oteen (GH No. 19) was constructed from the ground up and performed well, but the effort at GH No. 18, in Waynesville, was fraught with problems. Due to the "acute necessity" of the war, the Medical Department leased an old hotel and the surrounding buildings for conversion into a tuberculosis hospital.[120] Built in 1882, the hotel had three stories of brick construction, 80 rooms, and porches extending along the front and sides of the building. After several weeks of conversion work, the hospital opened in April 1918 with 250 beds inside, and 350 beds in tents. Members of Congress, such as Representative Zebulon Weaver of North Carolina, lauded the "splendid work" at GH No. 18, and welcomed the federal funds that came with the post.[121] The hospital, however, turned out to be a fire trap.

When Bruns visited in June, before the conversion was completed, he found littered grounds, buildings in need of paint, inadequate lavatories, and a poorly equipped kitchen attended by flies. He was so dismayed that the commanding officer, Charles E. Davis, felt it necessary to send him a long, explanatory letter. "The conditions you found distressed me more than you know," Davis wrote.[122] He attributed the deficiencies to lack of personnel and told Bruns that "I trust it will not be forgotten that when this Hospital opened and for a long period of time thereafter, there was not a single officer here who had had any previous military service whatever."[123] Coming from civilian life, Davis was also learning the art of command.

With additional personnel Davis was able to impose some order on the hospital, but in November the patient population exceeded capacity with 643 patients for 600 beds, and an inspector objected to tent wards on low ground that did not have suitable drainage. He recommended moving all of the patients in the tents to another hospital. On 5 December, however, Bushnell, mindful of the hospital bed shortage and the "exigencies of war," directed that the tents be moved to higher ground and provided more heat. The next day, however, the ubiquitous inspector Jere Clayton telegraphed the Surgeon General a dire warning: "Fire risk ominous" at GH No. 18. He described the main hospital building as "inadequate [and] dilapidated," and "tents so close together that if one takes fire all will burn." He ordered the immediate removal of every other row of tents to reduce fire danger, and required fire drills "in case of conflagration." Concluding that it was "not possible [to] adequately care for sick or their attendants [in] this institution," he recommended that "no more patients or enlisted men [from the] medical department be sent here and that the hospital be closed as soon as possible."[124] He confided to a colleague that the buildings and kitchens were "on a par with a dilapidated 'poor house' in a back woods county."[125]

When advised of this assessment the Surgeon General told Bushnell that "if loss of life should result there from after this recommendation has been made, the Medical Department might be justly blamed." The Surgeon General did not, however—perhaps could not—close the hospital, but instead approved Bushnell's plan to maintain the 600-bed capacity. Bushnell told Davis that "In view of the fact that the crest of the wave of tuberculosis patients is probably not yet reached…it would be inadvisable to give up this institution." Davis needed to make enough improvements to get the hospital through the winter.[126] With the press of patients, the hospital was forced to keep some on the second floor of the hotel, but added fire escapes and assigned only ambulatory individuals "who would be able to get up and leave the hospital without assistance."[127] Bushnell, acting more the military officer than physician, said that Waynesville had disadvantages but "they should not be magnified."[128] GH No. 18 avoided a conflagration, but in May 1919, when the training camp at Spartansburg, South Carolina, was no longer needed, the Medical Department closed the old hotel and transferred patients to a newly designated hospital at Spartansburg.

Not all of the tuberculosis hospitals were unsatisfactory. The Medical Department had a better situation at GH No. 20—Whipple Barracks, Arizona—perhaps because it was small and commanded by one of Bushnell's former medical officers, Major (Maj.) Carl Holmberg, who had been a patient and medical officer at Fort Bayard. The hospital opened in June 1918 with 150 beds, and for the next eighteen months it operated at capacity.[129] Holmberg established a standard of care for patients similar to that at Fort Bayard, instructed the medical officers in tuberculosis, and even held weekly medical seminars. Inspection reports were uniformly positive, ordering such minor changes as providing a sufficient number of fly swatters and providing lockers for enlisted men on duty.[130] However, even Whipple Barracks could not escape complaints about the food. But when a member of Congress forwarded such a complaint to the Surgeon General, the office responded with a petition signed by more than half of the Whipple Barracks patients stating that "this place is ideal in every respect for the care of tubercular patients."[131]

Even the ideal care of tuberculosis patients, however, could not ensure their survival. When Bushnell had told Rockhill of his plans to send Holmberg to Whipple Barracks, Rockhill informed him that Holmberg, who had been a patient at Fort Bayard two years earlier in 1916, still had "activity of the lungs." Bushnell replied, "I do not know how much to think of this." Holmberg, he noted, "has had rales for a long time. I do not think they amount to very much in his case. If that is the only ground on which the diagnosis is based, I should not pay any attention to it."[132] Carl Holmberg survived the war, but barely. Across the top of his efficiency report someone wrote in red ink, "Died 1-1-19." He was thirty-nine-years old.[133]

Race Relations

One of the ironic developments in the "War to Save Democracy" was that the increase in Army tuberculosis patients enabled the Medical Department to resegregate hospital wards by race. Before the war, as former Buffalo Soldier Charles Tyler had pointed out, social functions at Fort Bayard were often segregated or barred to African Americans. But medical services and benefits were not, in part because it was not practical in a hospital of only a few hundred patients already separated by rank and the severity of illness. In addition, the Buffalo Soldiers had shared duties with white soldiers in the West, and this tradition continued in the frontier environment of Fort Bayard. But with the wartime expansion the War Department renewed racial divides, which put it more in step with mainstream race discrimination. In March 1918, responding to complaints about integrated hospital wards, Surgeon General Gorgas circulated a memo to all Army hospitals stating that "it appears that it would be a better procedure, and for the best interest of all concerned, to arrange for the care of white and colored patients in separate wards or separate rooms, so far as possible." The memo added that, "It is appreciated that at times this might be difficult, if not impossible, as in the time of epidemic."[134]

Racial segregation and racism played out in several ways in the tuberculosis hospitals. One wonders, for example, about Gerald Webb's bedside manner with African American patients when he included racist jokes in letters to family and friends, even his son Gerry, age twelve.[135] GH No. 8, in Otisville, New York, ran segregated education and rehabilitation courses. The officer in charge, Matthew R. McCann, wrote that "from the beginning the presence of the two races has proved a source of embarrassment." When rehabilitation aides instructed black patients in English and arithmetic, they went to their segregated wards rather than teach them in the classroom because, McCann explained, "it was felt desirable to keep the races separate." Black and white patients also took separate daily walks, starting at different times "in order that colored men should not be at the rest house with white men." With no puzzlement or sense of irony, he concluded that the rehabilitation results for the black patients were unsatisfactory. "With the exception of two bright men who took up work in typewriting and bookkeeping classes with the white men," McCann wrote, "there was a general lack of interest and the classes were abandoned after eight weeks."[136] Jim Crow segregation was not conducive to a good rehabilitation program.

Most camps segregated social activities, too. While welfare organizations such as the Young Men's Christian Association (YMCA), Knights of Columbus, and the Red Cross provided recreational club facilities for patients at Army hospitals, African Americans at Fort Bayard did not get a club room until July 1919, and then representatives from the various organizations staffed the club "in rotation."[137] Black soldiers resented the second-class status at the hospitals, especially men who had served in the AEF in Europe and had risked their lives for their country. A hospital newspaper, *The Oteen*, of GH No. 19 at Waynesville, provides a glimpse of resistance to racism. When the newspaper began in 1918, it included a column called "A Dash O'Color," with a Sambo-stereotype cartoon as a header and contents including racist jokes and stories, perhaps written by white patients. By May 1919, however, a "Colored Americans" column replaced "Dash O'Color" with a drawing of a dignified, black Doughboy in salute (Figure 4-6). Instead of racist jokes, the column contained information of interest to the hospital's African American patients. One noted, for example,

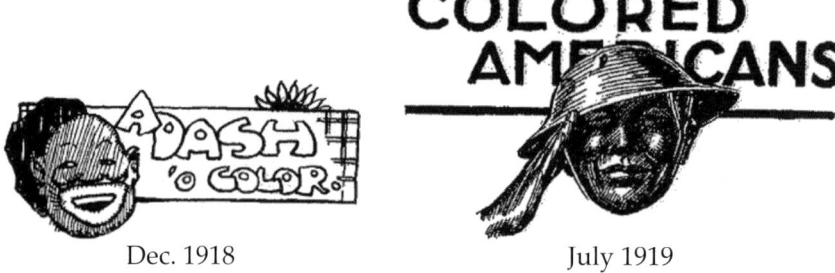

Dec. 1918   July 1919

Figure 4-6. Cartoons show African American patients asserting themselves at GH No. 19, at Oteen, North Carolina. The racist "Sambo" figure from December 1918 was replaced by the patriotic Doughboy in May 1919, in the hospital newspaper, *The Oteen*.
Courtesy of the National Library of Medicine, Bethesda, Maryland.

that "The Boys of [ward] E-9 wish to thank the Lt. Colonel for the carton of cigarettes which he gave them for the cleanliness of their ward."[138] Another column reported on entertainment that the Knights of Columbus offered African Americans. "This evening fills a long felt need and if we are to hope for further recognition of this sort, all should combine to shake the hand held out to us."[139]

The Influenza Epidemic

Unlike American society, tuberculosis recognized no color line. Nor did the influenza epidemic of 1918–19. In September 1918 the Army tuberculosis hospitals were hit by one of the worst pandemics in human history.[140] The first wave of influenza emerged in Army training camps in the spring of 1918 and traveled to Europe with the troops. There it flourished and mutated into a highly virulent second wave that exploded in early September in port cities in France, India, and the United States, and then swept the globe. Within months influenza sickened at least one-quarter of the world's population and killed an estimated 40 to 50 million people. Military and civilian physicians alike were appalled and helpless as the disease killed hundreds before their eyes. Normally, influenza is lethal only to the very old and very young, but this strain targeted young adults, ages 20 to 40, and could cause healthy immune systems to overreact, flooding victims' lungs with fluid and drowning them. It induced a deadly pneumonia against which medical treatment was impotent. Ultimately, influenza and related pneumonia killed more American soldiers and trainees during the war than did enemy weapons.

As influenza struck Army posts across the country, some institutions fared better than others. At Fort Bayard, Edward Rockhill identified Pvt. Cornie Gil as the hospital's first influenza patient. Gil had arrived from the military hospital at Ellis Island on 20 September and the next day had a temperature of 104.2 degrees, with the "typical symptoms" of vomiting, headache, backache, and sensitivity to light.[141] Within three days, six other patients fell ill and by the time the epidemic had passed, almost one-quarter of Fort Bayard patients (287 of 1,200) and one-fifth of the staff (115 of 595) had influenza.[142] To the west, at Whipple Barracks, about 27 percent (97 of 348) of tuberculosis patients got the flu, along with a staggering 42 percent (107 of 251) of staff.[143] Hospital commander Holmberg tried to quarantine the facility, but the war made that almost impossible. Whipple Barracks had to admit forty-seven patients and receive fifty-six new staff during the height of the epidemic, from 1 October 1918 to 14 November 1918.[144] "Of the fifty men who were sent here….during the quarantine," Holmberg told Bushnell, "nearly all developed the disease and six have died from pneumonia." And, he added, "so many of our nurses came down [with] the disease during the past week that we were obliged to go into the open market for temporary assistants."[145]

Some physicians expected the flu epidemic to be especially deadly for tuberculosis patients whose diseased lungs made them vulnerable, but Holmberg and others speculated that patients with tuberculosis in their lungs had "a sort of immunity against these strains" of influenza. The fact that medical staff was sometimes hit harder than patients seemed to support this view. At GH No. 16, in New Haven, medical officers observed that although 16 percent of the tuberculosis patients developed influenza, the rate among the corps men was twice as high.[146] The same was true at GH No. 17 at Markelton, Pennsylvania, where "almost no T.B. patients came down with influenza, whereas the healthy personnel of the same hospitals had many cases."[147] At GH No. 18 at Waynesville, North Carolina, only 5 percent (38 of 643) of tuberculosis patients had the flu, while 25 percent (72 of 263) of the healthy staff fell ill.[148]

Given the comparative isolation of many tuberculosis hospitals, some could keep their influenza rates down by prohibiting people from entering and leaving the posts. The chief medical officer at GH No. 21 in Denver explained that "during the height and severest intensity of the Influenza epidemic in this region, [November and December 1918] this reservation was kept under strict quarantine."[149] Incredibly, the hospital recorded zero cases of influenza among its more than 500 patients, and only six cases among the staff of some 400.

After the war, the Office of The Surgeon General studied the relation between influenza and tuberculosis, canvassing tuberculosis hospitals to learn whether influenza reactivated dormant tuberculosis or if tuberculosis patients were more liable to develop influenza than nontuberculous people. They found that less than 0.1 percent of influenza patients developed tuberculosis following their recovery from the flu.[150] A civilian physician reviewing studies from various sanatoriums reached a similar conclusion.[151] Some observers even speculated that influenza accelerated the decline in U.S. tuberculosis rates. In an editorial in the *American Review of Tuberculosis*, author Alfred Knopf noted that the tuberculosis rate declined 25 percent from 1900 to 1918, but that in the seven years following the epidemic the rate fell 41 percent. He attributed the reduction to improved standards of living and antituberculosis measures, but also he asked whether the influenza epidemic might have killed people quickly "who later might have developed [tuberculosis] and died of it."[152]

1919—More Trouble and Investigations

The warring nations signed an armistice as the influenza epidemic crested in the United States. With millions of fresh, well-fed American soldiers joining the Allied Army, the Central Powers of Germany and Austria knew they could not keep up the fight. The war ended on the 11th of November 1918. But despite the peace in Europe, the year 1919 would be one of the most chaotic in the United States' and world history.[153] As peace negotiators in Paris sought to remake the world, millions of people struggled with hunger, disease, and the wreckage of destroyed empires. A third wave of influenza swept much of the globe and typhus ravaged Eastern Europe. The major powers vied for control of colonies in Asia and Africa, and citizens sought to build new nations in the Baltic region, the Balkans, Eastern Europe, and the Middle East. Some regions fell into civil war, and after the 1917 overthrow of Russia's tsar, socialist revolution swept Russia, Hungary, and Germany, and threatened elsewhere.

The United States, relatively unscathed by the war, was not immune to the chaos. Antiforeigner hysteria and fear of Bolshevism fueled the first American "Red Scare." A newly elected Republican Congress refused to ratify the Treaty of Versailles or sanction President Wilson's beloved League of Nations. In September 1919, during a rail tour of the country to make his case for the League, the president collapsed in Pueblo, Colorado, and suffered a debilitating stroke that would incapacitate him for the remainder of his term as president. The economy staggered as the government cancelled war contracts and hundreds of thousands of soldiers returned home to reclaim their jobs. When corporations sought to roll back labor concessions won during the war emergency, workers resisted. Pressed by a tight labor market and wartime inflation that had outstripped wage increases, an unprecedented 20 percent of American workers—steel workers, miners, and transit workers, to name a few—struck in 1919 against increased hours and pay cuts. In addition to labor unrest, race riots wracked at least twenty-five cities and lynchings doubled between 1918 and 1919, to seventy-eight. Crowds murdered at least ten black veterans in their Army uniforms.[154]

In this time of anger and turmoil the Army opened its newest tuberculosis hospital in Denver, Colorado. During mobilization many cities had wanted military installations near them so they could benefit from the flow of federal funds. Community leaders in Denver believed that although posts, like training camps, might be temporary, a hospital for tubercular soldiers would be permanent.[155] The city therefore sent a delegation to Washington to make its case, and businessmen with the Denver Civic and Commercial Association raised $150,000 to purchase land east of Denver on which to build a hospital. When George Bushnell weighed locations for new tuberculosis hospitals, Colorado was a logical choice. For decades it had been a destination for health seekers and home to scores of tuberculosis sanatoriums, including the Navy's tuberculosis hospital at Fort Lyon. Some of the nation's best-known sanatoriums were in Denver, where Bushnell himself had sought treatment as a young officer. Before the war, some Coloradans had resisted the influx of tuberculosis patients into their state, worried about contagion and that the indigent sick could become dependent on local communities.[156] But patients in an Army hospital would be supported by federal benefits and the post could provide jobs to local residents. Denver had a climate comparable to Fort Bayard's, but located on national rail lines, it was less isolated. Given this, and the support of the local community, Bushnell chose Denver. In April 1918 the War Department signed a ninety-nine year lease with the Denver Civic and Commercial Association, and construction began in May. The Medical Department assigned Boulder physician William P. Harlow as commander to oversee construction and run the hospital.

Despite this goodwill, the new hospital, GH No. 21, got off to a rocky start. The hospital complex cost $3.2 million and soon comprised eighty-six stucco structures, with capacity for 1,400 patients. Buildings included approximately twenty open-air wards and infirmaries for officers and enlisted men, an isolation ward, quarters and barracks for medical personnel, and service structures such as kitchens, laundries, and the power plant. After the Armistice, the rapid demobilization reduced the military forces from more than four million to a little more than 200,000 by the end of 1919, generating a stream of tuberculosis patients found during discharge examinations. Patients began to arrive in October 1918, months before construction was completed.

In December 1918, inspector W. F. Lewis found fault with almost everything at the new hospital. He deemed "inadequate" the officers' quarters, the enlisted men's barracks, fire protection, the ambulance service, the laboratory equipment, the medical and surgical supplies, and the number and quality of the commissioned medical personnel. He also noted that the mess had been "inefficiently managed," and instructed the commander to "assure himself, by frequent inspections, that the meals served to patients …in wards are properly prepared and served in satisfactory condition."[157] In addition to material problems, morale had deteriorated across military hospitals because after the Armistice many patients and staff wanted to go home regardless of their illness or responsibility to care for the ill. Patient cartoonists at GH No. 42 in Spartansburg portrayed their frustration at having to pass numerous sputum tests before they could be discharged (Figure 4-7). Even Gerald Webb, who loved his job, told his wife in December 1918, "All I want is to get home and out now the war is over. I have no ambitions for promotion or anything else but to get back to you so quickly."[158] The morale problem among staff was so bad that in February 1919 Surgeon General Ireland advised all Army medical facilities that as far as the Medical Department was concerned, "the emergency is not yet over." He recognized that many medical personnel were anxious to be discharged from service and return home, but "you, who are not so fortunate as to have seen service overseas, have a deep obligation to those who fought and became casualties." He noted that "They have made their sacrifices; and yours is to be retention in the service until they have been made as fit as possible for return to civil life."[159] To drive home the point, Harlow, the GH No. 21 commander, began discharging "emergency men" according to their length of service and punishing poor behavior or neglect of duty with additional days in service. "This policy," the Army Medical Department observed, "notably improved the character of the services rendered."[160]

134   "Good Tuberculosis Men"

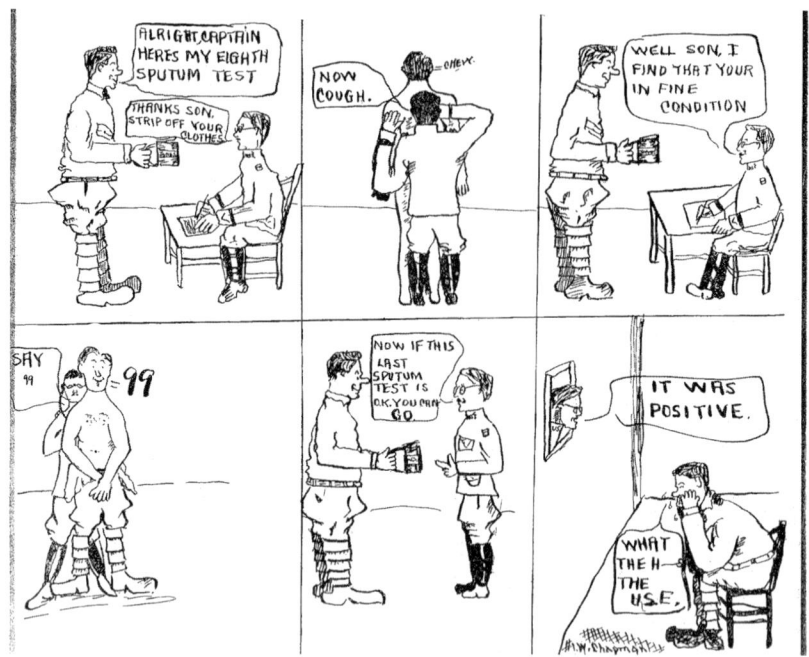

Figure 4-7. Cartoon portraying the frustration of sputum tests for tuberculosis at General Hospital No. 42 at Spartanburg, South Carolina, signed, I. W. Chapman, *Biand-Foryu*, 5 June 1919.
Image courtesy of the National Library of Medicine.

In even the best-run hospitals, tuberculosis patients had morale problems, resenting the rest treatment and confinement. But postwar military patients and their families were especially eager to get out of the hospital and vigorously asserted their rights and claim to benefits. The draft transformed the Army from a professional, volunteer organization to a conscripted army of "citizen soldiers," wherein men from all walks of life entered government service and demanded in return their rights and federal benefits.[161] Gone was the deference that patients and families had shown George Bushnell. Patients now argued with their physicians, challenged the chain of command, complained about the food, and demanded more access to their families. Some of the disgruntled went absent without leave, but others appealed to the media and elected officials for help.

To manage recalcitrant patients, GH No. 21 established a "disciplinary ward" for men sentenced to detention by court-martial or awaiting court-martial hearings. These wards posted guards to enforce rules of silence and bed rest. When several patients escaped or created a ruckus, medical officers resorted to putting them into straightjackets for twelve hours or more as punishment. Between December and February, medical officers put seven patients in the disciplinary ward into straightjackets.[162] Roy Parks, a mule driver in a coal mine before the war, arrived at GH No. 21 with tuberculosis in November and went absent without leave in December. He returned after a week with influenza and worsened tuberculosis symptoms. Sent to the disciplinary ward, Parks refused to use a throat spray and when a medical officer insisted, Parks cursed him and kicked his meal tray off the bed. The officer, Neill MacArtan, ordered Parks into a straightjacket. Patient John Evanka received the same treatment after escaping from the disciplinary ward and getting drunk with another patient. When a guard, Demet C. Sims, refused to put the jacket on Evanka, Harlow (the hospital commander) referred him to a court-martial for failure to obey an order. Staff also straightjacketed Joseph Willing for smuggling tobacco into the ward, Harold Bassett for having cigarettes in his possession, Charles Wilson for insubordination, William Morrisette for insubordination and refusing to take his medicine, and John Macon for assaulting a guard with a knife.[163] When an inspector—again, Jere B. Clayton—discovered this practice in February 1919, he stopped it immediately, but the matter soon became a public scandal that reverberated for months.

Patient Roy Parks was one of the first to go public. He reported the straightjacket incident to the hospital commander and inspector Clayton, and sent a six-page letter to his wife charging that his punishment had caused a pulmonary hemorrhage. She forwarded the letter to officials in Washington.[164] Several former patients, including E. R. McKee, collected letters from men who had witnessed the use of straightjackets and sent them to Senator George E. Chamberlain of Oregon, chairman of the Senate Committee on Military Affairs. Patients also complained about the food. McKee was particularly descriptive—the meat they served sometimes, he said, "had a kind of green tint, that looked like changeable silk: you looked at it sideways and it looked green and red, or all kinds of colors.... They also gave us milk that was blue and transparent: it had no appearance of milk that you would get any place else."[165] Another patient said, "We had stew all the time, and some of it was very poor; you could not eat it," while another told Harlow that "the coffee was bitter, and the milk was blue, and the eggs were not right."[166] The *Denver Times* began an investigative series on GH No. 21 in late May with headlines such as "Cruelty to Soldiers is Charged at Hospital 21" and "Yanks Say Bad Food is Served at Hospital 21."[167] Harlow responded clumsily to the criticism by putting guards at the hospital door to prevent outsiders from entering.[168]

Where once disgruntled tuberculosis patients were isolated on a remote plateau in New Mexico, now when they complained, they were heard. Just weeks after GH No. 21 received its first patients, at least six U.S. Senators and several members of the House of Representatives complained to the Medical Department about conditions at the hospital. A senator from North Dakota enclosed a letter from a Denver woman stating that, "The disciplinary ward of Hospital 21 under Col. Harlow's administration is a disgrace to the civilized world, no place on earth except in Siberia or Germany are such methods resorted to."[169] Other petitioners included Mrs. George Peabody of Petoskey, Michigan, who relayed her son's complaints about the food at the hospital to the Surgeon General, and William E. Hause, an infantry captain and patient at GH No. 21, who appealed to the Adjutant General of the Army for an investigation into conditions. Denver investment banker E. F. Powers sent *Denver Times* clippings about the poor hospital food to Secretary of War Newton Baker, demanding action "to the credit of the Government and the salvation of the boys."[170]

In response to the uproar, the Army Medical Department sent an investigator to GH No. 21 who confirmed so many of the problems at the hospital that the *Denver Times* claimed victory with the headline, "Charges at Hospital 21 are Upheld by Colonel."[171] But the inspector, E. R. Shreiner, minimized the problems in his memo to the Medical Department, believing that the food service was improving and that the use of straightjackets was "humane" and had been verbally approved by officials in Washington. He attributed much of the trouble to "sensationalism of the local press," and concluded that there was no reason to discipline any of the hospital officers.[172] The Medical Department, however, recognized that action was required and replaced Harlow with a career medical officer, Colonel Howard H. Johnson. This, and a transit workers' strike in Denver, seemed to take the wind from the scandal's sails. By 4 July 1919, the *Denver Times* reported: "Patients at Army Hospital Happy Now; New Commander Rooting out Abuses."[173]

But not everyone was satisfied. On 18 August 1919, Rep. William N. Vaile of Denver, to whom citizens and patients had sent their complaints, introduced House Resolution 245 calling for an investigation of conditions at GH No. 21. The resolution charged that the food served in the hospital "is insufficient in quantity, inferior in quality, and not properly adapted for the nourishment and sustenance of sick men," and that the treatment of patients was "inhumane, unnecessarily harsh, and of such nature as to retard recovery from disease."[174] Vaile asked the Select Committee on Expenditures in the War Department, which Congress had established to investigate war profiteering, to include this issue in its brief. The next month, Rep. Clarence Lea (D-CA), a member of the committee, and committee secretary B. A. Stuberg, while traveling to the West Coast to conduct committee hearings, stopped in Denver to hear testimony related to Rep. Vaile's resolution.[175] On 25 and 26 September, in proceedings at the hospital and the Brown Palace Hotel in Denver, they took testimony from more than thirty-five witnesses, including patients, medical staff, and several citizens about conditions at GH No. 21.

The hearings were anticlimactic. Most witnesses agreed that conditions had improved with the replacement of Harlow. The most contentious issue was whether the straightjacket had caused Roy Parks to hemorrhage. One of Parks' nurses, Margueritte Cunningham, testified that a straightjacket "would bring it [a hemorrhage] on."[176] But medical officer MacArtan testified that Parks had willfully punctured his nose with a pencil to induce bleeding, and two other physicians corroborated his assessment, one of them describing in detail for Rep. Lea the difference between bloody discharges from the lungs and the nose. This testimony, and the fact that a corpsman had seen Parks with a nosebleed, defused the argument that the use of straightjackets damaged patients' health. Some witnesses praised the hospital. Marine officer Kenneth Turner testified that he had been a patient in six American military hospitals and GH No. 21 "was the best institution I had come to"; and an American Legion investigating committee stated that "conditions in the hospital are ideal."[177] Witnesses also were unanimous that the food had improved with better-equipped kitchens and the employment of civilian cooks. Even Roy Parks said, "I have no kick on the food now."[178]

Patients did say that they left the hospital to eat when they did not like the meals. Stanley Ginther told the committee that he went out three or four times a week, as did Howard F. Kearns, who had been a tuberculosis patient in the hospital for ten months.[179] An astounding aspect of this hearing is that no one expressed concern that tuberculosis patients on leave or absent without leave could be a danger to others. Hospital commander Johnson did say that Army regulations required patients to stay in the hospital as long as they could benefit from treatment because of the National Tuberculosis Association's concern that patients who went home without proper care would result "in danger to the men and the community." The Secretary of War, he explained, approved the regulation "in order to cut down the spread of tuberculosis in the country."[180] But Johnson did not specify any medical criteria, nor did the congressman follow up on that point. The "tubercularization" theory of some tuberculosis infection providing immunity apparently informed the policy, eclipsing concerns about contagion. Not all patients, of course, would be infectious, but no one in the hearing discussed medical or scientific criteria—like a patient being sputum positive—as grounds for confinement to the hospital. The hospital approved passes in light of a patient's finances and his health. GH No. 21 medical director Thomas G. Clement said that leaves of absence "are all approved where the soldier has sufficient funds to pay his expenses while he is at home," and that a patient was generally allowed to go to the city "unless there is something in his [the patient's] physical condition or conduct as a patient which the ward surgeon states it might be detrimental for him to have a pass to go down town." Many patients, he said, had monthly passes.[181]

In the hospital's defense, Johnson pointed out that the problems at GH No. 21 were larger than the hospital itself, "the result of the lack of preparation for the war in the furnishing of proper hospital equipment and trained personnel."[182] The hospital survived the intense scrutiny and criticism of 1919, in part because many people recognized that the war emergency created conditions that would challenge even the best medical services. Congress took no action in the wake of these hearings, and the Republicans' eighteen-month investigation of the conduct of the war ended when Warren G. Harding became President in March 1921, and Republican control of the White House made criticism of the administration less attractive. As the Army decreased in size, public attention to conditions within the military diminished. The Medical Department was now committed to its new hospital in Denver.

End of an Era: Closing Fort Bayard and the Death of Bushnell

The tuberculosis hospital in Denver presented an alternative tuberculosis facility to Fort Bayard, which would soon become competition for the Army's first tuberculosis hospital. The Medical Department had greatly expanded Fort Bayard's patient capacity for the war emergency, but now had to consider the Army's long-term needs. In February 1919, Fort Bayard requested $900,000 to renovate existing buildings, increase the water supply, and improve utilities.[183] The Office of The

Surgeon General approved the improvements, but rumors of closure circulated. Col. E. M. Welles Jr., who had taken over command from Rockhill, sent a plaintive memo to the Surgeon General on 6 January 1919. "I have been informed by certain civilians in Silver City," he wrote, "that Fort Bayard is soon to be abandoned." If so, he needed to know ahead of time so he could sell the livestock "far enough in advance of the closing of the Hospital to get a good price."[184]

Like many rumors, this one had a kernel of truth. In 1919 the War Department assessed its postwar hospitalization needs. As the Army shrunk to prewar size it needed fewer hospital beds for soldiers, and more for the thousands of sick, wounded, and disabled veterans who would require hospitalization for months or years. The government therefore arranged to transfer some military hospitals to the Public Health Service for the continued care of veterans, abandoning other hospitals or returning them to the previous owners. In early 1919 the War Department operated fifty-five hospitals with about 64,000 beds.[185] Over the next year and a half it transferred twenty-five hospitals with about 23,500 beds to the Public Health Service, abandoned twenty-five more with 33,000 beds, and retained five hospitals with 3,700 to 7,000 beds. The Medical Department determined that the postwar Army needed only two tuberculosis hospitals, one in the East and one in the West. The choice for the East was one of the most successful tuberculosis hospitals, GH No. 19, at Oteen, North Carolina, "A city in itself," as described by one medical officer. "One year ago it was part corn field and part primeval forest. Today it has miles of cement roads, spacious lawns, flower gardens, a total of 97 buildings, its own power plant, laundry, garage, barber shop, post exchange, and houses 2,600 men."[186] But what about the western hospital?

In 1919, Fort Bayard lost its most powerful advocate, George Bushnell. His health deteriorated during his war service, and he experienced several lung hemorrhages in July 1919 and was forced to step down as head of the tuberculosis program in September.[187] After Jere Clayton's critical inspection of Fort Bayard in February 1919, Col. Roger Brooke, who would be Bushnell's successor, wrote, "I am strongly of the opinion that there are many reasons why the general hospital at Fort Bayard should not be continued or looked upon from this time on as a permanent hospital."[188] Although Brooke assured Welles that it would be "many moons" before the Medical Department abandoned Fort Bayard, the tide was turning.[189] At the end of the year, Brooke laid out for the Surgeon General the case for abandoning Fort Bayard. He argued: (*a*) the government had invested $3.3 million in the Denver location and only $1 million at Fort Bayard; (*b*) many of the buildings in Denver were "reasonably modern and well-constructed," whereas those at Fort Bayard were old and in poor condition; (*c*) Denver was "centrally located" near railroads that connected it to much of the country, while many of the staff and patients at Fort Bayard "object seriously" to the remoteness of its location; (*d*) labor and food supplies in Denver were "cheaper and more abundant" than at Fort Bayard; and (*e*) the Colorado climate had a "world wide reputation for promoting the cure of tuberculosis." Brooke concluded, "It is to the interest of the Government and of our personnel and patients to give up Fort Bayard as a hospital as soon as our patients are reduced sufficiently to be cared for at Denver or Oteen."[190]

A few months later, another senior medical officer, J. L. Chamberlain, went to Fort Bayard to evaluate the abandonment proposal and came back with a spirited defense. He noted that plans for a rail spur and a paved road from Silver City would ease the transportation problems. The hospital was growing its own food, and while the buildings needed repair, an investment of just $75,000 would modernize the site. Chamberlain stated that patient complaints had subsided and some of the earlier problems had been due to a "large number of emergency men who were continually clamoring to get out of the service." As for the isolation, he wrote, "[I]t is believed that removal from the temptations and attractions of a city constitutes a most valuable asset." Chamberlain reported that officers, enlisted men, and civilians "pleaded with tears in their eyes, that I would do everything possible to prevent a change, many of them stating that if they left there they would feel that they were going to their death." He recommended "urgently and unconditionally, that Fort Bayard as a tuberculosis sanatarium, be not abandoned."[191] Although Surgeon General Ireland was persuaded by Brooke's initial recommendation to abandon, Secretary of War Baker kept his options open, telling a congressional committee on 15 April 1920 that he was opposed to the recommendation, but "still studying it."[192]

In addition to the loss of Bushnell as an advocate, the War Department no longer considered Fort Bayard's isolation an asset. Bushnell had believed that proximity of family annoyed the staff and could excite the patient, slowing his recovery. As late as October 1917 he drafted a policy to prohibit patients from bringing their families with them to the hospital.[193] Surgeon General Ireland observed, however, that "great separation of a soldier from his family, particularly where prolonged treatment is required, as in tuberculosis, not infrequently depressed the patient—may even retard his recovery," and, he added, "frequently gives rise to complaints on the part of the family."[194] He therefore directed that the tubercular soldiers be transferred to Army tuberculosis hospitals near their homes.

Despite dissent within the Medical Department and opposition in New Mexico to the Army's abandonment of Fort Bayard, Secretary Baker acceded to the recommendation and the War Department transferred the hospital to the Public Health Service effective 15 June 1920.[195] The Office of The Surgeon General ordered Fort Bayard to transfer all enlisted patients and beneficiaries of the Soldier's Home to GH No. 21 in Denver, and convey responsibility for veteran patients at Fort Bayard to the Public Health Service. Army personnel began to pull out in May and on the 28th Fort Bayard threw a good-bye party that the *Silver City Enterprise* called "the most magnificent ever seen in the southwest."[196] As many as 5,000 people attended festivities that included band concerts, athletic events, a vaudeville program for bedridden patients, a banquet of roast turkey and young pig (most likely from Fort Bayard's stock), and dancing. The dinner program noted that the hospital had cared for more than 18,000 patients during its twenty years of service, and bade farewell with lines from a nineteenth-century poem, "You may break, you may shatter the vase if you will, But the scent of roses will cling round it still."[197]

The next month, on 26 June 1920, the Secretary of the Army issued an order renaming General Hospital No. 21, "Fitzsimons General Hospital," for Lt. William

Thomas Fitzsimons, a civilian surgeon serving as an Army medical officer and the first U.S. Army officer killed in the World War during an air raid at Dannes-Camiers, France, on 4 September 1917. The order noted that the name "also fittingly commemorates the eminent service rendered by the civil medical profession of America as members of the Medical Corps of the Army during the World War."[198] With its new name, Fitzsimons now joined the ranks of named Army hospitals in the country, along with Walter Reed in Washington, DC, Army and Navy Hospital at Hot Springs, Arkansas, Beaumont Hospital in El Paso, Texas, and Letterman in San Francisco.[199] With the transfer of Oteen hospital in North Carolina to the Public Health Service for veterans with tuberculosis in October 1920, Fitzsimons became the Army's sole tuberculosis hospital.

George Bushnell was not among the honored guests at Fort Bayard's closing ceremony. According to Earl Bruns, given the stress of war service, "he was in very poor health during most of the time."[200] Bushnell (Figure 4-8) had already reached the customary retirement age of sixty-four in September 1917, but Surgeon General Gorgas had immediately rehired him to continue running the

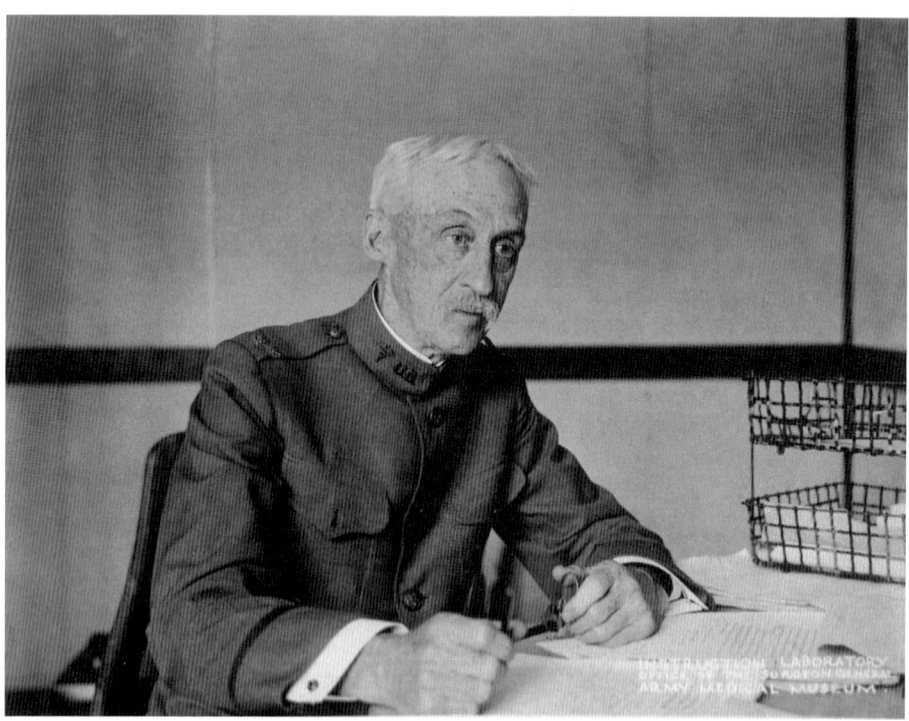

Figure 4-8. Colonel George Bushnell in his office while serving as head of the surgeon general's Office of Tuberculosis, showing the strain of war work and tuberculosis infection.
Photograph courtesy of the National Library of Medicine, Image #B03220.

tuberculosis program. When his health faltered, Bushnell stepped down from the post in January 1919, and retired on 15 October 1919. He returned to his home on a small farm in Bedford, Massachusetts, and wrote two books, *A Study of the Epidemiology of Tuberculosis* and *Physical Diagnosis of Diseases of the Chest*.[201] In July 1921, he traveled to London, appointed by Gerald Webb as the National Tuberculosis Association's representative to the "First International Union against Tuberculosis," and the next year lectured as Professor of Military Science and Tactics at Harvard University. In the summer of 1923, he and his wife Ethel moved to the more benign climate of Pasadena, California. The next spring, Bruns and other Fort Bayard alumni at Fitzsimons in Denver were looking forward to a visit by Bushnell when they received a wire that he was too ill to travel. Bushnell said he would visit when he felt stronger, but he did not recover from this tuberculosis breakdown. After several pulmonary hemorrhages, he died on 19 July 1924 at the age of 70 and was buried in Pasadena.[202]

Army Chief of Staff John L. Hines commemorated Bushnell and his tuberculosis work, noting, "His death removed one to whom many are indebted for their recovery from that dread malady in the past, and whose influence will be distinctly present in the future, wherever efforts are being made to overcome its ravages."[203] The Medical Department also honored Bushnell by naming roads, auditoriums, and an Army hospital after him. But the closure of Fort Bayard and the death of George Bushnell signaled the end of an era in treatment of tuberculosis. Instead of the isolation, rest, and the personalized care of Fort Bayard, medical officers contended with a modern, larger, more urban, and more bureaucratic institution, shaped by the demands of World War veterans and their advocates, and dedicated to more aggressive and invasive medical treatments. It was a new world of Army tuberculosis treatment, one where Bushnell's "good tuberculosis men"—some of whom who suffered from the disease themselves—would soon no longer be welcome.

Notes

1. On mobilization for the war see Robert H. Zieger, *America's Great War: World War I and the American Experience* (Lanham, MD: Rowman and Littlefield Publishers, 2000); Carol R. Byerly, *Fever of War: The Influenza Epidemic in the U.S. Army during World War I* (New York, NY: New York University Press, 2005); Jennifer D. Keene, *Doughboys, the Great War, and the Remaking of America* (Baltimore, MD: Johns Hopkins University Press, 2001 [hereafter cited as Keene, *The Doughboys*]); and Sanders Marble, "Professional Doctors but Amateur Soldiers: The US Army's Affiliated Hospitals Program, 1915–1955," *War & Society* 27 (May 2008): 39–58.

2. Charles B. Davenport and Albert G. Love, U.S. Army Medical Department Historical Unit, and U.S. Department of the Army, Office of The Surgeon General, *Statistics, Medical Department of the United States Army in the World War*, vol. 15 (Washington, DC: U.S. Government Printing Office, 1919, 1925 [hereafter cited as Davenport and Love, *Statistics*]); and Albert G. Love and Charles B. Davenport, *Defects Found in Drafted Men* (Washington, DC: Government Printing Office, 1920).

3. "Tuberculosis in France," *American Journal of Public Health* 7 (1917): 606–11; and "Tuberculosis in War," *New York Times* (28 April 1917). See also Halliday G. Sutherland, "Tuberculosis in the Fighting Forces of America," *American Medicine* 23 (1917): 305–7; Arthur Newsholme, "The Relations of Tuberculosis to War Conditions," *The Lancet* (20 October 1917): 591–95; Leslie R. Murry, "Tuberculosis and the War," *The British Journal of Tuberculosis* 2 (April 1915): 71–77; and R. Y. Keers, *Pulmonary Tuberculosis: A Journey down the Centuries* (London, UK: Bailliere Tindall, Cassell Ltd, 1978), 142–51.

4. For lower figures on tuberculosis among allied armies see James Alexander Miller, "Tuberculosis among European Nations at War," *Transactions of the National Tuberculosis Association* (1919): 179–96.

5. Editorial, "The Campaign against Tuberculosis in France," *American Medicine* 23 (1917): 287–88; on Rockefeller Foundation activities, see the annual reports on its website, http://www.rockefellerfoundation.org/about-us/annual-reports, accessed 24 August 2012; and Roy Porter, *The Greatest Benefit to Mankind: A Medical History of Humanity* (New York, NY: W. W. Norton and Company, 1997).

6. George E. Bushnell, "The Army in Relation to the Tuberculosis Problem," *Journal of the American Medical Association* 70 (15 June 1918): 1821–26. On tubercularization theory see Michael Worboys, "Before McKeown: Explaining the Decline of Tuberculosis

in Britain, 1880–1930," in Flurin Condrau and Michael Worboys, eds., *Tuberculosis Then and Now: Perspectives on the History of an Infectious Disease* (Montreal and Kingston: McGill-Queens University Press, 2010).

7. Arthur J. Myers, *Tuberculosis: A Half Century of Study and Conquest* (St. Louis, MO: Warren H. Green, Inc., 1970), 22.

8. George E. Bushnell, "Tuberculosis Bacteriemia and Massive Exogenous Tuberculosis Infection in Man," *Medical Record* 15 March 1919; Katherine Ott, *Fevered Lives*, 137–38; also George E. Bushnell, "Experimental Evidence as to Immunity from Tuberculosis Infection," *Medical Record* 18 January 1919. For similar views see William C. Pollock and James Hedges Forsee, "Tuberculosis among Doctors and Nurses at Fitzsimons General Hospital," *Military Surgeon* 75 (July 1934): 17–21.

9. William Osler, "The Tuberculous Soldier," *The Lancet* 2 (5 August 1916): 220.

10. G. E. Bushnell to Martha G. Ripley, 8 October 1910, Record Group112, Records of the Surgeon General of the Army [hereafter cited as RG 112], Entry 386, National Archives and Records Administration [hereafter cited as NARA]; and Andrew Anders to Chief Surgeon, American Expeditionary Forces, 31 December 1918, RG 120, Records of the American Expeditionary Forces, [hereafter cited as RG 120], Entry 2065, Box 5159, NARA.

11. Joseph F. Siler, U.S. Army Medical Department Historical Unit, and U.S. Department of the Army, Office of The Surgeon General, *Communicable and Other Diseases, Medical Department of the United States Army in the World War,* vol. 9 (Washington, DC: U.S. Government Printing Office, 1928 [hereafter cited as Siler, *Communicable and Other Diseases*]), 173. Before the development of virology in the 1920s and 1930s, medical scientists used the term virus to refer to a pathogen or disease agent.

12. G. E. Bushnell to A. E. Bradley, 5 November 1917, RG 120, Entry 2065, Box 5159, NARA.

13. Bushnell, "The Army in Relation to the Tuberculosis Problem," 1823.

14. Edward O. Otis, "Some Misleading Beliefs Regarding Pulmonary Tuberculosis," *Military Surgeon* 48 (February 1921). 164. See also Edward O. Otis, "The Soldier and Tuberculosis," *Transactions of the American Climatological Association* (1918): 160–67.

15. M.P., "The Nurse and Her Relation to Pulmonary Tuberculosis," *American Journal of Nursing* 20 (1919–20): 463.

16. See Siler, *Communicable and Other Diseases*, 191.

17. Leslie R. Murry, "Tuberculosis and the War," *The British Journal of Tuberculosis* 2 (April 1915): 71–77.

18. Maurice Fishberg, "Tuberculosis and War," *Journal of the American Medical Association* 68 (1917): 1796.

19. George Thomas Palmer, "Tuberculosis and War," *Journal of the American Medical Association* 69 (1917): 60.

20. Siler, *Communicable and Other Diseases*, 182.

21. Siler, *Communicable and Other Diseases*, 178.

22. G. E. Bushnell, "Lessons from the War as to Tuberculosis," *Journal of the American Medical Association* 70 (9 March 1918): 663.

23. Text of the circular may be found in Charles Lynch, F. W. Weed, and Loy McAfee, U.S. Army Medical Department Historical Unit, and U.S. Department of the Army, Office of The Surgeon General, *Surgeon General's Office, Medical Department of the United States Army in the World War,* vol. 1 (Washington, DC: U.S. Government Printing Office, 1923 [hereafter cited as Lynch, Weed, and McAfee, *Surgeon General's Office*]), 931–35; and Siler, *Communicable and Other Diseases*, 173–78. Bushnell describes the procedure in "The Diagnosis of Tuberculosis in the Military Service," *Military Surgeon* 40 (1917): 620–44, also published as "The Diagnosis of Tuberculosis in Military Service," *American*

Review of Tuberculosis 1 (1917): 325–52. For related correspondence on the article, see Commanding Officer, Fort Bayard to the Surgeon General, 5 May 1917, RG 112, Entry 23, NARA; and George Bushnell to Surgeon General, 5 May 1917, "Paper on the Diagnosis of Tuberculosis Camps in Military Service," RG 112, Entry 23, Box 466, NARA.

24. Unlike the technical preparations today, sputum tests involved simply looking at a stained sample through a microscope for tubercle bacilli.

25. Discussion regarding Jay Perkins, "What Shall be Done with Tuberculous Soldiers, Discovered in the Draft, in the Cantonments, Overseas?" *Transactions of the American Climatological Association* (1918): 176 [hereafter cited as Perkins, "What Shall be Done?"].

26. Lawrason Brown and Joseph H. Pratt, "Tuberculosis as an Army Problem," *Military Surgeon* 43 (August 1918): 157–59; and Siler, *Communicable and Other Diseases*, 179.

27. Siler, *Communicable and Other Diseases*, 193. On the history of X-ray technology see Bettyann Holtzmann Kevles, *Naked to the Bone: Medical Imaging in the Twentieth Century*, Sloan Technology Series (New Brunswick, NJ: Rutgers University Press, 1997); Joel Howell, *Technology in the Hospital: Transforming Patient Care in the Early Twentieth Century* (Baltimore, MD: Johns Hopkins University Press, 1995); and Barron H. Lerner, "The Perils of 'X-ray Vision': How Radiographic Images Have Historically Influenced Perception," *Perspectives in Biology and Medicine* 35 (1992): 382–97.

28. Mary C. Gillett, *The Army Medical Department, 1865–1917* (Washington, DC: Center of Military History, 1995), 99; and Vincent Cirillo, *Bullets and Bacilli: The Spanish-American War and Military Medicine* (New Brunswick, NJ: Rutgers University Press, 2004).

29. George R. Callender, "Roentegen Ray in Pulmonary Tuberculosis," *Interstate Medical Journal* June (1915): 598–603. See also Perkins, "What Shall Be Done?" 169.

30. F. E. Diemer and R. G. MacRae, "The Value of Chest Fluoroscopy," *Journal of the American Medical Association* 72 (18 January 1919): 172–74; and Ralph C. Matson, "The Value of Chest Fluoroscopy," *Journal of the American Medical Association* 72 (28 June 1919): 1893.

31. Siler, *Communicable and Other Diseases*, 194. In preparation for World War II, one medical officer supported the Bushnell policy because of the lack of resources and personnel trained in the use of X-rays. See William C. Pollack, "Tuberculosis in the Army," *American Review of Tuberculosis* 44 (1941): 659.

Chest X-rays are still considered but one of several means to diagnose tuberculosis, and the reliability of the analysis depends on the skill of the radiologist. See Michael D. Iseman, *A Clinician's Guide to Tuberculosis* (Philadelphia, PA: Lippincott Williams & Wilkins, 2000), 137–39.

32. Lynch, Weed, and McAfee, *Surgeon General's Office*, 468.

33. Clarence L. Wheaton, "Tuberculosis Control in Army Cantonment," *American Review of Tuberculosis* 3 (1919): 39–43.

34. Thomas McCrae, "Tuberculosis in the Soldier," *American Review of Tuberculosis* 2 (1918): 373, 375.

35. Discussion regarding Perkins, "Tuberculous Soldiers Discovered, What Shall be Done?" 177.

36. Hammond and Bushnell correspondence, January and February 1918, RG 112, Entry 31-J, Box 19, NARA.

37. Siler, *Communicable and Other Diseases*, 172.

38. John M. McDilly to Frank Billings, 15 January 1919, RG 112, Entry 31-J, Box 250, NARA.

39. Lynch, Weed, and McAfee, *Surgeon General's Office*, 950.

40. W. P. Chamberlain and various authors, U.S. Army Medical Department Historical Unit, and U.S. Department of the Army, Office of The Surgeon General, *Sanitation in the United States and Sanitation in the American Expeditionary Forces*, *Medical Department of the United States Army in the World War,* vol. 6 (Washington, DC: U.S. Government Printing Office, 1926 [hereafter cited as Chamberlain, *Sanitation*]), 431–73. See Siler, *Communicable and Other Diseases*, 182–85 for tuberculosis rates in each of the training camps. On the screening process at various training camps, see Francis E. Trudeau, "Special Tuberculosis Examinations in the Military Service," *Journal of the American Medical Association* 71 (7 September 1918): 818–22; Ralph C. Matson, "Examination of Recruits for Tuberculosis," *New York Medical Journal* 108 (1918): 199–203; and Lawrason Brown and Joseph H. Pratt, "Tuberculosis as an Army Problem," *Military Surgeon* 43 (August 1918): 139–59.

41. Matson, "Examination of Recruits for Tuberculosis," 201.

42. Gerald B. Webb to Varina Webb, 27 July 1917, Box 5, Gerald B. Webb Papers, Special Collections and Archives, Tutt Library, Colorado College, Colorado Springs, CO [hereafter cited as Webb Papers, Tutt Library].

43. Alexander Josewick to Gerald B. Webb, 28 December 1918, Box 5, Webb Papers, Tutt Library.

44. Earl H. Bruns, "The Tuberculosis Situation in the American Expeditionary Forces." Trier, Germany: Office of Civil Governor, American Area, Department of Sanitation and Public Health, 1919, RG 112, Entry 1011, Box 7, NARA [hereafter cited as Bruns, "Tuberculosis Situation in the American Expeditionary Forces"].

45. Siler, *Communicable and Other Diseases*, 198; and for a discussion of this process, see Siler, *Communicable and Other Diseases*, 587–609.

46. W. C. Gorgas, *Circular No. 24*, "Line of Duty," 11 September 1917, RG 112, Entry 10, Box 4614, NARA. See William S. Pollock, "Tuberculosis in the Army," *American Review of Tuberculosis* 44 (1941): 658–74, for a discussion of this matter.

47. J. H. Ford, U.S. Army Medical Department Historical Unit and U.S. Department of the Army, Office of The Surgeon General, *Administration: American Expeditionary Forces*, *Medical Department of the United States Army in the World War,* vol. 2 (Washington, DC: U.S. Government Printing Office, 1927 [hereafter cited as Ford, *Administration: AEF*]), 200, and Siler, *Communicable and Other Diseases*, 200.

48. Chamberlain, *Sanitation,* 515; and William H. Baldwin, "The Present Status of Soldiers and Draft Rejects with Tuberculosis," *American Review of Tuberculosis* 3 (1919): 322. See, for example, E. H. Bruns to H. M. Bracken, 5 July 1918, RG 112, Entry 31-J, Box 396, NARA.

49. Halliday G. Sutherland, "Tuberculosis in the Fighting Forces of America," *American Medicine* 23 (1917): 305–7.

50. Rep. Carl Hayden to W. C. Gorgas, 7 February 1918, RG 112, Entry 31-J, Box 20, NARA.

51. Siler, *Communicable and Other Diseases*, 199.

52. Chamberlain, *Sanitation,* 514.

53. Surgeon, Fort Ethan Allen to Surgeon General, 11 July 1917, RG 112, Entry 26, Box 91, NARA. On health in the training camps, see Nancy Bristow, *Making Men Moral: Social Engineering during the Great War* (New York, NY: New York University Press, 1996); Jennifer D. Keene, *World War I: The American Soldier Experience* (Lincoln, NE: University of Nebraska Press, 2011); and Allan M. Brandt, *No Magic Bullet: A Social History of Venereal Disease in the United States since 1880* (Oxford, UK: Oxford University Press, 1985, 1995).

54. Correspondence regarding George W. Troutman, RG 120, Entry 2065, Box 5159, NARA.

55. Louis Harris to Surgeon General, 14 January 1918, RG 120, Entry 2065, Box 5159, NARA; and "Disposition of Class D Patients," 24 June 1918, RG 1120, Entry 2130, Box 272, NARA.

56. Siler, *Communicable and Other Diseases*, 182.

57. Lynch, Weed, and McAfee, *Surgeon General's Office*, 376–77; Medical Department, U.S. Army, *Internal Medicine in World War II:* vol. 2, *Infectious Diseases* (Washington, DC: Office of The Surgeon General, Department of the Army, 1963), 331; and William H. Baldwin, "The Present Status of Soldiers and Draft Rejects with Tuberculosis," 323.

58. Memorandum, Office of The Surgeon General, "Discharge of Pulmonary Tuberculosis Patients," 15 April 1918, RG 112, Misc. Letters, Memos, etc., Box 18, NARA; and Siler, *Communicable and Other Diseases*, 193.

59. William C. Pollack, "Tuberculosis in the Army," *American Review of Tuberculosis* 44 (1941): 659; and Ford, *Administration: AEF,* 377.

60. Ford, *Administration: AEF,* 376 and 804.

61. See Siler, *Communicable and Other Diseases*, 185–90.

62. For more information on Webb, see Helen Clapesattle, *Dr. Webb of Colorado Springs* (Boulder, CO: Colorado Associated University Press, 1984); and Douglas R. McKay, *Asylum of the Gilded Pill: The Story of Cragmore Sanatorium* (Denver, CO: State Historical Society of Colorado, 1983), 58–64.

63. Gerald B. Webb, "The Effect of the Inhalation of Cigarette Smoke on the Lungs," *American Review of Tuberculosis* (March 1918): 25–27; and G. B. Webb, "Tuberculosis in the Army," *Journal of Laboratory and Clinical Medicine* 3 (1918): 137–39.

64. Gerald B. Webb to Varina Webb, 17 April 1918, Box 5, Webb Papers, Tutt Library.

65. Ford, *Administration: AEF,* 377; and Bruns, "Tuberculosis Situation in the American Expeditionary Forces."

66. Gerald B. Webb to Varina Webb, 2 May 1918, Box 5, Webb Papers, Tutt Library.

67. Clapesattle, *Dr. Webb of Colorado Springs,* 301. For a discussion of Webb's activities in the American Expeditionary Forces see pages 300–23.

68. Quoted in Clapesattle, *Dr. Webb of Colorado Springs*, 303–5.

69. Ford, *Administration: AEF,* 630–31.

70. R. J. Estill, "History of Base Hospital No. 8, U.S.A., July 17, 1917–March 6, 1919," RG 112, Entry 2130, Box 226, NARA.

71. Ford, *Administration: AEF,* 646–47; Morris Piersol, "History of U.S. Army Base Hospital #20," unpublished report, RG 120, Entry 2130, Box 270, NARA; and George Morris Piersol, "Internal Medicine as Observed at a Base Hospital in France," *Transactions of the American Climatological Association* (1919): 152–64. Several other hospitals had significant tuberculosis patient populations, including BH No. 86 at Mesves, BH No. 106 at Beau Desert, and BH No. 118 at Savenay.

72. Gerald B. Webb to George Bushnell, 20 July 1918, RG 112, Entry 31-J, Box 396, NARA.

73. George Bushnell to Gerald B. Webb, 7 August 1918, RG 112, Entry 31-J, Box 396, NARA.

74. Gerald B. Webb to William S. Thayer, 19 July 1918, RG 112, Entry 31-J, Box 396, NARA; and Gerald B. Webb to Varina Webb, 4 November 1918, Box 5, Webb Papers, Tutt Library.

75. A. R. Koontz, "War Gases and Tuberculosis: An Experimental Study," *Archives of Internal Medicine* 39 (1927): 832–64.

76. See, for example, Fort Bayard responses to Surgeon General inquiry, May 1919, RG 112, Entry 31-J, Box 20, NARA; and John L. Hankins and Walter C. Klotz, "Permanent Effects of Gas in Warfare," *Transactions of the National Tuberculosis Association* 18 (1922): 258–269.

77. Surgeon General memorandum, "Relation of Gassing to Tuberculosis," 14 May 1919, RG 112, Entry 31-J, Box 252, NARA. See also Hermann Harrison Cole, "A Clinical Study of Gassed Soldiers, with Special Reference to Pulmonary Tuberculosis," *American Review of Tuberculosis* 7 (1923): 230–55.

78. Editorial, "War Gases and Tuberculosis," *Journal of the American Medical Association* 89 (16 July 1927): 206.

79. Ford, *Administration: AEF,* 201; George R. Callender and James F. Coupal, U.S. Army Medical Department Historical Unit and U.S. Department of the Army, Office of The Surgeon General, *Pathology of Acute Respiratory Disease and of Gas Gangrene Following War Wounds, Medical Department of the United States Army in the World War,* vol. 12 (Washington, DC: U.S. Government Printing Office, 1929 [hereafter cited as Callender and Coupal, *Acute Respiratory Disease*]), 187–95. For more on pathology in World War I, see Cay-Rüdiger Prüll, "Pathology at War, 1914–1918," in Roger Cooter, Mark Harrison, and Steve Sturdy, eds. *Medicine and Modern Warfare* (Amsterdam: Rodopi, 1999).

80. Gerald B. Webb, "The Problem of Immunity to Tuberculosis," 25 December 1917, Webb Papers, Box 5, Tutt Library.

81. Gerald B. Webb, "Some Lessons of the War in Pulmonary Tuberculosis," *Transactions of the American Climatological Association* (1919): 114–28 [hereafter cited as Webb, "Some Lessons"]; and Clapesattle, *Dr. Webb of Colorado Springs,* 304.

82. E. H. Bruns to Henry A. Shaw, "Tuberculosis Immunity Investigation," 24 February 1919, RG 120, Entry 2065, Box 5159, NARA. Evidence suggests that a systematic review was never completed. See also G. E. Bushnell, "The Epidemiology of Tuberculosis in the Military Service," *Transactions of the National Tuberculosis Association* 15 (1919): 155 73.

83. Bruns, "The Tuberculosis Situation in the American Expeditionary Forces."

84. D. J. Glomsett et al., "What Can We Learn Regarding Pulmonary Tuberculosis from the Opportunity Afforded by the General Postmortem?" *War Medicine* 11 (1919): 993–94; and Webb, "Some Lessons."

85. Bushnell in discussion of Webb, "Some Lessons," 127.

86. G. E. Bushnell, *A Study of the Epidemiology of Tuberculosis, with Special Reference to Tuberculosis of the Tropics and of the Negro Race* (New York, NY: William Wood, 1920). See also a review by Edward O. Otis, *Military Surgeon* 48 (May 1921): 365–67.

87. G. E. Bushnell, "The Role of the International Union in Combating Tuberculosis," *American Review of Tuberculosis* 7 (September 1921): 602–10.

88. Edward R. Baldwin and Leroy U. Gardiner, "Reinfections in Tuberculosis: Experimental Arrested Tuberculosis and Subsequent Infections," *American Review of Tuberculosis* (1921): 510–13; and Edward Baldwin, *Tuberculosis, Bacteriology, Pathology and Laboratory Diagnosis with Sections on Immunology, Epidemiology, Prophylaxis and Experimental Therapy* (Philadelphia, PA: Lea & Febiger, 1927). For current discussion on immunity and tuberculosis, see Michael D. Iseman, *A Clinician's Guide to Tuberculosis* (Philadelphia, PA: Lippincott Williams & Wilkins, 2000), 63–96.

89. The following discussion is drawn from Jere B. Clayton, "Report of Sanitary Inspection of General Hospital, Fort Bayard, New Mexico, on February 19th, 20th, and 21st," RG 112, Entry 31-J, Box 20, NARA.

90. Clayton, "Report of Sanitary Inspection of General Hospital, Fort Bayard."

91. Surgeon General to Commanding Officer, Fort Bayard, 11 March 1919, "Recommendations made by Representative of Inspection Division, Surgeon General's Office," RG 112, Entry 31-J, Box 20, NARA.

92. Siler, *Communicable and Other Diseases*, 68.

93. *War Department Annual Report*, 1919, vol. 1, pt. 2, 2328. Syphilis also had high rates for days lost.

94. Christopher J. Juggard, "Copper Mining in Grant County, 1900–1945," in Judith Boyce DeMark, ed., *Essays in Twentieth-Century New Mexico History* (Albuquerque, NM: University of New Mexico Press, 1994), 47.

95. F. W. Weed, U.S. Army Medical Department Historical Unit and U.S. Department of the Army, Office of The Surgeon General, *Military Hospitals in the United States, Medical Department of the United States Army in the World War,* vol. 5 (Washington, DC: U.S. Government Printing Office, 1923 [hereafter cited as Weed, *Military Hospitals*]), 488–90; and "History of U.S.A. General Hospital, Fort Bayard, N. M., During World War," NARA, RG 112, Entry 31-J, Box 16.

96. Earl Bruns to George Bushnell, 4 July 1917, RG 112, Entry 31-J, Box 16, NARA.

97. Biographical information on Edward P. Rockhill from U.S. Army Surgeon General's Office Biographical Sketches of Medical Officers, Manuscript Collection 44, History of Medicine Division, National Library of Medicine.

98. Rockhill to Bruns, 10 June 1918, RG 112, Entry 31-J, Box 16, NARA.

99. General Orders No. 35, 19 October 1917, RG 112, Entry 31-J, Box 16, NARA; and Edward Rockhill to Bruns, 5 July 1918, RG 112, Entry 31-J, Box 16, NARA.

100. Surgeon General memo, "Women Physicians as Anesthetists," 12 March 1918, RG 112, Entry 31, Box 16, NARA.

101. G. E. Bushnell and Rockhill correspondence, June and July 1918, RG 112, Entry 31-J, Box 16. NARA. This could have been U.S. Representative Byron Patton Harrison (D-MS) or U.S. Representative Thomas Walter Harrison (D-VA).

102. Bruns and Rockhill correspondence, June 1918, RG 112, Entry 31-J, Box 16. NARA.

103. Correspondence regarding Anna Jamme inspection of Fort Bayard nursing personnel, February 1919, RG 112, Entry 31-J, Box 16, NARA.

104. Anna C. Jamme to Annie W. Goodrich, 15 February 1919 and Anna C. Jamme to the Surgeon General, 15 February 1919, RG 112, Entry 31-J, Box 16, NARA.

105. Dora Thompson memo, 7 March 1919, RG 112, Entry 31-J, Box 16, NARA. The Army Medical Department did not, however, take any action against the men—a captain and two sergeants—named in the complaint.

106. Correspondence between George E. Bushnell and the Department of Militia and Defense, Ottawa, July–August 1918, RG 112, Entry 31-J, Box 396, NARA.

107. For information on these hospitals see Weed, *Military Hospitals*; and for GH No. 16, see RG 112, Entry 31-J, Box 239; and *History and Roster of U.S. Army General Hospital No. 16, New Haven, Connecticut,* (New Haven, CT: Yale University Press, 1919); on GH No. 17, see RG 112, Entry 31-J, Box 244, NARA; and *The Star Shell* (1918–19) Markelton, PA, in the National Library of Medicine; on GH No. 42, see the *Biand-Foryu*, (1918–19), Spartanburg, SC, in the National Library of Medicine.

108. Surgeon General to Base Hospital, Camp Jackson, 1 February 1918, RG 112, Entry 10, Box 4614, NARA.

109. Weed, *Military Hospitals,* 516.

110. F. W. Weed, "Special Sanitary Inspection," 27 June 1918, RG 112, Entry 31-J, Box 208, NARA.

111. Memorandum, "Conditions at Army General Hospital No. 8, Otisville, N.Y. (Tuberculosis)," 6 January 1918, RG 112, Entry 31-J, Box 209, NARA [hereafter cited as Memorandum, "Conditions Otisville (Tuberculosis)"].

112. Memorandum, "Conditions Otisville (Tuberculosis)." Charles Eugene Perry also describes patient complaints at GH No. 8 in "The Rehabilitation of the Tuberculous Soldier," *Boston Medical and Surgical Journal* 181 (28 August 1919): 261–62.

113. Synopsis of Memorandum, "Conditions Otisville (Tuberculosis)," 11 January 1918, RG 112, Entry 31-J, Box 209, NARA.

114. 3rd Endorsement to Memorandum, "Conditions Otisville (Tuberculosis)," 16 January 1918, RG 112, Entry 31-J, Box 209, NARA.

115. J. B. Clayton, "Report of Sanitary Inspection of General Hospital No. 8 at Otisville, New York," 27 June 1919, RG 112, Entry 31-J, Box 209, NARA.

116. Merritte Ireland to Edmund Platt, 11 July 1919, RG 112, Entry 31-J, Box 209, NARA.

117. "Report of investigation concerning food and other conditions at U.S.A. General Hospital No. 8, at Otisville, N.Y.," 2 August 1919, RG 112, Entry 31-J, Box 209, NARA.

118. Paul C. Hutton, "Report of Sanitary Inspection of General Hospital No. 8 at Otisville, N.Y.," 16–19 August 1919, RG 112, Entry 31-J, Box 209, NARA.

119. Correspondence concerning GH No. 8, Otisville, August 1919, RG 112, Entry 31-J, Box 209, NARA.

120. Weed, *Military Hospitals,* 544-46.

121. Zebulon Weaver to Surgeon General Gorgas, 14 July 1918, RG 112, Entry 31-J, Box 247, NARA.

122. Charles E. Davis to E. H. Bruns, 2 July 1918, RG 112, Entry 31-J, Box 247, NARA.

123. Charles E. Davis to E. H. Bruns, 2 October 1918, RG 112, Entry 31-J, Box 247, NARA.

124. J. B. Clayton, "Report of Sanitary Inspector of General Hospital No. 18, Waynesville, North Carolina," 6 December 1918, RG 112, Entry 31-J, Box 247, NARA [hereafter cited as Clayton, "Sanitary Inspection Waynesville," 6 December 1918].

125. Correspondence concerning Clayton, "Sanitary Inspection Waynesville," 7 December 1918.

126. G. E. Bushnell to Davis, 16 December 1918, RG 112, Entry 31-J, Box 247, NARA.

127. Correspondence concerning Clayton, "Sanitary Inspection Waynesville," 6 December 1918.

128. G. E. Bushnell to Commanding Office, GH No. 18, 19 December 1918, RG 112, Entry 31-J, Box 247, NARA.

129. Weed, *Military Hospitals,* 556.

130. Inspection reports for August and December 1918, GH No. 20, Whipple Barracks, RG 112, Entry 31-J, Box 251, NARA.

131. Congressman William L. Nelson to Surgeon General, concerning complaint of L. E. DeVinna, September 1919, RG 112, Entry 31-J, Box 249, NARA.

132. George Bushnel to Edward P. Rockhill, 21 March 1918, RG 112, Entry 31-J, Box 19, NARA.

133. Efficiency Report of Carl Holmberg, RG 94, AGO, Box 5772, NARA.

134. Surgeon General, "Separation of White and Colored Patients," 22 March 1918, RG 112, Box 18, NARA. For more on segregation in the Army during World War I, see Gerald Astor, *The Right to Fight: A History of African Americans in the Military* (Novato, CA: Presidio, 1998); Arthur E. Barbeau and Lorette Henri, *The Unknown Soldiers: Black American Troops in World War I* (Philadelphia, PA: Temple University Press, 1974); and Mark Ellis, *Race, War, and Surveillance: African Americans and the United States Government during World War I* (Bloomington, IN: Indiana University Press, 2001).

135. Gerald B. Webb to Gerald B. Webb Jr., 5 May 1918, Box 5, Webb Papers, Tutt Library. For another example, see Gerald B. Webb to Benjamin C. Allen, 26 December 1917, Webb Papers, Tutt Library.

136. Matthew R. McCann, "Historical Sketch of Reconstruction Services, U.S.A. Gen. Hosp. #8, Otisville, N.Y.," April 1919, RG 112, Entry 31-J, Box 209, NARA.

137. "Colored Soldiers Get Club Room," *Silver City Independent*, 8 July 1919.

138. *The Oteen*, 9 November 1918, 16, National Library of Medicine.

139. *The Oteen*, 51 May 1919, 7, National Library of Medicine.

140. On the influenza epidemic, see Carol R. Byerly, *Fever of War*; Alexandra Minna Stern, Marin S. Cetron, and Howard Markel, guest eds., and David Rosner, contributing ed., "The 1918–1919 Influenza Pandemic in the United States: Lessons Learned and Challenges Exposed," *Public Health Reports* 125, suppl. 3 (April 2010); Nancy K. Bristow, *American Pandemic: The Lost Worlds of the 1918 Influenza Epidemic* (New York, NY: Oxford University Press, 2012); Alfred Crosby, *America's Forgotten Pandemic: The Influenza of 1918* (Cambridge, MA: Cambridge University Press, 1989; first published as *Epidemic and Peace, 1918*, Westport, CT: Greenwood Press, 1976) and John M. Barry, *The Great Influenza: The Epic Story of the Deadliest Plague in History* (New York, NY: Viking, 2004).

141. Edward Rockhill to Surgeon General, 27 September 1918, RG 112, Entry 31-J, Box 20, NARA.

142. Edward Rockhill, "Influenza," 17 April 1919, RG 112, Entry 31-J, Box 20, NARA.

143. Leopold Shumacker, "Influenza Report," 23 February 1919, RG 112, Entry 31-J, Box 252, NARA [hereafter cited as Shumacker, "Influenza Report"].

144. Shumacker, "Influenza Report."

145. Charles Holmberg to George Bushnell, 9 November 1918, RG 112, Entry 31-J, Box 251, NARA.

146. *History and Roster of the U.S. Army General Hospital No. 16, New Haven, CT* (New Haven, CT: Yale University Press, 1919), 17. See also H. J. Corper and E. D. Downing, "Laboratory Observations on the Influenza Epidemic in a Government Tuberculosis Hospital," *American Review of Tuberculosis* 3 (1919–20): 10–24 [hereafter cited as Corper and Downing, "Laboratory Observations"].

147. Roger Brooke, "Influenza," 15 February 1919, RG 112, Entry 31-J, Box 252, NARA [hereafter cited as Brooke, "Influenza"].

148. Walter Watterson to Surgeon General, 18 February 1919, RG 112, Entry 31-J, Box 247, NARA.

149. W. H. Bergtold, "Influenza," 14 March 1919, RG 112, Entry 31-J, Box 33, NARA. For a discussion of the impact of quarantine of a tuberculosis hospital see Howard Markel, et al., "Nonpharmaceutical Influenza Mitigation Strategies, US Communities, 1918–1920 Pandemic," *Emerging Infectious Disease* 12 (2006). Available at http://www.cdc.gov/ncidod/EID/vol12no12/06-0506.htm, accessed 24 August 2012.

150. Corper and Downing, "Laboratory Observations"; Siler, *Communicable and Other Diseases*, 162; and Brooke, "Influenza."

151. Maurice Fishberg, "Influenza and Tuberculosis," *American Review of Tuberculosis* 3 (1919–20): 543.

152. Editorial, "The Decline of Tuberculosis Mortality in the United States and the Influence of the Influenza Epidemic of 1918," *American Review of Tuberculosis* 13 (1926): 389. See also Roll H. Britten and Edgar Sydenstricker, "Mortality from Pulmonary Tuberculosis in Recent Years," *Public Health Reports* 37 (17 November 1922): 2843–58; and George Rosen, *Preventive Medicine in the U.S., 1900–1975: Trends and Interpretations* (New York, NY: Science History Publications, 1975), 32. The question of the impact of influenza on tuberculosis rates is still under examination today. See Andrew Noymer, "The

1918 Influenza Pandemic Hastened the Decline of Tuberculosis in the United States: An Age, Period, Cohort Analysis." *Vaccine* 29 (2011, Suppl. 2): B38–B41.

153. On the chaos of 1919, see Zieger, *America's Great War*; Cameron McWhirter, *Red Summer: The Summer of 1919 and the Awakening of Black America* (New York, NY: Henry Holt and Company, 2011); and Phyllis Lee Levin, *Edith and Woodrow: The Wilson White House* (New York, NY: Scribner, 2001).

154. On the events of 1919 see Joseph A. McCurtain, *Labor's Great War: The Struggle for Industrial Democracy and the Origins of Modern American Labor Relations, 1912–1921* (Chapel Hill, NC: University of North Carolina Press, 1997); Alan Dawley, *Changing the World: American Progressivism in War and Revolution* (Princeton, NJ: Princeton University Press, 2003); and Adriane Lentz-Smith, *Freedom Struggle: African Americans and World War I* (Cambridge, MA: Harvard University Press, 2009).

155. On the establishment of the new tuberculosis hospital at Denver, see Stephen J. Leonard, Thomas J. Noel, and Donald L. Walker Jr., "Honest John Shafroth: A Colorado Reformer," *Colorado History* 8 (2003); "Fitzsimons—The Story of a Hospital," *Military Surgeon* 65 (September 1929): 442–46; J. A. Wier, "The History of Fitzsimons Army Medical Center," *Denver Western Roundup* 36 (1980): 3–14; and Lyle W. Dorsett and Michael McCarthy, *The Queen City: A History of Denver*, 2d ed. (Boulder, CO: Pruett Publishing, 1986), 127.

The first official history of GH No. 21, Weed, *Military Hospitals,* 363, says it was located near Camp Miles, but there is no record of a Camp Miles in Colorado.

156. On resistance to tuberculosis patients, see Thomas A. Krainz, *Delivering Aid: Implementing Progressive Era Welfare in the American West* (Albuquerque, NM: University of New Mexico Press, 2005), 93–101; and a series of Public Health Service reports on "Interstate Migration of Tuberculous Persons," 1915, vols. 11–20.

157. W. F. Lewis, "Report of Sanitary Inspection of the Army General Hospital No. 21, Denver, Colorado," 22 December 1918, RG 112, Entry 31-J, Box 54, NARA.

158. Gerald B. Webb to Varina Webb, 9 December 1918, Box 5, Webb Papers, Tutt Library.

159. Memorandum, 11 February 1919, RG 112, Entry 31-J, Box 21, NARA.

160. Weed, *Military Hospitals,* 373.

161. Keene, *The Doughboys.*

162. Details on the use of straightjackets in GH No. 21 are found in U.S. Congress, *Hearings on H. R. 4474,* 68th Cong., 1st sess.; U.S. Congress, House Select Committee on Expenditures in the War Department, *War Expenditures*, 66th Cong., 1st sess. [hereafter cited as U.S. Congress, *War Expenditures*]; and E. R. Schreiner, "Special Report Relative to Complaint Submitted through Senator George E. Chamberlain," 3 June 1919, RG 112, Entry 31-J, Box 43, NARA [hereafter cited as Schreiner, "Complaint through Senator Chamberlain"].

163. U.S. Congress, *War Expenditures*, 189–90.

164. Schreiner, "Complaint through Senator Chamberlain."

165. U.S. Congress, *War Expenditures*, 743.

166. U.S. Congress, *War Expenditures*, 819 and 823.

167. "Cruelty to Soldiers is Charged at Hospital 21," *Denver Times*, 28 May 1919; and "Yanks Say Bad Food is Served at Hospital 21," *Denver Times,* 30 May 1919.

168. "Public Now Allowed in Hospital is New Order," *Denver Times*, 3 June 1919.

169. Letter forwarded to Senator Porter James McCumber (R-ND), "Dear Brother Elva," from "lovingly your sister, Edith," 11 June 1919; in RG 112, Entry 31-J, Box 43, NARA. Additional correspondence regarding problems at GH No. 21 can be found in RG 112, Entry 31-J, Box 43, NARA.

170. E. F. Powers to Newton D. Baker, 2 June 1919, RG 112, Entry 31-J, Box 43, NARA.

171. "Charges at Hospital 21 are Upheld by Colonel," *Denver Times*, 23 June 1919.

172. E. R. Schreiner, "Special Report Relative to Complaint Submitted through Senator George E. Chamberlain," 3 June 1919, RG 112, Entry 31-J, Box 43, NARA.

173. "Patients at Army Hospital Happy Now: New Command Rooting Out Abuses," *Denver Times* 4 July 1919.

174. U.S. Congress, *War Expenditures*, 4 September 1919, 177.

175. The Select Committee on War Expenditures also investigated complaints about conditions and the treatment of patients at Walter Reed, but these did not include tuberculosis patients.

176. U.S. Congress, *War Expenditures*, 721.

177. U.S. Congress, *War Expenditures*, 844 and 846.

178. U.S. Congress, *War Expenditures*, 819 and 698.

179. U.S. Congress, *War Expenditures*, 833 and 838.

180. U.S. Congress, *War Expenditures*, 858.

181. U.S. Congress, *War Expenditures*, 766–68.

182. U.S. Congress, *War Expenditures*, 857.

183. "U.S.A. General Hospital, Ft. Bayard, N.M., 1918," RG 112, Entry 31-J, Box 16, NARA.

184. E. M. Welles to Surgeon General, 6 January 1919, RG 112, Entry 31-J, Box 16, NARA.

185. The number of Army hospitals and beds changed almost every week because the Medical Department established additional hospitals during mobilization and the war, and then dismantled those hospitals during demobilization. These figures are drawn from Floyd Kramer, "The Year's Work in Military Hospitals and a Prospectus of the Future," *Military Surgeon* 47 (1920): 681–94; and "Memorandum for the Secretary of War," 14 April 1920, RG 112, Entry 29, Box 173, NARA.

186. Henry W. Hoagland, "The Treatment of Tuberculosis in the Army Hospitals," *Transactions of the American Climatological Association* (1919): 22.

187. Roger Brooke to Warfield T. Longcope, 14 August 1919, RG 112, Entry 29, 1917–27, Box 396, NARA; and "Obituary, George Ensign Bushnell," *Military Surgeon* 55 (September 1924): 423–24.

188. Roger Brooke, "Reply to Report of Sanitary Inspection of General Hospital, Fort Bayard, N.M., on February 19, 20, and 21, 1919, by Col. J. B. Clayton," RG 112, Entry 31-J, Box 20, NARA.

189. "Medical Department to Retain Hospital at Fort Bayard," *Silver City Independent*, 29 April 1919. See also "War Department to Retain Fort Bayard," *Deming Headlight* 7 May 1920.

190. Roger Brooke, "Memorandum for the Secretary of War," 11 December 1919, RG 112, Entry 31-J, Box 16, NARA.

191. Chamberlain memo for Chief of Staff, 13 April 1920, RG 112, Entry 31-J, Box 16, NARA.

192. Roger Brooke to Commander, Fort Bayard, 14 April 1920, RG 112, Entry 31-J, Box 20, NARA; and Congress, House Committee on Public Buildings and Grounds, "Public Buildings and Grounds," 15 April 1920, 66th Cong., 2nd sess., 4.

193. G. E. Bushnell to the Surgeon General, 22 October 1917, RG 112, Entry 31-J, Box 20, NARA. On the distribution of overseas patients to hospitals in the United States see Siler, *Communicable and Other Diseases*, 175–78.

194. Surgeon General to Adjutant General, 20 April 1920, RG 112, Entry 31-J, Box 16, NARA.

195. Under provision of Public Act 326, Section III, dated 3 March 1919. See congressional inquiries in RG 112, Entry 31-J, Box 16, NARA; and Carter Glass to Secretary of War, 5 April 1919, RG 112, Entry 31-J, Box 16, NARA; and Adjutant General memos, 12 May 1920, RG 112, Old Entry, 399, NARA.

196. "500 People at Bayard Farewell," *Silver City Enterprise,* 28 May 1920. See also *Silver City Independent*, "Military Stages Huge Celebration at Fort Bayard," 1 June 1920.

197. Program for the occasion of the Army's departure from Fort Bayard, May 1920, Silver City Museum. Poem may come from "Notes and Queries: A Medium of Inter-Communication for Literary Men, Artists, Antiquaries, Genealogists, Etc.," 17 November 1849, Gutenberg E-books.

In 1965, the Fort Bayard facility, comprising over 480 acres, was transferred to the State of New Mexico, which continues to operate the facility for various medical treatment programs.

198. General Order No. 40, War Department, 26 June 1920. For a biography on Fitzsimons, see Carol Byerly, "William T. Fitzsimons," in Sanders Marble, ed., *Builders of Trust: Biographical Profiles from the Medical Corps Coin* (Fort Detrick, MD: Borden Institute, 2011), 86–98.

199. Earl H. Bruns, "Colonel Bushnell: An Estimate of His Character and Work," *American Review of Tuberculosis* 11 (1925): 289 [hereafter cited as Bruns, "Colonel Bushnell"].

200. Bruns, "Colonel Bushnell," 289.

201. George E. Bushnell, *A Study of the Epidemiology of Tuberculosis with Especial Reference to Tuberculosis of the Tropics and of the Negro Race* (New York, NY: William Wood and Company, 1920); and Joseph H. Pratt and George E. Bushnell, *Physical Diagnosis of Diseases of the Chest* (Philadelphia, PA: Saunders, 1925).

202. Gerald B. Webb, "Colonel E. Bushnell, M.C., U.S.A.: An Appreciation," *Journal of the Outdoor Life* 21 (September 1924): 521–22.

203. Bruns, "Colonel Bushnell," 289.

Chapter Five
"A Gigantic Task": Treating and Paying for Tuberculosis in the Interwar Period

In May 1941, as the United States stood on the brink of another world war, Benjamin Goldberg, president of the American College of Chest Physicians, recited some stunning figures at the association's annual meeting in Cleveland, Ohio. He calculated that from 1919 to 1940 the Veterans Administration had admitted 293,761 tuberculosis patients to its hospitals. These patients had received government care and benefits for a total of 1,085,245 patient-years, at a cost of $1,185,914,489.56. These figures were "approximate," he added, because "many more millions of dollars have been utilized in the Army and in the Naval branch of the armed services, before members of those services having tuberculosis were invalided to the Veterans' Administration." As the nation faced another national emergency, he declared, tuberculosis specialists must advise the government on how to preserve the health of the nation and prevent a similar cost "in suffering and dollars."[1]

Goldberg's remarks reveal that although tuberculosis rates in the United States were declining 3 to 4 percent annually during the interwar years, the government's burden to care for tuberculosis patients remained heavy. The Army was only three-quarters the size it was before World War I (131,000 versus 175,000 strength) and experienced no major epidemics, so that suicide and automobile accidents became the leading causes of death in the peacetime Army. Although hospital admissions of active duty personnel for tuberculosis declined during the decade, tuberculosis admissions at Fitzsimons Hospital in Denver remained constant due to a steady stream of patients who were veterans of the war. Tuberculosis, in fact, became a leading cause of disability discharges from the Army and, with nervous and mental disorders, generated the greatest amount of veterans' benefits between the wars (Figure 5-1).[2] This phenomenon was generally the result of three factors. The first was the increasing complexity and cost of modern hospitals and medical and surgical practice. The Medical Department's tuberculosis program was decidedly bigger, busier, and more expensive at Fitzsimons Hospital than it had been at Fort Bayard. Located near a city rather than the

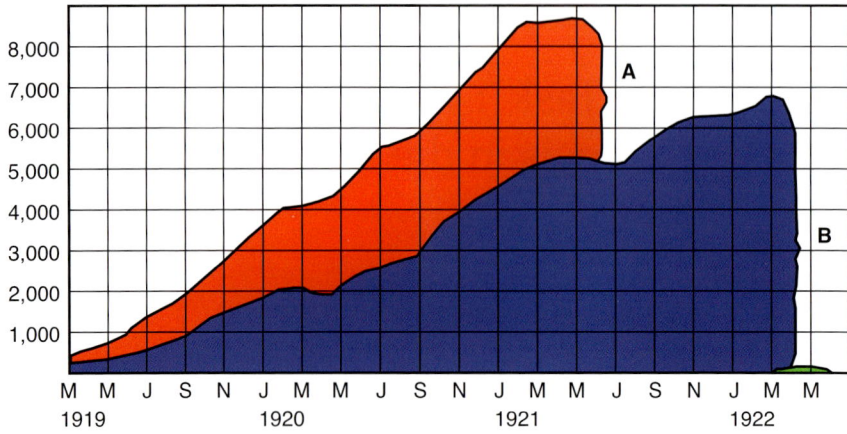

Figure 5-1. Chart showing increase in hospital care for tuberculosis veterans in the years immediately after the war, in Public Health Reports 37 (15 September 1922): 2248.
Available at http://www.ncbi.nlm.nih.gov/pmc/articles/PMC2000002/pdf/pubhealth rporig02581-0001.pdf.

mountains, Fitzsimons served as a general hospital for active military and veterans in the local region in addition to being a tuberculosis sanatorium, and it became a center of medical knowledge, skill, and technology. The second factor was a congressionally driven proliferation of veterans' benefits for tuberculosis in the 1920s and the large number of veterans seeking those benefits. Veterans comprised the majority of the patients at both Fort Bayard and Fitzsimons, but those at Fitzsimons faced a much more extensive and complex—indeed bewildering—array of benefits and programs that generated complicated administrative procedures and bureaucracy. The third factor contributing to the increasing cost of government care for tubercular soldiers and veterans was the development of new and more invasive therapies and rehabilitation programs that lengthened the already long hospital stays. The average length of the hospital stay for tuberculosis patients more than doubled from 148 days during the four-year time span of 1914–18, to 343 during 1929–31.[3]

Between World War I and World War II, the Medical Department also had to contend with tighter budgets. In the 1920s, Congress repeatedly expanded veterans' benefits but kept the War Department on a short rein, appropriating fewer funds than the department requested. These budget cuts made it more difficult for Fitzsimons and other Army hospitals to recruit and retain medical personnel and maintain the hospital plant and supplies. The story of tuberculosis in the Army after World War I, then, is one of increasing demand and decreasing resources, a dynamic that left Fitzsimons financially strapped even before the country entered the Great Depression. An examination of Fitzsimons' postwar environment—the modern hospital and technology, the ever-changing landscape of veterans' benefits, and new, invasive treatments for tuberculosis—illuminates these stresses.

Fitzsimons: A Modern Hospital in a New Environment

An Urban Community

Instead of standing on a remote mesa as did Fort Bayard, the postwar Army's tuberculosis program at Fitzsimons was embedded in American society. Denver at the time was buffeted by the turbulent social, economic, and political winds of the 1920s and after two decades of growth and the wartime economic boom, the city's economy staggered.[4] Fitzsimons also felt the impact of the tramway strikes in 1919 and 1920, for example, that cut the hospital off from the city until the commander made special arrangements for the transport of medical personnel. As the Ku Klux Klan gained strength across the country, fiercely defending native-born white Protestantism and punishing minorities, the *Denver Post* reported in 1924 that the "Invisible Empire" was the "largest most cohesive and most efficiently organized political force in the state of Colorado today."[5] It is not clear whether the Klan penetrated the hospital, but the religious life there was diverse. One of Fitzsimons' chaplains was Catholic, the other Protestant, and the post regularly offered Jewish religious services.

Less diverse racially, the War Department had retained few African American personnel during postwar demobilization and downsizing, and the Fitzsimons roster listed no more than one or two black enlisted men and no black nurses at all.[6] At the same time, however, Fitzsimons averaged about 100 African American male patients.[7] Unlike Fort Bayard, Fitzsimons maintained racially segregated wards, putting black officers and enlisted men together in the "colored" infirmary and ambulant wards with a separate recreation room, kitchen, dining area, and a sleeping porch. The Veterans' Bureau also established a hospital for black veterans at Tuskegee, Alabama. Despite such discrimination, African American soldiers and veterans had better access to healthcare than most black Americans. One study found that in 1928 in civilian society there was one hospital bed for every 139 white Americans, while 1,941 blacks had to "compete" for each available hospital bed.[8] This was not the case for black soldiers and veterans, however, because they were eligible for government hospital services, even if they were racially segregated. Fitzsimons did not segregate patients of other ethnicities. Mexicans and Mexican Americans, who worked in the post laundry, construction and maintenance, and on the hospital farm, were sometimes hospital patients and cared for in white enlisted wards.

Fitzsimons joined a host of tuberculosis hospitals in Denver, many established by ethnic and religious groups, including the National Jewish Hospital for Consumptives (1899); Agnes Memorial Sanatorium (1904); the Jewish Consumptives' Relief Society (1904); the National Swedish Hospital (1908); and the Evangelical Lutheran Sanitarium (1905).[9] This plethora of nearby hospitals allowed for close collaboration between Army physicians and other tuberculosis specialists. A medical officer told the Office of The Surgeon General that "our Fitzsimons pathologic presentations, I can say without exaggeration, attracted the attention of all the specialists throughout this section of the country."[10] Fitzsimons was certainly one of the most comprehensive sanatoriums in the region in terms of the services and programs it offered. It was the site for one of the first War Mothers' Homes, which offered accommodations to families who were visiting their loved ones in the hospital.[11] The American Red Cross was also on site, and showed Hollywood movies—two shows a night (the first for patients and the second for employees)—and set up radios in the wards to broadcast evening programs such as the baseball World Series. Other amenities included stables, a golf course, tennis courts, a baseball team, garage and service station, beauty shop, barbershop, restaurant, and newsstand. The hospital received national and international attention, with visits from President William G. Harding in 1924 and Queen Marie of Romania in 1926.

The Antituberculosis Movement

Very much a part of the bustling city around it, Fitzsimons operated in a world far less riven by tuberculosis than before the war. Although still a leading killer in the United States, the death rate from tuberculosis had halved in just twenty years, from almost 200 deaths per 100,000 people in 1900 to fewer than 100 deaths per 100,000 people in 1920, making the United States one of only three countries (with New Zealand and Canada) with rates below 100 per 100,000, or 0.1 percent.[12] These falling tuberculosis rates inspired redoubled efforts by the antituberculosis movement. Founded in 1904, the National Tuberculosis Association had chapters in every state by 1920 and ran annual Christmas Seal campaigns with the American Red Cross to raise funds and to tell the public that "tuberculosis is preventable and curable."[13] Governments at all levels promulgated antituberculosis measures, some of which were harsh. Arkansas barred schoolteachers with tuberculosis from the classroom, Alabama required that tuberculosis prisoners be segregated from the others, and Oklahoma refused to grant medical licenses to physicians with tuberculosis. At one point, the states of Washington and North Dakota prohibited people with tuberculosis from marrying.[14]

Most states required dairy herds to be tested for *Mycobacterium bovis*, the germ that causes tuberculosis in cattle, and by 1920 many large cities had outlawed unpasteurized milk. In 1925, no fewer than eight federal agencies were involved with tuberculosis control: (1) the Veterans' Bureau, (2) War Department, (3) Public Health Service, and (4) Office of Indian Affairs all managed hospitals for tuberculosis patients; (5) the Immigration Service screened newcomers for the disease; (6) the Department of Agriculture inspected cattle and swine for tuberculosis; (7) the Bureau of Mines investigated tuberculosis among miners; and (8) the Department of Labor and other agencies collected data on tuberculosis prevalence and control.[15] The interwar period was also the heyday of tuberculosis sanatoriums. Although in 1900 the United States had just thirty-four sanatoriums with 4,485 beds, by 1925 there were 536 institutions with 73,715 beds in the country. Many general hospitals ran tuberculosis wards as well.[16] These institutions produced so many journals and newsletters that they gave rise to an organization called Associated Editors of Tuberculosis Publications.[17] Despite the proliferation of sanatoriums, though, the vast majority of civilian tuberculosis patients (perhaps 90 percent) were treated at home.[18] This was not the case in the military, however, because Navy, Soldiers' Home, and Veterans' Bureau tuberculosis patients had access to hospital treatment, and many of them went to Fitzsimons.

A Modern Hospital

Cleaner and safer than ever before, by the 1920s the modern American hospital had become the preferred place for healthcare. By 1930, 65 percent of all births and 50 percent of all deaths in the United States occurred in hospitals.[19] National medical organizations moved to standardize hospitals in areas such as staffing credentials and levels, laboratory facilities, and operating equipment and procedures. The American College of Surgeons produced its first list of approved hospitals in 1919 and by 1925 had surveyed and accredited all government hospitals.[20]

The Army's new tuberculosis hospital stood as a center of modern medical expertise, technology, and training, and in the 1920s, was admitting and discharging 300 patients per month—almost the total patient annual capacity of Fort Bayard before the war. A complex of 160 buildings on 595 acres supporting 1,800 beds, Fitzsimons served as the Army's primary tuberculosis hospital and regional general hospital. The facility also offered outpatient services, delivering thirty to forty babies a year.[21] In addition to rest therapy, Fitzsimons' medical officers now treated tuberculosis patients with an array of new therapies, including physical therapy, surgery, and rehabilitation and vocational education. In 1929 Fitzsimons' laboratories completed 134,384 tests on patient blood, urine, feces, sputum, venereal lesions, and spinal fluid; produced 10,669 chest X-rays; and conducted 134 autopsies. Fitzsimons' surgeons performed 667 tonsillectomies, the dental department filled 1,663 cavities and extracted 2,169 teeth, medical personnel in the outpatient clinic conducted 601 physical examinations, hospital nutritionists prepared twenty different diets for patients, and the laundry washed three million pieces of dirty linen.[22] Fitzsimons was a big, modern, bustling facility (Figure 5-2).

Fitzsimons had twenty-three wards, seventeen of them for tuberculosis. Each tuberculosis patient admitted to Fitzsimons had a chest X-ray; a dental examination; an ear, nose, and throat examination; and submitted sputum, urine, blood, and stool samples to be tested for a variety of diseases and conditions.[23] Such procedures produced an increasing number of records and gave rise to new bureaucracy. Annual reports increased fivefold in length and ceased to mention medical personnel by name. Hospital correspondence referred to patients by number rather than name, and hospital management became so arduous that the commanding officer no longer had time to see patients.[24]

Not everyone welcomed the changes. George Bushnell's protégé Earl Bruns' career tracked the rise of the modern hospital. But as he assumed his mentor's mantle as the Army's tuberculosis specialist in 1921, he worried that large hospitals of more than 200 or 300 beds would be unmanageable and make it difficult for physicians to get to know their patients.[25] Born in Indiana in 1879, Bruns graduated from Miami Medical College in Cincinnati, Ohio, in 1903, and became an Army

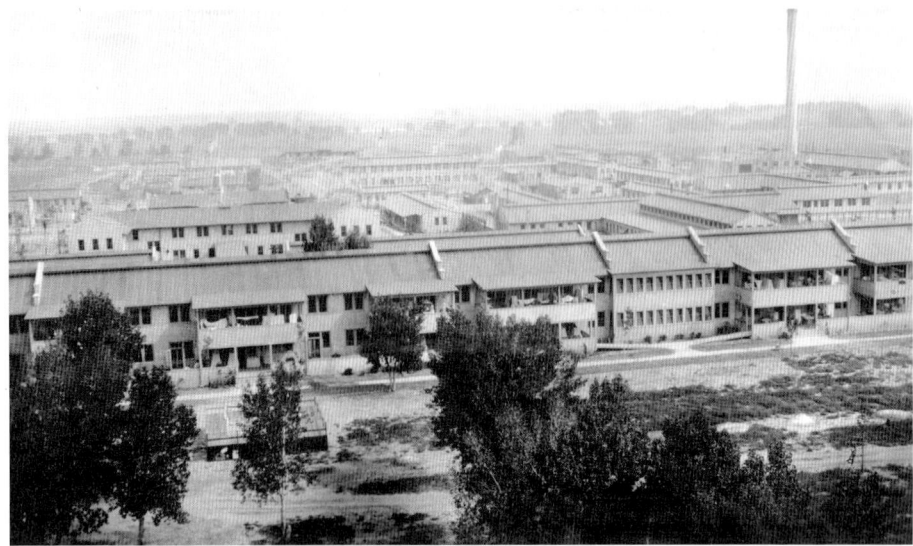

Figure 5-2. Overview of Fitzsimons General Hospital buildings in Denver, Colorado. 1920. Photograph courtesy of the Denver Public Library, Western Historical Collection, Image #Z-387.

physician in 1905.[26] He married Caroline Howard and after serving at several western posts, the couple went to the Philippines in 1906 where Bruns conducted research on tropical medicine until he fell ill in 1908. When Bruns and his wife arrived at Fort Bayard months later they both had tuberculosis. Bruns had active disease in both lungs, but after more than a year of complete rest he returned to light duty. Although his disease was "apparently arrested," records from 1913 and 1915 indicate that he still had tuberculosis bacilli in his sputum. Bruns eventually resumed full duty caring for patients and serving as Bushnell's deputy. After wartime service with Bushnell in Washington, the American Expeditionary Forces in Germany, and a course of instruction in tuberculosis in Switzerland, the Army Medical Department named him chief of medical services at Fitzsimons. There, Bruns (Figure 5-3) continued Bushnell's work, keeping the Medical Department at the forefront of tuberculosis treatment and research. He helped to structure, equip, and staff the Fitzsimons tuberculosis program, instructing medical officers in tuberculosis medicine, developing new therapies, and advocating the rehabilitation of tuberculosis patients to return them to a "productive way of life."[27]

Bruns recognized that the larger hospital could support specialists in fields such as orthopedics, urology, or neuropsychiatry, but he also believed that successful tuberculosis treatment depended on "the personality of the doctor in charge and the close personal contact between the physician and the patient." In 1923, therefore, he organized the Fitzsimons tuberculosis beds into seven 200-bed "units," each with one infirmary and two ambulant wards—to, in essence, transform a

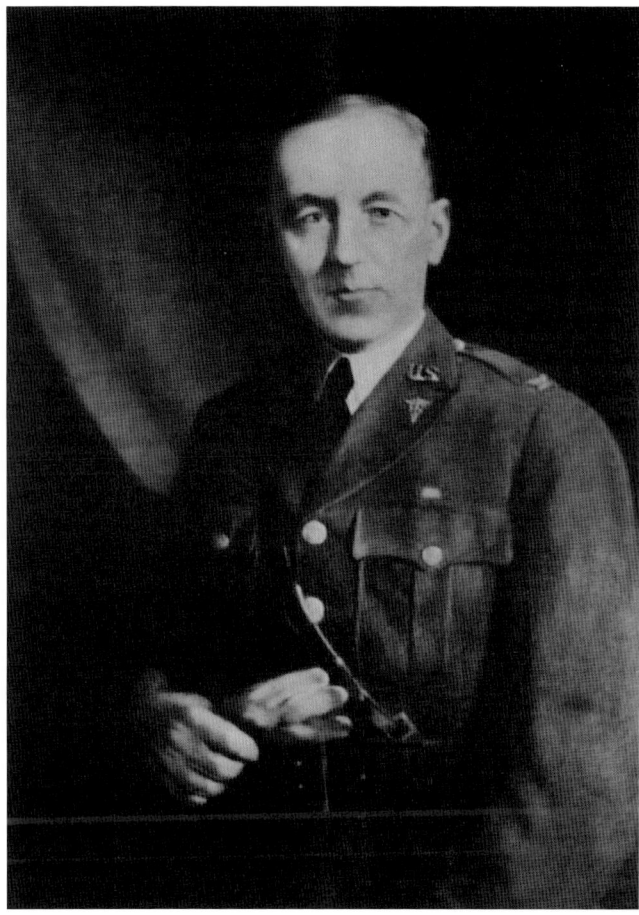

Figure 5-3. Portrait of Colonel Earl H. Bruns (1879–1933).
Photograph courtesy of the National Library of Medicine, Image #B03796.

large, impersonal institution into a collection of smaller, more intimate hospitals. Each unit operated as a separate sanatorium under the direction of one medical officer who would get to know each patient well and handle most of their tuberculosis treatments with support from specialists in other hospital departments. If, for example, a patient moved to the surgical ward for an appendectomy, or left the hospital and returned at a later date, he would return to his original unit and staff. Medical officers serving a four-year tour of duty would spend the first year assisting a ward officer and then the commander would select the most competent assistant to take over a ward. In 1926 Bruns reported that under the unit system "there is better cooperation and more kindly feeling between patients and doctors," and that it had succeeded because it was based on "the sound principle of continuity and individualization of treatment."[28] He believed such treatment afforded patients at Fitzsimons "the best opportunity" to get well compared to civilian patients, who had to contend with considerable "expense and privations" many could ill afford. "The treatment of tuberculosis is expensive," he noted, "because it means the best of food, the best of care, and the best of surroundings."[29]

Budget Woes in the New Army

Creating community, stability, and good patient care at Fitzsimons during the 1920s was not easy. After having four commanders in its first two years, Fitzsimons acquired more stable management in 1920. Colonel (Col.) William H. Moncrief Sr. (Figure 5-4) served as commander from September 1920 to August 1923, followed by Col. Paul C. Hutton (Figure 5-5), who ran Fitzsimons until September 1929.[30] Moncrief was a surgeon rather than a tuberculosis specialist, and never had active tuberculosis, but Hutton was intimately familiar with the disease. He had developed tuberculosis while on duty in the Philippines and went to Fort Bayard for treatment in 1905. Upon recovery, Hutton returned to duty as a medical officer at Fort Bayard. When transferred to Fort Seward in Alaska he investigated tuberculosis among Indian and Inuit peoples, in addition to his other duties. As a hospital in-

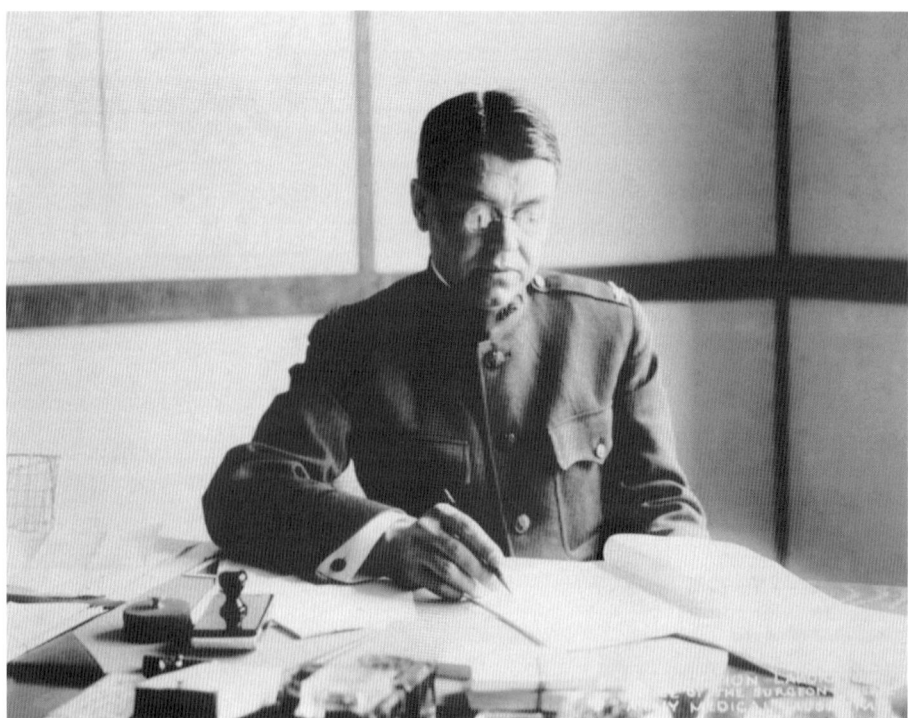

Figure 5-4. William H. Moncrief, commanding officer, Fitzsimons General Hospital, 1920–23. Photograph courtesy of the National Library of Medicine, Image #B019314.

spector after the war he visited Fitzsimons General Hospital seven times so that by 1923, according to the *Rocky Mountain News*, he was "perfectly familiar with every detail concerning it."[31] Also a student of Bushnell, Hutton carried on Bushnell's horticulture tradition, building greenhouses to furnish flowers for the hospital wards.

Moncrief and Hutton led Fitzsimons during a time of persistent budget and personnel shortfalls as Congress consistently reduced troop levels and cut War Department funding. The Department had proposed a peacetime Army of 500,000, but Congress—reflecting the nation's rejection of military and international involvement—was almost hostile to the military and authorized only 280,000 men in the National Defense Act of 1920 and further reduced troop numbers to 175,000 in 1922.[32] Army strength reached a low of 119,000 enlisted men and 12,000 officers in 1929 and stayed there for several years. The Medical Department shrank to a low of 11,535 in 1939 and the Surgeon General's staff fell from 2,100 during the war to only 177 people in 1934.[33] The National Defense Act of 1920 did promote the Surgeon General to the rank of major general, authorize relative military rank for members of the Army Nurse Corps, and create the Medical Administrative Corps to free physicians from paperwork. It also limited the Medical Department to only 5 percent of the strength of the Regular Army, below the 7 percent the Department recommended for peacetime. The Act based promotion on length of service instead of relative seniority, which meant that officers had to serve a certain number of years before promotion, regardless of vacancies in higher ranks.[34]

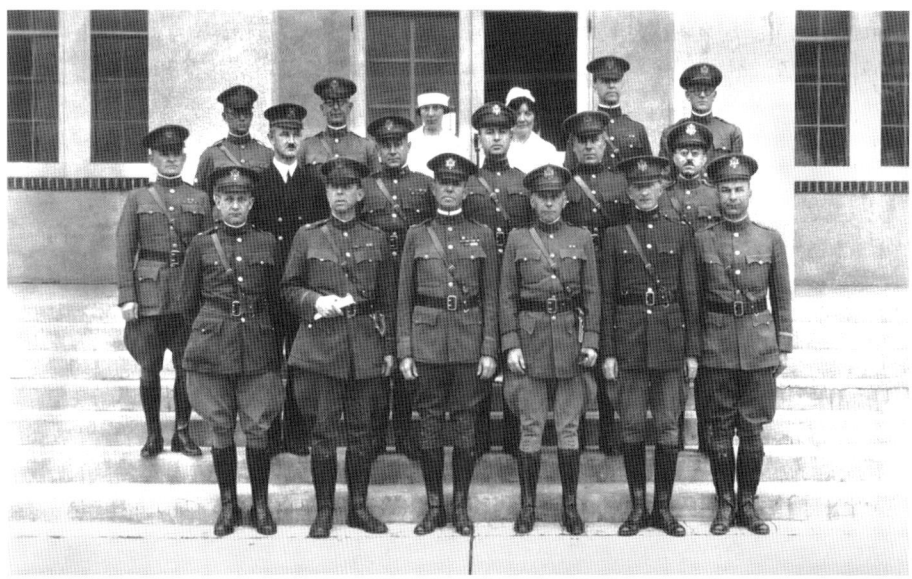

Figure 5-5. U.S. Army, Fitzsimons General Hospital, Denver, Colorado, Commanding Officer Colonel Paul C. Hutton (front row, third from left), and staff in the mid-1920s. Photograph courtesy of the National Library of Medicine, Image #A07785.

As private medical practice became increasingly lucrative during the 1920s, such provisions made it difficult to maintain a robust Medical Corps. Fitzsimons quartermaster Edgar W. Mumford told a Senate committee in 1921 that he had difficulty providing affordable housing to officers, and "I know a great many of these doctors will resign if their pay is reduced; they just can not get by."[35] Medical officers testified that they could not stay in the military service because they could not afford to send their children to college, maintain servants, or buy the requisite uniforms. Unmoved, Congress reduced the size of the Medical Corps, Medical Administrative Corps, Dental Corps, and Veterinary Corps to only 1,055, which required the Surgeon General to discharge more than 200 officers in 1922. Others resigned in response to the policy, leaving the department understaffed for years.[36] As historian Richard Ginn notes, "The department was held in high esteem by neither the civilian medical establishment nor the Army, and it experienced difficulty in recruiting qualified applicants."[37] In 1927 only thirty-five physicians took the entrance exam, and all but seventeen failed. Throughout the 1920s, Surgeon General Ireland struggled to maintain the personnel and resources he believed essential to meet the medical needs of the Army. One year he warned the Secretary of War, "In my opinion the Medical Department is less well prepared for field service than before the war with Germany."[38]

In 1922 congressionally mandated staff reductions required Fitzsimons to cut six of fifty-six officers. The Office of The Surgeon General told the commander, Moncrief, that fifty medical officers should suffice to meet the "minimum needs" of the hospital, adding superfluously, "we are expecting our officers everywhere to do more work."[39] Moncrief already faced a personnel shortage due to the recent arrival of 100 new Naval patients. He had three officers on sick report and others he considered unsatisfactory. In one case the hospital neurologist "is really not a neurologist, but a psychiatrist only, and Bruns tells me that he has not enough confidence in his judgement."[40] Staff cuts had made it "extremely difficult to maintain the desired morale," Moncrief reported in 1923. Without job security, medical officers "were not as keenly interested in the performance of their duties or in their professional advancement as would normally have been expected."[41] In 1926, laboratory personnel changed so often that they were not properly trained, and three years later Bruns warned Washington that "the shortage of medical officer personnel is interfering materially with the treatment of our patients."[42] This was compounded by the fact that the patient mix had become so much older and sicker that in 1929 Bruns had to reconfigure Fitzsimons tuberculosis units from one infirmary and two ambulatory wards to two infirmaries and one ambulatory ward. Bruns explained, "Most of the Veterans' Bureau tuberculous patients are far advanced cases who live in this vicinity and only come into the hospital when they have a flareup or an exacerbation of their disease." Consequently, "it is almost impossible for [a Fitzsimons medical officer] to supervise the treatment of all his patients, his time being devoted almost entirely to treating the very sick patients in the infirmary ward."[43] Enlisted personnel were lacking as well. In 1924 Fitzsimons was able to employ only 380 of the 450 employees they deemed necessary.[44] Funds for medical supplies and construction were also limited, though surplus war equipment and supplies lasted through the decade.

Staffing shortages and budget cuts required streamlining operations, adopting corporate management techniques, and cooperating with civilians.[45] In the medical field, Army hospitals such as Fitzsimons hired nurses from local areas and trained student nurses from three Denver area nursing schools in hopes of recruiting them for the Army Nurse Corps. In 1924 only 20 percent of the nursing staff was from the Army Nurse Corps and 8 percent from the Army Nurse Reserve Corps. The Fitzsimons chief nurse had to hire the remaining 72 percent from the local civilian nurse population and instruct them in military medical policy, procedures, and culture.[46] In 1929, to supplement its dwindling supply of medical officers, the Medical Department began requiring medical school graduates who held Army internships to remain in the Medical Corps for at least three years.[47]

In the postwar years, therefore, the U.S. Congress squeezed War Department budgets at a time when modern laboratory and surgical medicine made it increasingly expensive for the Army Medical Department to furnish and maintain hospitals. These budget pressures extended throughout the War Department and other branches of government, and when they hit the Veterans' Bureau, they intensified the Medical Department and Fitzsimons' problems.

Structuring Veterans' Benefits

Although Fitzsimons was an Army hospital, of its patients, a majority—74 percent in 1924—was veteran rather than active duty—a much larger percentage than any other Army hospital.[48] It was increasingly costly to provide tuberculosis care for these veterans, thanks to the legislative expansion of benefits for veterans with tuberculosis and expensive new forms of treatment available. Paying for those treatments, moreover, was complicated not only by the complexities of tuberculosis, but also by a continually changing and confusing government payment system.

Much of the historical attention to veterans' benefits during the interwar period has focused on the Adjusted Compensation Act of 1924, better known as the "Bonus Act" by which Congress awarded a lump sum payment to World War I veterans.[49] The bonus was in the form of a savings bond due to mature in 1945, but during the Depression economically suffering veterans launched a campaign demanding immediate payment from Washington, which culminated in the dramatic Veterans Bonus March of 1932. Although the bonus ultimately paid out in the 1930s, costing the U.S. Treasury $3.8 billion, the lesser known story is that the government spent more than two and a half times that ($10.2 billion) on medical and hospital costs and disability payments to World War I veterans during the interwar period.[50] In response to complaints and petitions from ailing veterans and their interest groups, Congress amended veterans benefits laws at least nineteen times in the decade following the war, generating a patchwork of benefits. Not surprisingly, much of the debate and legislation concerned tuberculosis, which was the single largest cause of disability payments for disease during the 1920s, claiming almost a quarter of all benefits.[51] The evolution of these tuberculosis benefits and their administration reveals the difficult if not impossible task of defining and legislating the circumstances under which veterans who developed tuberculosis merited government support.

The Medical Department had long avoided a heavy cost burden by simply discharging enlisted men with tuberculosis from the Army roster to the Soldiers' Home disability rolls so that the Home would assume payments and the patients could continue their hospitalization undisturbed. But by 1928 the Office of The Surgeon General told Hutton that "a great deal of pressure was [being] brought to bear from the Soldiers' Home authorities because of their lack of funds," so that Fitzsimons should retain tuberculosis patients—and the cost of their care— through their enlistment terms.[52] This practice added to the Medical Department's burden of tuberculosis treatment. At $4.50 a day, Fitzsimons' costs were comparable to those in other Army general hospitals. But this was about three times the cost of prewar tuberculosis hospital care.[53]

Administration

When the United States went to war in 1917 many in the Wilson Administration and Congress wanted to avoid a repetition of the late nineteenth-century situation whereby political parties competed for the veterans' vote by repeatedly expanding federal benefits for veterans and their families. By 1890 more than 40 percent of the federal budget went to Civil War veterans, and by 1915 virtually all veterans—93 percent—were receiving a federal pension.[54] Wishing to avoid similar long-term payments, the Wilson Administration did, however, recognize that a draft to build sufficient troop strength to fight this new war would lead to political expectations that the government would care for soldiers, sailors, Marines, and their families if military personnel were killed, wounded, or became sick in service. "It would be nothing less than a crime," Secretary of the Treasury William McAdoo told the Congress, "for a rich and just Government to treat its fighting men so heartlessly and to subject their dependent wives and children, who are unable to fight, to greater suffering than if they could fight."[55] The government thus sought to provide benefits based entirely on *compensation* for lost income and injury, and not *gratitude* for service to their country.[56] The United States would care for sick and injured veterans, but healthy surviving veterans should not expect long-term government support.

Congress began by passing the War Risk Insurance Act of 1917, which provided four kinds of benefits: (1) a family allotment of soldiers' pay to replace the loss of the breadwinner; (2) automatic compensation for death and disability; (3) additional, optional, government-subsidized life insurance of $10,000 per soldier; and (4) medical care in government hospitals. Army hospitals initially provided this last benefit because Congress failed to authorize or fund additional hospitals for this care. Congress also created the Federal Bureau of Vocational Education to provide rehabilitation training and payments to disabled soldiers. These programs did not include pensions, but, according to one historian, they "established unprecedented health care, disability, vocational rehabilitation, and survivors' benefits for World War I servicemen and their dependents."[57] After the war, thousands of these men remained in government hospitals; as of May 1921, the Bureau of War Risk Insurance was supporting 26,266 hospitalized patients, and at least 10,000 of them were suffering from tuberculosis.[58]

As thousands of sick and injured veterans overwhelmed Army and Navy hospitals, Congress turned to the Public Health Service (PHS) in March 1919 "to provide hospital and sanatorium facilities for discharged sick and disabled soldiers, sailors, and marines; Army and Navy nurses, male and female; patients of the War Risk Insurance Bureau; and other legal beneficiaries of the Public Health Service."[59] Established in 1798 for the care of sick and disabled seamen, the PHS had a long history of caring for sailors and members of the Merchant Marine, but it was not prepared for the scale of damage wrought by industrial warfare. Between March 1919 and June 1922 the PHS admitted 264,000 veterans for more than 14 million hospital days, and at a 1922 medical conference the PHS Surgeon General, Hugh S. Cumming, reported that approximately one-third of the patients in veterans' hospitals had tuberculosis.[60] Although the PHS operated twenty hospitals, it, too, was soon overwhelmed. Few had foreseen the magnitude of the tuberculosis problem. As two former Army medical officers, George T. Palmer and Henry W. Hoagland, wrote in 1921, "Neither in hospitals, sanatoria, nursing service nor competent medical personnel were we prepared for the great increase in recognized tuberculosis among our soldiers, sailors, marines and nurses." It was, they said, a "gigantic task," and the problem would endure "for perhaps twenty years to come."[61] The proliferation of agencies added to the confusing flood of patients. Because of Congress's patchwork approach to benefits, soldiers and veterans with tuberculosis had to go to the Bureau of War Risk Insurance for disability payments, to the Veterans Rehabilitation Bureau for disability training, and either the PHS or the Army or Navy medical departments for medical and hospitalization benefits. Veterans and their families complained to their government representatives about the bureaucratic nightmare. Veterans' benefits program administration was, one official later noted, "almost indescribably bad."[62]

Chaos reigned as to which agency was paying for what services for whom. In April 1920, Fitzsimons had about 800 vacant beds, but it could not admit several hundred discharged soldiers with tuberculosis because of bureaucratic red tape among various agencies.[63] Twelve hundred tuberculous veterans, in "a common battle against the life-sapping disease," converged on Tucson to compete for 278 tuberculosis beds available at the veterans' hospital there. The local newspaper headline read, "United States Red Tape Leaves Stricken War Vets to Die on the Streets of Tucson."[64] At the same time, some veterans received duplicate benefits. Fitzsimons commander Moncrief complained that it was unfair that veterans who received both Soldiers' Home and veterans' benefits could "pool their privileges and select the best from both sources," but the War Department avoided confronting that thorny issue.[65]

The Senate responded to the outcry by appointing a committee to investigate the administration of veterans' benefits, and it soon found that "unexplainable delays, confusion, red tape, complications, and intricate, slow-moving machinery have combined to increase the difficulties of the incapacitated ex-servicemen to the highest possible point in securing the compensation or aid to which they are entitled." The committee's July 1921 report described how the Federal Board for Vocational Education and War Risk Insurance conducted separate, duplicative physical examinations that confused veterans, and warned, "It would be unpardonable for Congress to tolerate a further continuation of the cumbersome, overlapping, haphazard methods under which this problem is being handled." The committee also stated, "we are convinced that there are not sufficient hospital facilities for attending to the two special cases of disease resulting from this war, neuropsychiatric and pulmonary tuberculosis."[66] A presidential committee had come to a similar conclusion, stating that because of the multiple government agencies, "There is no one in control of the whole situation."[67] Both committees recommended a single agency to handle veterans' benefits.

Congress responded by creating the Veterans' Bureau, and on 29 April 1922, the PHS transferred to the new agency fifty-seven hospitals (including Fort Bayard and several other Army tuberculosis hospitals), with 17,000 beds, 13,000 patients, 1,400 nurses, and 900 physicians and dentists.[68] The Bureau took over responsibilities of insurance, vocational education, and hospital care. Unfortunately, it began in scandal when the first director, Col. Charles R. Forbes, appointed by President William G. Harding, was convicted of fraud and sent to prison for selling off PHS surplus supplies and skimming funds from Veterans' Bureau accounts.[69] The appointment of former Army officer Frank Hines as Veterans' Bureau director in 1923 put the agency on more solid footing. In 1930, President Herbert Hoover consolidated all veterans programs, including Civil War pensions and the soldiers' homes, under one agency and renamed it the Veterans Administration, with Hines serving as director until 1945.

Eligibility

A single government agency, however, would not solve the problem of who was eligible for benefits and who was not. Regarding tuberculosis, the challenge was in determining whether soldiers and nurses who developed active disease after they had left military service had contracted it while in the Army—whether it was "service-connected." As with heart disease and some mental disorders, it was difficult, if not impossible, to determine the time and/or cause of onset of the tuberculosis infection.[70] At first the Medical Department ruled that men who developed tuberculosis in the first three months of service were not eligible for benefits because they most likely did not get the disease in the Army. But when trainees were discharged for tuberculosis without treatment several members of Congress protested this as an unfair denial of aid. The Medical Department reversed the policy and provided hospital and medical benefits to all military personnel diagnosed with tuberculosis, regardless of when they developed the disease, until they had received the maximum benefit of medical treatment. In 1918 Congress stipulated that every member of the Armed Forces should be presumed to be healthy upon entering the service and therefore entitled to compensation for subsequent illness or injury. During the war, therefore, the government discharged on disability about 20,000 men for tuberculosis and these men crowded the hospitals and depleted Medical Department resources.[71] After the Armistice, medical discharge examinations found several thousand more cases of active tuberculosis among outgoing soldiers who also required government hospitalization.[72]

But what of former soldiers who developed tuberculosis soon after discharge from the military? When government officials told such veterans that they were not eligible for benefits, some petitioned their congressional representatives for private compensation bills and Congress passed numerous bills awarding benefits to individuals who had been able to convince their senator or congressman of the merit of their particular case.[73] But this piecemeal and cumbersome approach lacked fairness, causing powerful interest groups such as the American Legion, Veterans of Foreign Wars, and Disabled American Veterans to take up the issue. The Legion was the largest, richest, and most influential of these groups, with some one million members in the 1920s. Awash in petitions and feeling the pressure, Congress sought a more efficient and equitable solution. In 1921 it stipulated that veterans with active tuberculosis or a neuropsychiatric disease causing a 10 percent disability within two years of service would be considered to have acquired it in the conduct of duty and be eligible for disability benefits. As the two-year time period expired, though, veterans with newly diagnosed tuberculosis or other ailments continued to accumulate, so Congress created a Committee on World War Veterans' Legislation to assess the problem. After holding thirty-one days of hearings and considering 200 amendments to the law, Congress passed the World War Veterans' Act of June 1924, expanding and bringing together into one program the various provisions governing veterans' benefits. As one observer put it, "The bill liberalizes the law in nearly every particular that we could liberalize it."[74] One key measure was a "presumption of service origin" stating that veterans who developed tuberculosis (or neuropsychiatric diseases, paralysis, encephalitis, or amoebic dysentery) between 6 April 1917, when the United States entered World War I, and 1 January 1925, were presumed to have contracted it during their military service and were eligible for government hospital and disability benefits.[75] One critic commented that the World War Veterans' Act amounted to "diagnosis by statute."[76] The measure added about 100,000 additional beneficiaries between 1926 and 1932, bestowing benefits, by one count, on a total of 328,658 veterans, almost 64,000 of them with tuberculosis.[77]

Disability

Determining who was eligible for benefits and which agency would provide them, however, did not solve the problem of how to calculate the degree of disability a veteran suffered or at what rate and for how long he should be compensated.[78] The World War Veterans' Act of 1924 directed the Veterans' Bureau to establish a table to calculate the extent of disabilities suffered by the nation's veterans, to create a rating system to calculate the degree of disability for various injuries and illnesses, and to award compensation accordingly. This table was heatedly contested by veterans and the federal government because it set out formulas that many people considered arbitrary. For example, a soldier who lost an arm was deemed 25 percent disabled while one who lost both arms or his sight was 100 percent disabled.[79]

But what about veterans with tuberculosis? Although a man could not recover an amputated arm or leg, some tuberculosis patients could recover their health. As with heart disease, tuberculosis could be mild, moderate, or severe; it could be aggravated by work or stress; and like mental illness, people could repeatedly recover and relapse. But did that mean that benefits should be terminated when a veteran's health improved? No, said Rep. Carroll Reece of Tennessee, who had a large number of tubercular ex-servicemen and a large tuberculosis sanatorium in his district. As he told his colleagues on the House floor, "Experts are agreed that there is no permanent cure for tuberculosis," Reece explained, but rather the disease is either "active or arrested." "By arrested is meant the germ is temporarily inactive, but will become active upon the slightest provocation." He argued therefore that "a system of permanent rating for the tuberculars must be adopted" to enable them to live peacefully with their disease quiescent. Reducing benefits when the tuberculosis was arrested would require the veteran to go back to work to support his family, even though it could shorten his life. "The conditions under which the tubercular patient may live," he said, "together with the resulting mental ease or mental disquietude, largely affect his power of resistance." Such work and worry could reactivate the disease, causing veterans who had been discharged as "arrested" to return to government hospitals as reactivated cases.[80]

Faced with such arguments, in January 1926 the Special Committee on World War Veterans Legislation considered provisions to determine disability payments for tubercular veterans, which included designations such as "temporary total disability" for patients in the hospital who were expected to recover or "permanent partial benefits" for patients who could regain only a portion of their health. The discussion revealed the difficulty of writing laws and setting benefits for such a complex disease.[81] Committee members tried to use analogies to understand tuberculosis, one member stating that "lung tuberculosis...cuts off a piece of that lung as definitely as an amputated limb, the amount depending on where the amputation takes place."[82] One witness, Dr. William LeRoy Dunn of Asheville, North Carolina, employed a horsepower metaphor, explaining that a healthy man operated at 100 horsepower, but a man who had active tuberculosis, even if he recovered, would never operate at full capacity again. "It may be 50, 70, 80, or 90 horsepower," he said. "He is safe at or under 90 horsepower, but you can not safely work him at 100 or 110...because he would get into trouble and burn out something."[83]

During one hearing committee members sparred verbally with tuberculosis specialists Dunn and Dr. Kenneth Dunham of the University of Cincinnati, both of whom worked with the American Legion and advised the Veterans' Bureau. The issue was the extent to which tuberculosis disabled an individual. When the physicians insisted that a 10 percent disability rating was too low, the committee tried to get them to recommend a single disability rating. They demurred. Every patient was different, they said, depending on the man, the extent of his disease, his occupation, and where he lived. Textile workers or miners, for instance, would be more likely to reactivate their disease than men working outdoors.[84] The witnesses agreed that tuberculosis disability typically exceeded 25 percent, but insisted that "it is almost impossible for the average doctor to exactly evaluate your disability in tuberculosis."[85] Members of Congress grappled with the difference between arrested and cured tuberculosis. One representative asked, "A man is never cured of tuberculosis?" to which the physician replied, "In a pathological sense he is never cured, practically speaking." The congressman therefore concluded, "If he is never cured he must have a handicap."[86] Another, Rep. John Rankin of Mississippi, asked, "Do you concede there is any such thing as a cured case of tuberculosis?" to which Dunn replied, "No, sir." "You never go further, then, than arrested?" asked Rankin. "No," replied Dunn.[87] Dunham finally suggested that Congress sidestep "a lot of intricate, difficult medical judgment" and simply to say that if a man had had tuberculosis, he should be given $50 [50 percent disability] a month.[88] Veterans' Bureau Director Hines quickly pointed out that "Now of course, a provision of a flat rate covering any disability is getting close to the pension system which I understand the ex-service men desire to avoid and most certainly we do."[89] He did not, however, oppose the proposal.

The spectre of thousands of veterans individually appealing to their elected officials for assistance caused Congress in July 1926 to approve a single standard for a permanent 50 percent disability for ex-servicemen with "arrested tuberculosis."[90] This provision, called the "statutory tuberculosis award," more than tripled the number of veterans covered from 12,019 in 1926 to 38,701 two years later, and increased the average payment to tuberculous veterans from $16.80 a month to just under $50.00 a month.[91] Military tuberculosis patients had become a "vast monetary expense" for the government.[92]

In 1930, twelve years after the end of the war, Congress awarded all disabled World War I veterans a new round of disability benefits in *gratitude* for wartime service. These non-service-connected benefits increased the pension rolls from 229,568 beneficiaries receiving $29.6 million in 1931 to 407,584 beneficiaries receiving $75.4 million in 1932.[93] Historian Walter Hickel has concluded that "despite the intentions of the War Risk Insurance Act's framers, compensation had become recompense for military service rather than for disability and its economic effect on veterans."[94] Veterans and their advocates were so successful that by the early 1930s more than 90 percent of federal social spending was on veterans' benefits.

Tuberculosis Rehabilitation

Veterans' rehabilitation programs also affected Army hospitals and government coffers by adding weeks or months to the time disabled soldiers were hospitalized.[95] Like many war wounds, tuberculosis robbed its victims of the energy and strength required for physical labor, long workdays, or simply living. Rehabilitation was intended to restore disabled men to productive work. It had nineteenth-century roots in efforts to educate and train freed slaves after emancipation and in Progressive Era efforts to retrain victims of industrial accidents for new occupations and help immigrants and the poor support themselves.[96] These programs did not require the labor market to make allowances for the needs of the disabled, but focused instead on helping the freedman, disabled worker, immigrant, or veteran adjust to the economy. Before the war, prevailing views held that disabled men were diminished individuals—but thousands of injured American war veterans (and millions in Europe) who were warriors and heroes challenged that view. Manpower needs did as well. During the war, the Army Medical Department sought to conserve military manpower by establishing convalescent camps in the United States and France to allow men temporarily disabled by illness or injury to recover and then return to active duty. Some medical officers suggested that such men could be employed in a "Limited Service Corps," working in fields such as telegraphy or photography, and thereby free up physically fit men for combat duty.[97]

Wartime rehabilitation programs also represented the government's commitment to help individual soldiers return to civil life as fit and productive as they could be.[98] To this end the Vocational Rehabilitation Act of 1918 provided rehabilitation training to soldiers eligible for disability compensation. The Act and subsequent amendments authorized up to four years of training and a monthly stipend during training. The program ran until June 1928; 25 percent of the almost 130,000 veterans who completed the training courses suffered from tuberculosis. (About half had orthopedic impairment or medical problems such as injuries to the lungs from chemical weapons, while 25 percent suffered from "shell shock" or other neuropsychiatric problems; only about 5,000 were amputees.)[99]

Earl Bruns was an early advocate of rehabilitation, writing in 1918 that, "the whole plan of reconstruction in tuberculosis, as well as other diseases and injuries, is to guide our disabled soldiers back to health and useful employment, imbued with the idea that they are still serviceable citizens and not candidates for soldiers' homes and an existence spent in idleness."[100] During Bruns' tenure at Fitzsimons, the hospital advocated a "Creed of the Disabled Soldier," which stated, "Once more to be useful—to see pity in the eyes of my friends replaced with commendation—to work, produce, provide, and to feel that I have a place in the world—a MAN among MEN in spite of this physical handicap."[101] Tuberculosis patients and other veterans with damaged lungs (generally from chemical weapons or severe pneumonia) needed exercise and physical therapy to help restore their breathing capacity. Fitzsimons had both a Physiotherapy Department and an Education Department that offered vocational rehabilitation and recreational activities (Figures 5-6 and 5-7).[102] During the 1920s, the physiotherapy department had eight to ten aides who provided more than 90,000 treatments annually, including massages, heat and light treatments, and electro- and hydrotherapy.[103] As medical chief at Fitzsimons, Bruns instituted a highly structured exercise program. When tuberculosis patients no longer had temperatures and were otherwise ready, they could begin to exercise in the wards for fifteen minutes a day, increasing up to an hour, after which they could join one of four walking classes progressing in length. Distances for each class were marked off on one of the hospital roads, as Bruns explained, with each class "walking at a certain

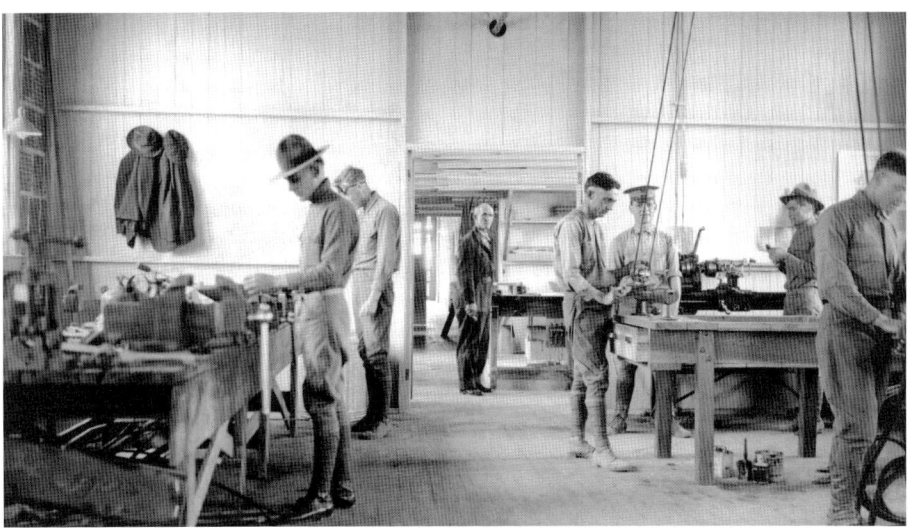

Figure 5-6. Interior view of vocational training classroom, Fitzsimons General Hospital, 1921, Scrapbook of L. E. Burns.
Photograph courtesy of the Denver Public Library, Western Historical Collection, Image #Z-385.

pace to a designated point, resting a stated number of minutes, and returning at the same pace to the starting point." Upon their return to the wards, nurses recorded a patient's temperature, pulse, and respiration. Patients could advance from one class to another on a weekly basis and complete all four in a month. Bruns believed that "the work done by this department is of great value" and would not allow any vocational or educational classes to interfere with patients' physical exercises.[104]

Vocational rehabilitation was intended to prepare Fitzsimons patients for life after discharge from the hospital, while the recreational activities were designed to keep them from being bored or depressed during their long months of rest treatment. As one medical officer remarked, "The brains of some of these men are very, very active. It is important for the man to forget the process going on in his lungs and divert his mind by some light occupational exercise."[105] The Education Department offered academic instruction in twenty-three subjects and vocational training in fields such as radio, cabinetry, mechanical and architectural drawing, agriculture, and raising poultry. In 1925, more than 700 patients took such courses. The Department proudly reported that colleges and universities accepted the academic courses for credit and that many patients "have perfected their talent to such an extent that they can, in cases of necessity, after leaving the hospital, use their knowledge in a business way."[106]

These programs all required additional space, equipment, supplies, and specially trained staff, all of which added to the cost of treatment. Decades later, a presidential commission evaluating veterans' programs concluded that the federal

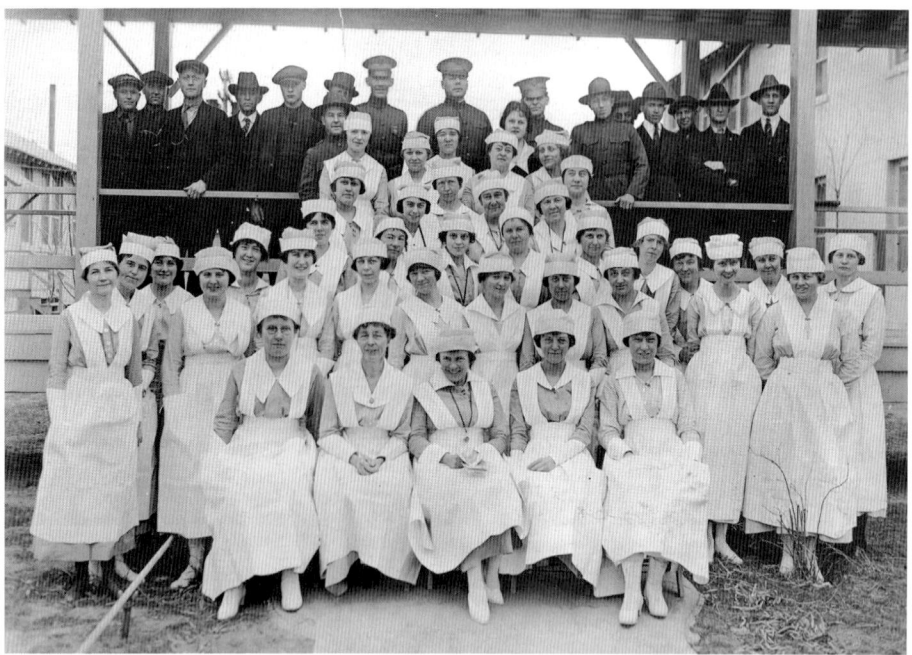

Figure 5-7. Rehabilitation Staff of the Education Department, Fitzsimons General Hospital, 1920.
Photograph courtesy of the Denver Public Library, Western Historical Collection, Image #Z-382.

rehabilitation program fell short of its goals because "the task of providing vocational rehabilitation to disabled veterans of World War I was much larger than anyone had estimated." If some benefited from rehabilitation training, "undue liberalization of the laws and lax administration permitted too many men to come under its provision and enroll in courses from which they could gain very limited, if any[,] benefits and increased the cost of the program to an unwarranted level."[107] Approximately 675,500 veterans applied for benefits, but federal officials deemed only about half of them eligible. Of those, 180,000 entered training, and 129,000 successfully completed their training courses. The program ultimately cost about $645 million.[108]

Invasive Therapies for Tuberculosis

In addition to rehabilitation, tuberculosis specialists developed a number of new therapies that increased the time and the cost of care for tuberculosis patients. By the end of the 1920s tuberculosis patients stayed in the hospital on average almost a year longer than those with any other diagnosis, including mental illnesses. Sexually transmitted diseases accounted for the greatest number of patient-days due to the high infection rates, but tuberculosis ranked second during much of the interwar period. During the years 1929 to 1931, for example, gonorrhea accounted for approximately 150,000 days lost in the Army annually compared to 100,000 days lost to tuberculosis each year. Sexually transmitted diseases, however, required only a few weeks of hospitalization, while the average days per tuberculosis case ranged from 267 to 327.[109]

Although tuberculosis rates in the United States were declining due to improved standards of living and control measures, treatment for those who contracted the disease proved frustratingly elusive to tuberculosis specialists—a generation of sanatorium and bed-rest therapy had failed to yield effective results. At the 1927 National Tuberculosis Association annual meeting PHS scientist William Charles White noted, "Because all the world longs for a cure for tuberculosis.... Not a year passes without at least one such claim." He dismissed as useless, for example, a drug called Sanocrysin, made of gold salts, as well as the "Spahlinger Cure," which involved twenty injections of a special compound. "One must draw a line of distinction between actual progress and the proclamation of progress," he observed.[110] Another speaker noted that because incipient or mild cases of tuberculosis had better recovery rates than serious cases, the current challenge to tuberculosis control was to "identify those incipient cases of tuberculosis."[111] Tuberculin was an important tool in this effort. Though it was a failure as a tuberculosis cure, tuberculin did provide an effective test to determine if someone was infected with tuberculosis bacteria. During the interwar period, colleges, universities, and medical schools began giving students periodic tuberculin tests to monitor the extent and spread of the disease within their institutions.[112] Under the New Deal during the 1930s, the PHS also launched a health surveillance program to identify people with active tuberculosis to isolate and treat them.[113]

But early detection did little for those who were already very sick. To treat those patients, physicians continued to pursue new therapies. At Fitzsimons, in addition to bedrest and rehabilitation programs, medical officers tried new drugs, electro- and hydrotherapy, prolonged exposure of parts of the body to the sun, and "collapse therapy," designed to help a diseased lung to heal itself through rest. These procedures, employed by civilian physicians as well as military, included "artificial pneumothorax," which involved the injection of air or some other substance outside the lining of the lung to collapse it temporarily; "phrenectomy," crushing or excising part of the phrenic nerve, which controls the movement of the diaphragm, to slow breathing; and "thoracoplasty," surgery that removed portions of ribs to enable the lung to collapse permanently.[114]

In the 1920s, all Fitzsimons medical officers attended a year-long course of instruction on tuberculosis and diseases of the chest taught by Bruns and others.[115] One of the students, Robert A. Bier, saved the mimeographed notes of Bruns' weekly lectures from 1926 and 1927 that profiled tuberculosis treatment at Fitzsimons during this time.[116] Bruns began his lecture series with an overview of the effects of tuberculosis on various parts of the body ranging from the characteristics of healed tuberculosis lesions on bones and soft tissues to the ultimate consumption of the lungs and other vital organs. He recommended conducting autopsies on every deceased patient because "no two cases were alike." Tuberculosis autopsies, he said, would make physicians "better diagnosticians, more accurate prognostiticians, and safer therapists" because the information would enable the physician to correlate symptoms and physical signs, identify errors in diagnosis, and help in the interpretation of shadows on chest X-rays.[117]

Bruns distinguished between tuberculosis infection and tuberculosis disease, noting that infection could be detected simply with a tuberculin test, while the disease diagnosis required X-ray findings, physical signs, positive sputum tests, and symptoms such as cough and fever. In the same lecture Bruns defined "quiescent" tuberculosis as the "absence of all constitutional symptoms, [though] expectoration and bacilli may or may not be present," and "arrested" tuberculosis whereby "all constitutional symptoms and expectoration with bacilli [are] absent for a period of six months." He asserted that although tuberculosis bacilli in the sputum usually suggested tubercular activity, "a patient may have an old fibrous lesion with a thick walled cavity throwing out tubercle bacilli and still be in good health." Such a case, he said, "should be considered inactive." Bruns further complicated the diagnostics for his students by including a new partner in the task: the federal government. As he told the legislators, after Congress determined that the Veterans' Bureau should compensate beneficiaries with "active" tuberculosis, it had to *define* "active." A special government committee therefore defined active pulmonary tuberculosis as involving two or more of the following six characteristics: (1) sputum positive for tuberculosis bacilli; (2) inflammation and fluid in the lining of the lungs; (3) a cavity or collapse of the lung tissue; (4) active tuberculous lesions detected by physical examination; (5) shadows or other indications on chest X-rays; or (6) symptoms suggesting tuberculosis such as fever, weight loss, and rapid pulse.[118] Given the complexity and difficulty of diagnosing tuberculosis this definition may have actually helped to clarify the process.

Bruns recognized the importance of X-ray, but believed that X-ray technology caused some physicians to neglect the extended, one-hour physical examination that was crucial to confirming radiological findings. Furthermore, X-ray machines and expertise were not always available and did not explain the origin or progress of the disease nor detect early or fresh lesions. Ever the Bushnell student, Bruns devoted four lectures to the physical examination of the chest, including one on the "Normal Chest" to provide a baseline of chest sounds to avoid erroneous diagnoses. He identified four kinds of cough—"dry, productive, paroxysmal, and emetic"—and offered a vivid description of sputum, noting "there is nothing typical about sputum in tuberculosis." It could be scanty or profuse, "usually odorless, but at times acquires a very disagreeable sweetish and nauseating odor." In far-advanced disease, it was "gray or greenish in color, made up of roundish and coin-shaped masses, which float around or sink to the bottom in the fluid mucous or saliva part of the sputum."[119]

Regarding treatment, Bruns noted that since the late nineteenth century, "Very little of importance has since been added to the treatment of tuberculosis, except tuberculin, pneumothorax, heliotherapy, and thoracoplasty."[120] But by the 1920s, the rest treatment appeared to have approached heroic proportions; Bruns recommended rest therapy from six months to "several years." Fitzsimons personnel taught patients to lay completely at rest with muscles relaxed. This "jelly fishing," as Bruns called it, allowed "respirations [to] become shallow and fewer. The patient scarcely breathes with the affected upper parts of his lungs, and thus quiescent, the activity of the lesions subsides and healing occurs." Such rest must, Bruns underlined, be in the open air. Mental rest was important as well, so "too much reading, studying and conversing should not be allowed." Regarding nutrition, he recommended vegetables such as spinach and carrots and "Bergundy [sic] or claret wines," but he also believed that "gain in weight is stressed too much," and that there was "nothing to be combated more energetically by the doctor than the tendency of tuberculosis patients to overeat."[121]

Bruns was skeptical of some new therapies: "I believe it is a mistake to introduce into our army sanatoria every new treatment that comes along."[122] Fitzsimons' medical officers, for example, rejected an "ozone treatment" developed in France and the so-called Holderness-Brunson treatment, which involved deep inhalations.[123] They did experiment with therapies such as a hotbox to heat patients' bodies and thereby kill germs, and X-rays to attack tubercular growths.[124] Fitzsimons personnel used codeine instead of morphine and heroin for the treatment of cough, and no longer prescribed creosote, arsenic, or mercury, which had been widely used in the nineteenth century. They did employ therapies such as intravenous calcium chloride for gastrointestinal tuberculosis, a "judicious combination of heliotherapy, bismuth paste, and tuberculin" to close tubercular sinuses, "intramuscular injections of iron and strychnine" to treat anemia, and electric cauterization of ulcers caused by tuberculosis laryngitis.[125] Bruns also counseled his students to maintain a positive attitude with their patients because the optimistic physician "by his own enthusiasm arouses the same hope and firm belief in the minds of his patients." This, Bruns believed, was the "keystone" that "leads to recovery in the end."[126] He also believed that good spirits were promoted by a healthy climate and plenty of sunshine.

Heliotherapy

In the nineteenth century, health seekers advocated the value of sunshine in the healing process and scientists observed that sunlight exposure could kill bacteria.[127] In 1903 Niels Ryber Finsen of Iceland received the Nobel Prize for his work on the effects of light on skin lesions, especially lupus vulgaris—tuberculosis of the skin.[128] At the same time, Swiss physician Augusto Rollier developed a method of applying sunlight to patients therapeutically, beginning with five minutes on the feet with patients lying on their stomachs and then five minutes while lying on their backs, moving up to uncover more of the body in five-minute intervals over succeeding days. Thus, after three weeks patients would lie completely exposed to the sun one hour or more on their backs and another hour on their fronts.[129] After Rollier's method was described at an international tuberculosis conference in Rome in 1911, Americans began to adopt the approach and were soon debating the length of time and amount of skin to be exposed and devising various lamps to use during cloudy weather.

Sunlight had always been a key component of treatment at Fort Bayard, but after the war medical officers began to employ it scientifically and call it heliotherapy. Bruns became a strong advocate. In 1922, he persuaded the Army to construct sun porches on the wards (Figure 5-8), telling his commanding officer that heliotherapy was "no longer in the experimental stage and cannot be considered a fad."[130] In his lecture on heliotherapy Bruns said, "One cannot help being impressed with the improved spirit among the patients on a heliotherapy ward. As their skin bronzes, their weight and strength increase, and they are able to expose themselves to the elements like the hardy and rugged races of centuries ago."[131] He acknowledged that it was not clear how heliotherapy worked, but that "the skin is said to be a great anti-body factory, and increased immunity results from a healthy and active condition."[132] Bruns speculated that the sun weakened the bacteria, eased pain, and that given such "remarkable results…the scientific reason is therefore of secondary importance."[133] Furthermore, patients "improve so markedly in general health and appearance that it is no wonder that they become enthusiastic over the sun treatment and cooperate so closely with their physician."[134] Fitzsimons' medical officers employed heliotherapy for nontubercular diseases such as diabetes, kidney disease, and depression, and to treat tuberculosis infections from one end of the body to the other.[135] For tuberculosis of the larynx

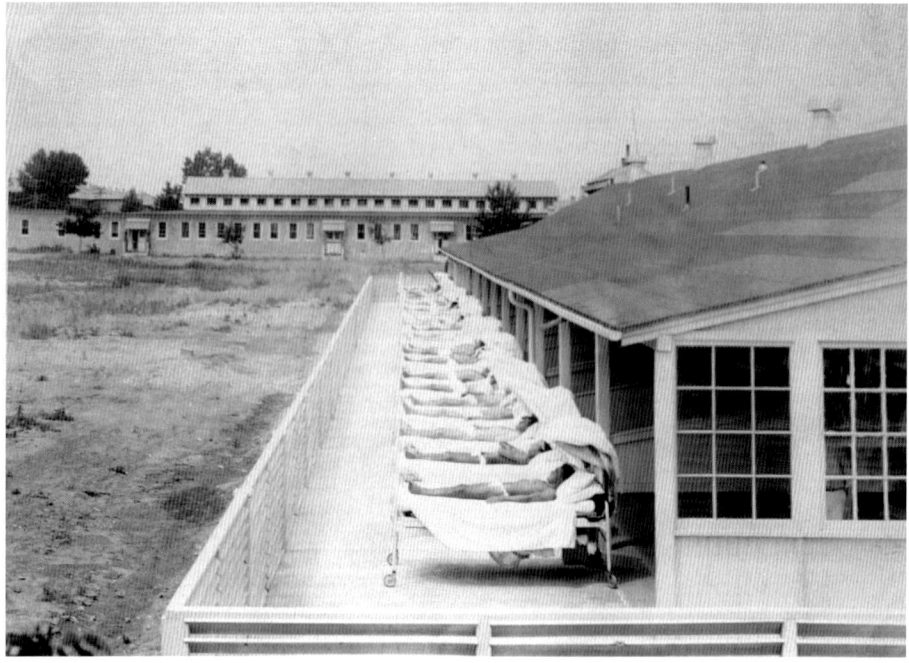

Figure 5-8. U.S. Army, Fitzsimons General Hospital, Denver, Colorado, exterior view, heliotherapy ward from south porch, n.d.
Photograph courtesy of the National Library of Medicine, Image #A05002.

or the middle ear (otitis media) they used metal mirrors to project sunlight onto the inner tissue, beginning with just thirty seconds, and continuing up to ten minutes of exposure. For tuberculosis of the testicles or anal region, Bruns instructed, "The patient assumes the knee chest position, separates his buttocks, and exposes the anal region to the sun."[136]

From 1922 through 1924 Bruns treated forty-five patients for Pott's Disease, or tuberculosis of the spine, with heliotherapy. Although many physicians performed surgery in an attempt to fuse deteriorated vertebrae, Bruns was reluctant to do so because "tuberculosis, no matter how it manifests itself, is a general disease and requires general treatment."[137] He required Pott's Disease patients to spend three years at Fitzsimons. During the first two years they stayed in bed with a plaster cast around the torso with a removable "trough" that allowed exposure of the spine to the sun. Patients could only lie flat on their backs or on their stomachs, resting on the elbows. Heliotherapy sessions ran two hours in the summer and three hours in the winter. In poor weather, patients rested under sunlamps (Figure 5-9). If X-rays showed that the spine had healed, usually after two years, Bruns put patients into a jacket with a metal brace for a year, during which time they

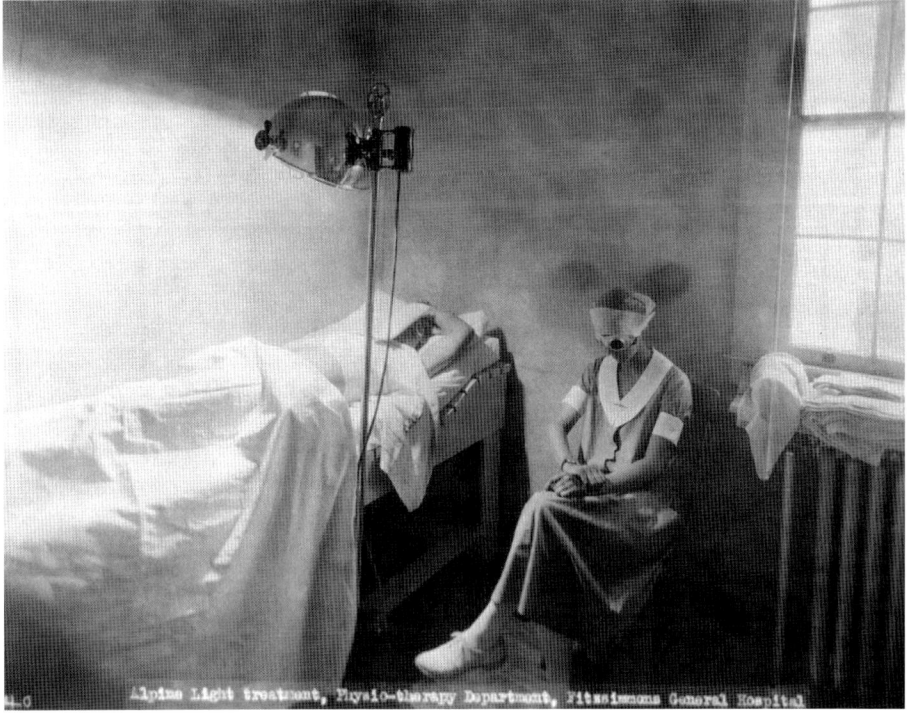

Figure 5-9. U.S. Army, Fitzsimons General Hospital, Denver, Colorado, alpine light treatment, Physiotherapy Department, patient attended by therapist, n.d.
Photograph courtesy of the National Library of Medicine, Image #A07799.

continued heliotherapy and began graduated exercise. Bruns was delighted with the results after three years. Of forty-five cases, six were "apparently cured," six were "arrested," twenty-eight were improved, two patients died, and the remaining patients had complications or acted "against medical advice," presumably leaving the hospital. With results like this, in 1924, Surgeon General Merritte Ireland noted that heliotherapy had been employed at Fitzsimons "with excellent results."[138]

Not all physicians were sanguine about the benefits of heliotherapy, and some cautioned that scientists did not yet understand how the sun acted on tuberculosis. A physician at the Jewish Consumptives' Relief Society sanatorium in Denver warned that heliotherapy could be as dangerous as tuberculosis if used "injudiciously," and another wrote that although heliotherapy might be valuable, "further investigation and many more scientific data are required before light should generally be prescribed" by physicians unfamiliar with the technique.[139] Such research did continue for decades and in the late 1980s, several groups of scientists were able to provide an explanation for why heliotherapy was effective: vitamin D. One group of researchers at the Webb-Waring Institute in Denver was able to "connect vitamin D, sunlight, and tuberculoimmunity and suggest that vitamin D should be considered a vital factor in the practical control of tuberculosis."[140] Fitzsimons' patients drank a lot of milk and often took cod liver oil, both of which contain vitamin D, so the sunlight could have activated the vitamin and supported the immune response against tuberculosis bacteria. Thus, as tuberculosis expert Michael Iseman writes, "Given what has subsequently been learned about the role of vitamin D as a potential enhancer of tuberculoimmunity, it is fascinating to consider that the physicians of this era may have stumbled onto early, valid forms of immunomodulation."[141] Bruns and other physicians practiced what appeared to work, even though they did not understand it.

Artificial Pneumothorax

Bruns devoted several weeks of lectures to "collapse therapy," which predominated in the interwar period.[142] Collapse therapy had two purposes. The first was to close lung cavities full of tuberculosis bacilli and thereby reduce the patient's bacterial load. As Bruns told his students, such cavities remained "as an active focus, excreting sputum swarming with tubercle bacilli, poisoning the lymph and blood with the products of the tubercle and mixed infection, and menacing the life of the individual."[143] The second purpose was an extension of the concept of rest therapy—if physicians could not get the patient to rest completely, they could at least "rest" the lung by reducing its size and/or retarding breathing. As historian Jack Spidle explains, "Instead of forcing the whole organism to rest in bed or on a chaise lounge, the diseased lung itself could be put at rest locally and allowed a chance to heal with the patient requiring much less extensive institutional care."[144] Collapse therapies were also intended to reduce the amount of dead and diseased tissue in the lungs and allow the beleaguered organs to recuperate. They involved a series of increasingly invasive procedures that ranged from temporarily collapsing the diseased lung (artificial pneumothorax); to crushing or severing the nerve that controlled the diaphragm, paralyzing it on one side (phrenectomy); to rib removal that would permanently collapse the lung (thoracoplasty).

In earlier centuries, people had observed that tuberculosis sufferers sometimes improved after they experienced a spontaneous pneumothorax, the collapse of a lung. In the nineteenth century, some European physicians began to induce the process by compressing the lung using different methods and substances such as air, oil, paraffin, or even ping-pong balls.[145] American physicians did not adopt such artificial pneumothorax procedures until the 1910s. Medical officers at Fort Bayard did their first artificial pneumothorax in January 1913, and in the next four years gave the treatment to forty-nine patients. Forty of the patients had successful collapses, twenty-three of them dramatically improved, two patients soon died of heart failure, and eighteen left the hospital, their fate unrecorded.[146] The pace picked up at Fitzsimons after the war, where medical officers did 12,700 pneumothoraces during the 1920s. In 1932, one Fitzsimons unit gave pneumothorax treatment to 46.7 percent of its patients.[147] Other Army hospitals performed some pneumothorax procedures but generally transferred all active-duty tuberculosis patients to Fitzsimons and veterans with tuberculosis to Veterans Administration hospitals.[148]

The pneumothorax was a familiar part of the landscape in tuberculosis sanatoriums between the wars. Patients with tuberculosis in just one lung were most suited for the procedure because their healthy lung could assume a greater burden. Physicians used only a local anesthetic to collapse the lung, but sought to minimize the pain because, as one team put it, "If the patient suffers at the first injection, he may not be persuaded to undergo the subsequent ones" and "may discourage other members of the same clinic from accepting the treatment."[149] With the patient lying on his or her side, arm raised overhead, the physician injected a needle between the ribs to insert air between the chest wall and the lung, thereby depressing the lung. The amount of air ranged from 500 to 1000 milliliters, and "refills" were required every few weeks as the air dissipated over time. Physicians used X-ray examinations to identify the section of lung to be collapsed and gauged improvement with subsequent X-rays and by observing changes in symptoms such as the reduction of fever or elimination of bacilli in the sputum. Many patients endured collapsed lungs (pneumothoraces) for a year or more. A woman at a civilian sanatorium wrote that "pneumothorax was a good friend to me," but after undergoing periodic injections for six years, she was "glad those days were gone."[150] Complications and dangers of the pneumothorax procedures included punctures of the lung, bronchial tubes, or lining of the lung, which could cause the lung to collapse completely or to rupture.[151] Bruns recommended using a "large blunt needle" for the initial puncture to avoid such problems.[152] Air embolisms, though rare, could be deadly, and cardiac failure could occur when one collapsed lung caused the other to enlarge and displace the heart.[153] Of Fitzsimons' 12,700 pneumothorax operations in the 1920s, medical officers reported sixteen cases of embolism and seven deaths during the procedure.[154]

Unlike heliotherapy, patients feared the pneumothorax. Fictional accounts of life in tuberculosis sanatoriums tend to portray it as torture. In *The Rack*, author A.

E. Ellis' protagonist, Paul, receives a pneumothorax refill: "The needle distended. It penetrated and, with a crunching sound traversed 2 inches of coriasceous tissue.... Paul spoke quietly and cautiously—he always feared that talking during the refill might lead to undue expansion and subsequent perforation of the lung, as if he had divined this Dr. Vernet pushed in the needle a little farther."[155] In *The Magic Mountain*, Thomas Mann describes patients "whistling through their pneumothorax hole," and one female character dies from an "overblown" pneumothorax.[156] In the novel, *Sanatorium*, Donald Stewart creates a tuberculosis physician who sadistically enjoys pneumothoraces, rewarding patients who agree to them and punishing those who refuse.[157]

An American Sanatorium Association survey in the 1930s found that physicians conducted "therapeutic" pneumothorax on anywhere from 1 to 68 percent of patients, with a national average of 10 percent.[158] Two-thirds of those patients had advanced disease lung cavitation and only about 38 percent had effective collapse procedures. The survey committee concluded that given the likelihood of problems and failure, pneumothorax should not be "undertaken lightly."[159] A British study of 2,100 professional papers on pneumothorax published between 1929 and 1939 found that only about one-third of the procedures were conducted under what the reviewers considered acceptable standards.[160] The number of patients with pneumothoraces at Fitzsimons was higher than in civilian sanatoriums, perhaps because a greater percentage of patients had moderate or advanced disease and were therefore candidates for the procedure, and because Fitzsimons surgeons generally underwent advanced training and were therefore skilled in the procedure. In 1935 Fitzsimons surgeons stated that "We believe that practically all cases of active pulmonary tuberculosis of recent onset.... should receive the benefit of artificial pneumothorax, particularly if the involvement is unilateral." By 1939, 65 percent of Fitzsimons patients with pulmonary tuberculosis had a pneumothorax.[161]

Phrenectomy

When efforts to induce artificial pneumothorax failed, physicians turned to other procedures. One of the greatest obstacles to successful pneumothorax was when the lining of the lung adhered to the chest wall due to tissue scarring, preventing the collapse. In such cases medical officers employed several procedures to effect collapse to close the cavities. One involved "unroofing" the tuberculosis cavity by incising and draining it of tubercular matter. Another was called the Jakobaeus operation, and involved cutting and cauterizing the adhesions that joined the lung to the chest wall to allow it to collapse. This could be painful and dangerous and was done rarely—only four times in 1929 at Fitzsimons and nine times in 1935.[162] A more common method was to crush or excise the phrenic nerve that runs from the neck to the chest and regulates breathing. Medical officers at Fitzsimons began this procedure in 1922, extracting 5 to 12 centimeters of the nerve to paralyze one half of the diaphragm, causing it to rise in the rib cage, pressing against the lung to thereby collapse and "rest" it on that side. In 1930, Lieutenant Colonel (Lt. Col.)

Alexander Cooper reported that in 16 percent of the ninety-six patients whose phrenic nerves were cut, the diaphragm successfully rose to reduce the thoracic cavity and partially collapse the lower lobe of the lung. Of the ninety-six patients, 40 percent had relief from coughing, and one-third generally improved after the operation. Fifteen of the ninety-six patients, however, died within a year of the operation, so Cooper concluded that the procedure could be valuable in "selected cases" where tuberculosis infected only one lung.[163] Phrenectomy peaked in the 1930s, but then declined after a 1936 Veterans' Bureau study concluded that the procedure "did not save or materially prolong life."[164]

Thoracoplasty

When patients did not improve with rest and pneumothorax, or adhesions prevented lung collapse, some specialists recommended more radical surgery. For years surgeons had been treating some forms of tuberculosis by cutting out tumors on the bone or joints, or cutting into and draining sinuses (i.e., fistulas, narrow elongated tracts that extended from a focus of infection, ultimately erupting through the skin and discharging pus).[165] But many physicians believed that pulmonary tuberculosis patients could not tolerate surgery due to their weakened condition. That changed after World War I. Wartime surgical experience with medical officers operating on hundreds of patients improved surgeons' ability to recognize and avoid shock in patients and to surgically clean infected wounds. Such advancements enabled the profession to develop new surgical procedures for a much wider range of patients and conditions than before the war.[166] The most drastic and disfiguring procedure used to treat pulmonary tuberculosis during the interwar period was to cut and collapse the ribs. Early thoracoplasty had involved the removal of the entire length of several ribs, but this left the chest exposed and allowed the lung to swing in and out, leading to gastrointestinal or breathing difficulties and pneumonia. The nineteenth-century German physician Ferdinand Sauerbruch pioneered thoracic surgery after treating a patient whose lung collapsed after being gored by a bull.[167] His procedure removed a small part of each rib where it connected to the spine, allowing the rib cage to fold down, thereby collapsing the lung while still protecting it.[168] Medical Corps surgeon John Alexander learned the procedure while serving in the American Expeditionary Forces during the war. When he developed tuberculosis of the spine and had to spend two years in a cast, he wrote one of the first textbooks on the surgical treatment of pulmonary tuberculosis—*The Collapse Therapy of Pulmonary Tuberculosis*.[169]

Medical officers at Fitzsimons began to employ thoracoplasty in 1922 and published several papers on their work.[170] Bruns and his colleague, Maj. Joseph Casper, reported on 120 such procedures. They observed that the surgery was most successful for young patients with strong, healthy hearts and tuberculosis in only one lung. Seriously ill patients were not good candidates, but, Bruns and Casper wrote, thoracoplasty could "give apparently doomed patients a chance, however slight, for recovery."[171] In fact, they wrote, patients often tended to "procrastinate and postpone the operation so that too often it becomes a desperate effort to save life."[172]

184 "Good Tuberculosis Men"

Thoracoplasty was a traumatic undertaking. Before the operation, nurses helped patients "empty their cavities" by coughing up as much tubercular material from their lungs as they could. Then, with the patient under general anesthesia and lying on his stomach or side, the surgeon would cut through the skin and muscles of his back, locating one rib at a time, freeing it from the connecting tissue, and removing about a half-inch of rib near the spine (Figure 5-10). Bruns and Casper cautioned, "it is much better to do too little than too much," and that physicians should remove only five to seven ribs at a time. The incision should be as large as required to work, but made gently, because it was not the length of the wound, but "the stripping and cutting of the ribs which causes shock." They instructed sur-

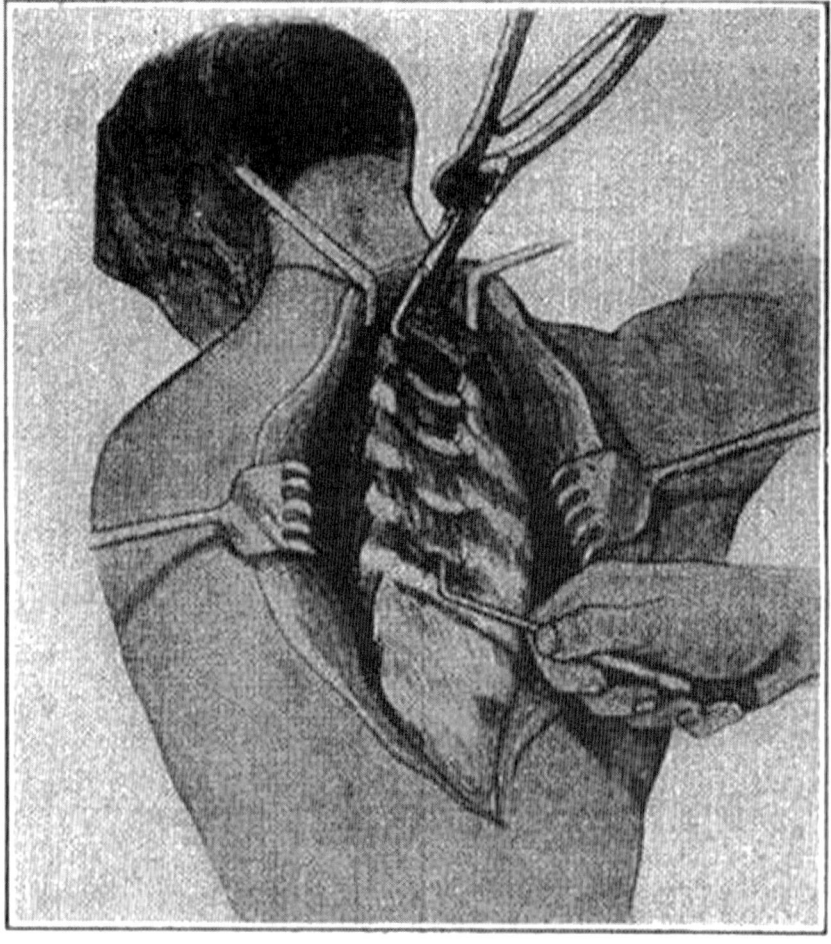

Figure 5-10. Illustration of thoracoplasty, in "The Nursing Care in Thoracoplastic Operations," *American Journal of Nursing* 29 (February 1929): 124–25.
Photograph used with permission of the *American Journal of Nursing*.

geons to remove any damaged tissue in the area, then sew up the muscles and the skin, close the wound, and apply a bandage strapped "firm enough to support the chest-wall and allow coughing."[173] After the operation, nurses watched for signs of shock such as a drop in blood pressure, rapid pulse, or clammy skin. "So much tissue is dissected at the time of operation," a civilian nurse explained, "that the whole wound weeps bloody serum much more freely than would be expected in an abdominal wound." After the operation she gave patients pain medication and a salt solution or whiskey and glucose intravenously. And because of the bleeding, "fluids should be forced....if the patient is not vomiting."[174] Some physicians did not prescribe narcotics for pain because the drugs would inhibit the coughing necessary to expel the tubercular material from the collapsed lung cavity. One nurse explained that a patient would need to indicate to the nurse if he had to cough, because if "the side, deprived of its bony framework is not supported, coughing causes more pain and may even result in hemorrhage or rupture of the lung and death."[175] Writing in the 1950s, Robert J. Gosling, a medical officer at Fitzsimons, provided a detailed and graphic description of the effect of thoracoplasty on a patient's body:

> With thoracoplasty a number of anatomical and functional patterns are altered. The balance of the neck is disturbed, allowing a lateral deviation of the head and neck towards the unoperated side. The shoulder on the operated side may be elevated and displaced anteriorly. The chest is deformed and may shift toward the operated side. A scoliosis may develop with the primary curve in the thoracic area, convex to the operated side, compensated by a secondary cervical curve above and a lumbar curve below. There is restricted movement and range of motion in the shoulder joint. There may be impingement of the scapula upon the uppermost remaining rib. There is a possibility of an anteriorly displaced head and neck with an accompanying kyphosis. The pelvis may be prominent laterally, anteriorly rotated and elevated on the unoperated side.[176]

Fitzsimons' medical officers did not, apparently, make great promises to their patients about the effectiveness of thoracoplasty. Casper wrote in 1932: "The surgeon has no miraculous power and his work here, as in other departments of surgery, is beset with pitfalls, filled with disappointments, and only occasionally crowned with conspicuous success." Even success, however, did not mean a cure for the underlying disease. "A patient must be made to realize that an operation for this condition is not curative," Casper wrote. "It may be necessary to operate again, and no matter what is done surgically the disease still remains a medical condition, and medical treatment is as much indicated after as before surgical intervention."[177]

Because thoracoplasty was reserved for the sickest patients, twenty of the 120 patients who received the operation at Fitzsimons between 1922 and 1930 died within three months, some from shock, others of heart failure or infection.[178] But in several articles Bruns, Casper, and another Fitzsimons surgeon, Major (Maj.) William Thearle, described the dramatic improvement some patients experienced as well as the drastic procedures they underwent. Perhaps the most impressive was that of "Colonel T." who developed tuberculosis in 1914, and arrived at Fitzsimons in 1924 at the age of forty-seven, in critical condition with tuberculosis in all lobes of both lungs as well as tuberculosis laryngitis, and producing two cups of sputum a day. He was "a seemingly hopelessly sick man and a truly desperate operator of risk." But after the removal of half of the ribs on the right side in November 1924, his "improvement was truly magical." The wound required five months to heal but after just three weeks the patient's voice was normal and he was producing less sputum. Surgeons removed the remaining ribs on the right side in June 1925, and by October his sputum was free from bacteria for the first time in ten years. Colonel T. gained forty pounds, could walk up to five miles a day, and even play golf. In April 1926 he developed tubercular meningitis and died within two weeks, but an autopsy confirmed that his lungs had healed dramatically.[179] Army records show that Col. T was actually Col. G. Soulard Turner (Figure 5-11), a cavalry officer who served from 1898 until his retirement on disability in 1920.[180]

Thearle also reported on a female patient at Fitzsimons, most likely an Army nurse, who, after three years of active tuberculosis, received a pneumothorax in her right lung. She improved at first, but then suffered a complete lung collapse in March 1924 and became very ill. Surgeons collapsed the ribs on her right side under local anesthesia, but the wound became infected, and they had to remove three ribs completely and insert a drain in her chest. When the patient did not improve, surgeons removed four more ribs, along with parts of three more, and subsequently performed "four minor procedures for infected rib ends." She finally improved. Her weight gradually rose from 83 to 120 pounds, and her coughing and sputum subsided. Although Thearle concluded that her tuberculosis was "apparently cured," she still had an opening in her chest from the drain, and her spine was curved from "the complete collapse of half the chest" (Figure 5-12). But, wrote Thearle, "such is scarcely apparent when she is dressed for out of doors."[181]

In 1929, *American Medicine* declared the surgical treatment of tuberculosis, "a pronounced achievement and an advance over earlier techniques. It has a definite effect in limiting the mortality among individuals for whom the prognosis had been most unfavorable."[182] However, these procedures were not free from controversy. In 1924, Watson Miller, chair of the American Legion Rehabilitation Committee, wrote to Surgeon General Ireland asking for information about pneumothorax and thoracoplasty because he had heard that some people believed that "a man suffering from pulmonary tuberculosis should not be operated upon to the extent required by the rib-sectioning incident to thoracoplasty."[183] Ireland sent him a reprint of Thearle's article, noting, "mortality in these operations is high," but "when one realized the hopelessness of this class of patients and their poor physical condition due to the advanced stage of the disease…the results appear to justify the operation."[184]

Not everyone followed the path toward more aggressive therapies. In New York, Saranac Lake sanatorium physician Lawrason Brown worried that "a new generation of physicians has entered the field of treatment of pulmonary

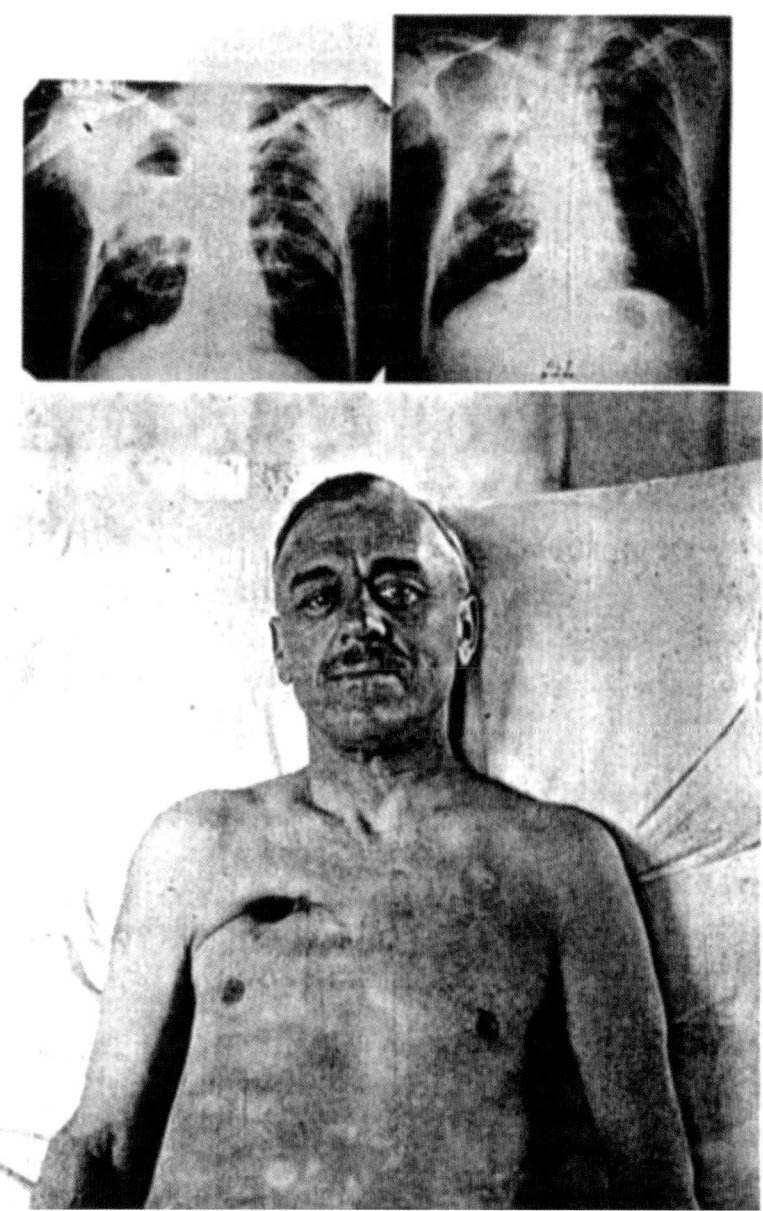

Figure 5-11. Photograph and X-ray images of Colonel G. Soulard Turner who underwent thoracoplasty at Fitzsimons General Hospital, in Earl Bruns and Joseph Casper, "Thoracoplasty in the Treatment of Chronic Tuberculosis," *American Review of Tuberculosis* 22 (1930): 753.

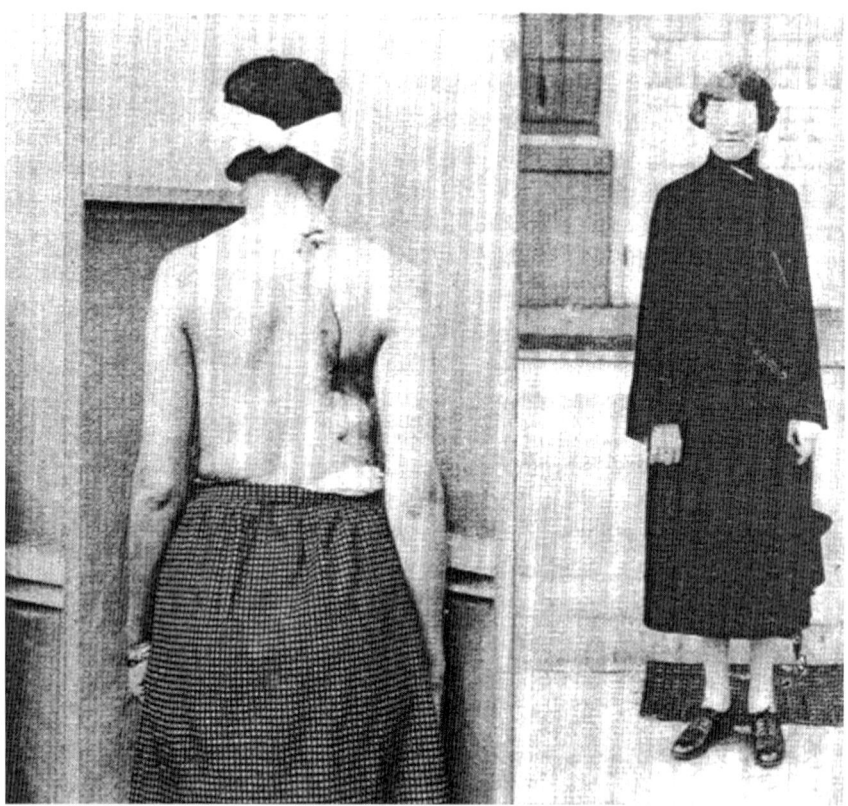

Figure 5-12. Photographs of a female patient at Fitzsimons General Hospital who underwent thoracoplasty described in William H. Thearle, "Extrapleural Thoracoplasty in Pulmonary Tuberculosis," *Southwestern Medicine* 10 (July 1926): 301.

tuberculosis. The rest treatment of Dettweiler, of Trudeau, of Walther, does not satisfy their desire for action."[185] Gerald Webb began to practice pneumothorax in 1912, but soon became wary of surgical interventions and did fewer and fewer.[186] Another specialist, James Waring of Denver, acknowledged that artificial pneumothorax was "a well-tried and proven procedure of incalculable benefit in properly selected cases."[187] But in 1934 he cautioned against "enthusiasm for surgery over the stethoscope," and lamented "this day of bold, well-nigh reckless surgery of the chest."[188] Physician and historian Thomas Dormandy has concluded that "despite all modifications and improvements, thoracoplasty remained a horrific operation; and it is not unreasonable to ask how it could have retained its popularity."[189]

It didn't for long. Never a popular procedure, in the following decade thoracoplasty gave way to lung resection—the removal of diseased lung tissue itself. Evarts C. Graham, a surgeon at Washington University, had served in the Medical

Corps during the war and gained extensive experience in treating patients with lungs damaged by chemical weapons, pneumonia, empyema, and tuberculosis. Continuing his investigations after the war, in 1933 he performed the first surgical removal of an entire lung for treatment of lung cancer.[190] In the following years, surgeons applied this procedure to tuberculosis and began to remove portions of the diseased lung (lung resection) or completely removed a lobe or lung (lobectomy and pneumonectomy) rather than ribs. As with lung collapse, this reduced the amount of diseased tissue, making it easier for antibiotics to fight the tuberculosis bacilli.[191] By the 1950s, the development of effective antibiotic therapy with streptomycin, isoniazid, and PAS (para-aminosalicylate), and the increasingly early detection of tuberculosis sidelined these surgical procedures in the United States. The resurgence of antibiotic-resistant tuberculosis in the 1990s, however, led physicians to return to lung resection and even thoracoplasty as the few tools available, absent effective antibiotics, to control the disease.[192]

Discharge on Disability

In 1923, Col. Joseph Siler of the Office of The Surgeon General informed Fitzsimons' commander William Moncrief that the hospital "will be used as a salvage hospital with the idea that Army officers who are ordered there will be salvaged and returned to a duty status, provided this can be done within a reasonable period of time." He noted that "[General Edmund] Munson, Hutton, Bruns and others are shining examples of this."[193] Moncrief had reservations, however. Fitzsimons was different from "the old days at Fort Bayard," he said, because "the amount of work to be done is large, and more is required of the individual than was the case at Bayard." Officers with tuberculosis had less time for rest, recreation, and recovery, so that although "admitting that we have saved shining examples," Moncrief recommended that the Army take the Navy's approach of retiring on disability all officers who had not recovered their health after one year of treatment.[194]

Throughout the 1920s, the Medical Department's policy regarding the discharge of personnel with tuberculosis was to retain enlisted men in the hospital for six months and officers and nurses for at least one year, until a retirement board determined whether they should be discharged for disability, or returned to full or partial duty.[195] Because the Army Medical Department generally sent tuberculosis patients to Fitzsimons for treatment, tuberculosis disability retirement policy was effectively determined by medical officers in Denver instead of Washington, and they considered it their responsibility to return as many patients as possible to active service. When tuberculosis patients appeared before retirement boards, they usually faced three officers who had been sick with tuberculosis themselves and were sympathetic with efforts to return them to active duty. In 1925, for example, the board consisted of Paul Hutton and Bruns, who had both been patients at Fort Bayard, and pathologist Maj. Shannon Van Alzah, who struggled with tuberculosis until his death in 1933. In 1931, Bruns even wrote about a method of thoracoplasty that "if successful, enables the patient to be returned to duty." It would be limited to resection of the upper five ribs, he explained, because "this sacrifices very little normal lung tissue, causing a minimum amount of deformity."[196] (Bruns' own heart disease and lung damage from years of active tuberculosis did not prevent Surgeon General Ireland from promoting him to lieutenant colonel in May 1931.)

After a new Surgeon General, Robert U. Patterson, took office in 1931, however, this approach shifted. Patterson, who had never had tuberculosis, nor served at Fort Bayard or Fitzsimons, moved to change the Medical Department's tuberculosis policy soon after taking office. He noted that tuberculosis caused "chronic invalidism" and rued "the large amount of time which is lost by each case."[197] He therefore issued a new disability policy similar to that advocated nine years before by Moncrief. Officers "who have been under treatment for one year…and who are considered to have little or no prospect of *prompt* return to unlimited duty will be considered permanently incapacitated and will be recommended for appearance before a retiring board."[198] Patterson did not consult with Fitzsimons officers; he simply sent them the policy in March 1932. "My office has felt for sometime," he advised, "that a too liberal policy was being followed as regards continuance on the active list of military personnel suffering from pulmonary tuberculosis." As physicians, medical officers may be interested in salvaging the tuberculous, he wrote, but as military officers they "must remember that the first object of military administration is to keep the Army effective as a combatant force." Retaining officers with tuberculosis "seriously interferes with the foreign service roster" and it was difficult to find "protected duty" for convalescent Air Corps officers who were "subject to the many strains of flying." He also objected to returning officers to duty when they were undergoing artificial pneumothorax, noting that the Veterans Administration rated such tuberculosis patients as totally and permanently disabled. Patterson's policy was therefore to "*govern* medical officers at Fitzsimons General Hospital regarding the disposition of patients with tuberculosis."[199] Under this new policy, although enlisted men and officers who recovered quickly and fully from their illness could return to duty, most could not.

A month after Patterson announced the new retirement policy Earl Bruns' health failed catastrophically. His service at Fitzsimons had been interrupted with a two-year stint (1926–28) on duty at Sternberg Hospital in the Philippines, but his health deteriorated there so he went on sick leave before returning to Fitzsimons (1929–30). On 29 April 1932 Fitzsimons admitted Bruns as a patient with an array of conditions that can all be attributable to tuberculosis. He had a dislocated shoulder incurred during convulsions most likely caused by blood poisoning (uremia) resulting from kidney disease. He also suffered from heart trouble, high blood pressure, and periodontal disease so severe that he had lost all of his teeth. As Bruns was recovering from his collapse and struggling with kidney failure, Col. W. P. Chamberlain in the Office of The Surgeon General sent Fitzsimons' commanding officer an extraordinary letter complaining that medical officers at the hospital were undermining the new policy on retirement of officers with persistent tuberculosis. He noted that one Air Corps officer, Captain (Capt.) Charles B. B. Bubb, told his retirement board that "Col. Bruns, who is conceded to be unquestionably the finest expert in the Army on tuberculosis," expected Bubb to fully recover and return to duty. Chamberlain wrote, "doubtless many junior officers have become indoctrinated with the same views. *It will be necessary to overcome this attitude*." He added that "General Patterson feels that Colonel Bruns has lost perspective regarding the administrative problems of pulmonary tuberculosis in the army."[200]

It was a measure of Bruns' stature that the Surgeon General believed an individual as sick as he was could undermine his policy. But the environment within which the Medical Department struggled with tuberculosis was changing. The falling tuberculosis rates in American society meant that the War Department could be more selective in who served and bar men with any signs of tuberculosis from the ranks. Furthermore, budget pressures and the increasing costs of tuberculosis care had made it more difficult to retain tuberculous enlisted men, nurses, and officers on the active duty rolls. Thus, in October 1932, despite the Fitzsimons commander's warning that "both [Bruns] and his wife will be heartbroken if it is necessary to separate him from active service," the Medical Department replaced Bruns as chief of the Fitzsimons medical service and retired him on disability.[201] Bruns went to Tucson to recuperate, and died within months on 16 March 1933 in Beaumont General Hospital at Fort Bliss, Texas.

Bruns received a soldier's burial in Arlington Cemetery and was honored in Denver a year later, on the anniversary of his death.[202] At a banquet, Governor (Gov.) Edwin C. Johnson declared that "the state of Colorado appreciates the contributions of Colonel Bruns to humanity," and the Denver Sanatorium Association presented the Army with a portrait of Bruns, which was hung in Fitzsimons (see Figure 5-3).[203] Perhaps referring to Bruns' forced retirement, Col. Robert M. Hardaway, who succeeded Bruns as Fitzsimons' chief of medical service, commented that "unfortunately we failed to honor him during his lifetime." The new congressman from Denver, Rep. Lawrence Lewis, did, however, celebrate Bruns, stating, "Although ultimately Colonel Bruns died of the disease with which he was afflicted...his career is an inspiring example to us all." Bruns, Lewis asserted, "surmounted physical disabilities and transformed what to a lesser man would have been a misfortune into an inspiration for greater achievement and service to humanity."[204]

But the time when one could pursue a productive and rewarding career in the Army after a serious bout with tuberculosis was coming to an end. Within a year Surgeon General Patterson retired Paul Hutton and several other ailing medical officers on disability and appointed Col. Carroll Buck, a medical officer who had not had tuberculosis, as Fitzsimons' commander. Buck would run Fitzsimons until 1941, struggling with the high cost and the politics of tuberculosis treatment during the dire years of the Great Depression. And when the country went to war again, recruits, trainees, and soldiers again showed up in its hospitals with tuberculosis, but this time the Army would have to look outside its own Medical Corps for "good tuberculosis men."

Notes

1. Benjamin Goldberg, "Presidential Address: War and Tuberculosis," *Diseases of the Chest* (October 1941): 322 and 324.

2. *Annual Report of the Surgeon General*, 1930 [hereafter cited as *ARSG*, year], 8.

3. The average hospital stay for all admissions during the 1920s ranged between three and eight weeks, with about six weeks for a gonorrhea patient, the most common diagnosis for Army hospitals. *ARSG*, 1934, 22; and *ARSG*, 1933, 52.

4. On the history of Denver see Carl Abbot, Stephen J. Leonard, and David Macomb, *Colorado: A History of the Centennial State*, rev. ed. (Boulder, CO: Colorado Associated University Press, 1982); Stephen J. Leonard and Thomas J. Noel, *Denver: Mining Camp to Metropolis* (Niwot, CO: University Press of Colorado, 1990); and Lyle W. Dorsett and Michael McCarthy, *The Queen City: A History of Denver*, 2d ed. (Boulder, CO: Pruett Publishing, 1986).

5. Abbot, Leonard, and Macomb, *Colorado: A History of the Centennial State*, 270.

6. Gerald Astor, *The Right to Fight: A History of African Americans in the Military* (Novato, CA: Presidio, 1998), 133; and P. S. Halloran, endorsement, 12 August 1930, "Accommodations for T. B. Patients—Female," Record Group [hereafter cited as RG] 112, Entry 31, 1928–37, Box 284, National Archives and Records Administration [hereafter cited as NARA]. In fact, national surveys of African American nurses counted only one in Denver in 1924 (named Vivian P. Lee), and another in 1940. See Darlene Clark Hine, *Black Women in the Nursing Profession: A Documentary History* (New York, NY: Garland, 1985), 57, 138.

7. P. S. Halloran, endorsement, 12 August 1930, "Accommodations for T. B. Patients—Female."

8. Pete Daniel, "Black Power in the 1920s: The Case of Tuskegee Veterans' Hospital," *Journal of Southern History* 36, no. 3 (1970): 368–88. See also Vanessa N. Gamble, *Making a Place for Ourselves: The Black Hospital Movement, 1920–1945* (Oxford, UK: Oxford University Press, 1995); Thomas J. Ward, Jr., *Black Physicians in the Jim Crow South* (Fayetteville, AR: University of Arkansas Press, 2003); and Susan L. Smith, *Sick and Tired of Being Sick and Tired: Black Women's Health Activism in America, 1890–1950* (Philadelphia, PA: University of Pennsylvania Press, 1995).

On blacks and tuberculosis see Marion M. Torchia, "The Tuberculosis Movement and the Race Question, 1890–1950," *Bulletin of the History of Medicine* 49 (1975): 152–68; Claudia Marie Calhoon, "Tuberculosis, Race and the Delivery of Health Care in Harlem, 1922–1939," *Radical*

History Review 80 (2001): 101–19; David McBride, *From TB to AIDS: Epidemics among Urban Blacks since 1900* (Albany, NY: State University of New York, 1991); and Tera Hunter, *To 'Joy My Freedom* (Boston, MA: Harvard University Press, 1997), chapter 9.

9. Jeanne Abrams, *Blazing the Tuberculosis Trail: The Religio-Ethnic Role of Four Sanatoria in Early Denver* (Denver, CO: Colorado Historical Society, 1991); Leonard and Noel, *Denver: Mining Camp to Metropolis*; and Meindert Bosch, *Bridges across the Years: A Ninety-Nine Year History of the Bethesda Hospital Association of Denver, Colorado* (Denver, CO: Bethesda PsycHealth System, 1988).

10. C. G. Snow to S. F. Siler, 9 March 1921, RG 112, Entry 31-J, Box 53, NARA.

11. Office of Public Affairs, Fitzsimons, *Fitzsimons Army Medical Center: The Life and History, 1918–1996* (Aurora, CO: Fitzsimons Army Medical Center, 1998).

12. *Public Health Service Annual Report,* 1923, 203; and Godias J. Drolet, "Tuberculosis Hospitalization in the United States," *American Review of Tuberculosis* 14 (1924): 623.

13. National Tuberculosis Association [NTA], *Directory of Tuberculosis Associations and Committees,* pamphlet No. 110 (New York, August 1919); and "Call Tuberculosis Worse than War," *New York Times* 14 September 1919. The NTA was the forerunner of the American Lung Association.

14. Katherine Ott, *Fevered Lives: Tuberculosis in American Culture since 1870* (Cambridge, MA: Harvard University Press, 1996); and James A. Tobey, "An Index to State Tuberculosis Laws," *Public Health Reports* 38 (1 June 1923): 1191–1200.

15. James A. Tobey, *The National Government and Public Health* (Baltimore, MD: Johns Hopkins Press, 1926), 107, 366–67.

16. Godias J. Drolet, "Tuberculosis Hospitalization in the United States: Results, Types of Cases, Facilities and Costs," *American Review of Tuberculosis* 14 (1926): 600–5.

17. See, for example, National Tuberculosis Association, "Directory of Sanatoria, Hospitals, Day Camps, and Preventoria for the Treatment of Tuberculosis in the United States," New York, NY, June 1923 and May 1934.

18. Ott, *Fevered Lives*, 80, n. 48.

19. Guenther Risse, *Mending Bodies, Saving Souls: A History of Hospitals* (New York, NY: Oxford University Press, 1999), 467; and Rosemary Stevens, *In Sickness and in Wealth: American Hospitals in the Twentieth Century* (New York, NY: Basic Books, Inc., 1989), chapter 5.

20. On standardization see Stevens, *In Sickness and in Wealth*, chapter 3.

21. *ARSG*, 1924.

22. *Fitzsimons Annual Report,* 1929 [hereafter cited as *FZAR,* year], RG 112, Fitzsimons General Hospital, Annual Reports, 1918–1930, Box 4, NARA.

23. *FZAR,* 1921.

24. Stevens, *In Sickness and in Wealth*, intro. According to Richard V. N. Ginn, the Medical Department hospitals lagged in the process of professionalizing hospital administration. See Ginn, *The History of the U.S. Army Medical Service Corps* (Washington, DC: Office of The Surgeon General and Center of Military History, 1997 [hereafter cited as Ginn, *Army Medical Service Corps History*]), 107.

25. See the discussion following Henry W. Hoagland, "The Treatment of Tuberculosis in the Army Hospitals," *Transactions of the American Climatological Association* (1919): 28–30; and Joseph F. Siler, U.S. Army Medical Department Historical Unit and U.S. Department of the Army, Office of The Surgeon General, *Communicable and Other Diseases, Medical Department of the United States Army in the World War,* vol. 9 (Washington, DC: U.S. Government Printing Office, 1928 [hereafter cited as Siler, *Communicable and Other Diseases*]), 196.

26. Biographical information from Esther E. Rohlader, "A Curriculum Vitae of Colonel Earl Harvey Bruns, MC, June 1965," RG 112, Biographical Background Files, Box 8, NARA; Walter Reed Army Medical Center, *Medical Officers Who Have Made Contributions of Worth to the Science of Medicine* (Washington, DC: Historical Unit, U.S. Army Medical Service, 1949); and RG 94, Records of the Adjutant General, Adjutant General's Office, Box 4073, NARA.

27. E. H. Bruns, "Reconstruction and Rehabilitation of the Tuberculous Soldier," *Journal of the American Medical Association*, 71 (3 August 1918): 373–75; and Earl H. Bruns, "The Unit System in Large Government Tuberculosis Hospitals," *U.S. Veterans' Bureau Medical Bulletin* 1 (January 1926): 7–9.

28. Bruns, "The Unit System in Large Government Tuberculosis Hospitals." For unit system of ward management as described by Earl Bruns, see *FZAR*, 1929, 30.

29. Earl H. Bruns, "The Climatic Treatment of Tuberculosis," *American Review of Tuberculosis* 26 (1932): 125.

30. William H. Moncrief Sr. died at Fitzsimons Hospital in 1961. His son, William H. Moncrief, Jr., also became a medical officer. See "William H. Moncrief," *Army Medical Bulletin* 50 (1939): 144–45; and the William H. Moncrief Papers, Military History Institute, Carlisle, PA. For biographical information on Hutton, see Association of Military Surgeons of the United States Biographical Sketch Collection, c. 1901–41, Manuscript Collection 142, Box 4, National Library of Medicine. During the war Hutton served in France with the 32d Division and on Pershing's general staff, and was awarded the coveted Distinguished Service Medal for his work.

31. "Lieut. Col. Paul C. Hutton, War Veteran, to be Fitzsimons Commander Sept. 1," *Rocky Mountain News*, 19 June 1923.

32. Lisa M. Budreau, *Bodies of War: World War I and the Politics of Commemoration in America, 1919–1933* (New York, NY: New York University Press, 2009); and Joseph W. A. Whitehorne, *The Inspectors General of the United States Army, 1903–1939* (Washington, DC: Office of the Inspector General and the Center of Military History, 1998), 325.

33. Ginn, *Army Medical Service Corps History*, 91.

34. "Promotions in the Army Medical Corps," *Army and Navy Journal*, 9 October 1926. Surgeon General Ireland was able to get Congress to approve an Army medical center, bringing together the various Army medical schools, and the Army Medical Museum on the campus of the Walter Reed General Hospital in Washington, DC. In 1920 the Medical Department also established the Medical Field Service School at Carlisle Barracks, PA, to train medical officers on the military side of their duties such as tactics, military organization, law, leadership, logistics, map reading, and medical field service (Ginn, *Army Medical Service Corps History*, 92).

35. U.S. Congress, Senate Special Committee on Readjustment of Service Pay, "Readjustment of Service Pay," November and December 1921, 67th Cong, 101. On reorganization see Ginn, *Army Medical Service Corps History*; and James A. Tobey, *The Medical Department of the Army: Its History, Activities, and Organization* (Baltimore, MD: The Johns Hopkins University Press, 1927), 46–50.

36. Tobey, *The Medical Department of the Army*, 48.

37. Ginn, *Army Medical Service Corps History*, 94.

38. *ARSG*, 1926, 15.

39. William Moncrief to Mahlon Ashford, 28 December 1922, RG 112, Entry 31-J, Box 24, NARA.

40. W. M. Moncrief to Charles R. Reynolds, 22 October 1921, RG 112, Entry 31-J, Box 24, NARA.

41. William Moncrief, *FZAR*, 1922.
42. J. A. Wilson to commanding officer, 16 September 1926, RG 112, Fitzsimons General Hospital Reports, Laboratory Services, 1918–39, Box 6, NARA; and Earl H. Bruns to J. F. Siler, 24 January 1929, RG 112, Entry 31-J, Box 280, NARA.
43. E. H. Bruns to J. F. Siler, 24 January 1929, RG 112, Entry 31-J, Box 280, NARA.
44. *ARSG*, 1924, 322.
45. Paul Kostinen has argued that such streamlining required greater cooperation and coordination with the private sector, laying the groundwork for the military-industrial complex, in Paul A. C. Koistinen, "The 'Industrial-Military Complex' in Historical Perspective: The Interwar Years," *Journal of American History* 56 (March 1970): 819–39. See also Whitehorne, *The Inspectors General of the United States Army*, 355; and Ginn, *Army Medical Service Corps History*, 94.
46. *FZAR*, 1924, 9.
47. *ARSG*, 1929, 8.
48. Surgeon General's Office [hereafter cited as SGO], "Monthly Per Diem Operating Expenses for Period January 1 to March 31, 1924," RG 112, Entry 29, Box 172, NARA.
49. On the bonus veterans, see D. Clayton James, *The Years of McArthur* (Boston, MA: Houghton-Mifflin, 1985); Jennifer D. Keene, *Doughboys, the Great War, and the Remaking of America* (Baltimore, MD: Johns Hopkins University Press, 2001); John W. Killigrew, "The Impact of the Great Depression on the Army," Ph.D. dissertation, Indiana University, 1979; and William Pencak, *For God and Country: The American Legion, 1919–1940* (Boston, MA: Northeastern University Press, 1989). An exception is Stephen Ortiz who discusses veterans' disability benefits policy in Stephen R. Ortiz, "The 'New Deal' for Veterans: The Economy Act, the Veterans of Foreign Wars, and the Origin of New Deal Dissent," *Journal of Military History* 70 (April 2006), 415–38.
50. Walter P. Dillingham, *Federal Aid to Veterans, 1917–1941* (Tallahassee, FL: University of Florida Press, 1952), 170–71 and 219–20.
51. *ARSG*, 1929, 3.
52. J. F. Siler to P. C. Hutton, 9 January 1928, RG 112, Entry 31, 1928–37, Box 271, NARA.
53. See SGO, "Monthly Per Diem Operating Expenses for Period January 1 to March 31, 1924"; and Merritte Ireland, Memorandum, 14 October 1924, RG 112, Entry 29, Box 172, NARA.
54. On the history of veterans' benefits see Stephen P. Ortiz, ed., *The Politics of Veterans' Policy* (Gainesville, FL: University Press of Florida, 2012); Larry M. Logue, "Union Veterans and Their Government: The Effects of Public Policies on Private Lives," *Journal of Interdisciplinary History* 22 (1992): 411–34; Theda Skocpol, *Protecting Soldiers and Mothers: The Political Origins of Social Policy in the United States* (Cambridge, MA: Belkap Press of Harvard University Press, 1992); Dillingham, *Federal Aid to Veterans*; Gustavus A. Weber and Laurence F. Schmeckebier, *The Veterans' Administration: Its History, Activities, and Organization* (Washington, DC: Brookings Institution, 1934); and Peter Karsten, *Soldiers and Society: The Effects of Military Service and War on American Life* (Westport, CT: Greenwood Press, 1978).
55. U.S. Congress, 65th Cong., 1st sess., Senate Document 81, W. G. McAdoo, "The Duty of a Just Government," August 15, 1917, 3.
56. Congress established an entirely new system based upon indemnity and compensation for World War I veterans, rather than gratuity. See Dillingham, *Federal Aid to Veterans*, 5.
57. K. Walter Hickel, "War, Region, and Social Welfare: Federal Aid to Servicemen's Dependents in the South, 1917–1921," *Journal of American History* 87 (March 2001): 1368.

58. According to a 1921 Bureau of War Risk Insurance study, on 5 May 1921, 26,266 patients were hospitalized, 10,266 of them for tuberculosis; 16,764 were in federal hospitals, the rest in contract hospitals. 10 June 1921, *Cong. Record*, 67th Cong., 1st sess., vol. 61, pt. 3, 2409–11.

59. Bess Furman, *Profile of the United States Public Health Service, 1798–1950* (Washington, DC: Government Printing Office, 1973), 328.

60. Hugh S. Cumming, "Tuberculosis Among the Ex-Service Men," *Journal of the American Medical Association* 79 (29 July 1922): 373–74; also published in *Public Health Reports* 37 (15 September 1922): 2241–52.

61. George Thomas Palmer and Henry W. Hoagland, "The Sanatorium Care of Tuberculous Soldiers by the Federal Government," *Transactions of the National Tuberculosis Association* 17 (1921): 471–72, and 475. For more on this situation, see Charles M. Montgomery, "The Medical Profession and the Tuberculous Ex-Service Patient," *Public Health Reports* 36 (2 December 1921): 2938–42; Cumming, "Tuberculosis Among the Ex-Service Men"; Philip P. Jacobs, "Tuberculosis as a War Problem," *Military Surgeon* 55 (1924): 498–514, 630–49, and 737–51; Godias J. Drolet, "Tuberculosis Hospitalization in the United States," *American Review of Tuberculosis* 14 (1924): 600–24; and Philip B. Matz, "The Tuberculosis Problem in the United States Veterans' Bureau," *American Review of Tuberculosis* 18 (1928): 776–93.

62. The President's Commission on Veterans' Pensions, *The Historical Development of Veterans' Benefits in the United States*, U.S. Congress, 84th Cong., 2nd sess., House Committee Print No. 244 ed. (Washington, DC: Government Printing Office, 1956), 43.

63. "400 Yanks Barred from Hospitals of Denver by Government Red Tape," *Denver Post* 21 April 1920.

64. Remarks by Rep. Carl Hayden, 30 March 1922, *Congressional Record*, 67th Cong., 2nd sess., vol. 62, pt. 5, 4814.

65. Correspondence regarding "Beneficiaries of the Soldiers' Home" February–May 1923, RG 112, Entry 31-J, Box 53, NARA.

66. Senate Report No. 233, 67th Cong., 1st sess., submitted 20 July 1921, *Congressional Record*, 67th Cong., 1st sess., 4092–95.

67. Report on "Consolidation of Government Agencies for Ex-Service Men," 19 April 1921, *Congressional Record*, 67th Cong., 1st sess., 458.

68. The American Medical Association opposed specialized hospitals for veterans, concerned that they would compete with other hospitals and limit their members' access to patients. AMA opposition intensified in 1924 when Congress extended veterans' benefits to non-service-related care, which some in the organization considered socialized medicine. Stevens, *In Sickness and in Wealth*, 127–29.

69. Furman, *Profile of the Public Health Service*, 344–47.

70. A. G. Crane, U.S. Army Medical Department Historical Unit and U.S. Department of the Army, Office of The Surgeon General, *Physical Reconstruction and Vocational Education*, and Julia C. Stimson, *The Army Nurse Corps*, vol. 13 (Washington, DC: U.S. Government Printing Office, 1923 [hereafter cited as Crane, *Reconstruction* and Stimson, *Army Nurse*]), 603–5. See also, for example, Administrator of Veterans' Affairs, *Annual Report*, 1932 (Washington, DC: Government Printing Office, 1932), 12–17.

71. Earl Bruns and others estimated that at war's end as many as 26,000 more soldiers and sailors might need hospitalization for tuberculosis discovered during their military discharge examinations and recommended 13,000 more tuberculosis beds in federal hospitals for demobilization. See letter from the Secretary of the Treasury, "Additional Hospital Facilities for Discharged Soldiers, Sailors, Marines, and Army and Navy Nurses," 1920, House Doc. 481, U.S. Cong., 66th Cong., 2nd sess., 24.

72. William H. Baldwin, "The Present Status of Soldiers and Draft Rejects with Tuberculosis," *American Review of Tuberculosis* 3 (1919): 328.

73. Members of Congress could—and still can—introduce private bills to address an individual's problem regarding a wide range of federal laws.

74. Remarks by Rep. Royal Cleaves Johnson (R-SD), on S. 2257, *Congressional Record*, 68th Cong., 1st sess., 10168.

75. The language reads, "Every commissioned officer, or enlisted man, or any other member of the military service who suffers a disability from disease contracted in line of duty shall be entitled to compensation, provided that the disease has not been caused by his own willful misconduct." Siler, *Communicable and Other Diseases*, 200.

76. Katherine Mayo, *Soldiers What Next!* (Boston, MA and New York, NY: Houghton Miffllin, 1934), 100.

77. Gustavus A. Weber and Laurence F. Schmeckebier, *The Veterans' Administration: Its History, Activities, and Organization* (Washington, DC: Brookings Institution, 1934), 459. See also William Pencak, *For God and Country: The American Legion, 1919–1940* (Boston, MA: Northeastern University Press, 1989), 185. On determining eligibility for hospital care and disability benefits for active-duty military personnel developing tuberculosis after 1925 see Alexander T. Cooper and Shannon L. Van Valzah, "Line of Duty in Pulmonary Tuberculosis," *Military Surgeon* 65 (July 1929): 53–58.

78. There is a small, but growing literature on the history of disabled veterans. See, for example, Beth O'Donnell Linker, *War's Waste: Rehabilitation in World War I America* (Chicago, IL: University of Chicago Press, 2011); Ana Carden-Coyne, "Ungrateful Bodies: Rehabilitation, Resistance and Disabled American Veterans in the First World War, *European Review of History* 14 (December 2007): 543–65; David A. Gerber, ed., *Disabled Veterans in History* (Ann Arbor, MI: University of Michigan Press, 2000); and Ortiz, *The Politics of Veterans' Policy*.

79. K. Walter Hickel, "Medicine, Bureaucracy, and Social Welfare: The Politics of Disability Compensation for American Veterans of World War I," in Gerber, *The New Disability History*, 245–46.

80. Rep. Carroll Reece remarks on S. 2257, 17 May 1924, *Congressional Record*, 68th, 1st sess., 8841.

81. U.S. Congress, House Committee on World War Veterans' Legislation, "World War Veterans' Legislation," pt 1., January 1926, 69th Cong., 1st sess. [hereafter cited as World War Veterans' Legislation].

82. World War Veterans' Legislation, 189.

83. World War Veterans' Legislation, 173.

84. World War Veterans' Legislation, 157.

85. World War Veterans' Legislation, 206.

86. World War Veterans' Legislation, 174.

87. World War Veterans' Legislation, 174.

88. World War Veterans' Legislation, 189.

89. World War Veterans' Legislation, 207–8.

90. H.R. 4474, and Dillingham, *Federal Aid to Veterans*, 49.

91. Dillingham, *Federal Aid to Veterans*, 50.

92. W. Paul Havens Jr., U.S. Army Medical Department Historical Unit and U.S. Department of the Army, Office of The Surgeon General, *Internal Medicine in World War II, Medical Department, United States Army in World War II*, vol. 2 (Washington, DC: U.S. Department of Defense, Department of the Army, Office of The Surgeon General, 1963): 331–32.

93. Dillingham, *Federal Aid to Veterans*, 54.

94. Hickel, "Medicine, Bureaucracy, and Social Welfare," 248.
95. William H. Baldwin, "The Present Status of Soldiers and Draft Rejects with Tuberculosis," *American Review of Tuberculosis* 3 (1919): 326.
96. Linker, *War's Waste*; and Beth O'Donnell Linker, "The Business of Ethics: Gender, Medicine, and the Professional Codification of the American Physiotherapy Association, 1918–1935," *Journal of the History of Medicine and Allied Sciences* 60 (July 2005): 320–54.
97. See, for example, Conrad E. Koeper, "Convalescent Hospital-Limited Service Corps," 10 March 1918, RG 112, Entry 10, Box 4603, NARA; and Estes Nichols, "Medical, Hospital and Social Aspects of Reconstruction for the Tuberculous," *Transactions of the National Tuberculosis Association* (1919): 174.
98. A. G. Crane, *Education for the Disabled in War and Industry. Army Hospital Schools: A Demonstration for the Education of Disabled in Industry* (New York, NY: Teachers College, Columbia University, 1921), 2.
99. Dillingham, *Federal Aid to Veterans*, 141.
100. E. H. Bruns, "Reconstruction and Rehabilitation of the Tuberculous Soldier," 375.
101. Fitzsimons General Hospital, *The Gift Book: Fitzsimons General Hospital, U.S.A* (Denver, CO: Wahlgreen Publishing, 1926).
102. Contemporaries and scholars refer to these activities by various terms including reconstruction, rehabilitation, occupational therapy, or vocational therapy. As Eliot Friedson has explained, "'Rehabilitation' is a vague and poorly delineated concept, and its concrete aims subject to a fair degree of variation. It has included physical training as well as vocational education, concrete surgical repair and correction as well as psychotherapy." Eliot Friedson, in Foreword, Glenn Gritzer and Arnold Arluke, *The Making of Rehabilitation: A Political Economy of Medical Specialization, 1890 to 1980* (Berkeley, CA: University of California Press, 1985), *xv*. I use the term rehabilitation for simplicity.
103. *FZAR*, 1927, 16; and *FZAR*, 1929.
104. *FZAR*, 1924, 13; and *FZAR*, 1922, 14–15.
105. Estes Nichols, "Medical, Hospital and Social Aspects of Reconstruction for the Tuberculous," *Transactions of the National Tuberculosis Association* (1919): 175. See also Harriet S. Lee and Myra L. McDaniel, *Army Medical Specialist Corps* (Washington, DC: Office of The Surgeon General, Department of the Army, 1968).
106. *FZAR*, 1927, 35; and *ARSG*, 1925, 382.
107. The President's Commission on Veterans' Pensions, *The Historical Development of Veterans' Benefits in the United States*, U.S. Congress, 84th Cong., 2nd sess., House Committee Print No. 244 ed. (Washington, DC: Government Printing Office, 1956), 132; Dillingham, *Federal Aid to Veterans*, 143; David R. Lyman, "The Limitations and Possibilities in the Federal Care of Tuberculous Ex-Service Patients," *Transactions of the National Tuberculosis Association* (1921): 83; and Mayo, *Soldiers What Next!*
108. Commission on Veterans' Pensions, *The Historical Development of Veterans' Benefits in the United States*, 130–32; and Dillingham, *Federal Aid to Veterans*, 141.
109. *ARSG*, 1934, 22–24.
110. William Charles White, "Progress in Tuberculosis Work," *Transactions of the National Tuberculosis Association*, 23rd annual meeting (1927): 62–64.
111. Hoyt E. Dearholt, "Progress in Public Education," *Transactions of the National Tuberculosis Association*, 23rd annual meeting (1927): 71.
112. Thomas D. Brock, *Robert Koch: A Life in Medicine and Bacteriology* (Madison, WI: Science Tech Publishers, 1988), chapter 18. On the more recent use of tuberculin testing see "Targeted Tuberculin Testing and Treatment of Latent Tuberculosis Infection," *Morbidity and Mortality Weekly Report* 49 (9 June 2000).

113. In a distinct departure from the theory of "tubercularization," a Public Health Service researcher, Wade Hampton Frost, proposed in 1937 that people with tuberculosis be identified and isolated and their contacts be tested for tuberculosis and also isolated and treated if infected. This established the principle of the Index Patient approach to epidemiology. See W. H. Frost, "How Much Control of Tuberculosis?" *American Journal of Public Health* 27 (August 1937): 759–66.

114. E. H. Bruns and Joseph Casper, "The Present Status of Chest Surgery in the Treatment of Pulmonary Tuberculosis," *American Review of Tuberculosis* 26 (1932): 665–87. See also E. H. Bruns and Joseph Casper, "Thoracoplasty in the Treatment of Chronic Pulmonary Tuberculosis," *American Review of Tuberculosis* 22 (1930): 739–56.

115. *FZAR*, 1921.

116. Bier donated his notes to the National Library of Medicine (NLM), "in memory of one of the Corps Finest Officers and Greatest Clinician, Colonel Edward [sic] H. Bruns." "Fitzsimons General Hospital, Denver, Lecture Notes, 1926–1927," NLM, WB 9 Y5 8L 1951 [hereafter cited as Lecture Notes, 1926–27].

117. E. H. Bruns, "Lecture IV, Pathology of Tuberculosis Autopsy," Lecture Notes, 1926–27, 1.

118. E. H. Bruns, "Lecture VI, Diagnosis of Pulmonary Tuberculosis," Lecture Notes, 1926–27, 2–3.

119. E. H. Bruns, "Lecture VI, Diagnosis of Pulmonary Tuberculosis," Lecture Notes, 1926–27, 7.

120. E. H. Bruns, "Lecture XVII, General Treatment of Tuberculosis," Lecture Notes, 1926–27, 1.

121. E. H. Bruns, "Lecture XVII, General Treatment of Tuberculosis," Lecture Notes, 1926–27, 3–6.

122. Earl Bruns to Paul Hutton, 1 March 1922, RG 112, Entry 29, Box 403, NARA.

123. Thomas E. Scott, "Holderness-Brunson Treatment for Tuberculosis," 30 June 1922, RG 112, Entry 29, Box 403, NARA.

124. *FZAR*, 1928, 26.

125. *FZAR*, 1931, 23; and E. H. Bruns, "Lecture XVII, General Treatment of Tuberculosis," Lecture Notes, 1926–27.

126. E. H. Bruns, "Lecture XIX, The Psychology of the Tuberculosis Patient," Lecture Notes, 1926–27, 9; and Earl H. Bruns, "The Climatic Treatment of Tuberculosis," *American Review of Tuberculosis* 26 (1932): 133.

127. For example, Charles Denison, *Rocky Mountain Health Resorts: An Analytical Study of High Altitudes in Relation to the Arrest of Chronic Pulmonary Disease* (Boston, MA: Houghton, Mifflin, and Co., 1880); Guy Hinsdale, "The Sun, Health and Heliotherapy," *Transactions of the American Climatological Association* (1919): 1–11; Horace LoGrasso and Frank C. Balderrey, "Heliotherapy in the Treatment of Pulmonary Tuberculosis," *American Review of Tuberculosis* 10 (1924–25): 117–31; and Samuel H. Watson, "Heliotherapy in Tuberculosis: A Scheme for Proper Selection of Cases, with a Word about Technique," *Southwestern Medicine* 10 (1925–26). Also on heliotherapy see Andrew McClary, "Sunning for Health: Heliotherapy as Seen by Professionals and Popularizers, 1920–1940," *Journal of American Culture* 5 (1982): 65–68; Carolyn June McQuien, "Tuberculosis as Chronic Illness in the United States: Understanding, Treating and Living with the Disease, 1884–1954," Ph.D. dissertation, University of Texas at Austin, 1993, 41–46.

128. The Nobel Foundation, see http://nobelprize.org/nobel_prizes/medicine/laureates/1903/finsen-bio.html, accessed 24 August 2012. Thomas Dormandy, *The White Death: A History of Tuberculosis* (New York, NY: New York University Press, 1999); and Henry W. Randle, "Suntanning: Differences in Perceptions Throughout History," *Mayo Clinic Proceedings* 72 (1997): 461–66.

129. U.S. General Hospital No. 20, Whipple Barracks, Ariz., "Rules for Sun Baths (Heliotherapy)," RG 112, Entry 31-J, Box 252, NARA and A. Rollier, "The Construction of an Institution for the Helio-therapic [*sic*] Treatment of Surgical Tuberculosis," *Tubercle* 2 (March 1921): 241–50.

130. E. H. Bruns, Memorandum, "Heliotherapy," 20 February 1922, RG 112, Entry 29, Box 403, NARA.

131. E. H. Bruns, "Lecture XIX, The Psychology of the Tuberculosis Patient," Lecture Notes, 1926–27, 7–8.

132. E. H. Bruns, "Heliotherapy in Tuberculosis," *Military Surgeon* 57 (1925): 383.

133. E. H. Bruns, "Heliotherapy in Tuberculosis Spondylitis," *American Review of Tuberculosis* 10 (1924–25): 136.

134. Bruns, "Heliotherapy in Tuberculosis Spondylitis," 137, 133.

135. Bruns, "Heliotherapy in Tuberculosis," 390.

136. E. H. Bruns, "Lecture XVII, General Treatment of Tuberculosis," Lecture Notes, 1926–27, 7; and Bruns, "Heliotherapy in Tuberculosis," 389.

137. Bruns, "Heliotherapy in Tuberculosis Spondylitis," 135. On Pott's disease, see also Linker, *War's Waste*, 36-52.

138. "Surgeon General Praises Work of Aides in Message," *The Re-Aides Post* (May 1924) in Estelle Angier, Medical Historical Unit, Personal Papers, Military History Institute, Carlisle, PA; and William C. Pollock, "Heliotherapy in Pulmonary Tuberculosis," *American Review of Tuberculosis* 14 (November 1926): 505.

139. I. D. Bronfin, "Heliotherapy in Advanced Pulmonary Tuberculosis," *American Review of Tuberculosis* 11 (1925): 96–111; and Edgar Mayer, "The Present Status of Heliotherapy in Tuberculosis," *Transactions of the National Tuberculosis Association*, 30th Annual Meeting (1934): 74.

140. Alfred J. Crowle, Elise J. Ross, and Mary H. May, "Inhibition by 1,25(OH)2-Vitamin D3 of the Multiplication of Virulent Tubercle Bacilli in Cultured Human Macrophages," *Infection and Immunity* 55 (December 1987): 2945–50. This research is explained by John Sbarbaro in a lecture, "Arts in Medicine," at the University of Colorado at Denver and Health Sciences Center, Denver, 2007, on DVD at the Denison Library, University of Colorado.

141. Michael D. Iseman, *A Clinician's Guide to Tuberculosis* (Philadelphia, PA: Lippincott Williams & Wilkins, 2000), 12.

142. On collapse therapies, see Dormandy, *The White Death*; Larry I. Lutwick, *Tuberculosis* (London, UK: Chapman and Hall Medical, 1995), 13–16; Ott, *Fevered Lives*; Linda Bryder, *Below the Magic Mountain: A Social History of Tuberculosis in Twentieth-Century Britain* (Oxford, UK: Clarendon Press, 1988), chapter 6; Godfrey L. Gale and Norman C. DeLarue, "Surgical History of Pulmonary Tuberculosis: The Rise and Fall of Various Technical Procedures," *Journal of Canadian Surgery* 12 (October 1969): 381–88; and R. Y. Keers, *Pulmonary Tuberculosis: A Journey Down the Centuries* (London, UK: Bailliere Tindall, Cassell Ltd., 1978), chapters 10 and 14.

143. E. H. Bruns and Joseph Casper, "Thoracoplasty in the Treatment of Chronic Pulmonary Tuberculosis," *American Review of Tuberculosis* 22 (1930): 739.

144. Jake W. Spidle Jr., *Doctors of Medicine in New Mexico* (Albuquerque, NM: University of New Mexico Press, 1986), chapter 4.

145. On the history of pneumothorax see James J. Waring, "The History of Artificial Pneumothorax in America," *Journal of Outdoor Life* 31 (1934): 16–18. On pneumothorax, see M. [Mary] E. Lapham, "The Treatment of Pulmonary Tuberculosis by Artificial Pneumothorax," *Stethoscopic Medicine Journal* 4 (1911): 742; Samuel Robinson and Cleaveland Floyd, "Artificial Pneumothorax as a Treatment of Pulmonary Tuberculosis," *Archives of Internal Medicine* (1912): 452–83; Roy W. Matson, Ralph C. Matson, and Mark Bascallion, "End Results of 600 Cases of Pulmonary Tuberculosis Treated with Artificial Pneumothorax," *American Review of Tuberculosis* (June 1923): 50.

146. Fort Bayard, "Annual Report for 1916," 6 February 1916, RG 112, Entry 26, Box 919, NARA; and Earl H. Bruns, "Artificial Pneumothorax in Treatment of TB," *New Mexico Medical Journal* (January 1915).

147. *ARSG*, 1932, 262–63, and 276.

148. *ARSG*, 1932, 262–63; and I. S. Kahn, "Artificial Pneumothorax Treatment of Pulmonary Tuberculosis at the Base Hospital Fort Sam Houston," *South Texas Medical Record* 14 (1920–21): 28–36.

149. Samuel Robinson and Cleaveland Floyd, "Artificial Pneumothorax as a Treatment of Pulmonary Tuberculosis," *Archives of Internal Medicine* (1912): 465.

150. Sudie E. Pyatt, "My Pneumothorax Days Are Over," *Journal of the Outdoor Life* 27 (1930): 344–45.

151. C. D. Parfitt and D. W. Crombie, "Five Years' Experience with Artificial Pneumothorax," *Transactions of the American Climatological Association* (1918): 52–80.

152. Abstract of E. H. Bruns, "Air Embolism as a Complication in Artificial Pneumothorax Therapy," *Colorado Medicine* 27 (1930): 237, in *Tubercle* 12 (December 1931): 126–27. See also Bruns, "Lecture XXI, Artificial Pneumothorax," Lecture Notes, 1926–27.

153. James L. Dubrow, "Effect of Permanent Pulmonary Collapse on the Heart," *Journal of the American Medical Association* 90 (28 April 1928): 1364.

154. Bruns, "Air Embolism as a Complication in Artificial Pneumothorax Therapy."

155. A. E. Ellis, *The Rack* (London, UK: Penguin Books, 1958, 1961), 277–78.

156. Thomas Mann, *The Magic Mountain* (various publishers, 1924), 48 and 301.

157. Donald Stewart, *Sanatorium* (New York, NY: Harper and Brothers, 1930), 81–82.

158. Ott, *Fevered Lives*, 99; and William C. Pollock, "Collapse Therapy in Pulmonary Tuberculosis," *American Review of Tuberculosis* 22 (1930): 780.

159. Andrew Peters, et al, "Survey of Artificial Pneumothorax in Representative American Tuberculosis Sanatoria, 1915–1930," *American Review of Tuberculosis* 31 (1935): 85–101.

160. Linda Bryder, *Below the Magic Mountain: A Social History of Tuberculosis in Twentieth-Century Britain* (Oxford, UK: Clarendon Press, 1988), 176–77.

161. *FZAR*, 1934, 20–21; and *FZAR*, 1939, 7.

162. *FZAR*, 1929 and 1935. See also Ralph C. Matson, "Surgical Treatment of Pulmonary Tuberculosis," *Transactions of the National Tuberculosis Association*, 23rd Annual Meeting (1927): 79–96; and Sam R. King and H. A. Patterson, "Severing Adhesions in Artificial Pneumothorax," *Southwestern Medicine* 19–20 (1935–36): 370–76; and *FZAR*, 1929.

163. Alexander T. Cooper, "Phrenicoexairesis in Pulmonary Tuberculosis," *American Review of Tuberculosis* 22 (1930): 779.

164. Philip B. Matz, "The End Results of the Surgical Treatment of Pulmonary Tuberculosis," *American Review of Tuberculosis* 33 (April 1936): 549.

165. See, for example, G. E. Bushnell, U.S. General Hospital, Fort Bayard, NM, 1904, "Surgical Report," RG 112, Entry 380, NARA; and Edward P. Rockhill, "Cases of Surgical Tuberculosis at Fort Bayard," 9 November 1918, RG 112, Entry 31-J, Box 20, NARA.

166. Ira M. Rutkow, *American Surgery: An Illustrated History* (Philadelphia, PA: Lippincott-Raven, 1998); Wilson Ruffin Abbot and F. J. Nordby, "The Prognostic Influence of Surgery upon the Sanatorium Tuberculosis Patient," *Southwestern Medicine* 9 (February 1925): 45–51; Matson, "Surgical Treatment of Pulmonary Tuberculosis," 79–96; H. G. Wetherill, "Surgery for Tuberculosis," *Journal of the American Medical Association* 80 (6 January 1923): 6–8; and Philip B. Matz, "The Surgical Treatment of Pulmonary Tuberculosis in the United States Veterans' Bureau," *American Review of Tuberculosis* 20 (1929): 809–32.

167. Dormandy, *The White Death*, 354–57.

168. Julia Irene Kemp, "Nursing Care in Thoracoplastic Operations," *American Journal of Nursing* 29 (1929): 123–24.

169. Herbert Sloan, "Historical Perspectives of the American Association for Thoracic Surgery: John Alexander (1891–1954)," *Journal of Thoracic and Cardiovascular Surgery* 29 (2005): 435–436; John Alexander, *The Collapse Therapy for Pulmonary Tuberculosis* (Springfield, IL: Clarence C Thomas, 1937).

170. *FZAR*, 1929, 28.

171. Bruns and Casper, "Present Status of Chest Surgery," 669.

172. Bruns and Casper, "Thoracoplasty in the Treatment of Chronic Pulmonary Tuberculosis," 742; and William H. Thearle, "Extra Pleural Thoracoplasty in Pulmonary Tuberculosis," *Southwestern Medicine* 10 (1926): 296–304.

173. Bruns and Casper, "Thoracoplasty in the Treatment of Chronic Pulmonary Tuberculosis," 748.

174. Kemp, "Nursing Care in Thoracoplastic Operations," 127. Also on nursing care, see Laura Ahrendt, "Thoracoplasty," *American Journal of Nursing* 38 (1938): 929–31.

175. Kemp, "Nursing Care in Thoracoplastic Operations," 128.

176. Robert J. Gosling, "Role of Physical Medicine in the Tuberculous Thoracic Surgical Patient," 1953, Medical Historical Unit Collection, Military History Institute, Carlisle, PA.

177. *ARSG*, 1932, 277.

178. Bruns and Casper, "Thoracoplasty in the Treatment of Chronic Pulmonary Tuberculosis," 750.

179. Thearle, "Extra Pleural Thoracoplasty in Pulmonary Tuberculosis," 299.

180. War Department, The Adjutant General's Office, *Army Register* (Washington, DC: Government Printing Office,) 1 January 1925, 798; and 1 January 1927, 829.

181. Thearle, "Extra Pleural Thoracoplasty in Pulmonary Tuberculosis," 304.

182. Editorial, "Surgery for Pulmonary Tuberculosis," *American Medicine* 35 (June 1929): 336.

183. Watson B. Miller to M. W. Ireland, 22 December 1924, RG 112, Entry 29, Box 403, NARA.

184. M. W. Ireland to Watson B. Miller, 14 January 1925, RG 112, Entry 29, Box 403, NARA.

185. Lawrason Brown and Homer L. Sampson, "The Fate of the 'Good Chronic' Case of Pulmonary Tuberculosis," *Transactions of the National Tuberculosis Association* (1934): 336.

186. Helen Clapesattle, *Dr. Webb of Colorado Springs* (Boulder, CO: Colorado Associated University Press, 1984), 249–59 and 396.

187. Patricia Paton, *A Medical Gentleman: James J. Waring, M.D.* (Denver, CO: Colorado Historical Society, 1993), 117.

188. James J. Waring, "The History of Artificial Pneumothorax in America," *Journal of the Outdoor Life* 31 (1934): 16.

189. Dormandy, *The White Death*, 358.

190. James S. Olson, *A History of Cancer: An Annotated Bibliography* (New York, NY: Greenwood Press, 1989), 233–34.

191. The major role played by surgery in the "conquest" of tuberculosis after World War II has been largely neglected. An exception is Barron H. Lerner, *Contagion and Confinement: Controlling Tuberculosis along Skid Row* (Baltimore, MD: Johns Hopkins University Press, 1998), 62.

192. Benjamin J. Pomerantz, et al., "Pulmonary Resection for Multi-Drug Resistant Tuberculosis," *Journal of Thoracic and Cardiovascular Surgery* 121 (2001): 448–53; R. K. Dewan, et al., "Thoracoplasty: An Obsolete Procedure?" *Indian Journal of Chest Disease and Allied Sciences* (1999): 83–88; and Lisa Belkin, "A Brutal Cure," *New York Times Magazine* (30 May 1999): 34–39.

193. J. F. Siler to William Moncrief, 12 February 1923, RG 112, Entry 31-J, Box 43, NARA.

194. William Moncrief to J. F. Siler, 13 March 1923, RG 112, Entry 31-J, Box 43, NARA.

195. William Moncrief, "Policy of Retaining Officers, Members of the Army Nurse Corps, and Enlisted Men, in the Service, after They Develop Manifest Tuberculosis," 13 March 1923, RG 112, Entry 31-J, Box 43, NARA.

196. *FZAR*, 1931, 39.

197. *ARSG*, 1931, 135.

198. Emphasis in the original. Robert U. Patterson, "Policy of the Surgeon General as Regards Military Personnel with Pulmonary Tuberculosis," 22 March 1932, RG 112, Entry 29, Box 108, NARA. The policy was slightly different for nurses who could return to duty after treatment for a "minimal lesion," but were then sent before a retiring board if they suffered a reactivation. Enlisted men who had been diagnosed with tuberculosis needed a special waiver to return to duty or reenlist.

199. Robert U. Patterson, "Policy of the Surgeon General as Regards Military Personnel with Pulmonary Tuberculosis," 22 March 1932, emphasis added.

200. W. P. Chamberlain to C. D. Buck, 7 October 1932, RG112, Entry 31-J, NARA. Emphasis in the original. Bubb was retired on disability in March 1934 but returned to duty during World War II as a colonel in the Army Air Corps, serving as chief of staff of the 8th Bomber Command and 8th Air Force in England, 1942–43.

201. C. D. Buck to S. J. Morris, correspondence, 10 August 1932, RG 112, Entry 31, 1928–37, Box 280, NARA.

202. "Col. Earl H. Bruns Expires in El Paso," *Rocky Mountain News*, 17 March 1933.

203. The portrait was done by artist J. I. McClymont, Colorado Springs, and has hung in the Bruns Conference Room of Building 500 on the site of the former Army hospital post, now called the Fitzsimons Life Science District.

204. Information on the Bruns Memorial comes from the scrapbooks and diaries of Lawrence Lewis, Lawrence Lewis Papers, 385 N11, C4, Colorado Historical Society, Denver. See also "Memory of Colonel Bruns is Eulogized at Banquet," *Rocky Mountain News*, 25 May 1934.

Chapter Six
"Good Tuberculosis Women": Tuberculosis Nursing during the Interwar Period

After eight-year-old Martha A. Hauch's mother died of pulmonary tuberculosis in 1904, Martha went to live with relatives in Virginia. Her father sent them money for her maintenance until his investments failed. To support herself as she became a young woman, Hauch tried teaching, working as a government clerk, and finally enrolled in the Army School of Nursing in January 1922 at the age of twenty-six. Like other nursing schools, the Army School of Nursing considered students an important source of labor. Instruction included coursework and hospital duty. Hauch trained at Walter Reed Hospital in Washington, DC, Fort McHenry in Baltimore, and an affiliated hospital in Philadelphia. At all three locations she cared for tuberculosis patients. In Philadelphia, she said that she worked "in the isolation ward in the obstetrical ward and cared for a very ill tubercular patient both before and after delivery." Many of her other patients "were in the advanced stages of the disease; a number of them were so ill that very close contact was necessary to care for them properly, such as helping them move, handling sputum cups, which all came under the general nursing care of the patient."[1]

In August 1923, Hauch spit up blood, or as she put it, had "a little color in my throat," but after a normal X-ray she returned to hospital duty. Five months later she had another hemorrhage, but the Medical Department reported "no definite diagnosis being made," so she continued to study and work. That August at Walter Reed Hospital, Hauch developed a cough and was finally diagnosed with tuberculosis and transferred to Fitzsimons for "chronic pulmonary tuberculosis, active, upper left lobe."[2] Because she had not yet completed her Army School of Nursing course, Fitzsimons put her on light duty status for the remaining three weeks required to complete her training. After graduation, she continued at Fitzsimons as a civilian patient/nurse until the end of 1924 when she became too ill to work.

Fitzsimons' physicians then tried to give the young woman a pneumothorax but could not because the lung adhered to the chest wall. Her condition deteriorated and from 6 April to 24 April she had twenty-three hemorrhages and was put on strict bedrest. As one of the fifty to sixty civilians treated at Fitzsimons every year, Hauch paid $1.50 per day for her care, but after eighteen months her resources were depleted. Not eligible for military benefits, Hauch and her relatives appealed to Congressman R. Walton Moore of Virginia for a private bill to pay her hospital costs. (Private bills are still used today to enable members of Congress to address the special needs of individuals.) Twenty months later Congress approved a private bill to keep Hauch as a patient at Fitzsimons. A congressional committee report stated that "according to the testimony, it appears that Miss Hauch was thrown into such intimate contact with advanced cases of pulmonary tuberculosis in the performance of her duties that it may be reasonable from the medical standpoint to assume that her present physical condition was probably caused by her occupation."[3] It is not known how long Hauch survived, but she struggled with the disease for several years, and by June 1928, her relatives were concerned that she would not live long enough to receive the congressionally mandated benefits.[4]

Hauch's case is but one of many examples of the perils of tuberculosis nursing. Modern hospitals and the increasingly aggressive treatment of tuberculosis in the 1920s, 1930s, and 1940s provided expanding job opportunities for nurses, but surgery and invasive procedures that drained wounds and chest cavities filled with purulent matter and tuberculosis bacteria also put them closer to sources of infection. The Army tuberculosis program was designed and directed by "good tuberculosis men," but medical officers may have been less vulnerable to tuberculosis infection than other hospital staff because they only saw patients intermittently during periodic examinations or procedures. Other personnel—hospital orderlies and civilian employees—cared for patients daily, working in the wards, helping to feed and bathe patients. Nurses perhaps were most directly exposed to tuberculosis infection because they cared for the sickest patients for hours at a time, day after day, and assisted physicians in medical and surgical procedures that probed infectious material.

Even though Congress recognized that Martha Hauch and other student nurses were contracting tuberculosis in the Army and authorized federal funds to compensate them, many nurses, doctors, and orderlies would die of the tuberculosis they contracted from their patients before medical institutions and the professions universally adopted appropriate measures to prevent the spread of tuberculosis bacteria from the sick to the well. Tuberculosis specialists, in fact, debated key issues regarding the disease for decades: How was tuberculosis transmitted? Did tuberculosis infection without active disease give an individual a certain degree of immunity to the disease? And what protective measures, if any, should hospitals and medical personnel adopt in caring for tuberculosis patients? In a 1994 article on healthcare workers' exposure to tuberculosis, Kent Sepkowitz stated that "a combination of genuine confusion, ignorance, and willful neglect conspired to keep the debate active and unsettled as late as the 1950s."[5] Sepkowitz suggested that the reasons for this inaction included hospitals' fears about discouraging young women from tuberculosis nursing, of being sued for transmission of tuberculosis to healthy people, and of losing patient clientele. But the delay in military and civilian hospitals' adoption of uniform protective protocols was also due to five unresolved issues concerning tuberculosis transmission at the time, specifically: (1) the difficulty in identifying sources of infection due to the ubiquity of tuberculosis in the population and the long and varying latency periods between infection and active disease; (2) the prevailing view that tuberculosis bacteria resided only in effluvia from the patient, especially coughed up sputum, and were therefore not transmissible through the air like measles or influenza germs; (3) the persistent theory that tuberculosis infection conveyed some immunity against the disease and was therefore not undesirable or dangerous; (4) the fact that measures to protect against tuberculosis transmission such as isolation, protective clothing, hand washing, and decontamination, were cumbersome and costly in time and money; and (5) human reluctance or refusal to adopt new ideas. An examination of tuberculosis nursing in the Army during the 1920s, 1930s, and 1940s reveals that although the Army Medical Department and other hospitals practiced rigorous aseptic and antiseptic protocols for surgery and infectious diseases such as diphtheria and scarlet fever, the same practices were not uniformly employed for tuberculosis patients and caregivers.

The Army Nurse Corps

Hauch had joined the second generation of Army nurses. The military had long resisted hiring female nurses, and in the first ten years after Congress established the Army Nurse Corps (ANC) in 1901, only about 100 female nurses served in Army hospitals annually, some of them at Fort Bayard. As the nursing profession grew, however, so did the ANC.[6] In the last half of the nineteenth century Florence Nightingale, advisor to the British Army, had led the effort to make nursing respectable and professional. In the United States middle-class women swelled the ranks of nursing because it was one of the few professions open to them that provided adequate income and useful work. Whereas in 1900 there were only 16 nurses and 173 doctors per 100,000 people in United States, by 1920 nurses outnumbered doctors 141 to 137 per 100,000 people.[7] At first the majority of nurses in the country worked in private duty, caring for sick people in their homes, but hospitals increasingly employed registered nurses, so that by the 1940s, hospital nursing became dominant over home care. Historian Barbara Melosh explains that hospital work was attractive to nurses because it provided more steady living and working conditions than private duty, and hospital technology and surgery supported nurses' interest in gaining professional expertise. The institutional setting also protected nurses against the tyranny of any one patient or doctor and provided social support.[8]

For members of the ANC, there was the added attraction of the opportunities for domestic and overseas travel on military assignments. Army nursing came of age during World War I, when the ANC grew to 21,480, but when Congress cut the War Department budget after the Armistice, Army nursing strength dropped dramatically.[9] During the interwar period the nursing staff, like the rest of the Medical Department, was "woefully short of personnel," according to then-Surgeon

General Merritte Ireland.[10] Only between 675 and 825 Reserve and Regular Army nurses were on active duty during any one year. As was the case at Fitzsimons, many Army hospitals had to employ civilian nurses to provide adequate care to patients.

Surgeon General Ireland was a strong supporter of nursing. He appointed Julia Stimson (Figure 6-1), with whom he had worked in the American Expeditionary Forces, as superintendent of the ANC in 1919. Stimson, of Massachusetts, graduated from Vassar College in 1901. She originally wanted to be a physician, but after her family discouraged her from pursuing that path, she studied medical illustration at Cornell and then entered the New York Hospital School of Nursing in 1904. Working at Children's Hospital in St. Louis, Stimson earned a master's degree from Washington University in 1917. When the United States entered the war, she joined the ANC as chief nurse of Base Hospital No. 21 out of St. Louis. By the end of the war she was chief nurse of the American Expeditionary Forces and received the Distinguished Service Medal for her service. As ANC superintendent,

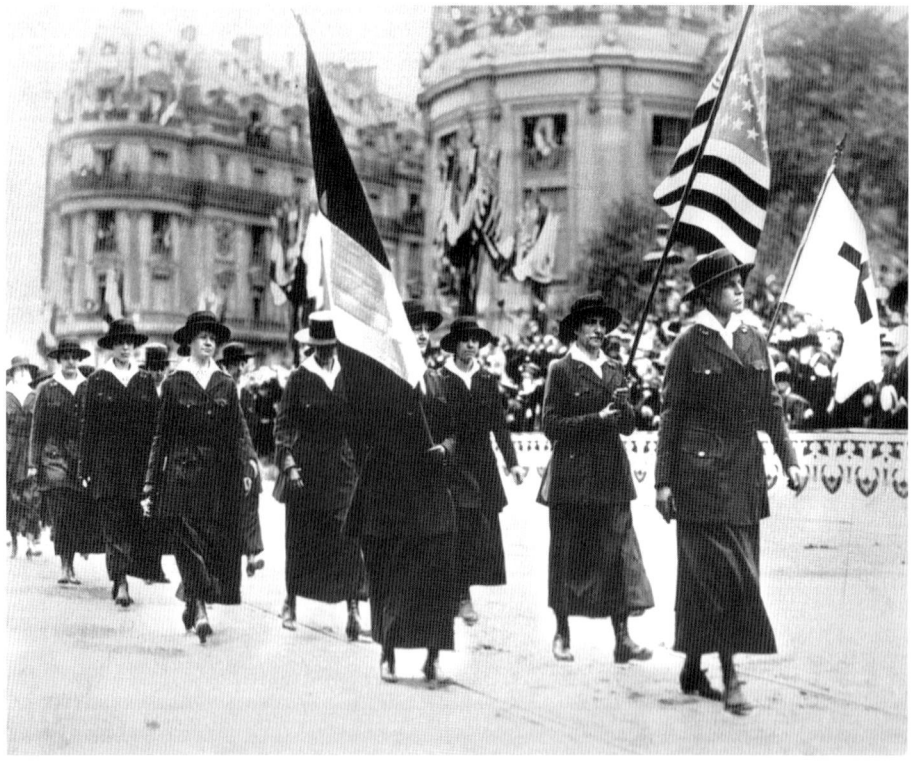

Figure 6-1. Julia C. Stimson, chief nurse of the American Expeditionary Forces, marching in the victory parade with other members of the Army Nurse Corps, in Paris, 1918.
Photograph courtesy of the National Library of Medicine, Image #B027286

Stimson was also dean of the Army School of Nursing, which graduated its first class in 1921. In 1920, she became the first woman to achieve the rank of major. Marlette Condé, an alumna of the Army School of Nursing, said Stimson "was direct in manner, forceful in speech. In uniform, appropriately enough, hers was a 'commanding' presence. But she was an approachable person"[11] (Figure 6-2). Stimson retired from the Army in 1937, and served as president of the American Nurses Association from 1938 to 1944. During World War II, however, she returned to service to recruit women to the ANC and advise federal agencies on nursing needs. The Army promoted her to colonel just weeks before she died in

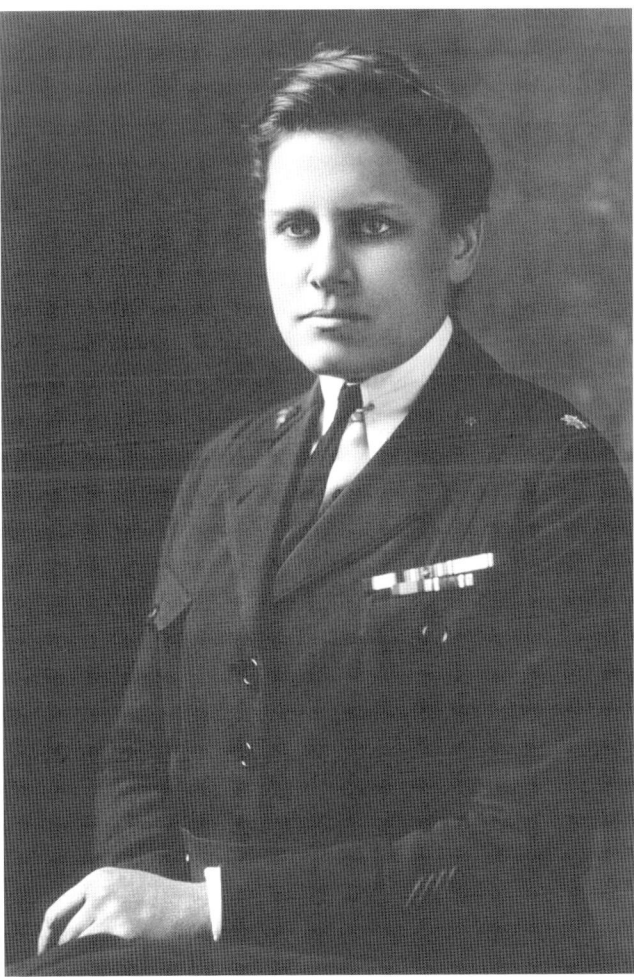

Figure 6-2. Julia C. Stimson as superintendent of the Army Nurse Corps, 1919–37. Photograph courtesy of the National Library of Medicine, Image #B08666.

1948 at age 67 of complications following surgery. Stimson always maintained high standards for Army nursing, and required the Medical Department, unlike many other hospitals, to hire only nurses who had graduated from certified schools of nursing.[12] During a national tour of Army posts in March 1932, Stimson reported that she was "well pleased with the high-efficiency which the nurse corps is maintaining at Fitzsimons hospital."[13]

Tuberculosis Nursing

Stimson knew that nursing care of surgical and bedrest tuberculosis patients was critical to recovery. Florence Nightingale, in fact, had believed that nursing was central to the healing process itself. "It is often thought that medicine is the curative process. It is no such thing," Nightingale wrote. Medicine and surgery could only "remove obstructions; neither can cure; nature alone cures.... And what nursing has to do in either case, is to put the patient in the best condition for nature to act upon him."[14] Nursing tuberculosis did require specific training, and during the interwar period nursing journals had numerous columns on the disease, its treatment, and special patient needs.[15] Army School of Nursing students received only general instruction on tuberculosis, so the Army's tuberculosis nurses were largely trained on the wards at Fitzsimons.[16]

Institutions like Fitzsimons were worlds unto themselves, and nurses were central to those worlds. Most sanatorium stays began with a journey, first by train and wagon, and increasingly in the 1920s and 1930s by car, to the sanatorium. Many arriving patients had suffered a lung hemorrhage and were quite ill and frightened by their breakdown. This first period was often a blur, but those who have written about their experience always remembered the nurses who come in and out of vision, taking their temperature, adjusting their bedclothes, and cautioning them not to get out of bed or to exert themselves. Tuberculosis specialist and author L. Fred Ayvazian described tuberculosis hospitals and sanatoriums as "highly structured and stable societies populated by individually precarious lives."[17] In their isolation from society, patients occupied themselves in various ways. After being fed and bathed by hospital staff they would sit outdoors or on sun porches, perhaps reading books and magazines, and writing letters, short stories, or newspaper articles. The *Journal of the Outdoor Life*, published by the civilian sanatorium at Lake Saranac, New York, provided a forum for some of this writing. By the 1920s, the radio entertained and provided a connection with the outer world. Phonographs were less desirable because one had to get out of bed to change the records. Other activities that could be done quietly in bed and required little exertion or assistance included stamp collecting, crafts, crossword puzzles, card games, knitting and sewing. A surprising number of tuberculosis patients—and nurses—smoked cigarettes.[18] Patients also spent their time following the disease course in other patients, tracking each others' weight gain and loss, and various medical and surgical procedures. Patients celebrated each others' bacteria-free sputum smears and successful lung collapses and mourned disastrous weight losses or lung hemorrhages. As Fred Ayvazian had noted, "Temperature fluctuations were watched

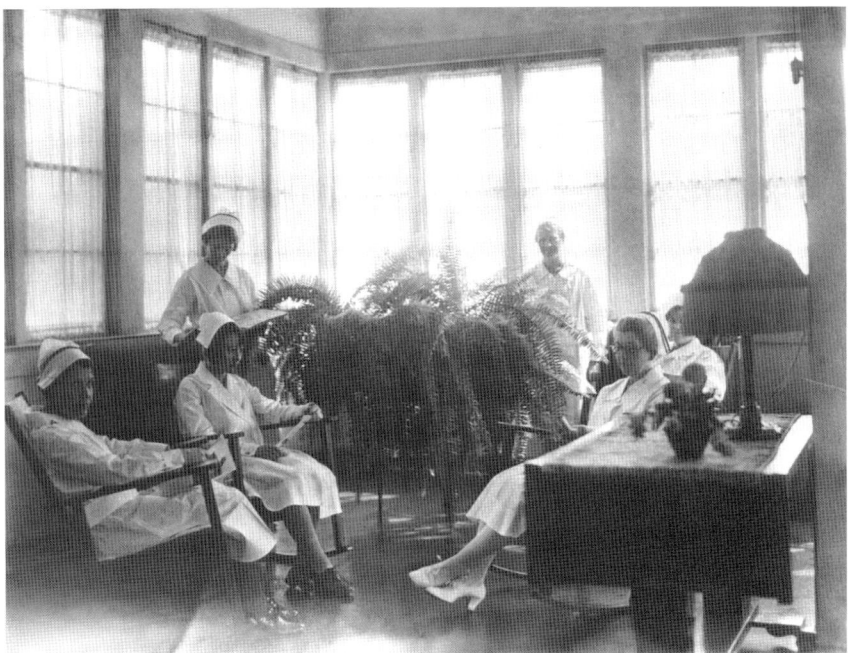

Figure 6-3. Interior view, solarium in nurses' quarters, Fitzsimons General Hospital, n.d. Photograph courtesy of the National Library of Medicine, Image #A016129.

with Dow-Jones attention....degrees of sputum positivity determined a castelike stratification with its own discriminatory practices."[19] By watching their roommates and ward mates, and the activities of hospital staff, patients could better gauge their own progress and treatment.

In this world physicians determined a patient's status and living conditions—whether they were confined to bed, what they could eat, and where. But patients had much more interaction—daily if not hourly—with the nurses. Fitzsimons employed at least eighty nurses at any one time during the interwar years, and, like many civilian and military nurses of the day, they lived on the post (Figure 6-3). Army nurses in the military environment had to adhere to strict regulations for behavior, such as minding curfews and not dating enlisted men or patients, and had their own dining room and Red Cross recreation hall. Nurses worked twelve-hour days, changing shifts at 7:00 a.m. and 7:00 p.m. They alternated night duty stints and were lucky to get one day off per month.[20] The Army instructed nurses to greet each patient individually at the beginning of each day shift; to take a patient's temperature, pulse, and respiration every four hours; feed those who could not feed themselves; provide the bedpan; bathe each patient; administer medications and treatments as ordered by the doctor; provide fresh drinking water; keep the bedside and patient's belongings orderly and clean; and notify the head nurse of any change in physical or mental symptoms. This care involved close, intimate contact with patients. Night nurses had similar duties, as well as preparing patients for bed and counting all opium and opium-derived medicines for the morning report.[21] They also made bed checks at 10:00 p.m., 2:00 a.m., and 6:00 a.m., and reported any patients not in their beds to the ward surgeon. Helene Sorensen, a Fitzsimons nurse, later remembered that "During the day, the patients rested on the building porches as part of their heliotherapy.... At night, they donned their stocking caps prior to sleeping on the porches or exposure to the fresh air."[22] Discipline remained a problem at Fitzsimons, however. Night nurses were responsible for fifteen patients, and one remembered how some patients would stuff their stocking caps with straw and pull up their bedcovers over a bundle of blankets so they could fool the night nurse and go out on the town.[23]

Perhaps the most illustrious patient during the interwar period was president of the Philippine Senate, Manuel Quezon, who had become friends with Gen. Douglas MacArthur in the late 1920s, when the latter commanded the Army's Philippine Department. When Quezon developed tuberculosis, then Army Chief of Staff MacArthur convinced him to take treatment at Fitzsimons, and Quezon arrived at the hospital in August 1930.[24] Like other patients, the Philippine leader no doubt had to learn the Fitzsimons protocols. He ultimately died of tuberculosis in 1944 in the tuberculosis sanatorium at Saranac Lake, New York, from where he led the Philippine government-in-exile.

About the same time Quezon was there, Helene Belanger had her first assignment in the ANC at Fitzsimons, from 1931 to 1934, and remembered that "we were responsible for tender loving care and nurturing of patients."[25] Nurses educated recently arrived patients on their new environment and regime—how to cover their mouths when coughing, spit into the sputum cup, and properly hold a thermometer in their mouths for five minutes. They also instructed them on how to relax in bed, how to avoid talking or laughing with too much animation, and how to totally relax in compliance with the rest cure. When tuberculosis specialist C. L. Minor spoke to nurses at the Army tuberculosis hospital in Oteen, North Carolina, he reminded them to treat patients as individual human beings and not as "cases." He advised that "the mind must be treated as well as the body," and that the nurse was crucial to that task. She must have "not only the confidence but the affection of the patient," and should be alert to the patients' worries, and encourage confidence in the doctor and obedience to his orders. "The doctor and nurse must be optimistic. Thus your radiating of optimism, cheerfulness…will make an optimist out of a pessimistic patient…. There is no such school of character building as tuberculosis bravely met by patient, doctor, and nurse."[26]

At the Army's Barnes General Hospital at Vancouver Barracks, Washington, nurse Lieutenant (Lt.) Midge Hall worked on the ward with thirty very ill patients and told a revealing story from the 1941 Christmas season. After the nurses had decorated the ward for the holidays she said, "I was bathing the patient when suddenly in the midst of his bath he sat up in bed, and before I knew what was happening he was kissing me on the cheek. I jumped back startled and very angry. He said, 'now now Lieut. you cannot get angry. Look at what you are standing under.' I looked up and there was a piece of mistletoe tied to the light cord. He said he had been waiting for days for some nurse to get under it. Well, I certainly could not be angry after that."[27]

Not all nurses held a romantic view of their work at Fitzsimons. Army nurse Major (Maj.) Edith A. Aynes, who wrote a memoir of her Army experience, *From Nightingale to Eagle,* began her career at Fitzsimons in late 1932. Aynes said her job was "to give nursing care to patients, to ride herd on the military's morning report and related records, to play policeman on the pass holders, to help check the property for the ward surgeon, and to assist the medical officers."[28] On her first day, Aynes swore to defend the Constitution and then received six white uniforms, six nurse caps, and an Army cape. The next day she began work on ward C-4 for African American patients, most of them World War I veterans. Chief nurse Mary Sheehan presented the ward to Aynes as a benefit for the new nurse because it was segregated by race rather than rank and would therefore give her experience caring for both officers and enlisted patients as well as veterans.[29] Aynes remembered that about twenty of the patients were in critical condition and could have died any moment. Another twenty patients were seriously ill, and "all a patient had to do to change from serious to the critical list was to have a sizable hemorrhage." Every man, Aynes wrote, "knew his symptoms, how he should progress, and what treatment would indicate which way he was headed... He measured his condition by the treatment he received: bedrest, and pneumothorax, repeated sputum tests or X-rays, narcotics for cough, or the appearance of blood."[30]

Aynes described the morning routine as an assembly line in which she was assisted by one of the 140 male attendants hired locally to staff the hospital. "When I entered the 25 bed ward to give baths that morning," she explained, "a white-suited civil servant preceded me down the ward, took the clothes and pajamas off patient after patient, filled the deep basins with water, produced washcloths, towels, and soap, and even warmed the bottle of alcohol for the backrub." As she bathed one patient he prepared the next one. "The man had been doing the same job for about 15 years and liked it. He was polite, quick, and willing, but he was one in a million."[31] Some orderlies were efficient and kind; others broke the rules. Aynes told of one corpsman who smoked marijuana on the wards, smuggling the cigarettes into the hospital in his gloves.[32]

Nurses also worked in the laboratories (Figure 6-4) and assisted in surgery, administering anesthesia and caring for patients before and after surgical procedures. In 1936 Fitzsimons surgeons performed 775 operations on tuberculosis patients.[33] "Collapse therapy, [was] very popular in those days," said ANC nurse Helene Belanger; so were more invasive procedures.[34] Rhoda Jahr arrived as a nurse at Fitzsimons in 1938 and reported that they "did thoracoplasties by the dozen! We did them by the ton!" Protective gloves were apparently used only in the operating room. Jahr remembered that "we would scrub our hands with this green soap, we dipped our fingers in iodine, and then in alcohol. Then we would put gloves on."[35] Another nurse explained, "[T]here were no disposable surgical gloves. After the surgeons used the gloves, the gloves would be washed and we would blow them up just like a balloon. That's how we check for leaks."[36]

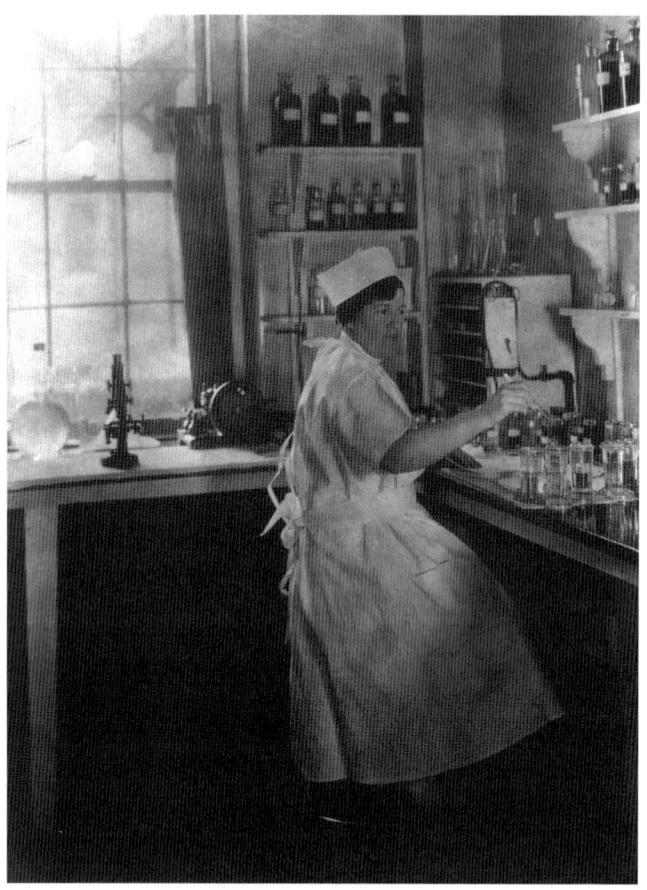

Figure 6-4. Nurse in laboratory, Fitzsimons General Hospital, n.d.
Photograph courtesy of the National Library of Medicine, Image #A016094.

Working with sick people always had its risks (Figures 6-5 and 6-6), and doctors and nurses caught a wide variety of illnesses. In 1935, for example, at least one-third of the Army's more than 600 nurses were ill enough to be admitted to the hospital. Although only five of them had tuberculosis, these women required much longer hospitalizations than nurses with other maladies and were less likely to recover.[37] Sick nurses could lose their jobs. Reta M. O'Brien served as a Reserve Nurse in the ANC during the war and again in 1921. That year ANC head Stimson evaluated O'Brien with the highest grade of numeral "I" for "work, conduct, and health good." But in 1923 Stimson graded her at numeral II, "as her health record was poor," and relieved her from duty "on account of having tuberculosis."[38] This was a problem not only for the individual nurse, but for the Medical Department. Years before, Florence Nightingale had understood this. "The

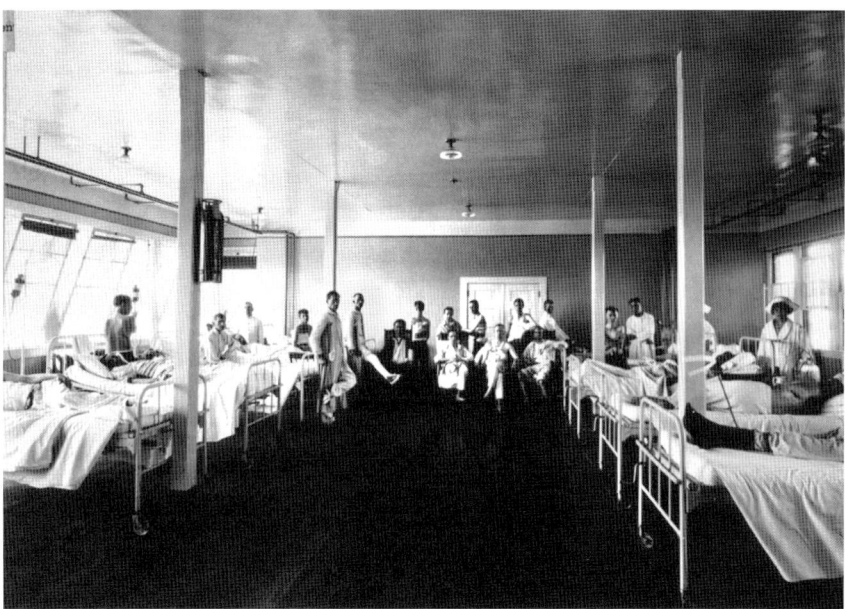

Figure 6-5. U.S. Army, Fitzsimons General Hospital, Denver, Colorado, interior view, Convalescent Room, Surgical Ward. Note the nurse standing at the right next to patient with open chest wound from thoracic surgery, which could be a source of tuberculosis infection.
Photograph courtesy of the National Library of Medicine, Image #A04992.

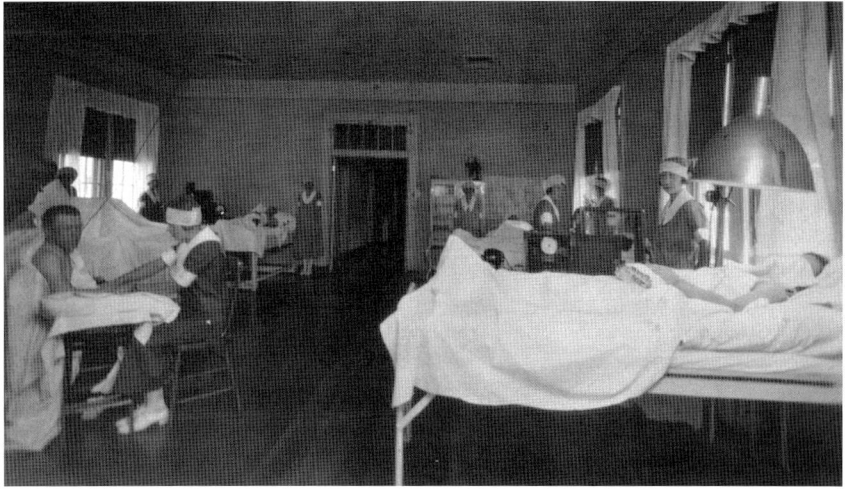

Figure 6-6. U.S. Army, Fitzsimons General Hospital, Denver, Colorado, general treatment room.
Photograph courtesy of the National Library of Medicine, Image #A07853.

loss of a well-trained nurse by preventable disease is a greater loss than is that of a good soldier from the same cause," she wrote. "Money cannot replace either, but a good nurse is more difficult to find than a good soldier."[39] After having to consider numerous private bills to help women like Martha Hauch, in 1930 Congress authorized formal disability retirement benefits for nurses with service-connected disabilities. From 1932 to 1936, ninety Army nurses retired on disability, eleven of them for tuberculosis. Other ailments included heart disease and digestive disorders, but although the average age of nurses who retired on disability was 46 years, that of nurses who retired with tuberculosis averaged only 29.4 years.[40]

Given the risks, some nurses were determined to avoid caring for tuberculosis patients. As one civilian nurse observed, "getting capable nurses that are not afraid of tuberculosis is most difficult. So many feel perfectly safe in the general hospital or in private practice who would not consider work in a sanatorium because of the supposed danger of infection" (Figure 6-7). The sad thing, she noted, was that "[tuberculosis] patients feel this keenly."[41] In 1919, Stimson dismissed five reserve nurses for misconduct when they refused to work at the Army tuberculosis hospital at Oteen, North Carolina. Even after a warning from the commanding officer, Zilpha Bartlett, Marion Ruth Ross, Alberta M. McHale, Mable Marie Rotzien, and Edyth M. Scott "refused to go on duty, stating the reason for such insubordination was the fact that they did not desire duty at a tuberculosis hospital."[42] Frances Lafaye Locke, a reconstruction aide, took a more judicious approach. When assigned to Oteen she asked for a transfer because she "feared to stay in a T.B. hospital," and after a month got her transfer.[43] Fear of tuberculosis transmission also hurt nurse training. A 1937 study found that only twelve of fifty schools offered nursing students instruction in tuberculosis nursing. Esta H. McNett, a nurse in Cleveland, Ohio, attributed this to "the fear of tuberculosis which now prevents administrators of schools of nursing from arranging affiliations for their students."[44]

Like many tubercular physicians, however, some nurses who had the disease saw it as an asset to their work. A civilian nurse who contracted tuberculosis in her first year in nursing school became a patient in the tuberculosis sanatorium, but after five years returned to school to finish her degree. "It was a hard undertaking," she wrote, because when she broke down again her friends and relatives advised her to give up nursing. "But I can't give up the thing I love," she explained, "I'm specializing in tuberculosis nursing because I understand the tuberculosis patients so well and I'm able to give them the encouragement that a nurse who has never been sick could not give."[45] For her, nursing had become a special calling.

Debate

By the late 1920s and early 1930s, some physicians began to notice higher rates of tuberculosis among nurses and nursing students than the general population and began to raise questions about tuberculosis transmission and hospital practices. This started a debate that continued without resolution for decades among military and civilian specialists regarding the nature of tuberculosis transmission

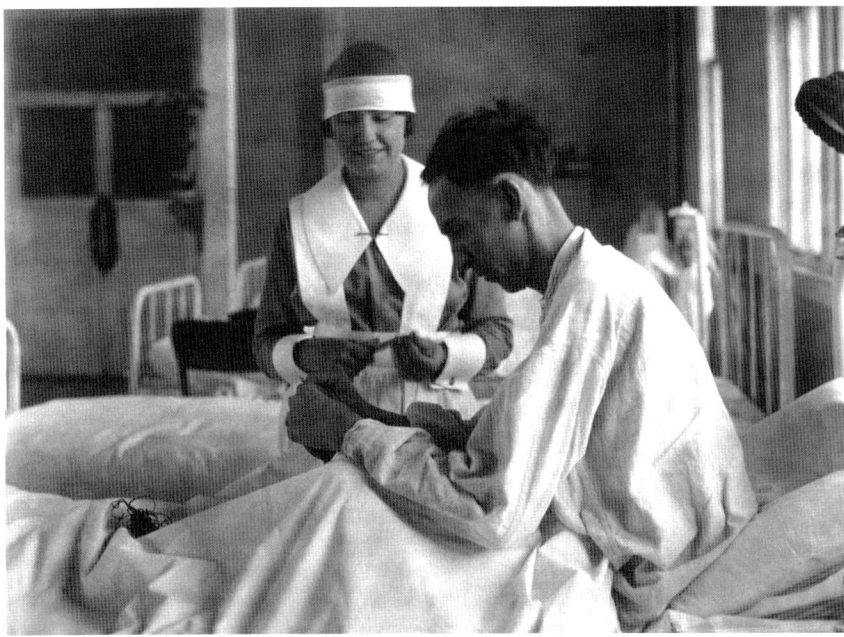

Figure 6-7. U.S. Army, Fitzsimons General Hospital, Denver, Colorado, Rehabilitation Aide giving bedside instruction, n.d.
Photograph courtesy of the National Library of Medicine, Image #A07798.

and to what degree individuals were susceptible or immune to active disease. Norwegian physician Johannes Heimbeck published a series of articles in which he tracked the high rates of tuberculosis infection among nurses compared to other groups. He found that 12 percent of student nurses developed active tuberculosis while they were in nursing school.[46] Others in the United States saw a similar trend. In 1928 Jessamine S. Whitney, statistician for the National Tuberculosis Association, pointed out that more than half of the nurses being supported by the American Nurses Association Relief Fund for invalid nurses had become disabled due to tuberculosis. She called for periodic physical examinations of nurses to monitor tuberculosis infection or the development of active disease and improved working and living conditions to help nurses resist the disease.[47]

Physician J. Arthur Myers at the University of Minnesota eagerly joined the debate, reinforcing Heimbeck's studies with his own observations of high rates of tuberculosis among student nurses, which in 1930 he called "one of the greatest problems in tuberculosis at the present time."[48] He waged a career-long campaign to convince hospitals to employ stringent contagious disease protocols with all tuberculosis patients. Called the "most prolific and influential writer on the subject of tuberculosis of his time in this country," Myers had earned a Ph.D. in anatomy at Cornell in 1914 but soon developed tuberculosis.[49] After he recovered, he joined the faculty of the University of Minnesota medical school and in the course of his career wrote some 700 papers, many of them on tuberculosis, as well as editorials, books, and obituaries. He also edited the British medical journal *Lancet* from 1930 to 1968, and, having vanquished his own tuberculosis, died in 1978 at the age of ninety. Concerned that the increased risks of developing active tuberculosis would discourage young women from tuberculosis nursing, Myers called for careful health surveillance of nursing school applicants and students to track any tuberculosis infections. He also advocated teaching nursing students to use "the same rigid technic [*sic*] as is employed in the prevention of such diseases as diphtheria and scarlet fever."[50] At the time such measures included isolating patients and requiring them to wear masks when receiving care, and masks, gowns, and gloves for medical personnel when caring for the patient. Myers published yearly on the issue in various medical journals, stressing the continued high rate of tuberculosis infection. In 1940, he wrote, "Hospitals and sanatoriums no longer have any excuse for permitting students of nursing to be exposed to tuberculosis.... Medical asepsis should be instituted and practiced continuously on the medical floors in every hospital and sanatorium."[51] But his words went unheeded.

Perhaps the biggest problem was that because tuberculosis infection was so widespread in the United States until the middle of the twentieth century, and because the latency period between infection and active disease was so variable, it was almost impossible for investigators to identify or fully understand the source of tuberculosis infection. Another problem was that for many years physicians and scientists failed to understand that tuberculosis was transmitted through the air. This was partly due to a desire to lay to rest the old concept that bad air or "miasmas" spread infectious diseases. In a 1928 article, Charles V. Chapin succinctly stated in his authoritative text, *The Sources and Modes of Infection*, that "Adherents of the miasmatic theory of disease must necessarily look to the atmosphere as the bearer of the poison, [and].... the demonstration by the early bacteriologists of the extreme smallness of bacteria served to strengthen this view." Subsequently, however, scientists learned that "the chief way in which living germs can get into the air is in the tiny droplets given off in loud talking, coughing, etc., and rarely did these float more than arm's length." "Thus," Chapin concluded, "the laboratory men have taught us that, under ordinary conditions, and except for a few feet around the coughing patient, the air is a negligible factor in the spread of infection."[52] This explanation shows that in place of miasmatic theory, physicians and scientists adopted a more material, physical concept of disease transmission that discounted unseen infections in the air, and looked instead to water, milk, blood, sputum, urine, feces, and insects as means of transmission of disease germs to humans. "It has become a comparatively simple matter to control contagious disease," wrote one Navy medical officer, "since it became known a few years ago that the infectious agent of communicable disease is not carried to any great distance through the air, and that the only danger of contracting these diseases is by coming in very close or actual contact with the patient or infected articles."[53]

Fear of sputum was one of the motivating forces behind the late-nineteenth-century movement to isolate tuberculosis patients in sanatoriums, as specialists began to distinguish between "open" cases in which patients had tuberculosis bacteria in their sputum, and "closed" cases in which they did not. (Scientists now believe that at least 15 percent of tuberculosis infection comes from sputum negative patients.[54]) Some writers argued that tuberculosis sanatoriums were safer than tuberculosis wards in general hospitals because all personnel and patients were specifically trained to take precautions against transmission, something not done in many hospitals.[55] Believing that sputum was the primary means of tuberculosis transmission, a nurse wrote in 1920, "It is a popular belief that the tuberculosis person is a constant source of infection to his associates. This is not true.... Even an advanced case whose sputum is full of bacilli, need not be isolated from the family except to have a separate bed, if he is educated to take...precautions." This meant he must cover his mouth when sneezing or coughing, spit into a receptacle, use separate dishes and utensils, and brush his teeth over the toilet. "The careless or ignorant patient with bacilli in the sputum," she warned, "is a real menace to his associates."[56] In 1922 medical officers Maj. T. E. Scott and Captain (Capt.) R. S. Loving also discounted the view that tuberculosis could be airborne, writing "The usual mode of infection is believed to be through the intestinal tract, by mouth."[57] Ernst S. Mariette, a tuberculosis specialist at the University of Minnesota School of Medicine and superintendent of a sanatorium, wrote in 1936 that in order to get tuberculosis "direct contact with the patient is unnecessary but contact with his sputum is."[58]

In the 1930s, the journal *Diseases of the Chest* even scolded perpetrators of "tuberculosis phobia," stating "tuberculosis is not a contagious disease in the sense that measles and scarlet fever are contagious diseases. It is a communicable disease and its incidence of communicability is in direct proportion to the lack of hygienic living." Families could care for tubercular loved ones in their homes if the patient took the proper precautions. Children should be kept away from direct contact with the patient, although "It is perfectly safe for them to come into the room."[59] In the 1940s Robert Lovell developed active tuberculosis while in medical school at the University of Michigan, and after a stint in a sanatorium wrote a guidebook for tuberculosis patients. He prescribed proper behavior in the sickroom. "You must always cover your mouth and nose with a wipe when anyone comes within 5 feet of you," he explained, "for the protection of the people who are taking care of you. Your mouth and nose, therefore, should be covered with a wipe when a doctor is examining or treating you, and when the nurse is bathing you or making the bed while you are in it."[60] Beyond the five-foot perimeter, however, he implied, the air was safe.

The third factor mitigating the adoption of preventive measures was the distinction between primary and secondary infection and the persistence of the theory articulated by George Bushnell and others that people who had been infected with tuberculosis early in life and had not developed disease were in some way immunized—"tubercularized"—and would not develop active disease. In 1922, Army physicians noted that "practically everyone who dies after the age of fifteen of other diseases than tuberculosis, will show evidence of past tuberculosis infection." This, they believed, indicated that these people carried "immune bodies against the disease."[61] For example, in 1924, responding to concern about the spread of tuberculosis among Filipino soldiers (Scouts) in the U.S. Army, one medical officer reported, "There is absolutely no danger to other Scout soldiers from keeping even active cases in the barracks as the Scout troops are thoroughly immunized against infection from the outside and will break down only from lesions that they already have and as a matter of fact had before their original enlistment."[62] Similarly, another medical officer wrote that he "thought it was doubtful if we should try for a bacillus-free world, but should rather work for subclinical natural vaccination," thus "training the tissues to meet an inevitable invasion" of tuberculosis.[63] Civilians shared this view. According to a civilian physician, "nearly all tuberculosis infection is acquired in childhood; that practically all active tuberculosis in adults originates from this childhood infection, and that adults themselves are practically immune to infection."[64] This belief seemed to exonerate medical institutions—and governments—from at least some blame for the spread of disease among nurses on tuberculosis wards, because many women had probably already been infected as children, rather than by their patients, and if they had not already been exposed, were therefore now "immune."

During the interwar period public health officials had developed a new tool to understand the level of tuberculosis transmission in the community at large. Tuberculin skin tests could detect tuberculosis infection before the disease advanced to the point of lung damage detectable by X-ray images or fluoroscopic examinations. By 1927, as many as sixty-five different tuberculin tests were available, facilitating health surveillance of civilian and military populations alike.[65] In the 1930s, for example, scientists Esmond R. Long and Florence B. Seibert tested 18,744 students at twenty colleges and found that positive tuberculin reaction rates ranged from 20 to 30 percent at colleges in the central states to 40 to 60 percent on the East and West coasts.[66] Hospitals that tested their nurses, nursing students, and other employees then faced the question of whether a positive tuberculin reaction made an individual more or less likely to develop active disease.

The other new tool to fight tuberculosis was a vaccine developed in 1921 known as Bacille Calmette-Guerin or BCG, which induced partial but not complete protection from tuberculosis. American medical scientists experimented with the vaccine with mixed results, and when in 1930, more than eighty-five babies of 249 died in Germany after receiving oral BCG vaccine, enthusiasm for BCG further subsided.[67] Many public health officials opposed BCG because it caused people to have positive tuberculin reactions and thus compromised the tuberculin test, a key tool in screening groups such as student nurses, other hospital staff, and military recruits for tuberculosis.[68] Ultimately BCG was (and still is) used predominantly in areas of high rates of tuberculosis where partial protection was valuable and where surveillance with tuberculin was rare.[69]

At Fitzsimons medical officers William Pollock and James Hedges Forsee used tuberculin testing to join the debate on immunity and tuberculization. They followed 755 physicians, dentists, and nurses at Fitzsimons over ten years and in 1934 reported that only thirteen had developed tuberculosis. Staying firmly in the "tuberculized" school, they cited Bushnell and argued that "individuals who present evidence of primary tuberculosis are classed as immunes, bearing in mind that their immunity is of a relative character." They called the body's response to tuberculosis "tuberculoallergy," and argued that it developed during the primary infection, and "when maintained at an optimum level, serves as a protective quality throughout life." Pollock and Forsee concluded that "officers and nurses may serve their tour of duty at Fitzsimons General Hospital without fear of contracting tuberculosis from exogenous [external] sources."[70] In an article the following year they acknowledged "the differences of views in regard to the character and quality of tuberculoallergy," but reiterated their opinion that an initial infection had a protective quality. Some of the thirteen people at Fitzsimons who developed tuberculosis may have already had the disease before they came to Fitzsimons, they suggested, and therefore had not been infected by a patient or colleague.[71] The key was to keep healthy and maintain a strong immune system so one did not break down. This approach put the onus on the individual to maintain a healthy lifestyle. As nurse Edith Aynes wrote, "Since Fitzsimons was primarily a hospital for tuberculosis patients, nurses were expected to eat all three meals so that they would not incapacitate themselves for duty by getting sick!"[72]

Steps to protect nurses and nursing students included screening them to eliminate tuberculin positive (or negative, depending on the hospital's policy) women, X-raying them every three or six months to detect new infections, isolating patients, and practicing communicable disease technique. In 1935, Jessamine Whitney called for *not* employing nurses with positive tuberculin tests.[73] The chief of the Fitzsimons medical service, Lt. Col. George Aycock, noted in 1939, however, that when assigning nurses to the wards, "no differentiation is made at Fitzsimons General Hospital between positive and negative [tuberculin] reactors in selecting them for assignment to duty on tuberculosis wards." He also said that "communicable disease technique is carried out by nurses on wards housing patients with open lesions" (those with tuberculosis bacterium in their sputum), but "such technique is relaxed on wards housing closed cases."[74] It is not clear just what "relaxed" meant.

Other evidence that Fitzsimons' physicians believed their staff was tubercularized and therefore protected from tuberculosis transmission comes via the pig farm on the post. Robert L. Black, a medical supply officer at the hospital (1929–30), told an interviewer that in addition to handling a number of administrative functions, he also managed the Hereford pig farm. "We had a big herd of pigs, and made lots of money off of them that went to the benefit of the hospital." He explained that "basically, the pig farm was designed to serve the very useful purpose of disposing of edible garbage without having to transport it to the dumps." But, Black continued, "It was later determined by the Veterinary Department that the pigs had picked up a good amount of tuberculosis, so we could not continue to sell them commercially."[75] The pigs most likely contracted tuberculosis from the cattle on the reservation rather than from the food scraps, but Black's statement suggests that hospital staff and patients continued to eat the pork, perhaps under the assumption that they had immunity.[76]

Another factor in delaying the universal adoption of effective measures to prevent the transmission of tuberculosis was that they were arduous and expensive. The most important and obvious precaution was to segregate tuberculosis patients from other hospital patients, which many hospitals did, despite the cost. Nursing administrators then began to calculate the time required to perform various nursing procedures in order to gauge the nurse staffing necessary to care for patients in isolation. One 1938 study found that while the average ambulant tuberculosis patient required only about one-half hour of care a day, a surgical tuberculosis patient confined to bed required 3.3 hours per day, and that "the hospitals included in this study were generally understaffed." The authors produced a table of nursing hours required for patients with various degrees of disease severity and concluded that "good nursing in the care of tuberculosis patients implies, first, good practice, second a sufficient number of nurses and a sufficient amount of time to put that practice into effect."[77] This study also showed that the sicker and presumably more infectious patients received more prolonged and intensive nursing care.

The next step hospitals could take to prevent tuberculosis transmission was to examine all incoming hospital patients with X-rays to identify and segregate those who had or might have tuberculosis. Specialists argued then as they do today that the unknown tuberculosis sufferer is more dangerous than the known one. But not all hospitals had the resources for such universal patient screening or even for basic anticontagion measures (Figure 6-8). Physicians at Bellevue Hospital in New York City stated in 1940 that "while it is most desirable to avoid tuberculous infection, we do not believe that this is entirely possible in large general hospitals at the present time." Nurses wore gowns and washed their hands, but "as a rule, nurses do not wear gloves or face masks."[78] At Fitzsimons, nurse Helene Belanger remembered, "We didn't wear gloves or masks but we did wash our hands a lot"; another nurse, Helene Sorensen, did "not ever remember wearing a mask, having the patient wear a mask, or wearing gloves for procedures."[79] At the Army's Barnes General Hospital at Vancouver Barracks, an inspection in January 1942 revealed that the precautions were incomplete. "Wards 15 and 13 have been set aside for contagious diseases wards [including tuberculosis] and although being very difficult to invoke enforced rigid isolation in this type of hospital, there has been no spread of communicable disease at any time."[80]

Such laxity had consequences. One physician reported in 1940 that twenty-five student or graduate nurses had developed tuberculosis at twenty-one different hospitals so that even if hospitals used precautionary measures, "To put a nurse in her teens or early twenties, on a tuberculosis service, or in a sanatorium, particularly one who is tuberculin-negative, is courting disaster."[81] A medical director at a civilian tuberculosis sanatorium wrote that because tuberculosis was a leading cause of death among nurses "it must be considered as an occupational disease as far as the nursing profession is concerned."[82] In 1942, the *American Journal of Nursing* sent a representative to eleven sanatoriums to study the wartime tuberculosis nursing shortage. The investigator, Dorothy Deming, observed that "probably the greatest variance exists in the practice of protective techniques during care." Whereas one hospital required all personnel caring for patients with posi-

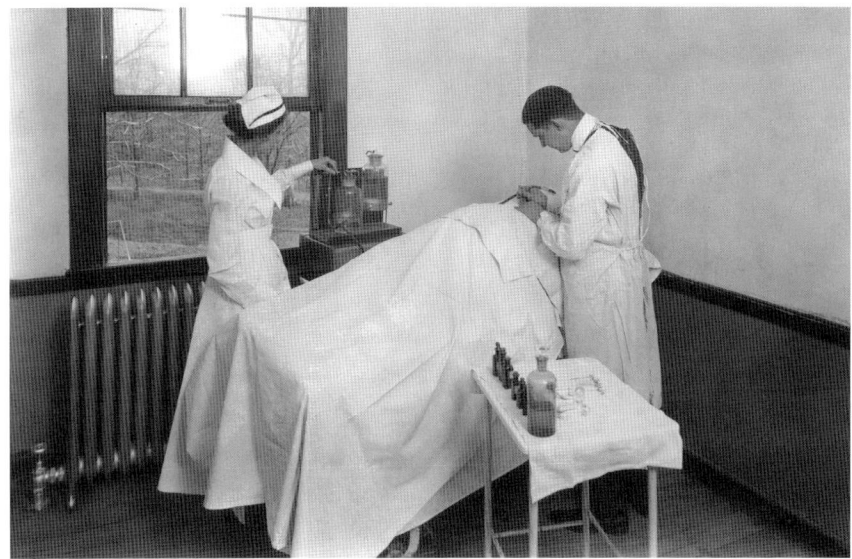

Figure 6-8. Photograph of pneumothorax procedure showing nurse and physician without contagious disease protection, Waverly Hills Sanatorium, Kentucky, n.d..
Photograph courtesy of the University of Louisville, Special Collections, Louisville, Kentucky.

tive sputum to wear protective gowns and masks, she found another institution where "masks and gowns are worn only when taking care of *non-tuberculous* patients!" Under such conditions, Deming wrote, "There is little wonder that nurses, especially those in the twenty-five to thirty-five age group, fear tuberculosis and are reluctant to nurse in tuberculosis hospitals."[83]

They had good reason. Myers and his colleagues in Minneapolis employed some of the most stringent measures in their tuberculosis wards, where the staff used gowns and masks and washed their hands for two minutes. In 1947 Myers credited such procedures at Fairview Hospital with a reduction in the conversion of student nurses from negative to positive tuberculin tests from 100 percent in 1932, to 33 percent in 1939, to their "ultimate goal" of zero nursing graduates becoming infected during their training in 1945.[84] But few hospitals at the time took such precautions.

Wade Hampton Frost

The beginning of the end of the theory of tubercularization arrived in 1937 with an article by Wade Hampton Frost, an epidemiologist with the Public Health Service, that transformed public health strategies toward tuberculosis and set the framework for the modern approach to infectious disease control. Medical historian Barron Lerner has called the article "seminal."[85] Frost gained a lifelong interest in tuberculosis after he contracted the disease as a young man. He went to Asheville, North Carolina, for treatment, and once recovered, pursued a career in epidemiology. His biographer, Thomas Daniel, believes that "Frost's greatest contributions to the understanding of a specific disease and to the field of epidemiology came from his studies of tuberculosis."[86] Frost's 1937 article reviewed the improvements in public health institutions and strategies and noted the declining tuberculosis mortality and morbidity rates in the United States. He challenged, however, the theory that childhood infection with tuberculosis rendered a measure of immunity to adults and questioned "the extremely pessimistic view of tuberculosis control" that supported universal infection of tuberculosis—the tuberculization theory. In an article published after his death from cancer Frost stated his challenge to the tuberculization theory most succinctly: "To have passed through a period of high mortality risk confers not protection, but added hazard in later life."[87] He argued instead for more strenuous efforts to prevent transmission: "if, in successive periods of time, the number of infectious hosts is continuously reduced, the end-result of this diminishing ratio, if continued long enough, must be extermination of the tuberculosis bacillus."[88] In other words, as the national population shifted from a majority of infected persons to a majority free from tuberculosis infection, public health officials could one day control the disease.

Frost also reasoned that "as the cases become fewer and fewer, preventive measures should be centered more and more upon the open cases."[89] He did not dismiss the role of immunity entirely; instead he argued that "one of the most important factors in the decline of tuberculosis has been progressively increasing human resistance." Therefore, the most powerful weapon against tuberculosis would be the "progressive improvement in the social order as a whole." Frost envisioned a new public health approach to tuberculosis whereby officials would identify, isolate, and care for the sick in sanatoriums and then identify and isolate their infected contacts to stop the spread of disease. He also called for more vigorous efforts to find and treat early cases of tuberculosis and special protection for groups most prone to the disease, which essentially meant improving the standard of living for the poor.[90] In sum, he proposed to *identify*, *isolate*, and *treat* all cases of tuberculosis in the country.

Other physicians began to adopt Frost's approach. In 1942, Ruth Rice Puffer, a biostatistician at the Tennessee Department of Public Health, cited his 1937 article and used the term "index case" to describe the first individual in a family or community suspected of having tuberculosis, around whom public health officials could test, isolate, and treat all others.[91] Arthur Myers described the transition: "The theory that it is dangerous to the future control of tuberculosis to prevent the young from becoming infected with tubercle bacilli has been replaced with the fact that the only safe procedure is to protect humanity everywhere, regardless of the age of individuals, against primary infection and reinfection with tubercle bacilli."[92] The Army's tuberculosis specialist during World War II, Esmond R. Long, also recognized the importance of Frost's views in tuberculosis epidemiology. He explained that a "new understanding" of tuberculosis was "reflected in a radically changed approach to the public health attack on the disease. Two principal procedures became recognized as the nucleus for tuberculosis control: case finding and isolation of discovered cases."[93] Frost's 1937 recommendations to reduce the tuberculosis exposure to the U.S. population would not reach the tipping point of consensus, however, until the late 1950s when tuberculosis had already yielded to heart disease and cancer as the leading causes of death in the United States.

Herein lies the fifth reason for the delay of the adoption of new control measures: People are often loathe to abandon long-held views and adopt new ideas. As Thomas Kuhn explains in *The Structure of Scientific Revolutions,* it requires the accumulation of a large body of evidence anomalous to a long-held scientific theory to change the way people think. Medical literature into the 1940s and 1950s shows that the tuberculization theory and the focus on sputum as the source of contagion endured as the prevailing understanding.[94] A nurse writing in 1947 about the importance of protective practices noted, "*This is a controversial subject*, but until there is proof that aseptic technique is unnecessary, it seems worthwhile."[95]

During World War II the Fitzsimons newspaper, *Stethoscope*, celebrated the hospital's twenty-fifth anniversary with a special edition showing eight pages of photographs comparing the facilities and equipment of "yester-year" with the modern, 1943 versions, including a new dormitory, mess hall, and recreation center for nurses.[96] A *Stethoscope* article the next year, however, showed medical staff performing a pneumothorax procedure on a patient without a protective mask.[97] Not until well after the war would tuberculosis treatment protocols require the strict isolation of patients, negative air-pressure rooms, and the use of respirators by medical personnel. During the interwar period, then, hospital and sanatorium workers, as well as family and friends caring for tuberculosis patients, continued to develop the disease. And nurses, who cared for the sickest patients day in and day out, would continue to fall ill at higher than average rates. The tuberculosis men and women of the Army Medical Department and in civilian institutions across the country would continue to struggle to defeat this insidious disease. They would also have to weather a Great Depression and another world war.

Notes

1. Martha A. Hauch to Civil Employees' Compensation Commission, 16 January 1928, U.S. Congress, House Rpt. No. 1173, Committee on Claims, to accompany S. 1368, 70th Cong., 2nd sess., 10. This discussion of the Hauch case is drawn from this committee report and documents in Record Group [hereafter cited as RG] 112, Records of the Surgeon General of the Army, Entry 31, 1928–37, Box 285, National Archives and Records Administration [hereafter cited as NARA].
2. U.S. Congress, House Rpt. No. 1173, 5.
3. U.S. Congress, House Rpt. No. 1173, 1.
4. May L. Campbell and Mrs. W. G. Campbell to Hon. R. Walton Moore, 26 June 1928, RG 112, Entry 31, 1917–27, Box 285, NARA.
5. Kent A. Sepkowitz, "Tuberculosis and the Health-Care Worker: A Historical Perspective," *Archives of Internal Medicine* 120 (January 1994).
6. On the history of military nursing, see Mary Sarnecky, *A History of the Army Nurse Corps* (Philadelphia, PA: University of Pennsylvania Press, 1999); Elizabeth A. Shields, "A History of the United States Army Nurse Corps, 1901–37," Ed.D. dissertation, Columbia University, 1980; Rita Chow et al., "Historical Perspectives of the United States Air Force, Army, Navy, Public Health Service, and Veterans Administration Nursing Services," *Military Medicine* 143 (July 1978): 457–63; and Connie L. Reeves, "The Military Women's Vanguard, Nurses," in Judith Hicks Stiehm, ed., *It's Our Military Too! Women and the U.S. Military* (Philadelphia, PA: Temple University Press, 1996).

On the history of nursing see Patricia D'Antonio, *American Nursing: A History of Knowledge, Authority, and the Meaning of Work* (Baltimore, MD: Johns Hopkins, 2010); Arlene W. Keeling, *Nursing and the Privilege of Prescription, 1893–2000* (Columbus, OH: Ohio State University Press, 2007); Susan M. Reverby, *Ordered to Care: The Dilemma of American Nursing: 1850–1945* (Cambridge, UK: Cambridge University Press, 1987); Darlene Clark Hine, *Black Women in White: Racial Conflict and Cooperation in the Nursing Profession, 1890–1950* (Bloomington, IN: Indiana University Press, 1985); Barbara Melosh, *"The Physician's Hand": Work Culture and Conflict in American Nursing* (Philadelphia, PA: Temple University Press, 1982); and Janet Wilson James, "Isabel Hampton and the Professionalization of Nursing in the 1890s," in Morris J. Vogel and Charles E. Rosenberg, *The Therapeutic Revolution: Essays in the Social History of American Medicine* (Philadelphia, PA: University of Pennsylvania Press, 1979).

7. Reverby, *Ordered to Care*, 159. The decline in doctors was due to the imposition of strict education and licensing requirements in many states during the early twentieth century.

8. Melosh, *"The Physician's Hand,"* 160.

9. Sarnecky, *A History of the Army Nurse Corps*, 135.

10. Merritte Ireland to Chief of Staff, memorandum, 18 April 1928, RG 112, Entry 29, 1928–37, Box 26, NARA.

11. "Superintendents and Chiefs of the Army Nurse Corps, 1901–1975," available at the Army Nurse Corps Association Web site: http://e-anca.org/ANCchiefs.htm, accessed 10 October 2012; and Washington School of Medicine, "Missouri Women in Health Sciences" Web site, http://beckerexhibits.wustl.edu/mowihsp/bios/index.htm, accessed 24 August 2012.

12. The Army did not commission male nurses until 1955.

13. *Stethoscope*, Fitzsimons General Hospital newspaper, March 1931, 24. From the files of the Office of Medical History, Office of The Surgeon General, Falls Church, VA.

14. Florence Nightingale, *Notes on Nursing: What It Is, and What It Is Not*, reprint ed. (Philadelphia, PA: J. P. Lippincott, 1860), 133.

15. See, for example, the December 1933 issue of the *American Journal of Nursing*.

16. 6th Annual Course of the Army School of Nursing, RG 112, Entry 283, 1923–24, Box 273, NARA.

17. L. Fred Ayvazian, "The 55 Trudeau Medalists (1926–1980)," *American Review of Tuberculosis* 55 (April 1980): 757. Ayvazian served as a captain in the Army at Fitzsimons during the Korean War, 1951–53. See "Dr. Levon Fred Ayvazian, Physician Writer," *Daily Hampshire Gazette* (3 November 2009).

18. Physicians did not agree on whether cigarette smoking was harmful to tuberculosis patients. See Editorial, "Cigarettes and Tuberculosis," *Diseases of the Chest* 2 (July 1936): 5–6.

19. Ayvazian, "The 55 Trudeau Medalists," 757.

20. Edith A. Aynes, *From Nightingale to Eagle* (Englewood Cliffs, NJ: Prentice-Hall, Inc., 1973), 42.

21. 6th Annual Course of the Army School of Nursing.

22. *Stethoscope* [published by Fitzsimons Army Medical Center], 1996, 3.

23. *Stethoscope*, 1996, 3.

24. John W. Martyn, "Memorandum for the Surgeon General," 18 August 1930, RG 112, Entry 31, 1928–37, Box 285, NARA.

25. *Stethoscope*, 1996, 8.

26. Della U. Knight, "Care and Treatment of Tuberculosis Patients," *U.S. Naval Medical Bulletin* 18 (1923): 121.

27. Margaret Elizabeth Gaule, "The Diary of an Army Nurse," unpublished manuscript, Okinawa, 1945, in possession of the author, 8.

28. Aynes, *From Nightingale to Eagle*, 41–42.

29. Aynes, *From Nightingale to Eagle*, 40.

30. Aynes, *From Nightingale to Eagle*, 37–42.

31. Aynes, *From Nightingale to Eagle*, 43.

32. Aynes, *From Nightingale to Eagle*, 48.

33. *Fitzsimons Annual Report*, 1936, 27–32. On nursing for surgical treatment of tuberculosis see Ralph Adams, Adelaide Joseph, and Ruth Pierce, "Chest Surgery," *American Journal of Nursing* 40 (August 1940): 893–902; Lisa Lincoln, "Thoracoplasty—Nursing Care," *American Journal of Nursing* 44 (November 1944): 1022–27; Vera Kezar, "Tuberculosis with Pneumonectomy," *American Journal of Nursing* 49 (March 1949): 188–90;

and Bess M. Ellison, "Nursing Care and Collapse Therapy," *American Journal of Nursing* 50 (August 1950): 473–75. See also Stephanie Kirby, "Sputum and the Scent of Wallflowers: Nursing in Tuberculosis Sanatoria 1920–1970," *Social History of Medicine* 23 (December 2010): 602–20.

34. *Stethoscope*, 1996, 3.

35. *Stethoscope*, 1996, 12.

36. *Stethoscope*, 1996, 13–14.

37. In 1935, tuberculosis accounted for 903 days lost per nurse compared to 528 for all diseases of the nervous system and 694 days lost for all diseases of the circulatory system. *Annual Report of the Surgeon General*, 1935, 120–21.

38. Julia Stimson to Ida F. Butler, 20 August 1923, RG112, Entry 29, 1917–27, Box 91, NARA.

39. Florence Nightingale, *Notes on Hospitals* (London, UK: Longman, Green, Longman, Roberts and Green, 1863), 21.

40. Julia C. Stimson to the Surgeon General, 17 July 1936, RG 112, Entry 29, 1928–37, Box 29, NARA.

41. Mary C. Campbell, "The Nurse's Problems in Sanatorium Management," *Journal of the Outdoor Life* 16 (1919): 339.

42. Julia C. Stimson to Clara D. Noyes, 5 August 1919, RG 112, Entry 29, 1917–27, Box 93, NARA.

43. Laura Brackett Hoppin, *History of the World War Reconstruction Aides* (Millbrook, NY: William Tyldsley, 1933), 63–64.

44. Esta H. McNett, "The Nursing Care of Tuberculosis Patients," *American Journal of Nursing* 37 (1937): 1031.

45. E. L. W., "The Right Nurse for Tuberculosis," letter to the editor, *American Journal of Nursing* 35 (1935). Also Claire Gilstrap, "An R. N. Takes the Cure," *American Journal of Nursing* 27 (1927): 629–31.

46. J. Heimbeck, "Immunity to Tuberculosis," *Archives of Internal Medicine* (1928): 336–42; and Heimbeck, "Tuberculosis in Hospital Nurses," *Tubercle* 18 (1936): 97–99.

47. "Tuberculosis among Young Women, with Special Reference to Tuberculosis among Nurses," *American Journal of Nursing* 28 (1928): 766–68.

48. J. A. Myers, "The Prevention of Tuberculosis among Nurses," *American Journal of Nursing* 30 (1930), 1361–72.

49. Julius L. Wilson, "Five Great Teachers in the Field of Tuberculosis," *American Review of Tuberculosis* (May 1981): 572.

50. Myers, "The Prevention of Tuberculosis among Nurses."

51. J. Arthur Myers, "Tuberculosis among Nurses," *American Journal of Nursing* 32 (1932): 1159–65; J. Arthur Myers and Harold S. Diehl, "The Student Nurse and Tuberculosis," *Journal of the American Medical Association* 102 (23 June 1934): 2086–88; Harold S. Diehl and J. Arthur Myers, "Tuberculosis and College Students," *Transactions of the National Tuberculosis Association* 32 (1936): 163–71; J. Arthur Myers, H. S. Diehl, Ruth E. Boynton, and Benedict Trach, "Development of Tuberculosis in Adult Life," *Archives of Internal Medicine* 59 (January 1937): 27–31; Willard B. Soper and J. Burns Anderson, "Pulmonary Tuberculosis in Young Adults," *American Review of Tuberculosis* 39 (1939): 9–32; and G. H. C. Joynt, "Tuberculin Tests on Student Nurses," *Chest* 5 (1939): 9–12.

Other studies included Ernest S. Mariette, "The Tuberculosis Problem among Nurses in Eight Tuberculosis Sanatorium," *American Journal of Nursing* 36 (1936): 605–17; Sidney J. Shipman and Elizabeth A. Davis, "Tuberculin Hypersensitivity and Tuberculosis Disease among Nurses: A Study of the Nursing Personnel of the University of California Hospital," *American Journal of Nursing* 28 (1928) 769; Everett K. Geer, "Tuberculosis among

Nurses," *Archives of Internal Medicine* 40 (1932): 77–87; Everett K. Geer, Earl J. Black, and H. E. Hilleboe, "Tuberculosis among Nurses—A 10-Year Survey," *Transactions of the National Tuberculosis Association* (1939): 253–57; and Paul Vincent Davis, "Tuberculosis among Nurses," *Chest* (1940): 214–20.

52. Charles V. Chapin, "The Science of Epidemic Diseases," *The Scientific Monthly* (June 1928): 485; and Charles V. Chapin, *The Sources and Modes of Infection* (New York, NY: John Wiley and Sons, 1910). See also Richard L. Riley, "Historical Background," in special issue, "Airborne Contagion," *Annals of the New York Academy of Sciences 353* (December 1980): 3–9; Chad J. Roy and Donald K. Milton, "Airborne Transmission of Communicable Infection—The Elusive Pathway," *New England Journal of Medicine* 350 (22 April 2004): 1710–12.

53. W. C. Newton, "The Care of Contagious Diseases," *U.S. Naval Medical Bulletin* Supplement No. 8 (January 1919): 7.

54. A. Tostmann et al., "Tuberculosis Transmission by Patients with Smear-negative Pulmonary Tuberculosis in a Large Cohort in the Netherlands," *Clinics of Infectious Disease* 48 (15 February 2008): 496–97; and Alka M. Kanaya, David V. Glidden, and Henry F. Chambers, "Identifying Pulmonary Tuberculosis in Patients with Negative Sputum Smear Results," *Chest* 120 (August 2001): 349–55.

55. W. H. Oatway, "Stop Spreading Tuberculosis!" *Modern Hospital* 53 (December 1939): 51–52; A. Myers, F. D. Herrington, and T. L. Streukens, "Personnel, Patients and TB," *Modern Hospital* 54 (January 1940): 58–60; and M. Pollack, "Do Our Hospitals Actually Spread Tuberculosis?" *Modern Hospital* 53 (August 1939): 44–45.

56. M. P., "The Nurse and Her Relation to Pulmonary Tuberculosis," *American Journal of Nursing* 20 (1919–1920): 463.

57. T. E. Scott and R. S. Loving, "Pulmonary Tuberculosis," *Journal of the Outdoor Life* 29 (June 1922): 167, 168. See also James G. Cumming, "Can the Tuberculosis Transmission Rate Be Reduced?" *Journal of the American Medical Association* 74 (17 April 1920): 1072.

58. Ernest S. Mariette, "The Tuberculosis Problem among Nurses in a Tuberculosis Sanatorium," *American Journal of Nursing* (1936): 605. On the role of sputum see Editorial, "Tuberculophobia," *Diseases of the Chest* 11 (July 1936): 6–7.

59. Editorial, "Tuberculophobia."

60. Robert G. Lovell, *Taking the Cure: The Patient's Approach to Tuberculosis* (New York, NY: MacMillan, 1948), 28.

61. T. E. Scott and Captain R. S. Loving, "Pulmonary Tuberculosis," *Journal of the Outdoor Life* 29 (June 1922): 167–68.

62. George R. Callender, "Tuberculosis and Filipinos," 17 May 1924, RG 112, Entry 29, Box 189, NARA.

63. Henry J. Nichols, "Some Medical Problems of the Day," *Military Surgeon* (September 1925): 261.

64. Robert B. Kerr, "The New Conception of Tuberculosis Infection," *American Journal of Nursing* 29 (November 1929): 1282.

65. Sociologist Paul Starr has argued that such testing encouraged a shift in public health policy and practice from improving social conditions and people's standard of living to focusing on individuals as the source of disease. Paul Starr, *The Social Transformation of American Medicine* (New York, NY: Basic Books, 1982), 191–92.

66. Esmond R. Long and Florence B. Seibert, "The Incidence of Tuberculous Infection in American College Students: Determination by Standardized Tuberculin on 18,744 College Entrants in 1935–1936," *Journal of the American Medical Association* 108 (22 May 1937): 1761–65. See also Esmond R. Long, "Tuberculosis and College Students,

with Special Reference to Tuberculin Testing," *Lancet* 55 (1937): 201–3; J. Arthur Myers, "Types of Tuberculosis Lesions Found in the Chests of Students of Nursing and Medicine," *American Review of Tuberculosis* 28 (1933): 93–117; and Heather Munro Prescott, "The White Plague Goes to College: Tuberculosis Prevention Programs in Colleges and Universities, 1920–1960," *Bulletin of the History of Medicine* 74 (2000): 735–72. See also Lee H. Ferguson, "Pulmonary Tuberculosis and Students," *American Journal of Public Health* 20 (1930) 955–62; H. W. Hetherington, F. M. McFedran, H. R. M. Landis, and E. L. Opie, "Tuberculosis in Medical and College Students," *Archives of Internal Medicine* 48 (1931): 734–43; Willard B. Soper and Julius L. Wilson, "Experience and the Detection of Pulmonary Tuberculosis in 3,000 Students Entering Yale University," *Transactions of the National Tuberculosis Association* (1932): 99–101; H. W. Hetherington, F. M. McPhedran, H. R. M. Landis, and E. L. Opie, "Further Study of Tuberculosis among Medical and Other University Students," *Archives of Internal Medicine* 55 (May 8, 1935): 709–26; Willard B. Soper and J. Burns Anderson, "Pulmonary Tuberculosis and Young Adults," *American Review of Tuberculosis* 39 (1939): 9–32; and Phyllis Q. Edwards and Lydia B. Edwards, "The Story of the Tuberculin Test from an Epidemiologic Viewpoint," *American Review of Tuberculosis* 81 (January 1960): 1–47.

67. Georgina D. Feldberg, *Disease and Class: Tuberculosis and the Shaping of Modern North American Society* (New Brunswick, NJ: Rutgers University Press, 1995), 64. On Bacille Calmette-Guerin (BCG) and tuberculosis see Michael D. Iseman, *A Clinician's Guide to Tuberculosis* (Philadelphia, PA: Lippincott Williams & Wilkins, 2000), 399–416; and Thomas Dormandy, *The White Death: A History of Tuberculosis* (New York, NY: New York University Press, 1999). Feldberg provides an analysis critical of U.S. policy; and Lee B. Reichman and Janice Hopkins Tanne argue, "Our feeling is that even a very effective strain of BCG does no more than protect infants and very young children against severe forms of TB," in *Timebomb: The Global Epidemic of Multi-Drug-Resistant Tuberculosis* (New York, NY: McGraw-Hill, 2002), 33. On BCG testing, also see Clifford Rosenberg, "The International Politics of Vaccine Testing in Interwar Algiers," *American Historical Review* 117 (June 2012): 671–97.

68. As Rene Dubos explained, Americans resisted BCG because "BCG induced a positive tuberculin reaction in the detection of asymptomatic disease." Such a view "was associated with the restrictive immigration policies of the 1920s and the related suspicion that immunization might hide otherwise detectable diseases," Rene Dubos and Jean Dubos, *The White Plague: Tuberculosis, Man, and Society* (New Brunswick, NJ: Rutgers University Press, 1952, 1987), *xxxii* and 60. Also J. Arthur Myers, "The Effects of the Diminished Incidence of Primary Infection on the Tuberculosis Control Program," *Diseases of the Chest* 22 (December 1952): 615–16.

69. On the more recent use of tuberculin testing see "Targeted Tuberculin Testing and Treatment of Latent Tuberculosis Infection," *Morbidity and Mortality Weekly Review* 49 (9 June 2000); and the Centers for Disease Control (CDC) and Prevention Web site, "Tuberculosis, Testing and Diagnosis," http://www.cdc.gov/tb/publications/factsheets/testing/skintesting.htm, accessed 24 August 2012.

70. William C. Pollock and James Hedges Forsee, "Tuberculosis among Doctors and Nurses at Fitzsimons General Hospital," *Military Surgeon* 75 (July 1934): 17–21 and the CDC Web site at http://www.cdc.gov/tb/publications/factsheets/testing/skintesting.htm, accessed 24 August 2012.

71. William C. Pollock and James Hedges Forsee, "Reinfection among Tuberculoallergic Doctors and Nurses at Fitzsimons Hospital," *American Review of Tuberculosis* 31 (1935) 203–16.

72. Aynes, *From Nightingale to Eagle*, 38. Exclamation in the original.

73. "Controlling Tuberculosis among Student Nurses," *Modern Hospital* 47 (October 1936): 53; Ernest S. Mariette, "Prevention of Tuberculosis among Nursing and Auxiliary Personnel," *American Journal of Nursing* 46 (December 1946): 825–27; and Benjamin W. Black, "Protecting Personnel against the Hazard of Tuberculosis," *Modern Hospital* 53 (November 1953): 63–64. On tuberculin positives, see Ernest S. Mariette, "The Tuberculosis Problem among Nurses in a Tuberculosis Sanatorium," *American Journal of Nursing* 36 (1936): 605–17.

74. G. F. Aycock memorandum to the adjutant, Fitzsimons General Hospital, 27 May 1939, RG 112, Entry 29, 1938–40, Box 66, NARA.

75. "Interview, Robert L. Black with Michael Baker, at FS in 1929–1930," in U.S. Army Military History Institute, Carlisle, PA, 1984, 19.

76. Thanks to Susan D. Jones, Ph.D., D.V.M. for her comments on this case.

77. Claribel A. Wheeler, ed., "A Study of the Nursing Care of Tuberculosis Patients," *American Journal of Nursing* 38 (1938): 1021–37.

78. H. McLeod Riggins and J. Burns Amberson Jr., "The Detection and Control of Tuberculosis among Nurses," *American Journal of Nursing* 40 (1940): 1141–42.

79. *Stethoscope*, 1996, 8. Simple cloth masks would have been ineffective in preventing inhalation of tuberculosis bacteria at any rate, but the absence of masks indicates a lack of concern about transmission.

80. Leslie N. Nunn, "Sanitary Report for the Month of December 1941," 1 January 1942, RG 112, Entry 31, 1938-44, Box 203, NARA.

81. Paul Vincent Davis, "Tuberculosis among Nurses," *Chest* 6 (1940): 218.

82. M. Pollack, "Don't Neglect Tuberculosis," *American Journal of Nursing* 44 (December 1944): 1133.

83. Dorothy Deming, "Nursing in Tuberculosis Hospitals," *American Journal of Nursing* 43 (December 1943): 1101–8; and Dorothy Deming, "We Couldn't Do without Aides," *American Journal of Nursing* 43 (October 1943): 891. Emphasis in original.

84. J. A. Myers, Ruth E. Boynton, and Harold S. Diehl, "Prevention of Tuberculosis among Students of Nursing," *American Journal of Nursing* 47 (October 1947): 665; and J. A. Myers, F. E. Harrington, and T. L. Steukens, "Minneapolis Proves its Case," *Modern Hospital* 54 (February 1940): 63–65.

85. Barron H. Lerner, *Contagion and Confinement: Controlling Tuberculosis along Skid Row* (Baltimore, MD: Johns Hopkins University Press, 1998), 70–73. See also Barbara Gutman Rosenkrantz, introductory essay, Rene Dubos and Jean Dubos, *The White Plague*, xxix.

86. Thomas M. Daniel, *Wade Hampton Frost, Pioneer Epidemiologist, 1880–1938: Up to the Mountain* (Rochester, NY: University of Rochester Press, 2004), 183; Thomas M. Daniel, *Pioneers of Medicine and Their Impact on Tuberculosis* (Rochester, NY: University of Rochester Press, 2000); and Kenneth Maxcyu, ed. *The Papers of Wade Hampton Frost, M.D.: A Contribution to Epidemiological Method* (New York, NY: The Commonwealth Fund, 1941).

87. Wade Hampton Frost, "The Age Selection of Mortality from Tuberculosis in Successive Decades," *Milbank Memorial Fund Quarterly* 18 (January 1940): 62. This article was republished as a historical paper with commentary by George W. Comstock, as "Invited commentary on 'The Age Selection of Mortality from Tuberculosis in Successive Decades,'" *American Journal of Epidemiology* 141 (1995): 3–10.

88. W. H. Frost, "How Much Control of Tuberculosis?" *American Journal of Public Health* 27 (August 1937): 759–66.

89. Frost, "How Much Control of Tuberculosis?"

90. Frost also raised the issue of tuberculosis eradication in Wade Hampton Frost, "The Outlook for the Eradication of Tuberculosis," *American Review of Tuberculosis* 32 (1935): 644.

91. Ruth Puffer et al., "Use of the Index Case in the Study of Tuberculosis in Williamson County," *American Journal of Public Health* 32 (1942); 601–4.

92. J. Arthur Myers, "The Effects of the Diminished Incidence of Primary Infection on the Tuberculosis Control Program," *Diseases of the Chest* 22 (December 1952): 611–13.

93. Esmond R. Long, chapter 14, "Tuberculosis," in *Communicable Diseases: Transmitted Chiefly Through Respiratory and Alimentary Tracts*, vol. 4, Preventive Medicine, In: *Medical Department, United States Army, Preventive Medicine in World War II*, John Boyd Coates, ed. (Washington, DC: Office of The Surgeon General, Department of the Army, 1958).

94. Thomas S. Kuhn, *The Structure of Scientific Revolutions,* 3rd ed. (Chicago, IL: University of Chicago Press, 1996).

95. Lavella Phelps, "Discussion on Paper by Mrs. Whitman," Mildred Whitman, "Today's Tuberculosis Control Program—a Challenge to Nurses," *Transactions of the National Tuberculosis Association* (1947): 396

96. *Stethoscope*, Fitzsimons Army Hospital, 15 October 1943, 11–18.

97. *Stethoscope*, Fitzsimons Army Hospital, 1 April 1944, 8.

Chapter Seven
Surviving the Great Depression: Fitzsimons and the New Deal

Congressman Lawrence Lewis, Democrat of Denver, was recovering from a bad cold as he and other state leaders worked over the weekend to prepare for President Franklin Roosevelt's visit to Denver on Monday, 12 October 1936. In this election year, the nation was mired in the depths of the worst economic depression it had ever seen. The Army Medical Department was, like most of the government, financially strapped, and Fitzsimons' future hung in the balance. As a cost-saving measure the Surgeon General wanted to close the facility and transfer patients to other government hospitals. Regardless of how effectively the Army's tuberculosis specialists could treat patients, they faced losing one of their most powerful weapons—their only tuberculosis center—if the Surgeon General had his way. The success of the Army's tuberculosis program was now a matter of politics and money as well as science and medicine.

Lewis, part of the Colorado contingent advising Roosevelt on his visit, was determined that the president should visit Fitzsimons. (Roosevelt had been there once before, during the 1932 campaign.) Lewis wrote in his personal diary that he had wired a White House assistant, Marvin H. McIntyre, who was traveling on the presidential train, stating, "I strongly urged the desirability of the President visiting Fitzsimons Hospital."[1] McIntyre told Lewis that the president had agreed, remarking that "the Secret Service doesn't want me to go to Fitzsimons hospital; but I'm going anyway. I've visited that hospital before and I want to see it again."[2] Lewis notified the local newspapers and then on the eve of the president's visit drove to Cheyenne, Wyoming, with Colorado Democrats Governor Edwin Johnson, Senator Alva Adams, and U.S. Representatives John A. Martin and Ed T. Taylor to meet the president's train and accompany him to Denver. Detailing his experience in his personal diary, Lewis wrote that about 10:00 p.m. he "went in to see the President who was working on the speech to be delivered tomorrow at Denver. He read part of it to us. He asked us about political conditions in Colo., etc. We were with him for about 1/2 hour." The visitors then returned to their sleeping cars on the train and before going to bed Lewis noted in his diary the berth that he occupied, referring to himself in the third person: "L. L. in Lower 10, Car G."[3]

On the morning of Roosevelt's visit to Fitzsimons, Lewis woke to find "a beautiful Colorado Autumn day." After breakfast he had another opportunity to speak to the president and "stressed again (as I did before) the fact that the strongest emotional appeal in Denver is his (the President's) favorable attitude toward Fitzsimons Hospital." Arriving in Denver midmorning, the party rode by car to the Capitol building, where Roosevelt recounted his administration's accomplishments on behalf of Colorado.[4] Lewis sat next to Eleanor Roosevelt on the platform and described the crowd as "very enthusiastic."[5] He then rode with Secret Service officers to Fitzsimons, where Mrs. Roosevelt visited a friend and tuberculosis patient, reporter Anna V. Herendee.[6] The president did not leave the car, but as was his custom, greeted people from the back seat (Figure 7-1). Wrote Lewis, "I stood by the President's car and talked with him about the Hospital and he asked various questions of me and Col. Buck, the commanding officer." Some

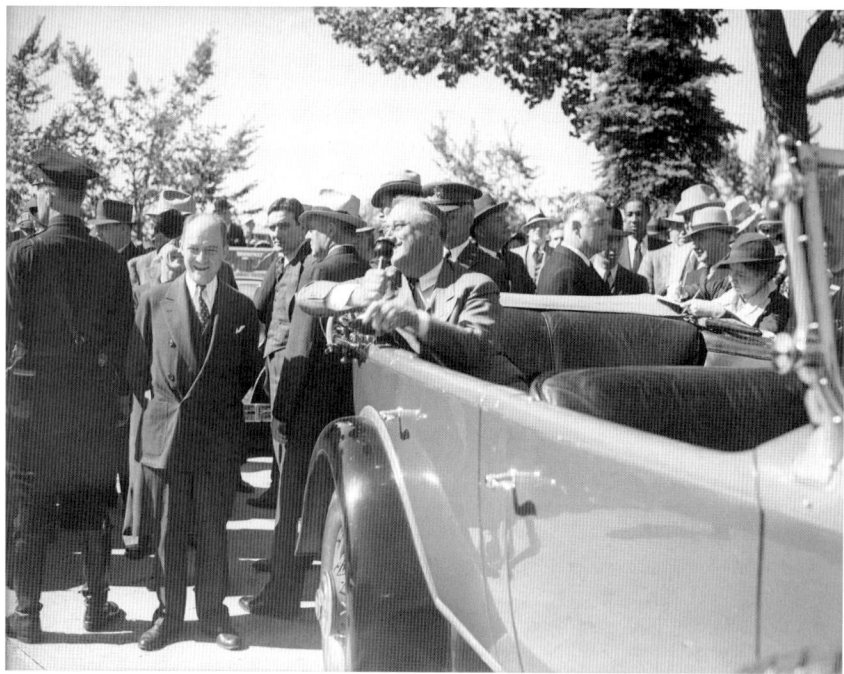

Figure 7-1. President Franklin Roosevelt makes a speech at Fitzsimons General Hospital, from his car, 12 October 1936 with Congressman Lawrence Lewis standing by.
Photograph courtesy of the Denver Public Library, Western History Collection, Image #Rh-221.

patients had come out to see the president, but Lewis suggested that he make some remarks, "explaining that his words would be carried to every bedside by a wiring system." Roosevelt spoke briefly of the good work of the hospital and gestured to the snow-clad mountains, announcing, "I am quite impressed with the beauty and value of this hospital and it will remain here as long as I am president of the United States."[7] That evening, Lewis recorded the president's words verbatim in his diary. He was so happy that "in violation of all rules of Secret Service L. L. [Lewis] tossed his hat high in the air and joined in the cheers."[8]

A successful presidential trip to one's hometown was certainly something to celebrate, but Roosevelt's promise of support for Fitzsimons was actually the coda to Lewis' four-year effort to keep the hospital alive. In the end, he more than succeeded. Instead of abandoning its primary tuberculosis hospital, as the Surgeon General had proposed, the Army transformed the post into the largest, most modern military hospital in the world. The rescue of Fitzsimons reveals the inner workings of Depression-era Washington and the War Department's efforts to take advantage of New Deal programs to maintain its military preparedness. During the Depression Congressman Lewis and the War Department learned how to secure funding from four different sources: annual military appropriations; patient benefits from various federal agencies; construction and work relief funding for specific projects on the Fitzsimons reservation; and dedicated federal funding for a new hospital building. The story of Fitzsimons during the Depression reveals the increasing role federal funds played in building the nation's medical infrastructure and the continuing demand that tuberculous soldiers, sailors, veterans, and government workers made upon the country. It also demonstrates what a single member of Congress could accomplish in the 1930s if he worked hard and played his politics right.

The Great Depression

The Great Depression in the United States began in the fall of 1929 and did not end until the United States entered World War II.[9] After the stock market crash of October 1929 the economy deteriorated with a breadth and depth never before seen. By the time of Franklin Roosevelt's inauguration in March 1933, stocks had lost 80 percent of their value; the gross national product had fallen 50 percent; more than 5,000 banks had failed; industrial production had fallen by 50 percent; and 15 million people—25 percent of the labor force in the United States—were unemployed. In Cleveland, Ohio, the unemployment rate was almost 50 percent, and in construction industries it was as high as 80 percent. After hitting bottom in 1933 the economy recovered slightly, only to collapse again in 1937. Economic calamity reached into the middle class to the point that in his second inaugural address Roosevelt noted that one-third of Americans were "ill-housed, ill-clad, and ill-nourished."[10]

As the economy failed after the crash, federal tax and tariff receipts declined and the Hoover administration (1929–33) cut government expenditures. In light of the economic crisis, peace on the U.S. borders, and a persistent isolationist and antimilitary public, Congress imposed deep budget cuts on the War Department. Following the tight budgets of the 1920s, these reductions cut military muscle and bone. Chief of Staff Douglas MacArthur, appointed in 1930, vigorously opposed the cuts, but in May 1931 he was forced to close fifty-three posts, and reduce headquarters and regional corps staff by 15 percent. He more successfully rejected proposals in 1932 to make Army tents and medical and mess facilities available to the Bonus Army protesters or to use Army barracks and surplus uniforms to house and clothe needy civilians. The Army, he believed, should not be used as a relief organization.[11] When the Roosevelt Administration came into office in 1933, it cut the War Department budget again by so much—20 percent—that MacArthur had to close another fifteen large Army posts and 200 smaller ones, cancel all military construction projects costing more than $20,000, limit training exercises, and even suspend target practice for all personnel except new recruits.[12] Such meager funding, MacArthur said, left him with "only a naked framework" of a national military force.[13]

Budget cuts also reached personnel. Advocates of increased Army air power, a motorized cavalry, and a modernized Navy wanted to shift funding from military personnel to machinery and thereby reduce the number of officers, including medical officers.[14] MacArthur and the War Department had set as an "irreducible minimum" 14,000 officers and 165,000 enlisted men for the Army, but in 1933 Congress funded only 12,000 officers and 118,750 enlisted men.[15] Congress passed a special retirement option to encourage officers in the World War I "hump" to retire, and in 1936 reduced the Medical Administrative Corps to only sixteen officers.[16] "It is a pity that we should have become so oblivious to the bitter lessons of the World War," wrote Secretary of War George Dern in 1935, "as to allow our defense to dwindle until, if another war should be forced upon us, we should, as usual, be unprepared for effective action." The normally soft-spoken former Utah governor continued: "In that event we should find that our so-called 'economies' have in reality been a hideously extravagant waste of money and lives."[17] General George C. Marshall, Army Chief of Staff (1939–45), later remarked that "during the postwar period, continuous paring of appropriations had reduced the Army virtually to the status of that of a third-rate power."[18] It was unclear whether the Army's first-rate tuberculosis hospital could survive in a "third-rate" budget environment.

As MacArthur struggled with issues of air power and mechanization, the burden of cutting the Medical Department budget fell to Surgeon General Robert U. Patterson (Figure 7-2). Appointed in June 1931, Patterson arrived at an unpropitious time, and unfortunately lacked the political acumen or finesse to maneuver effectively in Washington during a time of crisis. Born and educated in Canada, Patterson practiced medicine in Montana before entering the Medical Corps in 1901.[19] He served at a wide range of posts, from the Philippines and the Presidio in San Francisco, to the American mission in Cuba. During World War I, Patterson commanded an American Expeditionary Forces base hospital and received the Distinguished Service Medal, among other decorations, for his service. After

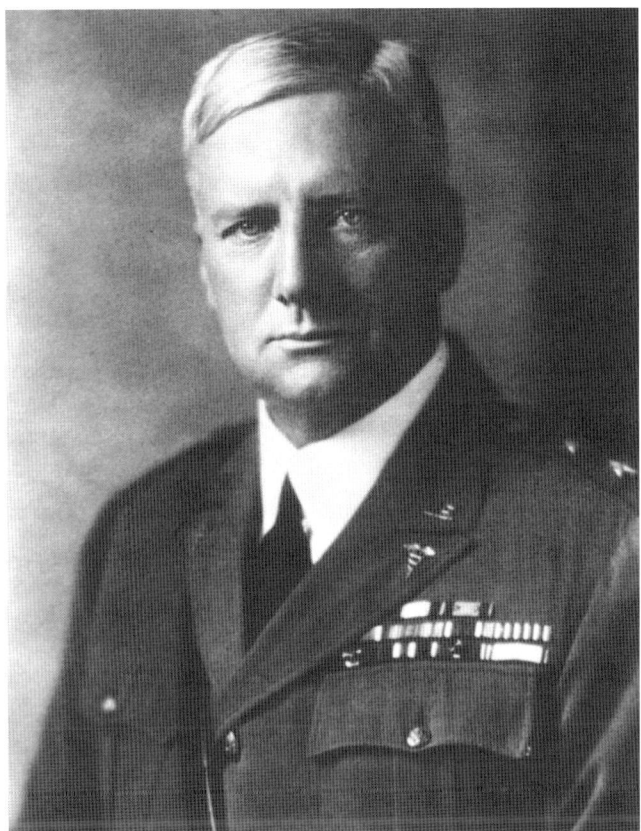

Figure 7-2. Robert Urie Patterson, Surgeon General, 1931–35.
Photograph courtesy of the National Library of Medicine, Image #B021105.

the war he worked in the Office of The Surgeon General (OTSG), advised the Veterans' Bureau on hospital administration, and commanded the Army and Navy General Hospital in Hot Springs, Arkansas, from 1925 to 1930. Serving as Surgeon General during the economic crisis, Patterson focused more on the *costs* of running a tuberculosis hospital than on the *needs* of tuberculosis patients—and it would cost him politically.

The Medical Department budget already had serious staffing shortfalls, so Patterson at first rejected deep reductions and instead proposed funding increases for staff and equipment, declaring "it was felt…that the view of this office should be on record." But the War Department did not even submit Patterson's request to Congress, and ordered him instead to cut.[20] One of his first austerity moves was to close the Army School of Nursing, a move that had been proposed by his predecessor, General (Gen.) Merritte Ireland, because of the low number—only 10 percent—of its graduates who subsequently joined the Army Nurse Corps (ANC).[21] Patterson did so clumsily, however, closing the school in January 1933, while ANC chief Julia Stimson was out of town and without consulting her. Stimson wrote, "I was given scant courtesy and told the matter was settled. So after 13 years the school is wiped out ruthlessly in two months."[22] At the same time that he implemented other painful budget and staff reductions, Patterson nevertheless allocated $2 million to rebuild the Army and Navy General Hospital in Hot Springs, Arkansas, a step that some people believed demonstrated favoritism for his former command.[23]

Roosevelt swept into office in March 1933 with a mandate to fight the Depression and took bold steps during his first 100 days. He quickly got Congress to pass legislation to restore confidence in the nation's banks, and then won approval of the Economy Act, which dramatically reduced federal spending, targeting the generous veterans' benefits, including those for tuberculosis, that Congress had passed in the previous decade.[24] The House of Representatives had tried to reduce veterans' benefits in 1931, but the American Legion was able to block any cuts.[25] But now, Roosevelt, ever the astute politician, knew that financially struggling Americans would object to the fact that veterans, who comprised only 1 percent of the population, received one-quarter of the federal budget in benefits. Telling Congress that "for three long years the Federal Government has been on the road toward bankruptcy," he called for immediately cutting $400 million in veterans' benefits and another $100 million through a 15 percent wage cut for federal employees, both military and civilian.[26] Facing a compliant Congress, catching veterans' organizations by surprise, and sweetening the legislation with a companion bill to legalize the sale of 3.2 beer, Roosevelt signed the Economy Act into law on 20 March 1933, less than two weeks after his inauguration. The bill stripped 500,000 veterans of government benefits—essentially all those receiving benefits for nonservice-connected illnesses or injuries, including the thousands who had presumptive benefits for tuberculosis—and cut benefit amounts by 25 to 80 percent for those veterans who retained them. Given the fact that as of March 1933, fully 60 percent of veteran patients were being treated for non-service-connected disabilities, the Economy Act set off the wholesale discharge of veterans—including tuberculosis patients—from federal hospitals.[27] The White House further accelerated the departure of patients from Fitzsimons and other Army hospitals with Executive Order No. 10, which required veteran patients to be cared for in Veterans Administration (VA) hospitals only, resorting to Army, Navy, and the Public Health Service hospitals only on an emergency basis.

In 1933, two main funding streams supported tuberculosis patients in Army hospitals like Fitzsimons: Congressional appropriations to the War Department for the physical plant, medical personnel, and supplies; and individual per capita benefits from the Army, Navy, VA, and the Soldiers' Homes to cover patients' hospital costs. As early as 1930, federal agencies scrambled to justify their budgets by maintaining high hospital occupancy rates. The VA and the Soldiers' Homes began to send more of their beneficiaries—and their benefits—to VA hospitals instead of Army and Navy facilities like Fitzsimons. The Economy Act cuts thereby caused government hospitals to seemingly fight over tuberculosis patients. It also left Patterson's Medical Department with hundreds of vacant hospital beds at the same time he wanted to build a new hospital in Hot Springs, Arkansas. With both funding streams—operating funds and veterans' benefits—slashed, the Surgeon General looked for places to cut.

The 1920s had been hard on Army hospitals, and like many of them, Fitzsimons, which in 1931 had more veteran patients than any other Army hospital—66 percent of its admissions—was falling into disrepair.[28] That year the Fitzsimons hospital commander, Colonel (Col.) Carroll S. Buck, advised the OTSG that the heating system of steam pipes was "rapidly reaching a point where extensive major replacements will be mandatory." In addition, "nearly all of the buildings of this hospital are of the semi-permanent type.... deteriorating rapidly, particularly as to the floors, and the cost of their proper maintenance increases from year to year."[29] Buck believed that certain repairs could prolong the life of the buildings, but War Department inspector Col. William S. Browning was less sanguine. In a November 1932 report he stated that while Fitzsimons was "efficiently and economically administered," he believed that "in view of the necessity for rigid economy in both funds and personnel during the depression, serious consideration should be given to the question of abandoning this hospital, as far as the Army is concerned, before becoming involved in a heavy outlay for repairs."[30] After receiving Buck's estimate for repair and renovation of the physical plant, which totaled $509,248, exceeding the Medical Department's construction and repair budget for the entire year ($497,232), the OTSG commented that "if the above required sum is reasonably correct, it is believed that this office must soon seriously consider the question of its ability to maintain the Fitzsimons General Hospital." Buck quickly pared the request to $113,000, but in March 1933, as Congress debated the Economy Act, another inspector was less circumspect than Browning and recommended "that this hospital be abandoned in so far as the Army is concerned."[31] This was not a new idea; as early as 1926, Surgeon General Ireland had considered in a "memo to file" transferring Fitzsimons to the VA and sending Army and Navy tuberculosis patients to Beaumont General Hospital in El Paso, Texas.[32] Nothing came of the idea, but now the economic crisis and the grim inspection reports offered Patterson a seemingly tidy way to cut his Medical Department's costs.

On 26 April 1933 Patterson asked Army Chief of Staff MacArthur for permission to abandon Fitzsimons "without delay," citing the declining number of active military tuberculosis patients, the reduction in veteran patients, and the cost of maintaining Fitzsimons' physical plant.[33] While MacArthur's staff recommended that he endorse the request and send it to the Secretary of War for approval, MacArthur asked for a detailed memo on the rationale for abandonment.[34] As Patterson's office developed the memo, the Surgeon General, perhaps assuming abandonment was a *fait accompli,* sent Fitzsimons' commander Buck two telegrams, the first advising him of the recommendation to abandon the facility and the second rather crassly inquiring about the feasibility of transferring Fitzsimons' equipment to other Army hospitals.[35] A week later, Patterson sent Buck a longer memo marked "confidential," and explained that "on economic grounds" Fitzsimons should be abandoned. But, he added, "[I]t is by no means certain that political pressure upon the Secretary of War and the president may not be so great as to force the retention of part of the hospital at least." He therefore asked Buck for a memo on the feasibility of maintaining a small hospital for 300 tuberculosis patients, adding, rather sanctimoniously, "as this is a confidential memo, please express yourself frankly, make your estimates from an unbiased standpoint, simply having in mind the best interests of the Army as a whole, and without allowing local sentiment or the personal feelings of military personnel on duty with you to influence you in any way whatever."[36]

Patterson, however, underestimated the power of local sentiment. When word of the proposed abandonment got out, Colorado State Representative Joseph Constantine of Denver protested to Patterson. The Surgeon General responded by outlining his reasoning, and noted that the Army might transfer the hospital to the VA. "But," he averred, "it is not in my province to decide that matter," and suggested that Constantine contact other high government officials, including the president. Patterson added a hand-written postscript to the state legislator, whom he had probably never met, noting, "this letter is confidential to you and not for publication—of course you are at liberty to use the information it gives."[37] That he trusted such secrecy also suggests Patterson's lack of political sagacity.

Patterson presented his rationale for abandoning Fitzsimons to MacArthur in a forceful twenty-one page document arguing that maintaining Fitzsimons for Army personnel was "financially indefensible," and that abandonment would save the Army money. Dated 10 May 1933, his memo opened by pointing out that the withdrawal of VA patients from military hospitals would leave some 2,000 beds vacant. This loss of patients and the supporting VA funds would "result in a marked increase in the cost of hospitalizing military personnel in Army hospitals unless the patients be concentrated in available military hospitals and one or more hospitals closed." Fitzsimons should be closed, he believed, because the majority of patients were veterans, not active military, and tuberculosis was declining in military patients, so that "there is no justification for the Army to maintain a separate hospital in a time of peace for the treatment of tuberculosis." In addition, Patterson argued, "Due to the lack of Army installations in the region and Denver's distance from national borders Fitzsimons has *no strategic* importance whatever." He also asserted that Fitzsimons maintenance and per diem costs per patient were the highest among Army hospitals and that Fitzsimons' patients could be accommodated at other Army facilities with tuberculosis patients going to the Beaumont General Hospital in Texas. Patterson closed cautioning that "for 15 years Fitzsimons General Hospital has meant a great deal of money in the pockets of the citizens of Colorado," so that "quite naturally the people of the State of Colorado and the City of Denver in particular, are anxious to have a large Government institution maintained by the State." If the VA took over Fitzsimons, he said, it "might help to satisfy the agitation in the State of Colorado if it were known that there is a possibility that a Government institution would probably not be entirely lost to the state of Colorado, although given up as an Army hospital."[38] The OTSG hand-delivered the memo to the chief of staff, but MacArthur did not immediately act.

The Gentleman from Colorado

Colorado officials would indeed agitate at the prospect of losing Fitzsimons. The hospital employed more than one-half of the 2,000 federal workers in Denver, and the city was struggling. The Depression had not hit Colorado immediately after the 1929 stock market crash, but falling farm prices and collapsing businesses and banks soon threw it into economic decline. The Dustbowl of 1933–39 would deepen the state's distress and even the number of Colorado millionaires fell from 181 in 1929 to twenty-nine in 1932.[39] Although a traditionally Republican state, in 1932 Coloradans voted Democratic across the board, making the congressional delegation—two senators, four U.S. representatives, and the governor—all Democrats for the first time in the state's history. One of those Democrats was Rep. Lawrence Lewis.

Lewis, a Denver lawyer, was an unlikely hero. Born in St. Louis, Missouri, in 1879, Lewis' family moved to Pueblo, Colorado, when he was a boy. After attending the University of Colorado, he worked as a reporter for the *Pueblo Chieftain,* and then returned to college. This time he attended Harvard, where he received a bachelor of arts degree and a law degree, and according to one colleague, was a "militant member of the Harvard Democratic Club."[40] Lewis returned to Colorado and started a successful law practice in Denver. During the war, he served on the Liberty Loan and Red Cross committees and volunteered for the Army. He was trained in field artillery, but did not go to France. Lewis ran unsuccessfully for Congress in 1930 but won in 1932 running on the Democratic ticket and in support of repealing Prohibition. Uniformly referred to as conscientious and hardworking, Lewis was by temperament quiet, courteous, and personally moderate—not a grandstander. As Senator Edwin Johnson of Colorado observed, "Midnight oil was his companion and every step he took was measured with meticulous study and care lest the slightest error creep in."[41] Never married, Lewis devoted his life to his work, and during his time in Congress carefully recorded his daily activities in large diaries, detailing how he traveled to and from work, where he ate meals, the various people he met, and what they talked about. These rich diaries reveal the tireless efforts he made on behalf of his district and state to win New Deal funds and jobs to keep Denver afloat during the Great Depression. Throughout the 1930s Lewis helped the silver mining industry, sugar beet farmers, and the budding aviation industry in the state, and he secured millions of dollars in public works and jobs programs for Colorado. His first and favorite client, however, was Fitzsimons Hospital.

Lewis began his efforts on behalf of Fitzsimons even before his election to Congress when he helped convince the Democratic candidate for president,

Franklin Roosevelt, to visit Fitzsimons during his 1932 campaign. Then, Roosevelt had amazed the obscure lawyer running for office because "without a word, he thanked me for my part in the victory fund drive [during World War I] and remembered the numerous instances where he had met me."[42] As both men faced the Depression, Lewis' challenge would be to support Roosevelt and advocate for his district at the same time. He therefore voted for the Economy Act, and then immediately sent a telegram to the Denver Chamber of Commerce warning that the number of patients at Fitzsimons "is likely to be reduced as a result of the economy program."[43] The message was superfluous, though, because local newspapers were already sounding the alarm. When the Economy Act cut Fitzsimons' salaries 15 percent the *Rocky Mountain News* warned that such reductions could be a prelude to closing the hospital, which would cost Denver $2 million in trade, and "come as a disastrous blow to Denver merchants and businessmen." Although city leaders protested, the newspaper suggested that such efforts were futile because the administration of the Economy Act was intentionally put in the hands of the president "largely for the purpose of blocking individual congressmen who might seek to protect their own constituents from what cuts would be made."[44]

But that was exactly what Lewis set out to do. With Fitzsimons as his new client, he quickly identified the levers of power in Washington regarding funding for the hospital; his diary shows that the freshman-congressman-but-seasoned-lawyer would talk about the hospital anytime, to virtually anyone in Washington. Lewis gathered a political team on behalf of Fitzsimons that included the Colorado congressional delegation, other state political leaders, and leaders of the Denver business community. Although Lewis rarely communicated directly with Fitzsimons' administrators or patients in 1933, newspaper reporters Charles O. Gridley of the *Denver Post* and Charles S. Holmes of the *Rocky Mountain News* functioned as conduits of information between Fitzsimons and the congressman.

As Lewis looked for support for Fitzsimons he at first got the runaround. He began with Secretary of War Dern, who referred him to MacArthur. The chief of staff had not yet received Patterson's May 1933 memo and told Lewis that the War Department was "most anxious to maintain Fitzsimons Hospital but that its continued operation depends in large measure upon whether Veterans' Administration patients are kept there," Lewis wrote in his diary. "MacArthur agrees that the veteran tuberculosis cases can be maintained at Fitzsimons. Suggested I bring pressure to bear on Gen. [Frank T.] Hines of Veterans' Administration."[45] On Saturday, 22 April, Lewis met with Hines who claimed that his hospitals could care for patients more cheaply than Army hospitals. When Lewis phoned Patterson, the Surgeon General's only suggestion was that Lewis "take the matter up with the President."[46] Lewis relayed these conversations to reporters Holmes and Gridley, who publicized his lobbying efforts. Then, with little sense of urgency in the matter, the congressman turned to other issues.[47] Four days later, however, Gridley shocked Lewis by reading to him Patterson's telegram to Buck on abandonment, which Lewis recorded verbatim in his diary: "'In view of immediate abandonment of Fitzsimons and transfer of all patients elsewhere you will report amount of money appropriated in construction and repair work at the hospital that you will not require beyond June 30. Funds not required up to June 30 to be transferred to Beaumont Hospital, El Paso.'" Feeling deceived and alarmed by the speed of developments, Lewis "got in touch immediately with [Colorado] Senators Costigan and Adams and newspaper men. Arranged for interview tomorrow morning (9:30 o'clock) with Surgeon General Patterson."[48]

The tense meeting at the Munitions Building between Patterson and the Colorado delegation prefigured Patterson's and Lewis' strategies on Fitzsimons for the next three years. Patterson based his argument for closing Fitzsimons on economics and the budget crisis, citing the possible savings to the Army, downplaying Denver's importance to the nation, and arguing that the Army should care only for active military patients in its hospitals. Lewis took a more political view, citing Denver civic pride, but also stressed the welfare of tuberculosis patients and the government's responsibility for them regardless of whether they were former military or on active duty. Lewis would also out-work Patterson on the issue. He opened the meeting at the Munitions Building recalling his telephone conversation with Patterson in which the Surgeon General gave Lewis the impression that there was no immediate danger of the War Department abandoning Fitzsimons. At this, "Patterson interrupted to say things had moved very fast since then and that he had sent late yesterday recommendation to Secretary of War that hospital be abandoned." Patterson denied sending the telegram to Buck about abandoning Fitzsimons, but "was very much flustered when L. L. asked him point blank about it." The Surgeon General then "gave a long monologue" saying that Fitzsimons was of "rather flimsy construction," and that the withdrawal of VA patients made it impracticable to run the hospital for Army patients only. Patterson said that "he would be glad to turn it over to Veterans' Admin." whereby "L. L. suggested removal of some T. B. Patients would be equivalent to a death warrant. Patterson denied this." The meeting ended with no resolution, but before the Colorado delegation left the War Department, they secured a promise from Dern and MacArthur that no definite decision would be rendered on Fitzsimons for at least ten days.[49]

Lewis then went to Postmaster General James A. Farley, a trusted Roosevelt political adviser, to warn him about the "political significance and disastrous results if Fitzsimons hospital is closed."[50] When Farley offered to deliver a letter to the White House, Lewis "burned the midnight oil" to complete it. Adolph F. Zang, Denver business leader and officer of the Denver Chamber of Commerce, was in Washington as part of the Fitzsimons advocacy group, and Lewis got him out of bed at the Willard Hotel to work on the letter. They revised and corrected the statement he had written and added an introduction. Then, after midnight Lewis woke up his congressional assistant to type the letter to Farley. Then, "To bed 2:20 a.m."[51] The next day Lewis appealed to Louis W. Douglas, Roosevelt's Director of the Budget, who had quickly become the power broker for government funding issues.[52] When the Colorado delegation finally got in to see the busy budget director, Lewis presented Fitzsimons as the most effective and economic means of treating tuberculosis and warned of the danger of transferring the very sick patients. Douglas was noncommittal but reassuring, expressing doubts about moving patients around to different government hospitals and stating that "he recognized the advantages of Colo. Climate for the treatment of T.B."[53] Douglas requested a "succinct memo" with evidence in support of Fitzsimons, as did Roosevelt's closest adviser, Louis M. Howe, when Lewis was able to get five minutes with him.[54] Lewis then turned to the memo.

Between committee sessions and meetings on other issues including help for the Colorado silver mining industry and repeal of the 18th Amendment on Prohibition, Lewis began developing an extended brief in support of Fitzsimons and collecting expressions of support from the Colorado legislature and governors of neighboring states, among others. But he had to scramble to keep up with events. When he learned on 9 May from *Denver Post* reporter Gridley that a hospital train had been ordered to transfer 100 veteran patients from Fitzsimons to the naval hospital at Fort Lyon, Lewis immediately did the rounds of officials. "Left at once in taxicab for [VA Administrator] Gen. Hines' office.... saw director of budget Lewis W. Douglas," he recorded that night. While the congressman waited, Douglas' assistant phoned Hines, Patterson, and MacArthur "asking that situation be held in status quo until complete study of hospital situation can be made. All agreed to this."[55] But when the meticulous congressman called Fitzsimons the next day to be sure that the transfer order had been rescinded, people there told him it had not. He again called the budget office and got assurances that Douglas "would do everything practicable to hold entire hospital situation in abeyance until whole hospitalization program can be studied."[56] Lewis redoubled his efforts on the brief, and on 10 May took his completed memo to Douglas and Louis Howe, and sent copies to a number of other government officials.[57]

In the brief, Lewis refuted Patterson's criticisms regarding the high cost of running Fitzsimons. He used Medical Department figures on the per diem costs of tuberculosis patients—not all patients—at the various Army hospitals, pointing out that treatment for tuberculosis patients at Fitzsimons cost $4.41 per diem, which was lower than VA hospitals ($4.83) or other Army hospitals, which ranged from $4.44 at Letterman in San Francisco to $5.26 at Walter Reed in Washington, DC. Lewis also dismissed Patterson's assessment of the high cost of maintaining the Fitzsimons plant, arguing instead that the government should conserve the $4 million it had already invested in the Denver facility. (He would later use aerial photographs of the Fitzsimons reservation to show the extent of government investment.[58]) He included a letter from Colorado tuberculosis specialists (including Gerald B. Webb) praising the medical care and cautioning against moving patients to other locations. He also recounted Fitzsimons' relative success in tuberculosis treatment, quoting the Surgeon General's own 1932 annual report that lauded the effectiveness of the rest treatment, heliotherapy, artificial pneumothorax, and thoracoplasty. Lewis cited commendations of other Army hospitals that sent tuberculosis patients to Fitzsimons, and Navy Surgeon General Percival S. Rossiter, who "deplored the removal of Navy tuberculosis patients from Fitzsimons Hospital" because "the Navy had no hospital suitable for treatment of tuberculosis;

that to send tuberculosis patients to [Navy hospitals in] Norfolk or Mare Island might be fatal to them." Perhaps most importantly, Lewis pointedly rejected Patterson's distinction between active military and veteran patients, reasoning that while the veteran population may decline over the years "the Army will continue on; and, in the case of war the existence of 'going concerns' of well-organized hospitals with efficient staffs will save many lives." Lewis closed his brief noting that Denver was situated centrally in the country and argued, "[I]f the government wishes to do everything possible to cure its tuberculosis patients, this institution should be saved for that purpose."[59] To Patterson's argument that closing Fitzsimons would save the War Department money, Lewis argued that maintaining Fitzsimons would save American lives.

A direct confrontation between the Surgeon General and the congressman in 1933 was diverted by the involvement of two other governmental bodies: an *ad hoc* committee and the Federal Hospitalization Board. In the face of such spirited opposition, Patterson finally sought advice and appointed what he called an "unofficial board" to compare the costs of caring for tuberculosis veterans at Fitzsimons and the "practicability and desirability of caring for these tuberculosis patients at the Soldiers' Home." He also asked for an assessment of "the possible psychological reactions that would result among these patients if moved to Washington, and…the possibility of criticisms from time to time, and the probable nature of them."[60] For its part, the White House placed the Fitzsimons issue within the larger question of national hospitalization policy. By May, Roosevelt was backtracking on the Economy Act, issuing a statement that benefit cuts for service-connected veterans had "been deeper than was originally intended." The government would therefore reconsider benefit levels and not close any hospitals "pending a careful, studious survey of the entire hospital situation." That, the president said, "will require considerable time."[61] The question of abandoning Fitzsimons therefore went to the Federal Board of Hospitalization, which had been established in 1921 to coordinate the activities of the various federal hospitals and included the Surgeons General of the Army, Navy, and Public Health Service, and the VA Director. With the problem bucked to these two boards MacArthur put Patterson's recommendation aside.

The freshman congressman from Colorado had fended off an attack on a tuberculosis hospital during the worst budget crisis in American history. The *Denver Post* rewarded Lewis by naming him to its May "Gallery of Fame."[62] The Roosevelt Administration recognized him as a significant player as well when it invited him to a White House meeting to discuss Senate efforts to rescind much of the Economy Act. On 4 June Lewis "jumped in taxicab and arrived just at 8:30, was informed Pres. Roosevelt was going to confer with some of the leaders of the House and I had been asked to be there." They met in the Oval Office until 11:00 p.m., and discussed the "Senate's amendment to independent offices appropriations bill limiting cuts and vets compensation of service-connected cases to 25 percent." Roosevelt was worried that reversing the budget cuts would undermine the gains since 4 March and warned that he would veto the revisions. Reporting on the meeting in his diary, Lewis recorded the names and titles of the men at the meeting, noting with pride that "of all 15 present L.L. only congressman who had not been in House for several terms and only one from Far West."[63]

Roosevelt was unable to stop the reversal of much of the Economy Act, but the Colorado freshman had apparently caught his eye because later that summer the *Denver Post* announced that the president was going to punish Colorado's senators Edward Costigan and Alva Adams for not supporting his programs and that "all patronage powers [would be] handed over to Lewis."[64] This meant that the Denver congressman would be given preference in such matters as recommending individuals for federal office and announcing federal funding for the state. The modest Congressman did not comment on this development in his diary. Two weeks later, however, he was less reticent after he had to stop two more efforts to transfer veteran patients from Fitzsimons to other hospitals—one on 12 June to remove VA patients and another on 15 June to remove Soldiers' Home patients.[65] Doubting by this time that VA director Hines was behind these moves, Lewis focused on Patterson, writing in his diary that he had "concluded to see Farley next week as to chances of having Surgeon Gen. Patterson removed."[66] Lewis would go to the mat for his tuberculosis hospital.

The Trials of Colonel Buck

During the hectic 1933 spring negotiations, Lewis had breakfast with Fitzsimons Hospital commander Col. Carroll Buck at the Army and Navy Club on 24 May. Buck was even more absorbed in Fitzsimons' trials than Lewis, but unfortunately Lewis did not report on their conversation in his diary. One of Patterson's first major appointments, Buck assumed command of Fitzsimons in August 1931. Born in Vermont, Buck attended medical school at the University of Minnesota before entering the Army as a contract surgeon in 1898 and later joining the Medical Corps. Buck served with Pershing in the 1916 Punitive Expedition into Mexico and during World War I ran medical supply depots in Philadelphia. He later told reporters that "the biggest disappointment of his life was that he was not sent overseas."[67] After the war, he was a surgeon at Schofield Barracks in Hawaii and studied hospital administration at the Army Industrial College.[68] Genial and soft-spoken, Buck described himself as a man with no hobbies other than his work. He soon found that keeping his hospital open was more than a full-time job.

Although the Army Medical Department did not abandon Fitzsimons, during 1933 the patient population fell from 1,125 to 699.[69] In an effort to manage these "seismic disturbances," as he called them, Buck sent a stream of letters to the Surgeon General's office reporting on the steps he was taking to implement budget cuts, repeatedly asking for competent staff, and seeking information about Fitzsimons' future.[70] In addition to cutting employee salaries by 15 percent, the Economy Act required Buck to cut civilian employees from 365 to 145. Given such drastically reduced staff levels, Buck told the VA not to send any more thoracoplasty cases to his hospital until its fate had been decided.[71] Economic hardship also caused the American Red Cross to discontinue many of its recreational programs, and when the First National Bank of Aurora, Colorado, closed in 1933, it froze the Fitzsimons Hospital Fund that held patients' cash for recreation and sundries.[72] And then there were Patterson's telegrams. Being in charge of Fitzsimons, Buck told a colleague, "was a fine job until the economy jolted us, now it is awful." Many of his employees appealed to him for assistance, and "drawing little wages and with dependents in most cases, many of whom are invalids, it is mighty hard to turn a deaf ear to their true stories."[73]

The word "embarrassed" appears often in Buck's letters as he struggled to maintain staff morale and provide proper care to the patients who could be transferred from the hospital at any time. On 7 July, Buck told the Surgeon General, "[W]e are further embarrassed by the uncertainty as to the policy to be followed in reference to the care of beneficiaries of the Veterans Administration. Practically no admissions are being made, and the slow attrition will soon leave us without many patients." His letter concluded that "the local situation is most unhappy, and any definite information on any of these subjects will furnish a certain amount of relief, even though the news is not good."[74] The same day, he asked the OTSG for a "definite date of the abandonment of this hospital," explaining "during the past three months the life of a hospital executive in the military service has been anything but a happy one, and I think that the amputations made at the other general hospitals are much more satisfactory than to have a re-amputation performed each month as seems to be the prospect for the undersigned." He confided, "In spite of the labor of Congressman Lewis in Washington, and the efforts of the *Denver Post* at home, I cannot figure that there is much prospect of the recovery of this hospital, and have been governing myself accordingly."[75]

As if Buck did not have enough problems, 1933 was a year of loss for him. In addition to the death of his leading tuberculosis expert, Col. Earl Bruns, in March 1933, Buck had to manage a staff that included Major Charles A. Shepard, a tuberculosis specialist who had been convicted of killing his wife Zenana with poison and sentenced to life in prison in 1931. The trial created quite a scandal, with sordid revelations such as a young woman's testimony that Shepard had proposed marriage to her before his wife died.[76] Shepard remained on duty at Fitzsimons with War Department approval pending his appeal, however, because he enjoyed the support of a senior Army officer's wife who was "a grateful patient of his in the Philippines." This situation led Rep. Fiorella LaGuardia (D-NY) to attach an amendment to the 1934 Army appropriations bill preventing commissioned officers from retaining their positions after being convicted of a felony, unless authorized to do so by Secretary of War.[77] When the Supreme Court overturned Shepard's conviction on a technicality in the summer of 1933, one can only wonder at the delicate social dynamics within the Fitzsimons community around the tainted medical officer.[78] Buck experienced another loss in July 1933 when one of Fitzsimons' best medical officers, Maj. Shannon Van Valzah, died of peritonitis, which Buck described as "a great shock to all of us."[79] But worse was to come. Buck's wife of more than thirty years, Ynez, went to Chicago to attend Van

Valzah's funeral and then traveled to Albany, New York, to visit their daughter. There she suffered a severe stroke and after several months of suffering, died on 12 November 1933.

During Congress' extended summer recess that year Lewis did what he could to help Buck and Fitzsimons. His approach was twofold: block the abandonment of the hospital and revise the language in Executive Order No. 10 that restricted veteran patients to VA hospitals. He stayed in Washington over the summer, as the *Denver Post* put it, "devoting his time principally to the retention of Fitzsimons General Hospital."[80] This time paid off because Lewis was again able to see the president. He wrote in his diary for 21 July, "To exec. offices at White House at 2:45 p.m. and after about 20 minutes wait saw Pres. Roosevelt (with [Colorado Governor Edwin] Johnson and [Denver businessman Jeffrey] Keating) for about 5 minutes. Talked of greater use of silver, world market for gold producers, Fitzsimons Hospital, special election in Colo. to submit repeal of 18th Amendment and special session of Colo. Legislature."[81] This brief meeting would prove crucial to Lewis because Roosevelt told him that concerning Fitzsimons "I could come back to him if I needed help to save it."[82]

Lewis got more good news when the Surgeon General's own "unofficial board" recommended against removing patients from Fitzsimons pending the review of national hospitalization needs. Lewis now turned to the Federal Hospitalization Board and met with most of the members to make his case. Lewis' statement to the board was more emotional than his brief to the Bureau of the Budget. The hospital was "the particular pride of our city," he explained, and "represents in the minds of our citizens the care and solicitude of the federal government for those who have had their health impaired or lost in the service of our country." Thus, he cautioned, "[e]ven the suggestion of its abandonment or its diminution in service is something that excites the public mind out there and creates grave public apprehension." While Lewis said he disliked "to deal in hyperbole," he believed Fitzsimons was "unsurpassed in any hospital for the treatment of tuberculosis in the world." With regard to economic issues he suggested that the government could save money if it opened all hospital facilities to all government patients. But, he added, they should consider issues other than money. "How about economy in human suffering and human lives? Fitzsimons has conserved and saved these. It should be allowed to carry on." He asserted that "after all, government is not merely a matter of dollars. It is dollars plus public sentiment and public support." Then, resorting to hyperbole after all, he stated that if Fitzsimons should be closed, "the public reaction among our people might be such as to imperil in Denver and vicinity the success of the Administration's entire program."[83]

The board, he wrote that night, "gave me a very courteous hearing at the outset of the meeting. L. L. talked for about 20 minutes and then withdrew."[84] He had read the board well, because it did pass a resolution stating that Fitzsimons should treat all government tuberculosis patients—military and veteran—until the board had time to examine the issue in greater depth.[85] When Roosevelt approved the recommendation days later, Lewis noted that Executive Order No. 10 was modified "to include all government hospitals thus permitting Veterans Administration within their discretion, to continue hospitalization [sic] their patients in Fitzsimons and other hospitals not controlled by Veterans Administration."[86] This was good news. A *Denver Post* 2 August 1933 headline read, "Lewis Announces Victory in Campaign to Save Fitzsimons."[87]

In the meantime, Congress continued to chip away at the Economy Act that had deeply cut veterans' benefits. In June 1933 it had rolled back $100 million in cuts by limiting benefits reductions to disabled veterans to 25 percent and creating review boards to which veterans could appeal. The following March 1934, Congress passed legislation to virtually repeal the Economy Act and, when Roosevelt vetoed the bill, both houses of Congress overrode the veto and handed the president his first congressional defeat.[88]

Round Two—1934

The year 1934 at first seemed to bode well for Fitzsimons. Congressman Lewis checked in with the Army Chief of Staff, recording in his diary that he "called on Gen. MacArthur who says he thinks Fitzsimons hospital is safe."[89] The same week Buck told a colleague in the OTSG that "I've gotten my head above water again" and that he had been "reassured by the Surgeon General personally that this hospital might be expected to continue under military administration."[90] But Buck soon felt neglected. "I do not get many direct replies to my letters," he told the OTSG.[91] Loy McAfee in the OTSG responded that he had a "lapful of letters" from Buck and was doing the best he could.[92] In early March Buck's worries were confirmed when the OTSG denied Fitzsimons construction and repair funds. Alarmed, Buck wrote Surgeon General Patterson a curious letter. Against his secretary's advice he addressed his superior officer as "Bob," and told him that "it looks as though open season would be declared on this institution each spring and that we should have to stand for a lot of gunning like the migratory fowl."[93] If Fitzsimons were indeed to be abandoned, he pleaded, "for the sake of patients and personnel that a definite decision be made promptly, as it is most demoralizing to everybody concerned to have the uncertainty hanging over them for a long period of time."[94] Patterson's response to this letter is unknown, but behind the scenes he was preparing to zero out the Fitzsimons budget, offer the facility to the Public Health Service, and obtain federal funds to construct a tuberculosis ward at Beaumont Hospital in El Paso.

Intent on his mission, and having to make deep cuts somewhere in the Army Medical Department, Patterson appeared before a closed-door meeting of the House Subcommittee on Military Appropriations on 7 March 1934 to recommend the abandonment of Fitzsimons "solely for economic reasons." He stated that "in time of peace there is no justification for a special hospital for tuberculosis in the Army." In a letter to subcommittee chairman Ross A. Collins (D-MS), Patterson conceded Lewis' point of the previous year that the Fitzsimons per diem patient cost was lower than other hospitals, but argued that it was due to the large number of patients there and that such benefit would accrue to Beaumont Hospital when its patient population increased.[95] Patterson also pointed out that fewer than 200 of the active duty patients at Fitzsimons had tuberculosis and that they could be cared for at Beaumont. He omitted the fact, however, that 451 veteran and 150 civilian tuberculosis patients were also at Fitzsimons at the time. According to the *Rocky Mountain News*, Patterson told the subcommittee that he would "be delighted if the Army could get rid of Fitzsimons."[96] The subcommittee approved the Surgeon General's request and included language in the military appropriations bill that would appall a Fitzsimons partisan: "Resolved: That no part of this or any other appropriation contained in this act shall be available for any expense on account of the Fitzsimons General Hospital beyond such an amount as may be necessary for the care of such hospital on a bare maintenance basis."[97]

That night Lewis wrote, "Chas. O. Gridley, correspondent for the 'Denver Post,' called up and directed my attention to the fact that on p. 29 of Army Appropriation bill is a provision for putting Fitzsimons Hospital on a 'bare maintenance basis.'" Then, "To bed after a hectic day and more hectic evening."[98] Two days later Gridley wrote a story suggesting that the proposal to abandon Fitzsimons was a "scheme...hatched by Texas and Arkansas representatives, with the aid of Surgeon Gen. Robert U. Patterson, in an effort to aid William Beaumont hospital at El Paso and the Army and Navy hospital at Hot Springs, Ark." Referring to the Army and Navy Hospital as Patterson's "pet institution," Gridley suggested that the Surgeon General needed to close Fitzsimons in order to justify building a new facility. He noted that one subcommittee member, Rep. Tilman B. Parks, represented the Arkansas district in which the Army and Navy Hospital was located and a Texas member, Rep. Thomas L. Blanton of Abilene, attached the offending amendment to the bill. According to Gridley, the plot was revealed when El Paso Congressman R. E. Thomason told a reporter that "he hopes by the plan to get 280 Fitzsimons patients and 52 Fitzsimons officers for William Beaumont."[99] The Army tuberculosis program—its patients, staff, and equipment—had become an object of pork barrel politics.

The collaborators still had to get by Lewis, however, and he launched into action, operating the levers of power he had identified in 1933 (Figure 7-3). "Spent all morning planning how to circumvent plans to abolish Fitzsimons hospital," he wrote in his diary.[100] The fight was now on a different playing field—the legislative branch of government—where Lewis could maneuver on his own turf. But as Holmes of the *Rocky Mountain News* wrote, "it is no light undertaking to amend any appropriation bill over the recommendation and report of the committee handling it."[101] Appropriations subcommittee chairmen were some of the most powerful members of Congress, so Lewis immediately went to the floor of the House and "saw a large number of friends in House and asked their support for amendment." These friends included Joe Burns of Tennessee, the powerful House majority leader. Lewis also called in his ace. "Went to White House executive offices and there saw Marvin H. McIntyre who remembered my conversation (in presence of Gov. Johnson) with President on July 21, 1933 concerning Fitzsimons and President's remark that I could come back to him if I needed help to save it." Lewis gave McIntyre his *Congressional Record* remarks on Fitzsimons and a "copy of Gen. Patterson's biography in 'Who's Who' in which he boasts of being a Republican." He then told subcommittee chairman Ross Collins that he wanted to offer an amendment to the appropriations bill to restore funding for Fitzsimons. Collins agreed to allow a debate on the amendment, but said that he would have to oppose it despite the fact that "he cared little about the matter one way or another." As Lewis wrote that evening, the chairman told him that "all he knew about Fitzsimons Hospital was what Gen. Patterson had told him. Collins admitted that Patterson is not open and above-board—(even said he is worse)."[102]

Lewis drafted his amendment to strike the offensive language and add $50,000 in hospitalization funds to cover Fitzsimons' expenses for the year.[103] The next day he phoned his colleagues to ask their support, tracking down senior members of Congress from the South who had influence with subcommittee chairman Collins.[104] The legislation moved quickly; the next day the full House considered the military appropriations bill and took up the Lewis amendment about two o'clock in the afternoon. Speaking for his provision, Lewis reiterated his previous arguments, adding that Patterson had misled the military appropriations subcommittee and the Congress by not telling them that the Federal Hospitalization Board sup-

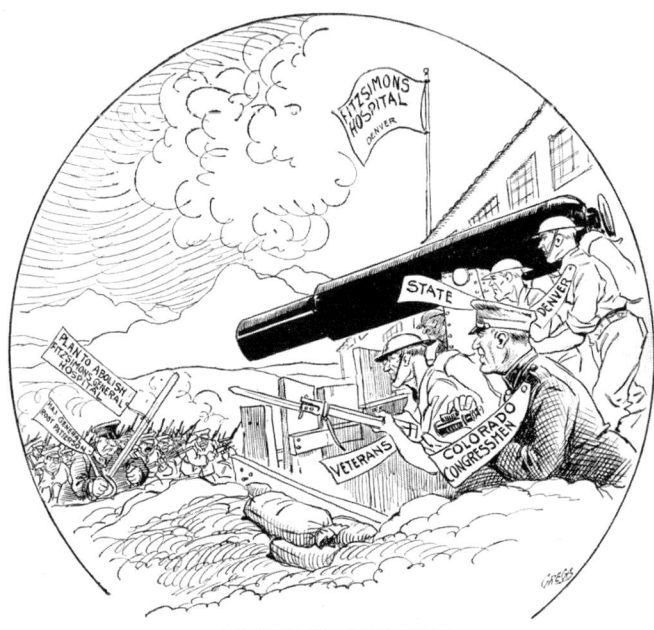

Figure 7-3. Denver Post cartoon dramatizing the local efforts to prevent the closing of Fitzsimons General Hospital, 7 March 1934, Lewis Scrapbook No. 4, 1933–34.
Image courtesy of the Colorado Historical Society, Denver, Colorado.

ported the continued care of government patients at Fitzsimons pending its review of national hospitalization requirements. More importantly, he said, "This is not a mere matter of dollars and cents—we are dealing with human lives." He told his House colleagues, "I wish we could visit the various wards, and see those fellows who reached out to me with fevered hands and said in hoarse whispers, 'Lewis, for God's sake are they going to take us away from here, are they going to break this hospital up and send us hither and yon to climates where we will not be able to live?'" A congressman from Missouri responded, "These are our men." Lewis agreed. "We represent not some bureaucrat who comes up secretly before a committee and says he wants such and such done," he argued, "but we represent the people at home and these poor boys that I have been describing."[105] The House applauded.

Chairman Collins dutifully cited the Surgeon General's arguments regarding the economies of closing Fitzsimons, and Rep. Thomason of El Paso extolled the benefits of treating tuberculosis in Texas, where the winters were milder than in Colorado. But Lewis rallied his supporters to the House floor, and after thirty minutes of debate the House agreed to his amendment. Not one to crow, Lewis simply recorded the vote noting, "Joe Byrns (majority leader), 'Billy' Bankhead, John McDuffie, Lindsay Warren, Mrs. Greenway, Mrs. McCarthy of Kansas, Mrs. Rogers of Mass, 'Ham' Fish of N.Y., the entire Colo. Delegation, Mrs. Jenckes of Ind. And many others (both Republican and Democrats) backed me up. House adjourned 4:02 p.m."[106]

A few days later Lewis visited Roosevelt's assistant Marvin McIntyre and "told him of the outcome of the fight in the House for Fitzsimons Hospital and of the obnoxious and clandestine conduct of Surgeon General Patterson and suggested his removal is in order."[107] He then repaid his Southern friends by gathering support for the cotton bill, noting in his diary that Congressman Billy Bankhead of Alabama had helped him on Fitzsimons and "we are reciprocating."[108] Lewis birddogged his Fitzsimons amendment through the Senate and it became law as part of War Department appropriations less than two weeks after Patterson's closed-door testimony. Wrote Fitzsimons commander Buck, "Fitzsimons is again on the map and those of us who are stationed here and interested in its future are delighted in consequence. We are very thankful that the annual Spring attack on the hospital only lasted two days, so that the morale was not wrecked and money not taken from us."[109] In April, however, the beaten-but-not-bowed OTSG sent Fitzsimons a curt memo advising that by the end of May the hospital would be downsized from 1,832 to 1,185 beds, a reduction of one-third capacity, and that the buildings and staff levels should be reduced accordingly.[110] To some extent this merely formalized patient reductions during the year, but it did not help morale.

The Fitzsimons fight had been good for Lawrence Lewis' reputation, though, as he approached his first reelection campaign. Despite his successes he faced opposition from the left of the Democratic Party, which wanted more help for the poor and the unemployed, and on the right from veterans who opposed Lewis' vote for the Economy Act. When he returned to Colorado in October Lewis was therefore "flabbergasted" when 500 people—more than twice the number he had expected—attended a Democratic dinner in his honor.[111] The state Democrats touted his successful campaign to save Fitzsimons as his crowning achievement and Lewis' campaign posters in English and Spanish did, too, stating "he saved Fitzsimons hospital from complete abandonment in 1933 and again in 1934."[112] Lewis visited Fitzsimons, dining with Buck in the patients' cafeteria, meeting with a women's committee on war veterans, presenting the hospital chaplain with an American flag, and visiting patients, including "about 100 or more men who came up to thank L. L. in person for having helped them to secure adjustment of their claims for compensation for service connected disabilities."[113] On election eve Lewis wrote, "The campaign is over—now for the election tomorrow!... I should not be surprised at anything. I may be defeated, I may be elected by a greatly reduced plurality, I may be elected by an increased plurality. We shall see."[114]

Benefiting from Coloradans' support for the New Deal and his own hard work, Lewis won by a greater margin than he had in 1932. But Fitzsimons' future was not secured. Plans to abandon it lived on in Patterson's office, which continued to plan the construction of a tuberculosis section at Beaumont Hospital. The week after the election, one of Patterson's assistants, Col. Roger Brooke, advised Patterson that the VA would probably be able to take over Fitzsimons in the near future if the hospital "could be transferred fully equipped." This, he was afraid, "would embarrass us somewhat down at William Beaumont" because they were expecting the Fitzsimons equipment. Brooke closed his memo on a lighter note. Having just returned from a hunting trip in North Carolina he told the Surgeon General he had "a big fat goose in storage at Walter Reed Hospital awaiting your pleasure."[115]

Round Three—1935

When Lewis returned to Washington for his second term, he occupied a strengthened position. The House Democratic Caucus rewarded him with a seat on the powerful Rules Committee, which determined what legislation reached the House floor and under what conditions each bill would be debated. The *Rocky Mountain News* proclaimed the appointment the first time "a representative of the Rocky Mountain region has been named to this powerful body."[116] Lewis' standing with the Administration remained strong. In January, MacArthur told him that his "fight for retention of Fitzsimons Hospital had been won and that I could now 'cease defensive tactics and assume the offensive' for improvement of the Hospital." MacArthur assured Lewis that he had "repeatedly over-ruled" the Surgeon General's efforts to abandon Fitzsimons, and confided, to the great interest of Lewis, that "Patterson's term will expire May 20, 1935 and that he will not be [re-]appointed."[117]

MacArthur's advice, however, was premature. On 2 February Lewis discovered that the Surgeon General had again asked the House subcommittee on military appropriations to eliminate funding for Fitzsimons. Doing his political homework, Lewis checked with the White House and MacArthur to confirm that they were not behind the Fitzsimons cuts, and then prepared to make his own statement before the subcommittee. At a hearing on 5 February he reminded them of the

Federal Board of Hospitalization's recommendation that government tuberculosis patients be treated at Fitzsimons, and told the subcommittee that Patterson's views "are not shared by his superiors. Authoritatively, I am assured that the General Staff is unalterably opposed to closing it." Lewis refuted Patterson's claims that the hospital was in poor condition and the weather not suitable for lung patients. When a member of the subcommittee cited Patterson's point that the War Department was bearing the cost of other departments' tuberculosis patients, Lewis countered with concern for the nation's military and veteran tuberculosis patients. "We, as Members of Congress, have to look at the whole picture. All the money comes from the Federal treasury—is raised by Federal taxes." The real question was "how and where can the Government most effectively and economically treat all Government patients afflicted with a certain disease—in this case tuberculosis?"[118] According to the *Rocky Mountain News* Lewis showed the committee that Patterson "was alone in recommending the abandonment of Fitzsimons."[119]

This time the subcommittee sided with Lewis and funded Fitzsimons. Taking nothing for granted, Lewis stood vigil on the House floor as his colleagues debated the military appropriations bill, and "stayed constantly in Chamber lest some attack should be made on Fitzsimons hospital to which if made, I am prepared to reply."[120] The next day he did the same, sitting in the front row, and was able to write that evening, "No effort made to amend bill so as to affect adversely Fitzsimons."[121] By the end of the week he wrote, "The Army Appropriation Bill passed as reported by the Appropriations Committee, with ample provision therein for Fitzsimons hospital."[122] The press began reporting that Patterson's "superiors in the War Department already have announced they will not recommend his reappointment," so as Lewis tracked the bill through the Senate the following week, he spoke to several senators about possible successors to Patterson.[123] By the end of the month Fitzsimons was secure for another year.[124]

On 10 May, two years after Patterson submitted his proposal to abandon Fitzsimons, the Secretary of War took his cue from Congress and rejected the recommendation. The following week he declined to reappoint Patterson to another four-year term as Surgeon General. Although six years short of mandatory retirement age, the sidelined Patterson chose to retire and become dean of the University of Oklahoma Medical School.[125] For Lewis, Buck, and Fitzsimons' patients and personnel, the battle against abandonment had been won. Now Lewis could, as MacArthur had suggested, take the offensive on improving Fitzsimons. This time the problem truly did turn on economics as much as politics and the solution would be to find additional streams of funding for the Army hospital. Therefore, on 10 May, the same day the Secretary of War chose not to abandon Fitzsimons, Lewis requested $2.25 million for a permanent building for Fitzsimons as part of a work relief projects proposal for Denver.[126] In June he asked for an additional $300,000 to fund more immediate repairs and construction at the hospital.[127]

Secretary of War George Dern appointed Col. Charles Reynolds as the new Army Surgeon General, who Lewis said "favorably impressed" him in their first meeting.[128] One of three brothers who were all medical officers, Reynolds' service history had not included tuberculosis work but he had successfully managed Army medical support for New Deal programs. He told Lewis that he would travel west to inspect both Beaumont and Fitzsimons hospitals to assess which one would be a better facility for tuberculosis treatment. Even before his visit, though, Reynolds told the General Staff, "It is my opinion that if funds can be made available a new general hospital should be built at Denver."[129] After an August trip during which Buck showed him around Fitzsimons, the new Surgeon General concluded that "from a standpoint of climate and transportation Denver affords decidedly the location of choice," and recommended the construction of "a modern 500 bed hospital building at an estimated cost of $2,250,000." Within a month Secretary Dern approved the request.[130]

From the Depression to the New Deal

Although Congress was still relentlessly cutting military spending, Lewis and the War Department came to realize that it was still willing to fund Army construction on civilian work relief projects at Fitzsimons and other hospitals. MacArthur, generally dubious of the New Deal, went after these funds to keep his department functioning.[131] The Public Works Administration (PWA) was created in 1933, and built bridges, dams, municipal buildings, port facilities, educational buildings, and hospitals across the country. A complementary relief program, the Works Progress Administration (WPA, later renamed the Works Projects Administration), established in 1935, put people to work on smaller construction projects building roads, schools, and airports, as well as projects in literature and the arts.[132] In the 1930s, then, the War Department took on nonmilitary activities such as laying down telegraph cable in Alaska, conducting the Nicaraguan interoceanic canal survey, lighting the Statue of Liberty, and engineering projects to control floods and improve harbors and waterways.[133]

Although no member of Congress from Colorado sat on the House military appropriations subcommittee from 1933 to 1950, and none on the Senate's counterpart until 1939, Lewis took advantage of the New Deal's focus on infrastructure construction to obtain federal appropriations for Colorado. He secured funding for Fort Logan in southwest Denver, convinced the government to build a new Air Corps Base at Lowry Field in southeast Denver, and saved Fitzsimons. These military facilities in turn increased Denver's strategic importance, which undercut one of Surgeon General Patterson's earlier arguments against the hospital. The WPA eventually spent more than $100 million in Colorado, and by 1936 the federal government was the largest single employer in the state with more than 43,000 workers.[134] State projects included sixty-three schools, more than 100 recreation buildings, twenty-six sewage disposal plants, and twenty-eight dams. A sign of Lewis' influence was that despite democratic Governor Johnson's refusal to provide matching state funds (he believed that federal grants were "unwarranted interference in local affairs and a waste of money besides") Colorado ranked tenth among states in per capita New Deal dollars.[135] And almost one in every six federal dollars coming to Colorado went to veterans who received treatment at Fitzsimons on both an inpatient and outpatient basis.[136]

By mid-1935, instead of Lewis petitioning the White House, the White House was calling him. In July he noted in his diary, "Rec'd phone message from [Louis] Howe that probably $282,200 for Fitzsimons Hospital improvements had been approved and announcement by President's Board would be made tomorrow."[137] This was the Administration's response to Lewis' $300,000 request, so later that year Lewis went out to Fitzsimons to view what was being done with the WPA funds. In addition to seeing renovated and repaired buildings, he noted, "Yesterday, total patients 865, of which 515 are Vet. Admin cases, 61 are CCC, 289 various branches of the Army and War Dept. employees."[138] More than bricks and mortar, the congressman understood the importance of maintaining the Fitzsimons patient census, and noted a new class of patients—"CCC" workers.

The Civilian Conservation Corps—the CCC—was perhaps the most popular New Deal jobs program.[139] It put healthy young men, ages eighteen to twenty-five, to work in the nation's parks and forests building trails and planting trees. If they became sick or injured the Army Medical Department took care of them, and by 1935 CCC workers accounted for 316,000 patient days, greater than VA veterans' 275,000 patient days in Army hospitals.[140] Although the CCC put a strain on hospitals such as Fitzsimons by increasing the demand on their limited resources, it was also a boon in generating additional patients at a time when government hospitals were struggling to defend their existence. Conceived during the New Deal's first 100 days, Roosevelt cobbled the CCC together using the resources of various federal agencies: the Labor Department recruited young men from state relief agencies; the War Department trained them and managed the camps; and the Interior and Agriculture departments supervised the conservation work. Through its existence from 1933 to 1942 the CCC employed 2.5 million men who developed more than 3 million acres of national, state, and local parkland; planted more than 4 million acres of trees; stocked almost a billion fish; and built a network of forest-fire lookout towers.[141] A 1936 Gallup poll found that 82 percent of the public supported the program; Wayne N. Aspinall, Speaker of the Colorado House of Representatives and later congressman, called the CCC "one of the great political institutions of Colorado."[142]

At first resistant to managing civilian projects, Dern and MacArthur soon gave the CCC their full support, suspending other activities to mobilize for the program. They saw the camps as an opportunity to recruit and train Army reserve personnel and, during a time when Congress was slashing officer positions, demonstrate "the value of the officer corps to the public and Congress."[143] The War Department's first victory came when it met Roosevelt's goal of signing up 250,000 CCC workers by the Fourth of July, 1933. The Medical Department screened CCC applicants for disabilities and diseases, inoculated enrollees against smallpox and typhoid, and provided camps with physicians to oversee sanitation and provide routine healthcare. Accidents and car wrecks were the leading cause of death for CCC workers, and respiratory infections and sexually transmitted diseases the most common illnesses. Most ailing CCC workers were cared for in their quarters or camp infirmaries, but seriously injured men and those suspected of having infectious diseases, including tuberculosis, went to Army hospitals, and sick and injured CCC workers who were veterans went to VA hospitals.[144] Tuberculosis specialists repeatedly recommended that all CCC enrollees be screened by X-ray for the disease, but the War Department decided that such screening was impractical because "the amount of equipment, personnel, both professional and unskilled, would be enormous and out of all proportion to the benefits accrued."[145] Medical officers did reject hundreds of CCC applicants for tuberculosis, but by 1939 the CCC camps had reported 1,758 cases of active tuberculosis among its workers.[146]

Supporting the CCC camps at first depleted the Army medical staff. In 1933 when Patterson needed forty medical officers for the CCC camps, he took fifteen of them from Fitzsimons citing "the anticipated loss of veteran patients and the consequent abandonment of the hospital."[147] Soon, however, CCC enrollees began to occupy beds vacated by veterans so that by November 1933 fifteen medical officers were transferred back to Fitzsimons, and the War Department eventually called on Medical Reserve officers to serve as CCC camp physicians. In the mid-1930s, the OTSG authorized the hospitals to hire one civilian doctor and dentist for each thirty CCC and VA patients, and one civilian nurse for every ten such patients.[148] Roosevelt also directed the War Department to lift its restriction on black officers and employ African American medical officers and chaplains to care for African American workers in the CCC camps.[149]

In the mid-1930s the CCC, the VA, and other federal agencies like the PWA and WPA, which also sent patients to military hospitals, began to pay the Medical Department per capita reimbursements for maintenance and repair costs at the rate of $0.20 per patient day. Years of deferred maintenance caused the Medical Department to seek these funds, explaining, "the maintenance cost of a hospital increases each year. New scientific developments, modern equipment, appliances, etc., place great demands on the hospitals built twenty years or more ago, and many of our hospitals are not fire resistant."[150] By 1938 maintenance credits for construction and repair of hospitals tallied $228,000 from the CCC, $59,000 from the VA and $2,000 each from the Navy and the WPA.[151]

In 1936 Fitzsimons admitted 486 CCC patients—more than 10 percent of its 4,100 admissions that year. Although CCC tuberculosis cases were low, several patients had long hospital stays.[152] As late as June 1943—a year after the program ended—fourteen CCC enrollees were still in government hospitals, half of them at Fitzsimons. CCC tuberculosis patients Joe R. Gonzales, Agustín Tovar, Lucio G. Rodriguez, and Davies Gonzales were all at Fitzsimons—Joe Gonzales and Tovar had been at Fitzsimons for almost four years.[153] It took time for the staff to locate suitable facilities to which to transfer the men, because, as Buck explained, "it was felt that it would have done an injustice to the individual and to the community where they reside, to release them without arrangements for their continued care."[154]

A fan of the CCC, Roosevelt recommended to Congress in 1939 that it be made permanent, but it gave him only a three-year extension. As war broke out in Europe and Asia and the United States began to increase its military forces, the CCC became a burden rather than a welcome jobs program, and camps fell into disrepair. Congress allowed the CCC to expire in 1942, but some camps would serve new federal missions—troop training and prisoners of war detention.

Building a New Hospital

Public health trends during the Depression were complex. Widespread, persistent poverty increased the sickness rates for some groups of people, but to the surprise of many, mortality rates for many diseases, including tuberculosis, continued to decline due to public health improvements and surveillance. As part of the New Deal, for example, the Public Health Service conducted a "health inventory" and launched public health campaigns to reduce diseases such as pellagra, polio, heart disease, sexually transmitted infections, and tuberculosis.[155] With regard to the latter, public health officials warned that death rates were no longer "an adequate criterion of the extent of sickness and impairment," because if fewer people were *dying* of tuberculosis, more people were *living* with tuberculosis.[156] While Franklin Roosevelt is known for the March of Dimes campaign against polio, he and Eleanor also joined the fight against tuberculosis. The First Lady addressed a meeting of the National Tuberculosis Association in 1935 and kicked off its 1936 Christmas seal campaign. Tuberculosis took such a toll on the country, she said, that "we cannot look upon any money which is spent to prevent it as really amounting to anything in comparison with what it costs us if we let it go on and continue unchecked."[157]

Despite such efforts, the Depression was unequivocally hard on hospitals. In 1934, the *Journal of the American Medical Association* observed that private hospitals "have seen a considerable proportion of their paying patronage reduced to such financial straits as to be forced to enter the tax-supported institutions."[158] This trend pressured government hospitals at all levels by increasing their patients and reducing their income. Although the Roosevelt Administration expanded the social safety net with Social Security for the elderly and disabled, it stopped short of national health insurance. Hospital construction, however, was one way of supporting the national healthcare infrastructure. The New Deal provided construction grants across the country for hospitals, medical schools, and medical clinics, and as historian Rosemary Stevens shows, the $77 million in PWA and WPA funds for medical facilities provided the foundation for the Hill-Burton Act of 1946, which subsidized postwar hospital construction.[159]

Although there was no national health planning, the Federal Board of Hospitalization's study of national government hospital needs ultimately determined Fitzsimons' fate. In July 1936, the Board expanded on Surgeon General Reynolds' call for a new 500-bed hospital at Fitzsimons, noting the need for "a modern, fireproof hospital particularly adapted for the treatment of tubercular patients in this area, not only for the Army and the Veterans' Administration but at times for patients of the Navy and other Government agencies." It therefore recommended to the President the construction of a 600-bed hospital at the Fitzsimons site "at a cost not exceeding $2,250,000."[160] This was the amount requested by both Lewis and Reynolds. The Board adopted the resolution unanimously and sent it to the Bureau of the Budget for funding approval. By 1936 War Department staff had changed their posture and, after attending Bureau of the Budget meetings observed that "in view of the fact that Fitzsimons Gen. Hospital is to be retained as an Army hospital, it appears advisable that it be included in the Army authorization bill that is to be presented to Congress."[161]

Congressman Lewis then set to work acquiring the funding. This task was much less politically contentious but still involved a long, sustained effort as Lewis pursued the two-step process of securing congressional authorization for the project and then obtaining congressional appropriations for construction. His activities also included helping to transfer the title of the land from the Denver Chamber of Commerce to the War Department, getting the VA to commit to funding 250 beds for tuberculosis patients at Fitzsimons, shepherding hospital blueprints through the War Department, and requiring that Colorado marble be used in construction. Congress easily approved the funding for a new building at Fitzsimons in 1937. The next year Lewis turned to New Deal construction programs rather than War Department monies to secure congressional appropriations for the building by adding the words "and hospitalization" in the public works bill for 1938.[162] That legislation authorized $4,050,000 for Fitzsimons' new building, $3,750,000 from PWA and $300,000 from WPA programs.[163] Charles Gridley called the measure "a triumphant climax to a five year fight by the *Denver Post* for the preservation and expansion of Fitzsimons General Hospital."[164]

Fitzsimons won the lion's share of the Army Medical Department's hospital construction budget for fiscal year 1939—$4 million of $7 million. Groundbreaking for the new building began in August 1938, and in December the War Department contracted with the Great Lakes Construction Company of Chicago, Illinois, for a 608-bed hospital to be completed after 600 days of work, for $2,999,035.79.[165] Buck and the OTSG had been developing plans for a new building since 1933 so by 1937 architects and engineers had reams of blueprints. These plans abandoned the dispersed pavilion style of the World War I era for a multiple-story building that required less land and saved medical personnel steps between departments and wards.[166]

In his 1939 annual report, the Surgeon General said that the new building "will be the largest single hospital structure ever built by the Army." With nine stories, a basement and subbasement, it would measure 554 feet long by 156 feet deep with the wider section at the center, comprising 404,500 square feet (Figure 7-4). Outfitted for tuberculosis patients, it included nine heliotherapy decks, as well as outpatient, clinical, and dining facilities, and 608 beds, which would increase Fitzsimons' capacity to a pre-Patterson level of 1,185 beds. The largest wards had only five or six beds per room, and there were 173 single rooms. The Surgeon

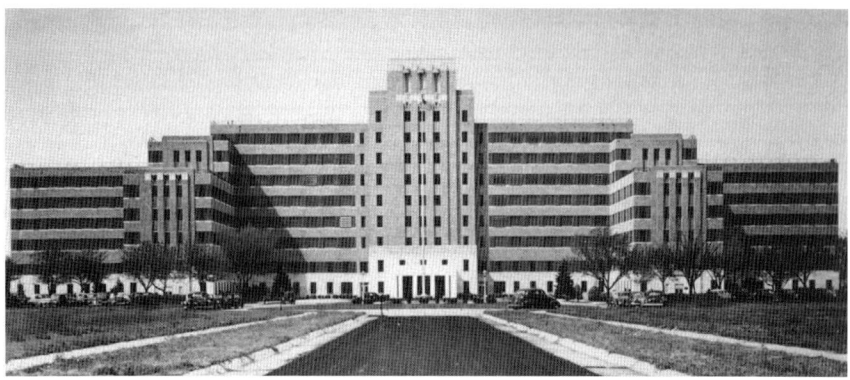

Figure 7-4. The new building at Fitzsimons General Hospital, c. 1941. Photograph courtesy of the National Library of Medicine, Image #A07858.

General explained that this facilitated not only the segregation of patients by rank, sex, and disease, but also "permits the same separation of patients who have some type of tuberculosis according to types of lesions," that is, pulmonary patients with serious tuberculosis in one room and those with less serious in another.[167] The building was equipped for wheelchairs and the hearing impaired and some rooms had outlets to provide oxygen from a central supply.[168] As one reporter wrote, the equipment in the new hospital "includes everything from cages for experimental rats and guinea pigs to a machine for sterilizing operating room air that is the very latest development of alert medical science."[169]

The expanded capacity also suited Fitzsimons' increasingly broad mission. Its 1940 annual report noted that although the chief purpose of the hospital was to care for patients with tuberculosis, "due to a greater military population in this vicinity, the hospital has widened its scope of professional work and serves this military community for the definitive treatment of general medical and surgical cases."[170] On a visit to Fitzsimons in late 1940, the new Surgeon General, Major General James C. Magee, welcomed the additional beds because the growing Army would generate new medical cases. "Presently, Fitzsimons hospital treats an average of 900 cases daily," he told reporters, "with the opening of the new unit, the load can be extended to 1,500."[171]

Dedication

In the fall of 1936, Lewis had run as a proud ally of President Roosevelt, and both men won their elections by wide margins. By 1937, however, Lewis, like Roosevelt, had lost some of his shine. As the economy continued to languish, many Coloradans became frustrated or disillusioned with the New Deal. Lewis had also voted against some key legislation, including the Wagner Act, prized labor legislation that established minimum wages and maximum hours for millions of workers. A Washington newspaper observed that "Lewis is [the] only Rules Committee Democrat member north of Mason Dixon line against [the] wages and hours bill." It complained that he "Votes NO on all New Deal measures except pork. Regarding this, his one conviction is that all pork should go to Denver."[172] The "pork," however, did not offend many Colorado voters, because when another Lewis—John L.—president of the American Federation of Labor, put Congressman Lewis on his 1938 blacklist, the Colorado American Federation of Labor endorsed him nonetheless—its members voted for the congressman who brought jobs to their state.[173] In 1940 Lewis again retained his seat even though he campaigned little, staying in Washington due to the wartime emergency, and despite the fact that much of Colorado voted Republican, electing a Republican governor and supporting Wendell Wilkie for president over Roosevelt.[174]

In late 1941, as work on the new building at Fitzsimons neared completion and Army Medical Department officials prepared for the dedication, they asked Lewis to do the honors. Col. Frederick Wright, the Fitzsimons director of surgery, had assumed command after the retirement of Carroll Buck in June 1940.[175] Congressman Lewis happily accepted, and in his usual formal manner recorded in his diary, "Colonel Frederick S. Wright, of the Medical Corps, Commanding Officer at Fitzsimons General Hospital at Denver, called and discussed with me plans for the 'dedication' of the new building at the hospital at which he wishes me to speak."[176] To prepare his remarks, Lewis reviewed the *Congressional Record* and his diaries on his work for Fitzsimons.[177]

On a cold 3 December day whipped by prairie winds, 500 invited guests gathered outside the imposing entrance of the shiny new structure. They included Army Surgeon General James Magee; the governor of Colorado; the mayor of Denver; numerous other federal, state, and city officials; and a sister, brother, and nephew of William Thomas Fitzsimons, the hospital's namesake. According to the *Rocky Mountain News,* Col. Wright "turned to Representative Lewis, who sat with his hat pulled down and his coat rolled up about his ears," saying "Without Mr. Lewis, this new building would not be possible."[178] Amidst applause, Lewis took the podium to recount the story of saving Fitzsimons, beginning with the establishment of the tuberculosis hospital during World War I: "I know many ex-service men with arrested cases of tuberculosis who are now engaged in useful civil occupations who owe their recovery of relatively good health to having been treated at Fitzsimons [H]ospital," he observed. In spite of this good work, though, "there were some in the Congress and elsewhere" who wanted to abandon the hospital. While he said, "I shall pass lightly over many exciting episodes during the anxious days and nights between 1933 and 1936," he did read the text of his 1934 amendment to restore funding for Fitzsimons. He saluted the members of the U.S. Congress who had supported his amendment, naming more than twenty individuals, and adding slyly, "none of the influential persons who actively advocated abandonment of Fitzsimons are now connected with the government." Then Lewis recalled how "one beautiful Indian summer day, October 12, 1936, President Roosevelt came to Denver....and so Fitzsimons was definitely saved from abandonment."[179]

It was a triumphant day for Lewis, but the ribbon-cutting ceremony was one of the last public events he attended. He was exhausted. He had striven to execute his duty to the fullest with a perfect attendance record in Congress.[180] But his diaries suggest the cost. In the late 1930s his handwriting became smaller, so that he could fit all of his activities on one daily page, but by end of the decade, he began to leave whole weeks and months blank. At times he simply stapled committee reports to pages to document his work. As Hitler began his rampage across Europe, Lewis' writing—when he wrote—grew even smaller, covering the pages and margins with his work and news of the Battle of Britain. The 1941 diary includes the *Congressional Record* vote on the draft, news of Hitler's blitzkrieg against Russia, and notes on trips to the dentist. In April he checked into Walter Reed General Hospital—more for a rest than medical treatment—and although he mustered his energy to attend the Fitzsimons dedication, he did not record the event in his diary. It stands silent until a single entry for Sunday, 7 December 1941: "Attack by Japs on Pearl Harbor."[181] Lawrence Lewis' diaries end there. In March 1942 the Capitol physician ordered him to bed rest due to high blood pressure and "dental troubles," which were likely infections that were taxing his body.[182] While Lewis recuperated his staff carried on the work of his congressional office.[183] Colorado voters were not inclined to change horses during wartime, and despite his absence from the House, they reelected Lewis in 1942. In Florida for his health, he missed the swearing in and most official business in 1943, as well as President Roosevelt's visit to Fitzsimons in April 1943.[184] By September Lewis returned to the Congress, but his health did not hold. In early December he checked into Walter Reed, and died of a heart attack on 8 December 1943 at age sixty-four.[185]

The *Denver Post* attributed Lewis' death to "overwork on congressional duties."[186] So did his colleagues upon hearing the news on the House floor. "Lawrence Lewis is a casualty just as truly as if he had lost his life in actual conflict," said Rep. John Chenoweth, (R-CO). Said John McCormack (D-MA), "Lawrence Lewis died in the line of duty."[187] Members praised his good manners and graciousness. Rep. Robert F. Rockwell said that "Lawrence Lewis did not seek fame—he preferred to accomplish what he thought was best for his people in a modest manner; he sought no reward—except the personal satisfaction of a job well done."[188] After funeral services in Washington, Lewis was buried next to his parents in a cemetery in Cincinnati, Ohio. The new Fitzsimons hospital building stood as his memorial. Like him, it was quickly swept into wartime service, but unlike the congressman, the hospital thrived. Among the first patients admitted to the new building on 17 December 1941 were victims of the Japanese attack on Pearl Harbor.

As it had over the centuries, war would foster disease. Tuberculosis would again flourish in war-torn regions, and Fitzsimons and the Army Medical Department would be called upon to care for the sick. After years of haggling over fifty beds here and fifty beds there the Army Medical Department now quickly increased Fitzsimons' capacity to 3,000 beds. In 1942 Congress authorized

American military hospitals to admit tuberculosis patients from Allied nations as well, and Fitzsimons cared for soldier-patients from Britain, Canada, Norway, the Netherlands, the Philippines, China, and even enemy soldiers with tuberculosis from Germany, Italy, and Japan.[189] The next world war brought a new globalism to Fitzsimons. "The geographic area served by this hospital," remarked its commander, Brig. Gen. Omar H. Quade, "has been extended to include the greater part of the world."[190]

Notes

1. Lewis Diaries, 12 October 1936, Lawrence Lewis Papers, 385 N11, C4, Colorado Historical Society, Denver [hereafter cited as Lewis Diaries]. This story of Roosevelt's visit to Denver in October 1936 is drawn from articles in the *Rocky Mountain News* and *Denver Post* and the scrapbooks and diaries of Lawrence Lewis. Available sources do not indicate whether the Secret Service's concern had to do with the president's security or with fears of disease transmission.

2. "Secret Service Men Say President Will Not Visit Fitzsimons Hospital but His Secretary Indicates He Will," *Denver Post*, 10 October 1936; and Lawrence Lewis, "Address of Hon. Lawrence Lewis, of Colorado, at Dedication of a New Building at Fitzsimons General Hospital," 15 June 1942, *Congressional Record*, 77th Cong., 2nd sess., A2614.

3. Lewis Diaries, 12 October 1936.

4. Franklin D. Roosevelt, "Campaign Address at Denver, Colo. 'We Have Sought and Found Practical Answers to the Problems of Industry, Agriculture, and Mining,'" 12 October 1936, *The Public Papers and Addresses of Franklin D. Roosevelt, with a Special Introduction and Explanatory Notes by President Roosevelt* (New York, NY: Random House: 1938–50), vol. 5, 433–49.

5. Lewis Diaries, 12 October 1936.

6. "A Visit by Mrs. Roosevelt," *New York Times*, 13 October 1936.

7. "Support of Fitzsimons Promised by President," *Denver Post*, 12 October 1936.

8. Lewis Diaries, 13 October 1936.

9. On the Depression see David M. Kennedy, *Freedom From Fear—The American People in Depression and War, 1929–1945* (New York, NY: Oxford University Press, 1999); and Robert S. McElvaine, *The Great Depression: America 1929–1941* (New York, NY: Times Books, 1984).

10. Franklin Delano Roosevelt, Inaugural address, 20 January 1937, *Inaugural Addresses of the Presidents of the United States* (Washington, DC: U.S. G.P.O., 1989); Bartleby.com, 2001. www.bartleby.com/124/, accessed 18 October 2012.

11. John W. Killigrew, "The Impact of the Great Depression on the Army," Ph.D. dissertation, Indiana University, 1960, IV-23. On the War Department during the Depression see also Mary C. Gillett, *The Army Medical Department, 1917-1941* (Washington, DC: Center of Military History, United States Army, 2009); Elias Huzar, *The Purse and the Sword: Control of Army by*

Congress through Military Appropriations, 1933–1950 (Ithaca, NY: Cornell University Press, 1950); D. Clayton James, *The Years of MacArthur* (Boston, MA: Houghton-Mifflin, 1985); and Joseph W. A. Whitehorne, *The Inspectors General of the United States Army, 1903–1939* (Washington, DC: Office of the Inspector General and the Center of Military History, 1998).

12. James, *The Years of MacArthur*, 430; and Huzar, *The Purse and the Sword*, 226–27.

13. Killigrew, "The Impact of the Great Depression on the Army," X-20–21.

14. James, *The Years of MacArthur*, 356.

15. Huzar, *The Purse and the Sword*, 143.

16. Richard V. N. Ginn, *The History of the U.S. Army Medical Service Corps* (Washington, DC: Office of The Surgeon General and Center of Military History, 1997), 97.

17. *War Department Annual Reports,* 1935 [hereafter cited as *WDAR,* year], 1.

18. Huzar, *The Purse and the Sword*, 137.

19. For biographical information on Patterson see "The Surgeons General," Office of Medical History, U.S. Army Medcal Department,Web site, http://history.amedd.army.mil/surgeongenerals/R_Patterson.html, accessed 24 August 2012; and Gillett, *The Army Medical Department, 1917–1941*, 507–8

20. *Annual Report of the Surgeon General*, 1932 [hereafter cited as *ARSG*, year], 10.

21. Mary T. Sarnecky, *A History of the Army Nurse Corps* (Philadelphia, PA: University of Pennsylvania Press, 1999), says this contributed to a nursing shortage during World War II, 154.

22. Sarnecky, *A History of the Army Nurse Corps*, 445, 153–54.

23. *ARSG*, 1931, 378–79; and "Texas and Arkansas Plot to Close Fitzsimons," *Denver Post*, 8 March 1934.

24. See Chapter 5 in this volume on veterans' benefits for tuberculosis.

25. Walter P. Dillingham, *Federal Aid to Veterans, 1917–1941* (Tallahassee, FL: University of Florida Press, 1952), 55–56.

26. Kennedy, *Freedom From Fear*, 138–39. The bill was formally titled "Bill to Maintain the Credit of the United States Government." For more on the Economy Act, see Stephen R. Ortiz, "The 'New Deal' for Veterans: The Economy Act, the Veterans of Foreign Wars, and the Origin of New Deal Dissent," *Journal of Military History* 70 (April 2006), 415–438; Dillingham, *Federal Aid to Veterans, 1917–1941*; Michael B. Wallerstein, "Terminating Entitlements: Veterans' Disability Benefits and the Depression," *Policy Sciences* 7 (1976), 173–82; and William Pencak, *For God and Country: The American Legion, 1919–1940* (Boston, MA: Northeastern University Press, 1989).

27. Patterson memo, "Abandonment of Fitzsimons General Hospital," 8 May 1933, Record Group 112, Records of the Surgeon General of the Army [hereafter cited as RG 112], Entry 31, 1928–37, Box 280, National Archives and Records Administration [hereafter cited as NARA].

28. On average out of 4,620 patients, 3,086 were veterans. See *Fitzsimons Annual Report* [hereafter cited as *FZAR*], 1931, 15.

29. *FZAR*, 1931, 1–2, and 4.

30. Excerpt included in 1933 inspection report, RG 112, Entry 31, 1928–37, Box 280, NARA.

31. "Annual Estimate, C & R, FY 1934," February 1933, and February1933 endorsements, RG 112, Entry 31, 1928–37, Box 283, NARA; and 1933 inspection report, p. 8., RG 112, Entry 31, 1928–37, Box 280, NARA.

32. Merritte W. Ireland, "Memorandum to File," 16 June 1926, RG 112, Entry 29, 1917–27, Box 378, NARA.

33. R. E. Callan, "Memorandum for the Chief of Staff: Abandonment of Fitzsimons General Hospital," 28 April 1933, summarizing the Surgeon General's memo of 26 April 1933; original memo not in file, RG 112, Entry 31, 1928–37, Box 280, NARA.

34. Callan, "Memorandum for the Chief of Staff: Abandonment of Fitzsimons General Hospital."

35. C. D. Buck, "Reduction of Personnel," 13 April 1933, and radiograms of 5 April 1933, RG 112, Entry 31, Box 278, NARA; and "U.S. to Abandon Army Hospital Here by June 30," *Rocky Mountain News*, 26 April 1933.

36. Patterson memo, "Reduced Use of Fitzsimons General Hospital," 3 May 1933, RG 112, Entry 31, 1928–37, Box 280, NARA.

37. Joseph P. Constantine to Robert U. Patterson, 6 May 1933, and Robert U. Patterson to Joseph P. Constantine, 10 May 1933, RG 112, Entry 31, 1928–37, Box 280, NARA.

38. Patterson, "Abandonment of Fitzsimons General Hospital," 8 May 1933, RG 112, Entry 31, 1928–37, Box 280, NARA. Emphasis in the original.

39. Stephen J. Leonard, *Trials and Triumph: A Colorado Portrait of the Great Depression, with FSA Photographs* (Boulder, CO: University Press of Colorado, 1993), 260. Also on the Depression in Colorado, see Phil Goodstein, *From Soup Lines to the Front Lines: Denver during the Depression and World War II, 1927–1947* (Denver, CO: New Social Publications, 2007); and Carl Abbot, Stephen J. Leonard, and Thomas J. Noel, *Colorado: A History of the Centennial State*, 4th ed. (Boulder, CO: University of Colorado Press, 2005).

40. Remarks by Rep. Willliam S. Hill, quoting a letter from John O'Connor, former Member of Congress, dated 16 December 1943, Appendix to the *Congressional Record*, 78th Cong., 2nd sess., 31 May 1944, A2680.

41. Quoted by Rep. John R. Murdock, Appendix to the *Congressional Record*, 78th Cong., 2nd sess., 31 May 1944, A2691.

42. "30,000 Denverites Turn Out to Welcome Gov. Roosevelt," *Rocky Mountain News*, 16 September 1932. See also "Rousing Denver Welcome Awaits Roosevelt Today," *Rocky Mountain News*, 15 September 1932.

43. Lewis Diaries, 11 April 1933.

44. "Salaries Cut $5,000 Month at Fitzsimons," *Rocky Mountain News*, 9 April 1933.

45. Lewis Diaries, 20 April 1933; and "Denver Post Battle to Save Fitzsimons is Bringing Results," *Denver Post*, 20 April 1933.

46. Lewis Diaries, 22 April 1933.

47. Lewis Diaries, 23 April 1933. See also "Fight to Prevent Abandonment of Fitzsimons Opens," *Rocky Mountain News*, 27 April 1933.

48. Lewis Diaries, 26 April 1933.

49. Lewis Diaries, 27 April 1933.

50. Lewis Diaries, 29 April 1933.

51. Lewis Diaries, 2 May 1933.

52. Huzar writes that both the War Department and Congress "have regarded the voice of the budget bureau as that of the president," Huzar, *The Purse and the Sword*, 137.

53. Lewis Diaries, 3 May 1933.

54. Lewis Diaries, 9 May 1933; and "Budget Chief is Given Case on Fitzsimons," *Rocky Mountain News*, 4 May 1933.

55. Lewis Diaries, 9 May 1933. See also Lawrence Lewis, "Address of Hon. Lawrence Lewis, of Colorado, at Dedication of a New Building at Fitzsimons General Hospital, 15 June 1942, *Congressional Record*, 77th Cong., 2nd sess., A2613.

56. Lewis Diaries, 10 May 1933.

57. Lewis Diaries, 3 June 1933.

58. Remarks of Rep. Lawrence Lewis of Colorado, "Memorandum Concerning Fitzsimons Army Hospital in Denver Colo.," 73rd Cong., 1st sess., *Congressional Record*, 3 June 1933, 4932–34.

59. "Lewis Invited to Fitzsimons Conference," *Denver Post*, 22 July 1933.

60. "Outline of Data Desired in Report of an Unofficial Board for the Soldiers' Home, Washington, DC," and other correspondence, RG 112, Entry 31, 1928–37, Box 284, NARA.

61. John T. Woolley and Gerhard Peters, "The American Presidency Project," Santa Barbara, CA: University of California, available at: http://www.presidency.ucsb.edu/ws/index.php?pid=14637, accessed 24 August 2012.

62. "May Gallery of Fame" *Denver Post*, May 1933.

63. Lewis Diaries, 4 June 1933.

64. "New Threat against Fitzsimons Seen in Order to Move Patients,"*Rocky Mountain News*, 15 June 1933.

65. Lewis Diaries, 12 June and 15 June 1933.

66. Lewis Diaries, 16 June 1933.

67. "Col. C. D. Buck Quietly Arrives to Take Charge of Fitzsimons," *Denver Post*, 2 August 1931; and "Col. C. D. Buck New Head of Fitzsimons Hospital," *Rocky Mountain News*, 22 May 1931.

68. Veterans of Foreign Wars, John S. Stewart Post No. 1, "The Story of a Great Institution, 1918–1938, Fitzsimons General Hospital," 1938, Colorado Historical Society, Denver.

69. *ARSG*, 1934, 159.

70. *FZAR*, 1933; Buck memo, "Care of BSH [Beneficiary of the Soldiers' Home] cases," 13 June 1933, RG 112, Entry 31, 1928–37, Box 284, NARA; Buck to McAfee, 3 August 1933, RG 112, Entry 31, 1928–37, Box 280, NARA, and similar correspondence in this file.

71. Patterson to Medical Director, Veterans Administration (VA), 2 May 1933, RG 112, Entry 31, 1928–37, Box 284, NARA.

72. "Fitzsimons Hospital Patients Follow a Variety of Activities," *Denver Post*, 4 February 1934.

73. C. D. Buck to J. B. Huggins, 11 July 1933, RG 112, Entry 31, 1928–37, Box 280, NARA.

74. Buck to Patterson, "Prospects of Fitzsimons General Hospital," 7 July 1933, RG 112, Entry 31, 1928–37, Box 280, NARA.

75. Buck to McAfee, 7 July 1933, RG 112, Entry 31, 1928–37, Box 280, NARA.

76. See "Major Shepard is Given Life Imprisonment," *Rocky Mountain News*, 23 December 1930; "Major Shepard Gets Life Term," *Rocky Mountain News*, 4 February 1931.

77. McAfee to Buck, 11 April 1933, RG 112, Entry 31-K, Box 280, NARA. The identity of the officer is unknown.

78. U.S. Supreme Court, Shepard v. United States, 290 U.S. 96, (1933); and Buck, "Report of Annual Examination of Major Chas. A. Shepard," 6 January 1934, RG 112, Entry 31-K, Box 280, NARA.

79. "Denver Surgeon Dies," *Nevada State Journal*, 10 July 1933.

80. "Lawrence Lewis Will Remain Two Weeks in Capitol," *Denver Post*, 23 July 1933.

81. Lewis Diaries, 21 July 1933.

82. Lewis did not mention this in July 1933, but referred to the conversation when he reminded Marvin McIntyre of it the following spring. See Lewis Diaries, 7 March 1934.

83. "Remarks Made before the Federal Board of Hospitalization, July 25, 1933, by Congressman Lawrence Lewis of Colorado Regarding Fitzsimons General Hospital," RG 51, Records of the Bureau of the Budget, Entry 4, Box 9, NARA.

84. Lewis Diaries, 25 July 1933.
85. Federal Board of Hospitalization, "Resolution Adopted by the Federal Board of Hospitalization," and other correspondence 25 July 1933, RG 112, Entry 1928–37, Box 280, NARA; and Lewis Diaries, 25 July 1933.
86. Lewis Diaries, 2 August 1933.
87. "Lewis Announces Victory in Campaign to Save Fitzsimons," *Denver Post*, 2 August 1933.
88. While many people welcomed the action, veterans' organizations, especially the Veterans of Foreign Wars, launched an urgent campaign to reverse it. See Stephen R. Ortiz, *Beyond the Bonus March and the GI Bill: How Veteran Politics Shaped the New Deal Era* (New York, NY: New York University Press, 2009).
89. Lewis Diaries, 10 January 1934.
90. Buck to L. B. McAfee, 6 January 1934, RG 112, Entry 31, 1928–37, Box 280, NARA.
91. Buck to McAfee, 21 January 1934, RG 112, Entry 31, 1928–37, Box 280, NARA.
92. McAfee to Buck, 3 March 1934, RG 112, Entry 31, 1928–37, Box 280, NARA.
93. Floyd Kramer memo, "Veterans' Administration Reimbursement," 5 March 1934, RG 112, Entry 31, 1928–37, Box 280, NARA.
94. Buck to Patterson, 8 March 1934, RG 112, Entry 31, 1928–37, Box 280, NARA.
95. Robert U. Patterson to Ross A. Collins, 8 March 1934, RG 112, Entry 31, 1928–37, Box 280, NARA.
96. "Congressman Fighting Hard to Save Hospital for Denver," *Rocky Mountain News*, 8 March 1934.
97. Debate on amendment to the military appropriations bill for fiscal year 1935, *Congressional Record*, 73rd Cong., 2nd sess., 8 March 1934, 4024. See also "Report Criticizes Department," *New York Times*, 6 March 1934.
98. Lewis Diaries, 5 March 1934.
99. "Texas and Arkansas Plot to Close Fitzsimons, *Denver Post*, 8 March 1934.
100. Lewis Diaries, 6 March 1934.
101. "Congressmen Fighting Hard for Hospital," *Rocky Mountain News*, 8 March, 1934.
102. Lewis Diaries, 7 March 1934.
103. Lewis amendment *Congressional Record*, 73rd Cong., 2nd sess., 8 March 1934, 4024.
104. Lewis Diaries, 7 March 1934.
105. "Fitzsimons to Remain in Operation—House Votes Ample Funds," *Denver Post*, 8 March 1934.
106. "After 30 minutes debate, on division 70 ayes and 22 noes for amendment. On Teller Vote, 74 ayes and 51 noes." Lewis Diaries, 8 March 1934; and comments regarding an amendment to the military appropriations bill for fiscal year 1935, *Congressional Record*, 73rd Cong., 2nd sess., 8 March 1934, 4024–29; Lewis Diaries, 8 March 1934. See comment on page 24.
107. Lewis Diaries, 12 March 1934.
108. Lewis Diaries, 15 March 1934.
109. Buck to McAfee, 13 March 1934, RG 112, Entry 31, 1928–37, Box 280, NARA.
110. Roger Brooke, "Operating Capacity of Fitzsimons General Hospital," 2 April 1934, RG 112, Entry 31, 1928–37, Box 280, NARA.
111. Lewis Diaries, 14 October 1934.
112. Lewis scrapbook, No. 6, Manuscript 385, Lawrence Lewis Papers, Colorado Historical Society, Denver.

113. Lewis Diaries, 24 October 1934.

114. Lewis Diaries, 5 November 1934.

115. Roger Brooke to Patterson, 12 November 1934, RG 112 and 331, 1927–38, NARA.

116. "Lawrence Lewis Receives a Seat on Rules Committee," *Rocky Mountain News*, 11 January 1935.

117. Lewis Diaries, 11 January 1935. Historian Mary C. Gillett writes that "a new policy forbidding the reappointment of general officers eliminated the possibility of dissension about whether he should remain as surgeon general longer than four years." See Gillett, *The Army Medical Department, 1917–1941*, 508.

118. "Statement of Hon. Lawrence Lewis," 5 February 1935, War Department Appropriations bill for 1936, Subcommittee of House Committee on Appropriations, U.S. Congress, 74th Cong., 1st. sess., 675; and remarks by Rep. Lewis, "Fitzsimons General Hospital at Denver, Colo.," 22 February 1935, *Congressional Record*, 74th Cong., 1st sess., 2504–7. See also Lewis Diaries, February 1935.

119. "Lewis Repeats Role as Savior of Fitzsimons," *Rocky Mountain News*, 20 February 1935.

120. Lewis Diaries, 20 February 1935.

121. Lewis Diaries, 21 February 1935.

122. Lewis Diaries, 22 February 1935.

123. Lewis Diaries, 25 February 1935.

124. "Final Attempt to Block Funds for Fitzsimons is Voted Down," *Denver Post*, 15 February 1935.

125. In 1942 Patterson became dean of the School of Medicine of the University of Maryland in Baltimore. He died at Walter Reed General Hospital in 1950 and was buried in Arlington National Cemetery. Available at: http://history.amedd.army.mil/surgeongenerals/R_Patterson.html, accessed 24 August 2012.

126. "$13 Million Asked for Denver Projects; Lewis Backs Huge Plan of Work Relief," *Denver Post*, 10 May 1935.

127. "$300,000 Fund Sought for Fitzsimons Repairs," *Denver Post*, 30 June 1935.

128. Lewis Diaries, 7 June 1935.

129. Reynolds memo, "Fitzsimons General Hospital," 8 July 1935, RG 112, Entry 31, 1928–37, Box 283, NARA.

130. C. R. Reynolds memo, "Fitzsimons General Hospital," 21 August 1935, and endorsement, 16 September 1935, RG 112, Entry 31, 1928–37, Box 280, NARA; and "Three Million May be Spent on Fitzsimons," *Denver Post*, 5 August 1935, Lewis Scrapbook No. 7, 1935–36.

131. James, *The Years of MacArthur*, 364 and 431.

132. McElvaine, *The Great Depression, America, 1929–1941*, 152–53, 265–75.

133. James, *The Years of MacArthur*, 363–64. For a partial list of Medical Department construction financed by nonmilitary New Deal programs see C. M. Walson, "Permanent New Military Department Construction," *U.S. Army Medical Bulletin* 35 (1936): 52–58.

134. Abbot, Leonard, and Noel, *Colorado: A History of the Centennial State*, 282.

135. Abbot, Leonard, and Noel, *Colorado: A History of the Centennial State*, 275; and Lyle W. Dorsett and Michael McCarthy, *The Queen City: A History of Denver*, 2d ed. (Boulder, CO: Pruett Publishing, 1986), 231 and 286.

136. Leonard, *Trials and Triumphs*, 108–9.

137. Lewis Diaries, 12 July 1935.

138. Lewis Diaries, 3 December 1935. Examples of federal construction at Fitzsimons: In 1934 federal workers paved roads, built sidewalks, and brought about eighty acres of the 595-acre reservation under cultivation with irrigation and drainage ditches (*FZAR*, 1934, 3–7);

in 1937 Work Projects Administration appropriations funded 133,931 square feet of road, 11,799 linear feet of curb and gutter, and 15,333 square feet of sidewalk (*FZAR*, 1937, 4); and in 1940 federal workers renovated eighteen buildings on the post, painted eleven other buildings, and expanded twenty-five sets of quarters by enclosing the open porches (*FZAR*, 1940, 2–3).

139. John C. Paige, *The Civilian Conservation Corps and the National Park Service, 1933–1942: An Administrative History* (National Park Service, available at: http://www.nps.gov/history/history/online_books/ccc/ccc1a.htm, 1985, accessed 24 August 2012); Joseph M. Speakman, *At Work in Penn's Woods: The Civilian Conservation Corps in Pennsylvania* (University Park, PA: Pennsylvania State University Press, 2006); and Robert J. Moore, *The Civilian Conservation Corps in Arizona's Rim Country: Working in the Woods* (Reno, NV: University of Nevada Press, 2006).

140. *ARSG*, 1935, 134.

141. William E. Leuchtenburg, *Franklin D. Roosevelt and the New Deal, 1932–1940* (New York, NY: Harper Colophon Books, 1963), 174; and Paige, *The Civilian Conservation Corps*, chapter 5.

142. Speakman, *At Work in Penn's Woods*, 1 and 170; and Leonard, *Trials and Triumphs*, 61. On the Civilian Conservation Corps [hereafter cited as CCC] in Colorado see the Colorado State Archives Web site, http://www.colorado.gov/dpa/doit/archives/ccc/cccscope.html, accessed 24 August 2012.

143. James, *The Years of MacArthur*, 420.

144. Adjutant General to the administrator of the Veterans' Administration, 20 February 1935, Record Group 407, Records of the Adjutant General's Office [hereafter RG 407], CCC, Box 933, NARA. Correspondence regarding the disposition of veteran-members of the CCC, January–March 1935, RG 407, CCC, Box 933, NARA.

145. War Department letter to Civilian Conservation Corps, 28 August 1940, RG 407, CCC, Box 934, NARA. Specialists recommending X-ray screening of CCC employees included Esmond Long and H. E. Kleinschmidt, "Desirability of a Tuberculosis Survey of Applicants for the CCC," 23 July 1935; Henry C. Pillsbury, "Mass Radiography of Selectees, Civilian Conservation Corps," 17 April 1936; and related correspondence in RG 407, CCC, Boxes 937 and 938, NARA.

146. *ARSG*, 1939, 266.

147. Buck and McAfee correspondence, October 1933, RG 112, Entry 31, 1928–37, Box 280, NARA.

148. E. C. Jones memo, "Employment of Doctors, Dentists, Nurses and Other Civilian Employees for the Care of CCC and VA Patients, Fiscal Year 1938," 3 July 1937, RG 407, CCC, Box 1018, NARA.

149. Charles Johnson, "The Army, the Negro and the Civilian Conservation Corps: 1933–1942," *Military Affairs* 36 (October 1972), 85–86; and John A. Salmond, "The Civilian Conservation Corps and the Negro," *Journal of American History* 52 (June 1967): 82.

150. *ARSG*, 1936, 142–43.

151. *ARSG*, 1937, 166.

152. C. D. Buck, "Reimbursement for Subsistence," 16 October 1934, RG 112, Entry 31, 1928–37, Box 284, NARA.

153. Adjutant General's Office, "Continued Medical Attendance and Hospitalization for Former CCC Enrollees Hospitalized at Present," 15 June 1943, RG 407, CCC, Box 933, NARA.

154. *FZAR*, 1942, 5.

155. John Duffy, *The Sanitarians: A History of American Public Health* (Champaign,

IL: University of Illinois Press, 1990), 256–66.

156. Edgar Sydenstricker, "Health and the Depression," *The Millbank Memorial Fund Quarterly Bulletin* 11 (October 1933): 273–80. On tuberculosis during the Depression see Natalia Molina, *Fit to Be Citizens? Public Health and Race in Los Angeles, 1879–1939* (Berkeley, CA: University of California Press, 2006), 134, 244–45; and Emily K. Abel, *Tuberculosis and the Politics of Exclusion: A History of Public Health and Migration to Los Angeles* (New Brunswick, NJ: Rutgers University Press, 2007).

157. "First Lady Urges Tuberculosis War," *New York Times,* 31 March 1935; and "Seal Sale Opened by Mrs. Roosevelt," *New York Times,* 27 November 1936. Eleanor Roosevelt died in 1962 at the age of 78 of complications of tuberculosis she had contracted in her youth. Available at: http://www.gwu.edu/~erpapers/abouteleanor/erbiography.cfm#yr1953, accessed 26 November 2012.

158. "Hospitals in 1933," *Journal of the American Medical Association* 102 (31 March 1934): 1084; and Rosemary Stevens, *In Sickness and in Wealth: American Hospitals in the Twentieth Century* (New York, NY: Basic Books, Inc., Publishers, 1989), 148.

159. Stevens, *In Sickness and in Wealth,* 163–70.

160. Federal Board of Hospitalization, "Minutes," 28 July 1936, Record Group 51, Records of the Office of Management and Budget [hereafter RG 51], Entry 3, Box 8, NARA.

161. George R. Spalding, "Hearing on the Bureau of the Budget in Connection with the Future of Fitzsimons Hospital," 19 October 1936, RG 112, Entry 31, 1928–37, Box 283, NARA.

162. "Fitzsimons Building Authorization Also is Voted by House," *Denver Post,* 19 July 1937; and "Way Cleared for Grant of PWA Funds to Fitzsimons Hospital," *Denver Post,* 14 May 1938.

163. United States Housing Act, Amendments of 1938, approved 21 June 1938; and *ARSG,* 1939, 186.

164. "Fitzsimons Will Get Almost 4 Millions," *Denver Post,* 20 June 1938.

165. *FZAR,* 1939.

166. The late nineteenth century development of the elevator and antiseptic and aseptic protocols enabled hospitals to abandon the pavilion style. See Allan Brandt, "Of Bed and Benches: Building the Modern American Hospital," in *The Architecture of Science,* Peter Gailson and Emily Thompson, eds., (Cambridge, MA: MIT Press, 1999); and Charles E. Rosenberg, *The Care of Strangers* (New York, NY: Basic Books, 1987).

167. *ARSG,* 1939, 186.

168. "Army to Train Hospital Aides at Fitzsimons," *Denver Post,* 30 March 1941.

169. "World's Best Equipped Hospital Soon Ready for Patients," *Rocky Mountain News,* 30 March 1941.

170. *FZAR,* 1940, 1.

171. "Fitzsimons New Building Wins Praise," *Denver Post,* 25 October 1940.

172. *Washington Times,* 2 December 1937, Lewis scrapbook, No. 10, 1937–38, Lewis Papers.

173. "Lewis Launches Congress Purge, Issues Blacklist," *Philadelphia Inquirer,* 13 July 1938, Lewis Scrapbook, No. 10, 1937–38.

174. Scrapbook No. 11, Lewis Papers.

175. "Colonel Buck to Retire from U.S. Army June 30," *Denver Post,* 25 April 1940. Due to the wartime emergency, within weeks Buck returned to duty at Letterman Hospital in San Francisco; "Fitzsimons Training Program is Speeded," *Denver Post,* 6 September 1940.

176. Lewis Diaries, 24 November 1941.

177. Lewis Diaries, 22 November 1941.

178. "Fitzsimons Dedication Marked by Simplicity,"*Rocky Mountain News*, 4 December 1941; and "Fitzsimons' Kin Present at Dedication," *Denver Post*, 4 December 1941.

179. Lawrence Lewis, "Address of Hon. Lawrence Lewis, of Colorado, at Dedication of a New Building at Fitzsimons General Hospital," 15 June 1942, *Congressional Record* 77th Cong., 2nd sess., A2613; and *Rocky Mountain News*, 4 December 1941.

180. "Four Congressmen Have Perfect Record," *Denver Post*, 23 June 1936.

181. Lewis Diaries, 7 December 1941.

182. Some researchers have linked dental and periodontal disease to a number of health complications. See National Institutes of Dental and Craniofacial Research, "Periodontal (Gum) Disease: Causes, Symptoms, and Treatments, NIH publication 12-1142, August 2012; http://www.nidcr.nih.gov/OralHealth/Topics/GumDiseases/, (accessed 23 October 2012).

183. "Rep. Lewis Rests on Doctor's Orders," *Rocky Mountain News*, 26 March 1942 and "Doctor Orders Rest for Lawrence Lewis," *Denver Post*, 26 March 1942.

184. Phil Goodstein, *From Soup Lines to the Front Lines: Denver during the Depression and World War II, 1927–1947* (Denver, CO: New Social Publications, 2007), 431–32.

185. "Lawrence Lewis Back on Job After Illness of a Year," *Denver Post*, 8 September 1943.

186. "Lawrence Lewis Dies at Capital," *Denver Post*, 9 December 1943.

187. *Congressional Record*, 78th Cong., 1st sess., 9 December 1943, 10539–43; and Appendix to the *Congressional Record*, 78th Cong., 2nd sess., 31 May 1944, A2680–A2691, *passim*.

188. Appendix to the *Congressional Record*, 78th Cong., 2nd sess., 31 May 1944, A2680–A2691, *passim*.

189. Jack Carberry, "Miracle Worked on Wounded Man at Fitzsimons," *Denver Post*, 31 March 1943.

190. *FZAR*, 1942, 2.

Chapter Eight
Camp Follower: Tuberculosis in World War II

President Franklin Delano Roosevelt proclaimed a "limited national emergency" on 8 September 1939, a week after Germany invaded Poland. But due to underfunding during the interwar period, one observer wrote that, "to prepare for war the Medical Department had to start almost from scratch."[1] Given the lean years of the 1920s and 1930s and the Army Medical Department's policy of discharging officers with tuberculosis from duty, Surgeon General James C. Magee had to turn to the civilian sector for a tuberculosis expert. He recruited Esmond R. Long, M.D., Ph.D., director of the Henry Phipps Institute for the Study, Prevention and Treatment of Tuberculosis in Philadelphia. He could not have made a better choice. Long was also professor of pathology at the University of Pennsylvania, director of medical research for the National Tuberculosis Association, and the youngest person to be awarded the Trudeau Medal at age forty-two years (in 1932) for his tuberculosis research.[2] He would now become the Army's point man on the disease and stand at the front lines of the Medical Department's struggle with tuberculosis beginning before Pearl Harbor to well after V-J (Victory-Japan) Day.

His mission to reduce the effect of tuberculosis on the Army differed from that of Colonel (Col.) George Bushnell in the previous war because disease was less of a threat. In fact, World War II would be the first war in which more American personnel died of battle wounds than of disease. Of 405,399 recorded fatalities, battle deaths outnumbered those from disease and nonbattle injuries more than two to one: 291,557 to 113,842.[3] Malaria, sexually transmitted diseases, and respiratory infections did sicken millions of soldiers, sailors, Marines, and airmen, but most survived. Thanks in part to sulfa drugs and, beginning in 1943, penicillin to treat bacterial infections, the Army Medical Department had only 14,904 deaths of 14,998,369 disease admissions worldwide, a 0.1 percent death rate.[4] Tuberculosis declined, too, representing only 1 percent of Army hospital admissions for diseases—1.2 per 1,000 cases per year—a rate much lower than the 12 per 1,000 cases per year during World War I. The Medical Department concluded that "tuberculosis was not a major cause of non-effectiveness during the war."[5]

But Sir Arthur S. McNalty, chief medical officer of the British Ministry of Health (1935–40), called tuberculosis "one of the camp followers of war." War abetted tuberculosis, he explained, because of the "lowering of bodily resistance and increased physical or mental strain or both."[6] It also found fertile ground in crowded barracks and camps, and ran rampant in the World War II prison camps and Nazi concentration camps. And just one active case of tuberculosis per thousand in the Army meant thousands of tuberculosis sufferers among the 11 million Americans in uniform, each of whom consumed Medical Department resources: the average hospital stay per case during the war was 113 days.[7]

But if tuberculosis was a camp follower, Esmond Long (Figure 8-1) was a tuberculosis follower.[8] He tracked it down, studied it, and tried to prevent its spread at every stage of American involvement in the war. With war looming in 1940, the National Research Council asked Long to chair the Division of Medical Sciences, Subcommittee for Tuberculosis, to advise the government on preventing and controlling tuberculosis in both civilian and military populations during war mobilization. Once the United States entered the war, Long received a commission as a colonel in the Medical Corps and moved his family from Philadelphia to Washington, DC. Working out of the Office of The Surgeon General, Long set up a screening process with the Selective Service to keep tuberculosis *out* of the Army and then traveled to more than ninety induction camps to ensure adherence to the procedures. He also oversaw the expansion of tuberculosis treatment facilities in the United States, inspected Fitzsimons and other Army tuberculosis hospitals, advised medical officers on treating patients, kept abreast of research developments in the labs, monitored outbreaks of tuberculosis in the theaters of war, and wrote articles for medical and lay periodicals to publicize the Army's antituberculosis program. In 1945 Long traveled to the European theater to inspect hospitals caring for tubercular refugees and liberated prisoners of war (POWs). There he saw the horrors of the concentration camps at Buchenwald and Dachau where Army medical personnel cared for thousands of former prisoners sick and dying of typhus, starvation, and tuberculosis. After the war Long organized the tuberculosis control program for the Allied occupation of Germany, and returned annually in the 1950s to assess its progress. He split his time between the Army Medical Department and the Veterans Administration (VA) to supervise the transition of the federal tuberculosis treatment program from the War Department to the VA. He also helped organize and evaluate the antibiotic trials, which ultimately led to an effective cure for tuberculosis. After returning to civilian life Long continued to study tuberculosis in the Army, and he wrote the key tuberculosis chapters for the Army Medical Department's official history of the war.

With Long as a guide, this chapter shows how war once again served as handmaiden to disease around the globe. This time the Army Medical Department assumed not only national but international responsibilities for the control of tuberculosis in military and civilian populations, among friend and foe. Long and the Army Medical Department did succeed in demoting tuberculosis from the leading cause of disability discharge for American World War I personnel (13.5 percent of discharges), to thirteenth position during the years 1942–45 (1.9 percent

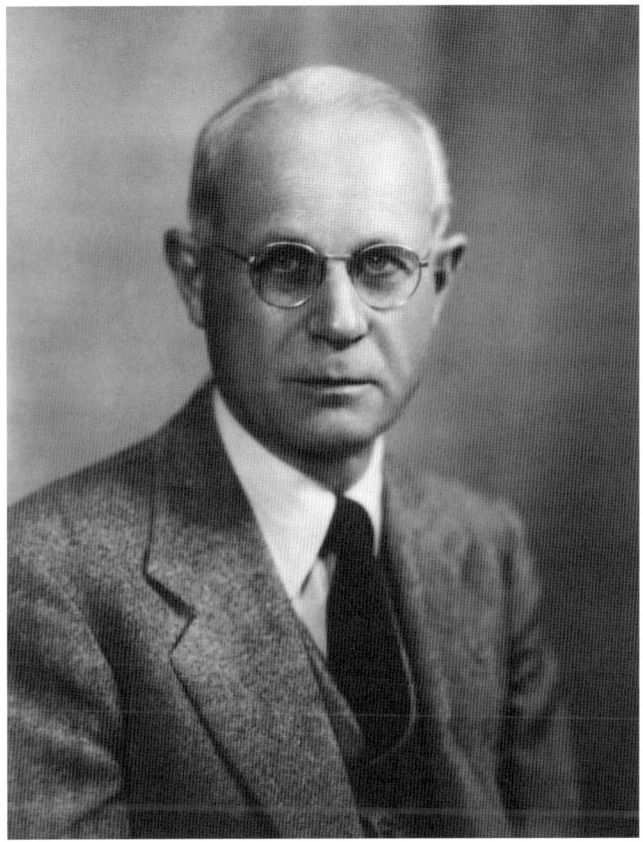

Figure 8-1. Esmond R. Long, who directed the Army tuberculosis program during World War II. Photograph courtesy of the National Library of Medicine, Image #B017302.

of all discharges), behind conditions such as psychoneuroses, ulcers, respiratory diseases, arthritis, and other diseases.⁹ But this achievement required continued vigilance, an Army-wide surveillance program, and dedicated personnel and resources. The first step was to keep tuberculosis out of the Army.

Screening Redux

After war broke out in Europe, Congress passed the National Defense Act of 1940, which established the first peacetime military draft in U.S. history, increasing Army strength eightfold from 210,000 in September 1939 to almost 1.7 million (1,686,403) by December 1941. This resulted in a 75 percent rise in the number of patients in military hospitals, straining the Medical Department, which had only seven general hospitals and 119 station hospitals in 1939.¹⁰ The year and a half before Pearl Harbor, therefore, was hectic, and while Congress was soon appropriating freely, pledging "all of the resources of the country" to meet the crisis, the War Department was constantly readjusting to meet the escalating emergency.[11]

The National Research Council Committee on Medicine, Subcommittee on Tuberculosis, chaired by Long, met for the first time on 24 July 1940 and prioritized its responsibilities: first, develop recommendations on how to screen draft registrants for tuberculosis; second, screen civilians in federal service and wartime industries; third, figure out how to care for people rejected by the draft for the disease; and finally, help civilian and military agencies prepare for tuberculosis in war refugee populations. In its first nine-hour meeting, the subcommittee decided on centralized tuberculosis screening centers at 200 recruiting stations and generated a list of tuberculosis specialists nationwide to evaluate recruits and interpret X-rays at those centers. Subcommittee members stressed the importance of maintaining good records for processing any subsequent benefits claims and, most importantly, called for X-ray screening of all inductees—not just those who looked like they might have tuberculosis.[12]

The War Department leadership initially rejected such comprehensive screening of inductees as expensive and time-consuming. The fact that tuberculosis death rates in the country had fallen two-thirds from 140 per 100,000 people in 1917 to 45 per 100,000 people in 1941, and in the Army from 4.6 per 1,000 in 1922 to 1.4 per 1,000 in 1940, may have led to complacency. But Long, his colleagues, and the national tuberculosis community, mindful of the cost to the nation in sickness, death, and disability benefits in the previous war, persisted.[13] The American College of Chest Surgeons asked in July 1940, "Shall We Spread or Eliminate Tuberculosis in the Army?" and their president, Benjamin Goldberg, reported that the VA had spent almost $1.2 billion on tuberculosis patients through 1940.[14] One medical officer calculated that 31 percent of all veterans who died as a result of World War I service and whose dependents received benefits, had died of tuberculosis.[15] Even the lay press chimed in with a TIME magazine article, "TB Warning," that stressed the importance of chest X-rays.[16] Advocates pointed out that X-ray technology was more available and less expensive than in the previous war, and radiologists were more plentiful and skillful.[17] They were also confident that new technology, such as the development of a lens that allowed the direct and rapid photography of a fluoroscopic image and new 4 x 5 inch films, which made storage and transport easier than that of the 11 x 14 inch films, rendered screening more practical than in 1917–18.[18]

The Army Medical Department agreed with the National Research Council subcommittee. Since 1934 it had required X-rays for all Army personnel assigned overseas, but it had not yet convinced the War Department on universal screening.[19] In June 1941, Brigadier General (Brig. Gen.) Charles Hillman, Chief, Office of The Surgeon General Professional Service Division, told the National Tuberculosis chairman, C. M. Hendricks, that "the desirability of routine X-rays had long been recognized by the Surgeon General's Office," but "considerations other than medical entered the picture and the character of induction examinations had to be adapted to the limitations of time, place, and available equipment."[20] When Fitzsimons informed Hillman later that new recruits were arriving at the hospital with tuberculosis, he responded almost plaintively. "I am working with the Adjutant General to devise some method by which *every* volunteer for enlistment in the Regular Army will have a chest X-ray and serological test before acceptance." He asked for all available evidence of sick recruits, explaining that "data on Regular Army men of short service now in Fitzsimons with tuberculosis will help me get the thing across."[21] As the data and advice accumulated, in January 1942, the Adjutant General required that all voluntary applicants and reenlisting men be given chest X-rays. Finally, on 15 March 1942, mobilization regulations made chest X-rays mandatory in all induction physicals.[22]

With universal screening in place, Long, as chief of the tuberculosis branch in the Office of The Surgeon General, oversaw the screening process and faced a task similar to that of George Bushnell in 1917–18, finding that fine line between excluding as much tuberculosis as possible from the Army without rejecting too few or too many men. Conscious of his predecessor's miscalculations, Long was careful not to criticize Bushnell's tuberculosis program, at one point noting that World War I medical officers were "not to be reproached for not having knowledge that came into existence only later, any more than the chief of the Army air service in 1917 is to be reproached because more efficient airplanes are available now than then."[23]

The wartime emergency produced a public health campaign regarding tuberculosis and other disease threats. A War Department pamphlet, *What Every Citizen Should Know about Wartime Medicine*, presented the issue as one of maintaining troop health and limiting public costs. "The strenuous activity of soldiering is likely to cause extension of an incipient (early) tuberculous invasion of the lungs, or to precipitate the breakdown and reactivation of arrested cases," it explained. Such illness could result in disability "and the necessity of providing long care of these patients in military hospitals where they must remain isolated from nontuberculous patients."[24] The Public Health Service also created a tuberculosis office to handle the expected increase in tuberculosis, and, as the National Research Council Subcommittee recommended, gave war industry workers chest examinations.[25]

As military and civilian screening boards found thousands of people with active tuberculosis and sent many of them to tuberculosis sanatoriums and hospitals, they generated what a public health nurse referred to as "potentially the greatest case finding program that workers in tuberculosis control have ever known."[26] At the same time, however, war mobilization drew civilian medical personnel into the military, reducing staffing in home front institutions. Army medical personnel ultimately numbered more than 688,000, including 48,000 physicians in the Medical Corps, 14,000 dentists in the Dental Corps, and 56,000 nurses in the Army Nurse Corps—a large portion of the nation's medical professionals.[27] To maintain his nursing staff, VA Director Frank Hynes even asked the Army Nurse Corps in May 1942 not to hire VA nurses away from his hospitals.[28] Given the shortage of tuberculosis specialists for the local induction boards, Esmond Long requested names of qualified physicians who had been discharged from the Army because of tuberculosis to serve on those boards. But George F. Aycock, director of medical services at Fitzsimons, told him that most such officers were "physically unable to carry on any work which would be of value to state public health offices."[29]

Army tuberculosis rates during World War II, while lower than during World War I, did show a similar "U" curve with high rates at the beginning of the war as the Selective Service built up the military forces and cases that had eluded screening became active during training or combat (Figure 8-2). Tuberculosis rates fell as radiologists became more proficient at identifying tuberculosis infections, and then another sharp, higher increase in cases at the end of the war as discharge examinations found people who had developed active tuberculosis during their service. Postwar studies also revealed a seemingly paradoxical phenomenon that during the war military personnel serving overseas had lower tuberculosis rates than those serving in the United States, yet higher rates when they returned home. Long attributed this to rigorous physical exams military units received prior to

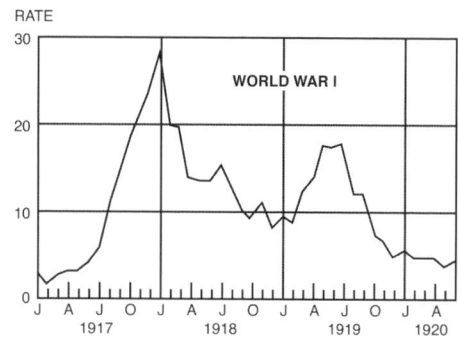

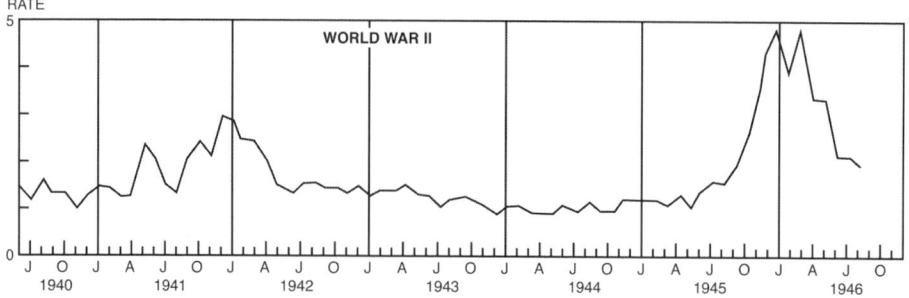

Figure 8-2. Chart comparing the incidence curves of tuberculosis in the Army during World War I and World War II. From Esmond R. Long, "Tuberculosis," in John Boyd Coates, Robert S. Anderson, and W. Paul Havens, eds., *Internal Medicine in World War II, Medical Department, U.S. Army in World War II*, vol. 2, *Infectious Diseases* (Washington, DC: Office of The Surgeon General, Department of the Army, 1961), chart 17, p. 335. Available at http://history.amedd.army.mil/booksdocs/wwii/infectiousdisvolii/chapter11chart17.pdf.

overseas deployment, which eliminated many cases of tuberculosis, and the subsequent lack of surveillance opportunities and skilled diagnosticians in the theaters of war. As a result, troops who developed tuberculosis were not discovered until their separation examinations, conducted when they were once again in the United States.[30]

In the end, the screening process rejected 171,300 men for tuberculosis as the primary cause (thousands more had tuberculosis in addition to the disqualifying condition), and Long calculated that this saved the government millions of dollars in hospitalization costs.[31] After the war, however, Long identified two factors that allowed tuberculous men into the Army: the failure to screen all inductees until March 1942, and the 4 x 5 inch stereoscopic (fluorographic) films, which were used in the interest of speed but which Long believed caused examiners to miss about 10 percent of minimal tuberculosis lesions in recruits. To better understand the latter problem he had two radiologists read the same X-rays and found substantial disagreement between their findings. Long therefore concluded that "if the induction films had each been read by two different radiologists, undoubtedly many more of the men who had tuberculosis at entry could have been excluded from service."[32] The Army ultimately discharged 15,387 enlisted men for tuberculosis during the war, which earned it thirteenth position as a cause of disability discharge.[33] As one medical officer said, "Evidently our record, in spite of the many difficulties and delays experienced, is not too bad."[34]

Tuberculosis in the Theaters of War

American military forces fought in nine theaters of war—five in the Pacific and Asia, the other four in North Africa, the Mediterranean, Europe, and the Middle East. The Allies gave priority to defeating Germany and Italy in Europe beginning with operations in North Africa and the Mediterranean. After fighting in Tunisia in 1942–43, the Allies invaded Sicily on 10 July 1943, and moved up the Italian peninsula. By April 1944—in preparation for the D-Day invasion on 6 June 1944—the United States had more than 3 million soldiers in Europe, supported by 258,000 medical personnel managing a total of 318 hospitals with 252,050 beds.[35] The war against Japan got off to a slower start as U.S. military forces developed the means to execute an island war across vast expanses of ocean. After fighting began in the Southwest Pacific, military forces grew from 62,500 troops in March 1942 to 670,000 in the summer of 1944 with 60,140 medical personnel.[36] Even though military personnel developed tuberculosis in all of the nine theaters, the numbers were not high and tuberculosis was not a major military problem. In the Southwest Pacific theater, for example, only sixty-four of more than 40,000 hospital admissions were for the disease.[37]

Tuberculosis was of the greatest consequence in the North Africa and Mediterranean theaters, in part due to poor screening early in the war, but also because, according to historian Charles Wiltse, it was the theater "in which the lessons of ground combat were learned by the Medical Department as much as by the line troops."[38] In general, medical personnel learned the importance of treating battle casualties as promptly as possible and keeping hospitals and clearing stations mobile and far forward to shorten evacuation and turnaround times. With regard to tuberculosis, the Medical Department had to relearn the World War I lesson of the importance of having skilled practitioners—or "good tuberculosis men"—in theater. They also ascertained which treatments were appropriate close to the battle lines and which were not, and when and how best to evacuate tubercular patients to the United States.

When soldiers with tuberculosis began to appear at Army medical stations in North Africa in late 1942, Major General (Maj. Gen.) Paul R. Hawley, chief of medical services for the European theater of operations, called for a tuberculosis specialist. On Long's recommendation, Hawley appointed Col. Theodore Badger (Figure 8-3) as a senior consultant in tuberculosis on 2 January 1943. A professor of medicine at the Harvard School of Medicine, Badger had served in the Navy during World War I, and then attended Yale and Harvard where he earned his medical degree.[39] Chief of medical service of the 5th General Hospital (GH), organized out of Harvard, Badger would play a role similar to that played by Gerald Webb during World War I—medical specialist, teacher, and troubleshooter.[40]

Assessing the tuberculosis situation in the Mediterranean theater, Badger identified five hazards: (1) the development of active disease in American troops who had not been X-rayed upon induction; (2) association with British troops and civilians who had not been screened for tuberculosis; (3) drinking of nonpasteurized and possibly infected milk that could transmit tuberculosis; (4) battlefield conditions that could activate soldiers' latent infections; and (5) the undetermined effects of other respiratory infections.[41] Badger soon got the Army to use pasteurized milk and to establish X-ray centers with the proper equipment and trained staff, but he was not able to examine the thousands of American soldiers in the war zone. To gauge the extent of the tuberculosis problem he therefore arranged for a mobile X-ray unit to conduct spot surveys of troops in the field. Three examinations of some 3,000 troops each found only about 1 percent with signs of tuberculosis. To avoid losing manpower, Badger reported in mid-1943 that "up to the present time no individual has been removed from duty because of X-ray findings, and follow-up study has, so far, not indicated the necessity for it."[42] Instead, Badger planned to recheck those with suspicious films every few months to see if the signs had advanced. Follow up, however, was easier said than done in an army on the move, so Badger and Hawley finally decided in February 1944 that all patients with active or suspected tuberculosis would be evacuated back to the United States.[43] Badger recommended that patients with pleural effusion, the accumulation of fluid between the layers of the membranes that line the lungs and chest cavity that often indicates tuberculosis, be evacuated back to the United States. He also ended the practice of transporting some tuberculosis patients sitting up, insisting that they be transported as litter patients on bed rest.[44]

In late 1943, dissatisfied with the way in which many Army hospitals were handling tuberculosis, Hawley established "tuberculosis reception centers" at various general hospitals, designating the 6th GH from Massachusetts General Hospital,

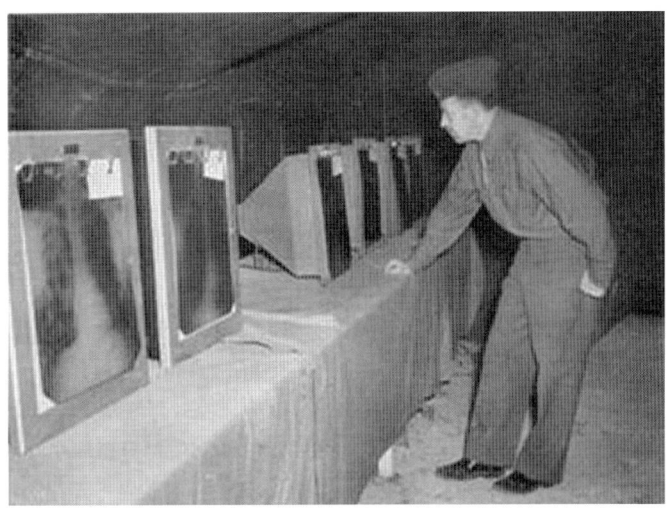

Figure 8-3. Theodore L. Badger, senior consultant on tuberculosis for the U.S. forces in Europe and North Africa. Photograph in W. Paul Havens and Leonard D. Heaton, eds., *Internal Medicine in World War II, Medical Department, U.S. Army in World War II*, vol. 1, *Activities of Medical Consultants* (Washington, DC: Office of The Surgeon General, Department of the Army, 1961), 409. Available at http://history.amedd.army.mil/booksdocs/wwii/MedConslt1/figures/figure138.jpg.

Boston; the 17th GH from Henry Ford Hospital, Detroit; the 24th GH from Tulane University, New Orleans; the 26th GH from the University of Minnesota, Minneapolis; and the 46th GH Oregon School of Medicine, Portland, as such centers.[45] Although the number of tuberculosis patients was small, knowledgeable medical officers took any tuberculosis case seriously, because, as one wrote, "a single soldier with an open tuberculosis lesion can infect a great many others in a short period of time."[46] Col. Donald S. King and Captain (Capt.) George T. McKean treated tuberculosis patients in the North Africa and Mediterranean theaters and reported on a situation whereby eight of fifty-seven men in a medical battalion developed tuberculosis. King described how the problem slowly unfolded in early 1943 after a battalion cook showed symptoms. Medical personnel X-rayed the rest of the kitchen staff in April and found another open case. Two men developed symptoms in September 1943, another cook in January 1944, and after the sixth case was discovered in November 1944, medical staff X-rayed the entire battalion and found two more sick men.[47] King and McKean calculated that the 383 patients they treated for tuberculosis had an average hospital stay of 58.5 days, which amounted to "a total of 22,405 overseas hospital days."[48]

The experience of another hospital in North Africa illustrates the pitfalls of tuberculosis treatment close to the front lines. The 46th GH served there for eight months—November 1943 to August 1944—admitting 8,995 patients, but only

171 for tuberculosis.[49] Maj. Samuel L. Diack cared for many of these patients who included four British servicemen, a Norwegian sailor, nine members of the Merchant Marine, and a Yugoslav civilian who had spent two years in a German labor camp. Treatment included bed rest, fresh air when possible, and good nutrition, which was difficult in wartime. Diack gave eighteen patients artificial pneumothoraces, fourteen of which were successful. Of six patients who were evacuated from the hospital, however, three "undoubtedly suffered setbacks due to prolonged train travel and much handling," he reported. He gave another patient phrenic exeresis (removal of part of the phrenic nerve), but after the patient developed complications and almost died, Diack wrote "it was probably an error in judgment to do the operation in the first place."[50] He ended up evacuating most American patients to the United States, but discharged to full duty the Yugoslav civilian, whom he considered healed, and put sixteen patients also considered healed on limited duty, telling them to get X-rayed again in two or three months.

Tuberculosis cases appeared in the later years of the war, too. During the Allied bombing of Germany, several members of Air Corps units stationed in England succumbed to active tuberculosis. In the 56th Fighter Group, Eighth Air Force, eight men developed the disease between August 1943 and September 1944. When medical officers found an acute case in the 78th Fighter Group, Eighth Air Force, they X-rayed the entire unit, taking more than 3,600 chest films in late 1944, and evacuating seven men to the United States. When the medical investigators could not find a common source of infection among the airmen they concluded that all of the cases were reactivations of previous infections.[51]

Some medical officers in the United States complained to Long's office that more tuberculosis patients should be given artificial pneumothorax before they were evacuated out of the field to begin their treatment sooner, but given experiences like Diack's, Badger disagreed. It would be better to wait until they arrived in the United States, he asserted, due to the lack of experts in the field, the inevitable delays in transport, and the fact that "emphasis in the active theater is on immediate wartime emergencies, without a disproportionate amount of time spent on the individual soldier."[52] Long agreed, saying that he had "great confidence" in Badger's advice.[53] Badger's recommendations, however, were not always approved. In 1944, as the Allies moved into Germany, he warned that military personnel would be coming into contact with tuberculous civilians and recommended spot checks of personnel in Army hospitals. With Hitler in his sights, Gen. Hawley responded, "I am sorry but we are fighting a very rapid war at this moment and such surveys will have to wait until this thing slows down a bit."[54]

If troops could contract tuberculosis in the war theater, medical personnel faced a high risk of exposure in the hospitals as well. Long recognized this, noting that "fortunately, the senior consultant in tuberculosis in the area, Col. Badger, was aware of the possibility of contagion."[55] Indeed, in the 1930s, Badger wrote that "the greatest responsibility of the hospital lies in the observation of rigid medical asepsis where cases of open tuberculosis are under medical and nursing care."[56] But military hospitals in the field rarely function under optimal conditions, and anticontagion technique required supplies and time that were in short supply. Still, hospitals under Badger's purview, such as the 46th GH, took measures such as prohibiting nurses from working long hours, giving them extra days off, and requiring chest X-rays every two months.[57] In spite of these precautions, four nurses in the Mediterranean and European theaters developed active tuberculosis in 1943, thirty in 1944, and thirty-eight in 1945, a rate 3.8 times greater than that for the troops in theater.[58]

As the war progressed, more of these patients returned home by air rather than by sea. As the first true air war, World War II saw the introduction of air evacuation when Army aeromedical squadrons deployed in early 1943. After successful trials in the Pacific and North Africa, air evacuation increased so that during the Battle of the Bulge (1944–45), some patients arrived in U.S. hospitals within three days of being wounded.[59] Some medical officers were concerned about the effects of transporting tuberculosis patients by air where they would be exposed to high speeds, jolting, and reduced air pressure. Tuberculosis specialists in New Mexico and Colorado therefore studied 143 white, male military patients, twenty-two-years old to twenty-eight-years old, with active tuberculosis flown to Army hospitals in nonpressurized air ambulances for any signs of trouble. Fearing the worst, they instead found that "severe discomfort, pulmonary hemorrhage, and spontaneous pneumothorax did not occur in the series either during or following the flight," and concluded that air transport up to 10,000 feet was safe and preferable to time-consuming travel by water. By the end of the war the consensus was that rapid air evacuation to the United States also reduced the need to give a tuberculosis patient a pneumothorax in the field.[60] As the war progressed, therefore, the burden of caring for tuberculosis patients fell increasingly on the hospitals in the United States.

"A City of 10,000"—Fitzsimons during the War

From the roof of Fitzsimons' new building in April 1943, *Rocky Mountain News* reporter John Stephenson could see the Rocky Mountain Arsenal, the Denver Ordnance Plant, and Lowry Field, "places where the Army studies how to kill people." But, he wrote, "The Army is merciful. It lets the right-hand of justice know what the left hand of mercy is doing at Fitzsimons General Hospital." The largest Army hospital in the world, Fitzsimons had 322 buildings on 600 acres, paved streets with traffic lights, a post office, barbershop, pharmacy school, dental school, print shop, bakery, fire department, and chapel. It was, wrote Stephenson, "a city of 10,000."[61] No longer a liability, Fitzsimons was the pride of the Army Medical Department. One Army inspector reported that "it is apparent that no expense has been spared in this extraordinary building or in the general equipment and maintenance of the whole hospital plant."[62] As Congressman Lawrence Lewis had hoped, Fitzsimons' mission now extended beyond caring for tuberculosis patients to meeting the general medical and surgical needs of the wider military community in the Denver region. The modernized hospital also received a promotion with the appointment of a general to command—Brig. Gen. Omar H. Quade—in April 1943. During the war the hospital maintained about 3,500 beds, reaching its highest daily patient population after the war—3,719 on 3 February 1946. The annual occupancy rate, calculated in patient days, increased from 603,683 in 1942 to a high of 1,097,760 for 1945, about 85 percent capacity.[63]

With the reduction of tuberculosis in the Army over the years, the percentage of tuberculosis patients among all those at Fitzsimons had declined from 80 percent to 90 percent in the 1920s to 40 percent to 50 percent in the late 1930s. As the Army grew it now rose again. During the war Fitzsimons admitted more than 8,100 patients with tuberculosis. In fact, in 1943, only eighteen patients had battle injuries; the rest were in the hospital for illness and noncombat injuries. Unlike during the previous war, however, this Medical Department had a network of more than fifty veterans' hospitals to which it could transfer patients too disabled by tuberculosis or other disease or injury to return to duty. Now, instead of allowing patients to stay in the service and receive the benefit of hospitalization with the hopes that they would recover and return to duty, the Medical Department discharged patients to VA hospitals as soon as they were determined to be unfit for military service, thereby reserving capacity for active-duty personnel.[64]

Fitzsimons' staff did, however, employ a number of medical advances to return an increasing number of sick and wounded officers and enlisted men to duty and in 1943 invited reporters in to show them some of their victories. They showcased patients like Private (Pvt.) Virgil E. Stratton of Montana whose arm was severely damaged when he was strafed at Dutch Harbor in the Aleutian Islands. Army medics had immediately given Stratton sulfa to prevent infection and blood plasma to replace the blood volume he had lost, but the bullet had severed an important nerve in his arm so that by the time he arrived at Fitzsimons his arm was so flexed that his hand was resting on his shoulder. Surgeons were able to reattach the nerve endings, though, and with physical therapy and three operations to lengthen the nerves, Stratton was able to use his arm and hand well enough to return to duty and to study business at the University of Denver.[65] The hospital newspaper, *Stethoscope*, reported in October 1943 on the most exciting medical development during the war when medical researchers met at Fitzsimons to discuss a "sensational new drug still in the experimental stage."[66] Maj. D. P. Greenlee had returned from a training course in penicillin therapy at Bushnell General Hospital in Utah to supervise the administration of the new drug on a variety of infections.[67] He soon reported a cure rate of 93 percent.[68]

There were fewer victories in tuberculosis treatment. In 1943, Gen. Quade noted that "[r]est is still stressed as the basic treatment for pulmonary tuberculosis. Collapse procedures are frequently used as additional measures but not as substitutes for a well regulated rest regime."[69] During the war about one-quarter of all tuberculosis patients were treated with pneumothorax.[70] In the 1930s surgeons had begun pulmonary resection, removing parts of the lung (lobectomy) or entire lungs (pneumonectomy) for the treatment of cancer and lung ailments such as abscesses. During the war Fitzsimons surgeon Col. John B. Grow and other surgeons tried lung resection to treat tuberculosis, with few patient deaths.[71] In 1946, however, when Grow's staff contacted thirty patients who had had such surgery, they found that half of them were doing well, but three others had died, seven were seriously ill, and the rest were still under treatment. Grow concluded that "because of these relatively unsatisfactory results, it was felt that pulmonary resection in the presence of positive sputum was extremely hazardous and the indications were consequently narrowed down."[72]

Outside the operating rooms, the "City of 10,000" had a rich social life with people arriving at the post from all corners of the country. With Congressman Lewis's acquisition of the School for Medical Technicians, Fitzsimons assumed the role of medical trainer, offering six- to twelve-week courses in technical training for dental, laboratory, X-ray, surgical, clinical, and pharmacy assistants. By 1946 the School had graduated more than 28,000 such technicians to serve around the world.[73] The Women's Army Corps arrived at Fitzsimons in February 1944 when 165 women attended the medical technicians school as part of the first coeducational class.[74] Members of the Women's Army Corps, rehabilitation aides, Education Department staff, dietitians, as well as nurses increased the female presence at Fitzsimons, as did activities of welfare organizations such as the Gold Star Mothers, the Red Cross, and the Junior League. Fitzsimons' patients and staff also enjoyed visits from celebrities, including Jack Benny, Miss America, Gary Cooper, Dorothy Lamour, and other entertainers such as the big band leader Fred Waring and his Pennsylvanians, the Denver Symphony Orchestra, and an African American Methodist Church children's choir from Denver.[75] Like communities across the country, the hospital participated in war bond campaigns and had a huge war garden that produced thousands of ears of sweet corn and bushels of other vegetables.[76] In February 1944, patient Cleveland Green, of Texas, made the front page of the *Stethoscope* when he bought $5,000 in war bonds. The African American soldier who had fallen ill during his service in the New Hebrides Islands said, "I know that the money I have saved and put into war bonds will now help the fellows who are still battling to get this thing over with sooner."[77] For spiritual guidance the chaplain's office offered Catholic and Protestant services on Sundays, and a rabbi from Denver or Lowry Field provided Jewish services. The chaplain's office also relied on civilian clergy and "chaplain-patients" to assist in comforting and counseling patients and their families. In 1944 alone chaplains conducted more than 1,500 services, made more than 115,000 hospital visits, and held a small service to honor each deceased patient.[78]

Despite national mobilization and generous congressional funding, the Army could not escape the strain on its hospitals. By July 1944, Fitzsimons had reached capacity so the Medical Department designated two more hospitals as specialty centers for tuberculosis. Earl Bruns' widow Caroline, who lived in Denver at the time, was no doubt pleased when the department named Bruns General Hospital in Santa Fe, New Mexico, in honor of her husband. Bruns along with Moore General Hospital in Swannanoa, North Carolina, cared for enlisted patients with minimal or suspected tuberculosis. Enlisted patients with questionable tuberculosis diagnoses and most officers and women patients would still go to Fitzsimons. Brig. Gen. Larry B. McAfee, who had worked in the Office of The Surgeon General during the 1930s, took command at Bruns Hospital and soon had 750 tuberculosis beds with the requisite staff and equipment, but the hospital struggled. On inspection, Long noted that McAfee "had a difficult task" because "frequent changes in personnel, inevitable under the circumstances, interfered seriously with the efficiency of the treatment given."[79] Patients drinking on the wards or going absent without leave increased, and Long attributed the low morale to Bruns' isolated location and "patients who had not seen their families for months or years."[80] Patients also complained about the food. Hazel L. Roundtree of New Orleans wrote to McAfee about her brother's treatment. He had developed tuberculosis while fighting in Germany and was undergoing thoracoplasty in "a series of operations." Her mother had been visiting the hospital for two months caring for her brother and other patients. While the doctors and nurses were wonderful, she wrote, "something has to be done about the food." Bruns was serving "goat meat, creamed meats, and even ribs—for boys who have had operations such as these." They send the food back, she said, "especially when the ribs are served."[81] Esmond Long visited Bruns the same week Roundtree wrote her letter and also observed problems with the food service. He recommended forty electrically heated food carts to make meals more palatable, but did not mention anyone serving ribs.[82]

Enemy Prisoners of War with Tuberculosis

Bruns Hospital's burden increased in 1945 when it began to receive tubercular enemy POWs. To relieve pressure on Allied resources in Europe and the Pacific, the Americans interned thousands of Italian, German, and Japanese prisoners of war in the continental United States.[83] The importation of prisoners began with a trickle in May 1942 and reached a peak population as recorded by the Army Medical Department of 425,871 in May 1945, the vast majority of them Germans—371,683—followed by 50,273 Italians and 3,915 Japanese POWs.[84] The federal government held them in 150 base camps and 340 branch camps across the country ranging in capacity from 250 to 3,000 men and repatriated them by the end of 1946 per the requirements of the Geneva Convention. Under the terms of the Convention, prisoners could be made to work in military, agricultural, and industrial operations if treated well and provided decent living conditions. Some POWs could not work, though, because they were sick or injured. Wary of prisoners bringing infectious diseases or parasites into the United States, medical personnel screened them for infections, vaccinated them against smallpox and typhoid, disinfected their clothing, and transferred those who needed medical care to hospitals designated to care for POWs. When a spot survey found that five of 525 Italian officers and enlisted men had active tuberculosis with bacteria in their sputum and twenty-five had X-rays suggestive of tuberculosis, Long recommended X-raying all incoming prisoners of war. This time the War Department agreed.[85]

At first the War Department sent prisoners with tuberculosis to a POW camp hospital in Florence, Arizona, but they posed a danger to other prisoners and their military guards.[86] After ten prisoners contracted tuberculosis in the hospital, to avoid violating Geneva Convention provisions protecting POW health, in January 1944 the War Department transferred tubercular prisoners to specialized tuberculosis facilities, sending German POWs with tuberculosis to Glennan General Hospital in Oklahoma, Italian POWs to Bruns General Hospital, Santa Fe, New Mexico, and Japanese POWs to the station hospital in Camp McCoy, Wisconsin.[87] Fitzsimons received POWs of all three nationalities.

When representatives from the French Embassy and the U.S. Department of State inspected the Fitzsimons POW facility in June 1944 it had 100 German, seventy-five Italian, and three Japanese POW patients with tuberculosis. The POW spokesman, German Lieutenant (Lt.) Wolfgang Hagenmeister, told the inspectors that the prisoners had "no complaints whatever concerning any phase of the care being given to them."[88] But he apparently did not speak for everyone. The three Japanese sailors—Saburo Nakagawa, thirty-six-years old, Kuzunori Makino, twenty-eight-years old, and Sadamu Okada, twenty-five-years old—were not satisfied. Captured in the South Pacific, they arrived at Fitzsimons in May 1944, and were confined in Ward B, a separate building housing POW patients. On 11 August, all three attempted to commit suicide by hara-kiri, cutting their wrists, necks, and stomachs with a sharpened table knife before medical personnel could stop them.[89] After Fitzsimons' physicians treated their wounds, they refused to eat for ten days. When that failed, they sought another method—death by mutiny. At 9:00 pm on 29 October 1944 ward attendant Pvt. Casey handed the prisoners a bottle of milk through the barred door of their section, and one of them threw it back at him, breaking the glass. When Casey told them to clean it up, they refused and became so belligerent that he called for support about 9:25 pm. The Corporal of the Guard arrived with Pvts. Rohmiller and Rogers, armed with clubs. Col. Francis E. Howard of the War Department's Prisoner of War Division reported what happened then:

> When they arrived at the ward, they were informed by Pvt. Casey, the guard on duty, of the throwing of a milk bottle by one of the prisoners. Casey showed them the mess caused by the broken bottle. The three soldiers thereupon opened the door which led into the Japanese prisoners section, gave a broom to one of the Japanese and told them to clean up the mess. Nakagawa said something to the prisoner in Japanese, whereupon he refused to clean up the mess. Nakagawa then grabbed Rohmiller's club and the other two prisoners "rushed" Rogers. Rogers broke his club "over their heads." The Japanese grasped him by the throat and were "trying to strangle him." Casey fired a shot into the floor in order to frighten the prisoners, but they continued their attack upon Rogers, who asked Casey for his gun. Upon receiving the gun, Rogers ordered the prisoners to "get back into their section." Nakagawa "rushed" Rogers and Rogers fired upon him. Nakagawa fell to the floor and the other two prisoners rushed Rogers "one of them circling around in front of the gun and the other attacking from the side." Rogers fired at them both. Makino fell and Okada ran into his room.[90]

When Lt. Col. Dennis E. Kelley, the executive officer, arrived "he found all three prisoners dead." Each had been killed by a single gunshot. Pvt. Rogers suffered a head injury "caused by some blunt object 'used with considerable force.'" The War Department and the State Department both investigated the incident, interviewing thirteen people at Fitzsimons who had knowledge of the events. The War Department board determined that Rogers "'was acting in the execution of his duty as a sentinel' when he inflicted the fatal injuries, and that the shootings were in self defense." Getting wind of the story, the *Denver Post* reported that "Enemy Patients Precipitated Row to Get Selves Shot after Previous Hara-Kiri Attempt Was Foiled."[91]

The Fitzsimons incident was the only time American guards killed Japanese prisoners of war on U.S. soil. Other Japanese POWs had caused trouble for Allied guards, though. According to historian Arnold Krammer, "The average Japanese soldier was molded to prefer death to surrender."[92] Scores of Japanese POWs attempted suicide or incited guards to shoot them during the war. In 1943 guards killed forty prisoners and wounded fifty at Camp Featherstone, New Zealand, and in 1944 twenty-three Japanese POWs committed suicide by slitting their throats at an American camp in New Caledonia.[93]

Although the Medical Department proudly reported that the health of POWs in 1944 was better than that of U.S. military personnel in the country, even the tuberculosis centers designated for POWs had difficulty meeting Geneva Convention standards.[94] A representative of the International Committee of the Red Cross inspected Bruns Hospital in February 1945 and found the 145 Italian POW tuberculosis patients clad in blue pajamas and red velvet dressing gowns confined to their beds. The prisoners had no complaints about the food or the medical care and each received three packages of cigarettes a week. But "aside from excellent medical care and first-class food," the inspector concluded, "there is much to be desired." The hospital was administered by members of the Medical Corps and "no one, not even the staff officers knew the regulations concerning prisoners." Furthermore, none of the hospital rooms had copies of the Geneva Convention, there were no Italian newspapers, and "convalescent prisoners should be authorized to enjoy the fresh air in a garden which should be specially prepared for them."[95] Regardless of these shortcomings, the treatment of tubercular POWs in the United States was humane—complete with velvet robes. Allied troops captured overseas, however, often encountered horribly different situations.

Recovered American Prisoners of War and Others

As Allied troops liberated France in 1944 and crossed into Germany they encountered thousands of refugees or "displaced persons"—escaped prisoners from Nazi concentration camps, exhausted and terrified Jews, slave laborers, political prisoners, Allied POWs, and other victims. The Nazi camps that held these people served as incubators for diseases such as tuberculosis and typhus, and the frightened, sick, and starved refugees inundated Army hospitals in late 1944 and early 1945. Theodore Badger reported one of the first waves that arrived on 18 December

1944 when 304 men, most of them Russians, came to the 50th GH in Commercy, France. They had been in the Nazi labor camps for the mines and heavy industries, where thousands died and survivors were malnourished and sick. All of the 304 had tuberculosis, 90 percent with moderate or advanced disease. Four were dead on arrival, eight more died in the first week, and one-third of the patients would die by May.[96] Alarmed, Gen. Hawley, Chief Surgeon of the European Theater of Operations, ordered that all displaced civilians and recovered military personnel be examined for signs of tuberculosis "to establish the gravity of the situation."[97] The situation was dire. At one time the 46th GH had more than 1,000 tuberculosis patients, all recovered Allied POWs, causing Esmond Long to remark that the hospital "had the largest number of tuberculosis patients of any Army hospital in the world."[98]

The 46th GH from Portland, Oregon, which had cared for tuberculosis patients in the Mediterranean theater, also stood on the front lines of the tuberculosis problem in Europe. Serving at Besancon, France, the hospital would receive the Meritorious Service Unit Plaque and Col. J. G. Strohm, the commanding officer, the Bronze Star Medal for service during the liberation of France. During the spring of 1945, the 46th GH admitted 2,472 Russians, forty-one Poles, and 128 Yugoslav POWs and former slave laborers freed by American forces. The influx began on 12 March and within four days the 46th GH had admitted 1,200 such patients. "The hospital staff was agast [sic] at the terrible physical condition of these people," reported the hospital commander.[99] When Badger visited the 46th GH in March 1945 he said the patients "constitute one of the most seriously affected groups with tuberculosis and malnutrition that I have ever seen," explaining that most of them suffered "acute fulminating, rapidly fatal disease, mixed with chronic, slowly progressive, fibrotic tuberculosis." Medical personnel (Figure 8-4) cared for these patients as best they could, comforting many of them as they died. They began the rest treatment with some men but, as Badger reported, convincing Allied POWs to submit to absolute bed rest after months of confinement was "practically impossible." He explained that "[t]he concept of bedrest was foreign to these men under any circumstances, and with the Russians, it was against their principles of treatment of tuberculosis, which commanded exercise and sunshine." Consequently, "[t]he severity of the problem of contagion is magnified by the ignorance of the patients, the complete absence of all sense of personal hygiene, and unwillingness to obey orders, and complete lack of discipline both military and professional." Despite these difficulties Badger was able to report that after a month "those men who did not die of acute tuberculosis showed marked improvement."[100]

In late 1944 Hawley requested 100,000 additional hospital beds for the displaced persons and POWs he expected to encounter after the German surrender, but Gen. George Marshall and Secretary of War Henry L. Stimson denied the request, believing they could not spare resources of that magnitude. The European Theater, they decided, must use German medical personnel and hospitals to care for the prisoners.[101] Only after the war did American hospital units transfer their equipment and supplies to German civilians and Allies for their use.

290 "*Good Tuberculosis Men*"

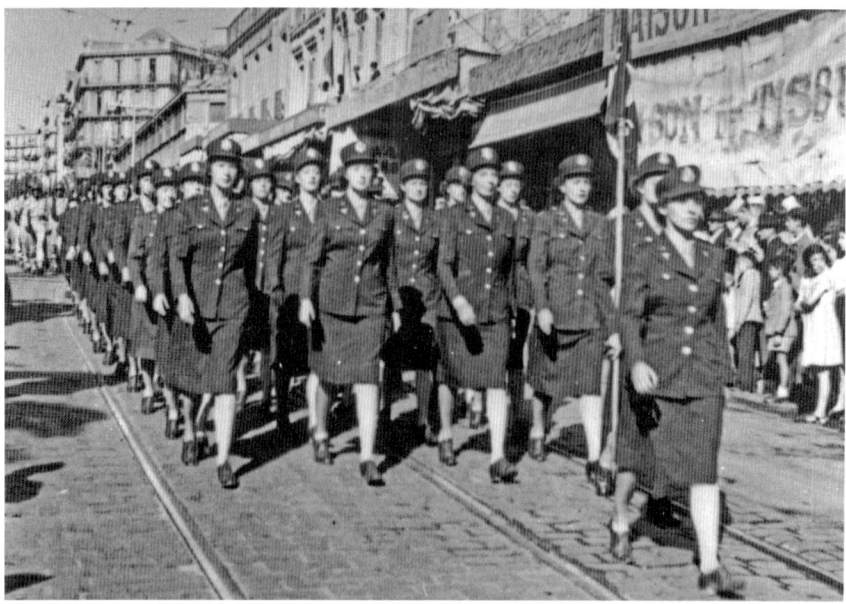

Figure 8-4. 46th General Hospital nurses who cared for former prisoners of war.
Photograph courtesy of Oregon Health Sciences University, Historical Collections and Archives, Portland, Oregon.

The liberation of Europe also freed American POWs, who, not surprisingly, had higher rates of tuberculosis than other American military personnel. Captured British medical officer Capt. A. L. Cochrane cared for some of them in the prison where he was confined and noted sardonically that imprisonment was "an excellent place to study tuberculosis; [and] to learn the vast importance of food in human health and happiness." German prison guards gave POWs only 1,000 to 1,500 calories per day, so Red Cross food parcels, which provided an additional 1,500 daily calories per person, were critical to preventing malnutrition and physical breakdown. Cochrane observed that the American and British POWs received the most parcels and had the lowest tuberculosis rates in the camp, while the Russians received nothing at all and had the highest rates. During the eighteen months that French POWs received the Red Cross parcels, he noted, just two men of 1,200 developed tuberculosis but when parcels for the French ceased to arrive in 1945, their tuberculosis rate rose to equal that of the Russians. The situation, he concluded, showed the "vast importance of nutrition in the incidence of tuberculosis."[102] Not all Americans got their parcels, though. William H. Balzer, with an American artillery unit, was captured in February 1943, and remembered how German guards stole the Americans' packages. He also described a half-hearted German effort to screen for tuberculosis in which medics X-rayed some of the prisoners, but "only two-hundred and some men, out of nearly two-thousand got this opportunity. And, the ones who got the X-ray, that was the last they heard of it." Balzer survived imprisonment but never recovered from the ordeal. Severely disabled (70 percent), he died in 1960 on his forty-sixth birthday.[103]

Exact tuberculosis rates among American POWs are not known because the rush of events surrounding the liberation of prisoners from German and Japanese control prevented a systematic X-ray survey. Rates did appear to be higher, though, for prisoners of the Japanese than for prisoners of the Germans. Long reported that about 0.6 percent of recovered troops from European POW camps had tuberculosis, whereas data from the Pacific theater suggested that 1 percent of recovered prisoners had tuberculosis. Moreover, an analysis of the chest X-rays done at West Coast debarkation hospitals revealed that 101 (or 2.7 percent) of 3,742 former POWs of the Japanese showed evidence of active tuberculosis.[104] John R. Bumgarner was a tuberculosis ward officer at Sternberg General Hospital in Manila, the Philippines, before the war. A POW for forty-two months after the Japanese invasion, he described his experience in *Parade of the Dead*.[105] Bumgarner did what he could to care for many of the 13,000 prisoners in the camp, but knew that "my patients were poorly diagnosed and poorly treated." The Japanese had an old X-ray machine with which he tried to identify and isolate tubercular prisoners in a makeshift hospital. But given the otherwise complete lack of staff and resources he worried that he would unknowingly put uninfected patients into the tuberculosis ward. The narrow cots were so close together, he wrote, "the crowding and the breathing of air loaded with this bacilliary miasma from coughing ensured that those mistakenly segregated would be infected."[106]

Bumgarner was able to stay relatively healthy throughout his imprisonment. His luck ended, however, because "on my way home across the Pacific I had the first symptoms of tuberculosis." Severe chest pain and subsequent X-rays at Letterman Hospital in San Francisco revealed active disease. "I had gone through more than four years of hell—now this!" Once back in the United States the Army Medical Department moved him from hospital to hospital, and he described the next three years as a story of "sad miscalculations by me and the Army Medical Corps." He was transferred from Letterman in San Francisco to a hospital in North Carolina, back west to Bruns in Santa Fe, New Mexico, then back to North Carolina, and finally to Fitzsimons in Denver, Colorado. By then, he wrote, "I felt I was the most traveled patient in the armed services." Discharged on disability for tuberculosis in September 1946 he began to work at the Medical College of Virginia but soon had a lung hemorrhage. This time it took eight years of rest, with surgery and new antibiotic treatment for him to recover. By 1956, however, Bumgarner had married his sweetheart, Evelyn, and begun a medical career in cardiology that lasted for thirty years.[107] He was more fortunate than James E. Neuman, who survived the Bataan Death March but after three years of imprisonment was starved from 170 to 92 pounds on his 6'2" frame and had tuberculosis of the lungs, throat, and stomach. Doctors at Bruns Hospital warned his parents that Neuman could not survive a trip home, but loathe to have their son die in the hospital, they arranged to fly him home to Fort Worth, Texas, where he was greeted as a hero before he died one week later at age twenty-five.[108]

Tuberculosis continued to take its toll on POWs for years after the war. The VA followed POWs as a special group because, explained Long, of "the hardships that many of these men endured, and the notorious tendency for tuberculosis to make its appearance years after the acquisition of infection."[109] A follow-up study published in 1954 reported that for American POWs during the six years after liberation tuberculosis was the second highest cause of death, after accidents.[110]

From Concentration Camp Prisoners To Sanatorium Patients

If the challenges Army medical personnel faced in caring for sick and starving POWs and refugees were unprecedented, the scale of disease and suffering they encountered in the Nazi concentration camps was almost unimaginable. Allied troops had heard about secret and deadly camps but were not prepared for what they found. As the Allies converged on Berlin from the East and the West, the Nazis evacuated thousands of prisoners—most of them Jews seized from across Europe, as well as POWs—to interior camps to hide their crimes and prevent the inmates from falling into Allied hands. These evacuations became death marches as SS (abbreviation of *Schutzstaffel,* which stood for "defense squadron") guards beat and murdered people, and failed to feed them for days on end. Survivors were crowded into camps such as Buchenwald and Dachau making them even more chaotic and deadly. Americans, therefore, liberated camps that were riven with disease, especially typhus, tuberculosis, and malnutrition.[111] An examination of Army Medical Department activities in one of these camps, Dachau, where evacuation hospitals spent the most time and confronted large numbers of people with tuberculosis and typhus, brings the American experience to light.

The Allies liberated Buchenwald on 11 April 1945. The following day the world learned that Franklin Roosevelt had died. Americans then liberated Dachau on 29 April, the day Italian partisans executed Mussolini in Milan, and the next day Hitler killed himself in his bunker. Dachau (Figure 8-5) had been the first of hundreds of concentration camps in the German Reich to which the Nazis sent political enemies, the disabled, people accused of socially deviant behavior, and, increasingly after the Kristallnacht pogroms of 1938, Jewish men, women, and children. In January 1945 Dachau held 67,000 prisoners, but with troops of the Seventh U.S. Army approaching the SS began evacuating and killing prisoners. Capt. Marcus J. Smith, a medical officer in his thirties, arrived at Dachau on 30 April 1945, the day after liberation, part of a small team trained to treat persons displaced by the war. Horror greeted him outside the camp in a train of forty boxcars loaded with more than two thousand corpses. Smith called the frost that had formed on the bodies in the intense cold, "Nature's shroud."[112] Inside Dachau he encountered more grotesque piles of naked, skeletal bodies of prisoners and scattered, mutilated bodies of German guards. His job, he wrote to his wife in Chicago, was to "survey the medical condition of the inmates, the medical facilities (and manpower), environmental conditions, such as waste disposal, water supply, living conditions, insect control, foodhandling, and anything else pertaining to health and sanitation."[113]

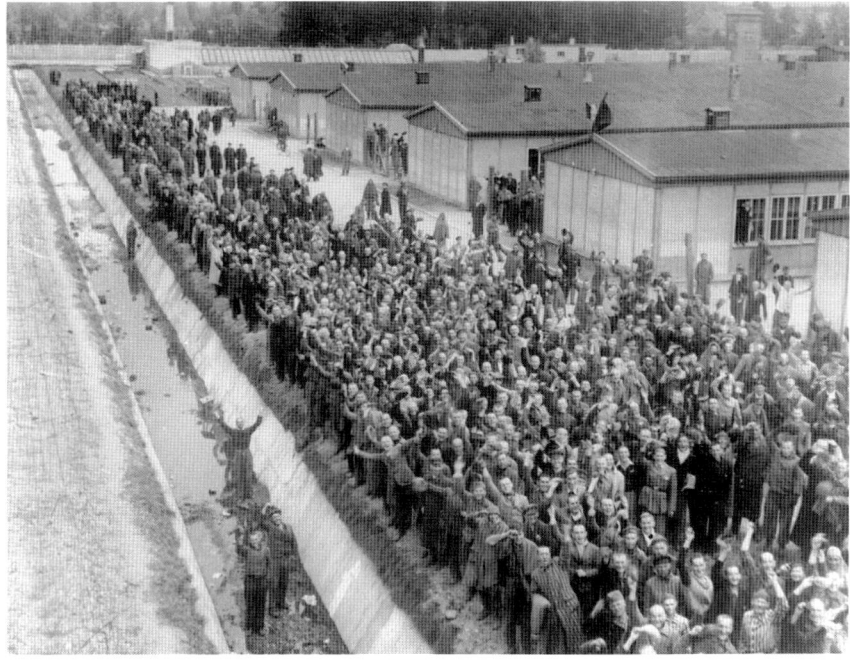

Figure 8-5. Dachau survivors gather by the moat to greet American liberators, 29 April 1945. Photograph courtesy of the United States Holocaust Memorial Museum, Washington, DC.

Smith found more than 30,000 prisoners, mostly Jews of forty nationalities, and all men except for about 300 women the SS had kept in a brothel. They were in desperate condition. Typhus and dysentery raged, at least half of the prisoners were starving, and hundreds had advanced tuberculosis. "The well, the sick, the dying, and the dead lie next to each other in these poorly ventilated, unheated, dark, stinking buildings," Smith told his wife. The men were "malnourished and emaciated, their diseases in all stages of development: early, late, and terminal."[114] He wondered, "What am I going to write in my notebook?" and then started a list of needed supplies: clothes, shoes, socks, towels, bedding, beds, soap, toilet paper, more latrines, and new quarters. He almost despaired. "What are we going to do with the starving patients? How will we care for them without sterile bandages, gloves, bedpans, urinals, thermometers, and all the basic material? How do we manage without an organization? No interns, no nursing staff, no ambulances, no bathtubs, no laboratories, no charts, and no orderlies, no administrator, and no doctors.... I feel helpless and empty. I cannot think of anything like this in modern medical history."[115]

What Americans such as Marcus Smith did in the weeks following the liberation of the camps is little known, eclipsed by histories of the Nazi regime and the postwar sagas of camp survivors building new lives. The reference to the days before liberation as the "Last Days" of Dachau or Buchenwald is a misnomer, though, because the suffering did not end. Thousands of prisoners who had survived the camps would die just days after liberation; thousands more spent months in the hospital; for others it was a time for revenge, grief, joy, hope, fear for the future, or all combined. The Army Medical Department mission was both altruistic and self-interested. At risk to their own health, Americans provided life-saving care for thousands of victims, but they also wanted and needed to prevent the liberated prisoners from spreading disease to Allied troops and civilians throughout Europe. Not all of their policies and practices were welcome. Prisoner-patients were suspicious or fearful of many medical practices and resented quarantines that deprived them of their liberty. American efforts did prevent a deadly typhus epidemic from sweeping postwar Europe and helped contain tuberculosis rates in Germany, but the Nazis had created a human catastrophe so immense that even the most dedicated efforts would at times fall short.

Faced with horror on such a scale, Smith and other Army Medical Department personnel assigned to the concentration camps threw themselves into the work of cleansing, comforting, treating, and nurturing their patients. American commanders called in at least six Army evacuation hospitals (EH) to care for the sick and dying in the liberated camps. EH No. 116 and EH No. 127 began arriving at Dachau on 2 May with some forty medical officers, forty nurses, and 220 enlisted men.[116] Consulting with Smith and his team, the units set up in the former SS guard barracks. They tore out partitions to create larger wards, scrubbed the walls and floors with Cresol solution, sprayed them with dichloro-diphenyl-trichloroethane (DDT), and then set up cots to create two hospitals of 1,200 beds each. Medical staff also discovered physician-prisoners who had cared for the sick and injured as well as they could, and could now advise and assist, and in some cases translate for the medical staff. Other able-bodied prisoners worked in the barracks as well. In two days the hospitals were ready to admit patients by triage, segregating them by disease and prognosis. Laurence Ball, the EH No. 116 commander, noted that more than 900 patients had "two or more diseases, such as malnutrition, typhus, diarrhea, and tuberculosis."[117] Staff bathed and deloused them, gave them clean pajamas, and put them to bed.

The prisoner-patients' reactions to their American doctors and nurses ran from joy and gratitude to terror and resentment. Many were too ill to respond or were shocked beyond belief that they were actually free (Figure 8-6). Witnesses described how some inmates were in a daze, oblivious to the dead bodies around them.[118] Elizabeth May Craig, a *Portland News Herald* reporter, described the scene as she walked through a ward of 110 beds in EH No. 116. "Rows of skeletons, shaved heads, great eyes looking at you; a few able to stagger around.... Some are huddled completely under drab blankets; they look like little children, they are so emaciated. Some lie in stupor; they are far gone, or the high temperatures of typhus, as much as 105, hold them."[119] Some patients, she wrote, "are frightened and will not take treatment."[120] Another observer wrote of "prisoners who could not get it through their heads that things had changed, who hid in terror at sight of the uniform."[121] Some resisted showers, perhaps fearing the gas chamber, while others were terrified of hypodermics of penicillin because Nazi doctors had at times executed inmates by injection.

While the hospitals were setting up, other personnel provided food to the malnourished prisoners. But starving people cannot eat too much too soon without danger, and some individuals had no internal regulator. Dachau survivor Nerin Gun, a Turkish journalist in Budapest arrested by the Nazis for reporting on the concentration camps, observed with horrible irony that some inmates "died of over eating because they had gorged on the cans of Spam the generous American soldiers had—open handedly but unwisely—given them."[122] Aware of this problem, medical personnel warned against overeating and at first provided thin soup, then military rations, food from the SS larder, and "French pasteurized milk." One of the Americans' joys at Dachau was to watch people fill out and regain their strength after a week or two of adequate nutrition. By the end of May an Army nutritionist arrived with one million frozen eggs, which were kept under guard and would feed the camp for forty days.[123]

Death by overeating was but one of the dangers that the prisoners faced. The physician-prisoners warned the Americans that "nearly all of the inmates had

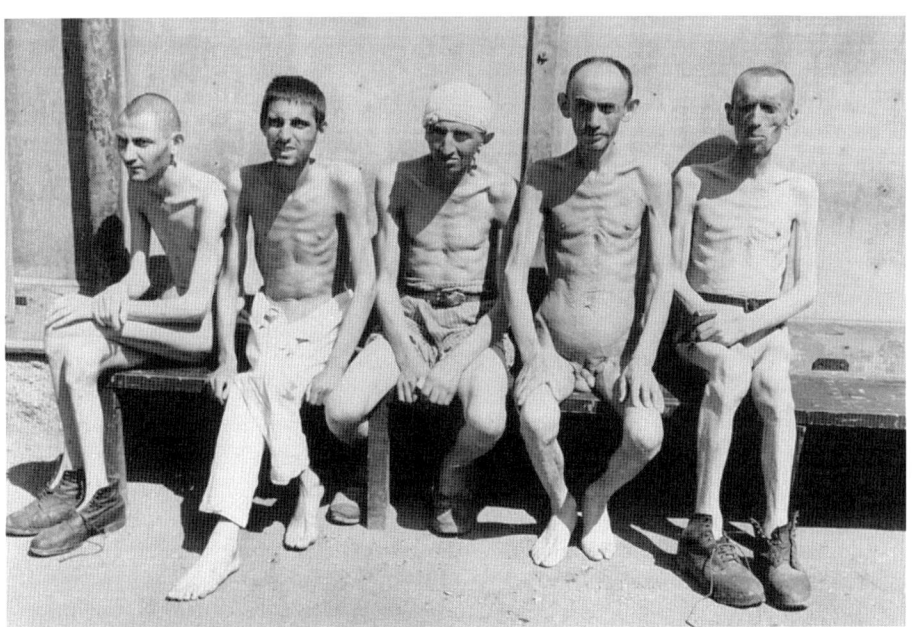

Figure 8-6. Survivors in Dachau, 1 May 1945.
Photograph courtesy of the United States Holocaust Memorial Museum, Washington, DC.

typhus, and contact with them must be avoided."[124] During May 1945, American hospitals at Dachau had more than 4,000 typhus patients and lost 2,226 to typhus and other diseases.[125] Typhus, a rickettsial disease transmitted by body lice, had a mortality rate as high as 40 percent. With no medical cure, treatment consisted of supportive care—keeping patients clean and nourished—to mitigate effects of prolonged fever, such as the breakdown of tissue into gangrene.[126] The Americans knew that typhus had taken three million lives in Eastern Europe after World War I, but now they had a means of prevention and better weapons—a typhus vaccine and DDT. On 2 May, the day the evacuation hospitals arrived, the commander of the Seventh Army imposed quarantines for typhus and tuberculosis, and summoned the U.S. Typhus Commission, which had controlled a typhus outbreak in Naples, Italy. A typhus team arrived the next day and began to immunize American personnel and dust them with DDT. On 7 May staff began to vaccinate inmates but kept typhus patients isolated for at least twenty-one days from the onset of illness to prevent transmission to others.[127] This meant that the Americans did not immediately enter the inner camp barracks—the worst, most typhus-infested part of the camp—nor did they quickly relieve crowding there for fear of spreading typhus-bearing lice. It took over a week for personnel to prepare more spacious and clean quarters. Inmates were bewildered and angry to find that they could not leave. One survivor wrote, "Liberation was merely a changing of the guard."[128]

Starving people could be fed and restored, lice could be controlled, and people with typhus either lived or died, but the management of tuberculosis was not so simple.[129] When the Nazis took office in 1933 they had set the eradication of tuberculosis as one of their highest goals, but in 1938, after public education efforts failed to control the disease, the government began to authorize the confinement of tuberculous people, sending many of them to concentration camps.[130] Ironically, instead of eradicating tuberculosis, the Nazi regime created ideal environments for tuberculosis to thrive in the concentration camps. As Army medical officer Abner Zehm wrote, "The conditions under which the prisoners lived were conducive in every way to the development and spread of tuberculosis."[131] Malnutrition, heavy labor, and harsh treatment activated tuberculosis in thousands of other prisoners and the intense crowding and lack of ventilation ensured its dissemination.

Shocked and frightened by the disease and suffering they saw, American medics redoubled their efforts. Medical officer Maj. E. G. Lipow of Montana methodically conducted triage in the dirty, crowded, lice-ridden barracks, deciding who should and who should not go to the hospital. "I take the sickest, who have a chance to live," he told a reporter.[132] Smith wrote his lists, reported to his wife, and kept track of the daily death toll, finding comfort as the number of people who died daily fell from 200 during the first week to twenty by the end of May. Another medical officer performed autopsies. He chose ten of the dead bodies, five from the death train and five from the camp yard, to see what had caused their deaths. All had typhus and extreme malnutrition, eight had advanced tuberculosis, and some bodies had signs of fractures and head injuries.[133]

Survivors held vivid memories of the Americans. Steve Ross, a Polish Jew, survived ten concentration camps between 1940 and 1945 before he was liberated at age fourteen. He had been one of 1,800 prisoners living in barracks for about 100 people, isolated by Nazi doctors for medical experiments. The guards had stopped feeding them two weeks before liberation, so when the Americans arrived, Ross called them "God's Army." "I was so overwhelmed with joy and happiness when I saw such strong men who had saved my life." Sick and starving, "hospitalization," he remembered, "was the first English word I learned."[134] Ross spent six months in the hospital for tuberculosis and later immigrated to the United States, becoming a psychologist in Boston. Nerin Gun, the Turkish journalist, called the arrival of American soldiers, "The Gift" and described the first soldier who walked into the compound as "upright, stalwart, unafraid…the very incarnation of the American hero."[135] But Gun deeply resented the quarantine. "The drastic measures taken by the Americans to arrest the epidemic seemed unfair to us at the time.…not only could we not leave the camp but we were restricted to our own barracks, the healthy along with the sick. We were still sleeping two or three to a palette or on the ground; the food was still horrible."[136] Closing the camp was "an idiotic precaution," and prisoners got out anyway. "Even if we had spread a few germs among those good, kind, handsome Germans, would that have been such a catastrophe?"[137]

By the end of May, conditions at Dachau had improved. Typhus was abating and American officials began to release groups of inmates by nationality. Beyond Dachau, the U.S. Typhus Commission tracked down new cases of typhus in civilian and military populations, deloused one million people, sprayed fifteen tons of DDT, and created a *cordon sanitaire* on the Rhine requiring all who crossed from Germany to be vaccinated and dusted to prevent the spread of disease. Thus the Army averted a broader typhus epidemic.[138] The tuberculosis situation was more complicated and presented the Americans with a conundrum. What to do with thousands of people suffering from a long-term, infectious, and deadly disease? Tuberculosis treatment required months, if not years, of bed rest. When EH No. 127 medical officer A. D. Piatt analyzed X-rays of 2,267 Dachau patients, he found that more than 30 percent of them had signs of tuberculosis, and predicted that tuberculosis incidence would increase in Europe "as a result of the return of numerous persons with undiagnosed active disease from concentration camps to their homes."[139]

Esmond Long arrived in the European theater in April 1945, and following tuberculosis, traveled in May to Buchenwald and Dachau. He believed that the prognosis for most tuberculosis patients was poor and that those who did recover would require long-term care. Such long-range care, he told the Surgeon General, "cannot be accepted as a responsibility of the U.S. Army. It will have fulfilled its mission when it has effected a suitable transfer for continued care." The best course would be to return patients to their native homes, but given their weak condition and the postwar situation, that was impossible. In line with the War Department approach to caring for Allied POWs and refugees, Long recommended that non-American medical staff assume responsibility for providing care and that German physicians "who have proper training and recognize a medical obligation" be employed. He also identified a German hospital in a nearby town that, supplied with Army laboratory facilities and equipment, could serve as a sanatorium. "Blankenheim hospital," he concluded, "all things considered, offers a satisfactory solution to the problem."[140] One can imagine, however, that some former concentration camp internees were appalled by the idea of being sent to a German hospital and cared for by German staff.

As with the American POWs, tuberculosis continued to follow Dachau survivors into their new lives. Thousands of Jewish survivors emigrated to what would become the state of Israel. Fifteen years after liberation, the Israeli Minister of Health reported that although concentration camp survivors comprised only 25 percent of the population, they accounted for 65 percent of the tuberculosis cases in the country.[141] Tuberculosis continued to thrive in Europe as well.

Aftermath

Army Medical Department responsibilities did not end with the Allied defeat of Germany and Japan but involved caring for war casualties for many more months and years. The tuberculosis problem, in fact, increased in some ways with demobilization, posing three challenges: (1) high rates of tuberculosis in postwar Germany threatened to spread it to U.S. occupation troops; (2) separation X-rays of soldiers as they demobilized revealed thousands of cases of tuberculosis, generating the upward surge on the "U" curve in tuberculosis patients in Army and VA hospitals; and (3) in their eagerness to get home, many tubercular veterans left government hospitals while still contagious, risking the spread of the disease to their families and communities. None of this surprised Long and his colleagues, but all of the issues required government resources and thoughtfully crafted policies.

Tuberculosis had thrived during the war years. Before Hitler invaded Poland, Germany's tuberculosis death rate had been among the lowest in Europe, fewer than 60 per 100,000, but during the war it increased dramatically, peaking in 1945–46 at 260 per 100,000 in the city of Berlin.[142] Tuberculosis rates increased in other major European cities as well. Amsterdam, with the lowest prewar rate, increased from 35 to 83 deaths per 100,000; London, which had a well-organized antituberculosis program under the British National Health Service, went from 60 to 100 per 100,000; Rome from 84 to 188; Vienna from 109 to 257; and in the worst situation of all Europe—a consequence of the Nazi regime—Warsaw tuberculosis death rates rose from 155 to 500 per 100,000 during the war.[143] American journalist Edward P. Morgan wrote ominously that "the dread white plague, spawned and spread for a decade in German concentration camps, is increasing and it threatens to do more lasting damage than any other one disease." In the "bedlam of liberation," former prisoners were spreading the germs to the outside world, so that "the Germans cannot say in truth that they never employed germ warfare," he declared. "The delayed-action spread of tuberculosis will probably do more damage to Europe than could have been done by any horror bomb load of bacilli."[144]

Long more temperately characterized the post-World War II tuberculosis situation in Germany as "a grave public health problem" due to "unmistakable evidence that the incidence of the disease, and its mortality, are rising."[145] He attributed the increase to the breakdown of public health programs during the war, the use of tuberculous persons in war industries, the importation of laborers from conquered countries with little or no health screening, and the virtual incubation of tuberculosis in the concentration camps. Now that U.S. troops were in Germany, Long pursued recommendations by Badger and others to develop a comprehensive plan to monitor and control the disease in civilian and military populations. The first step, which he had in some ways instituted at Dachau, was to restore the German public health infrastructure so that it could assume responsibility for tuberculosis control and care of patients. This process was part of the larger American effort to locate experienced medical and public health personnel (under the denazification rules aimed at excluding former Nazi officials) so they could care for the displaced persons. The program then focused on identifying, isolating, and treating people with active disease.[146]

After his 1947 visit to Germany, Long recounted a case that illustrates the suffering and heartache tuberculosis could cause. A routine chest X-ray examination had found an American soldier in the early stages of tuberculosis, and after a few months in the hospital he returned to active duty. Working in Heidelberg, Long wrote, the soldier "was intimate at this time with a young Polish girl and applied for permission to marry her." Under Occupation Forces rules medical personnel gave the young woman a physical examination, including a chest X-ray, and discovered advanced tuberculosis, so "permission to marry was refused." The couple, however, arranged for a healthy woman to be X-rayed in her place at another Army installation, and with a clean bill of health the couple married. Medical personnel discovered the falsified X-ray when the newlywed woman fell seriously ill and was hospitalized in Frankfurt. They also found that her husband's tuberculosis had flared, and the sick young man was court-martialed and dishonorably discharged for his deceit. The young woman, wrote Long, "remained in the hospital, a case with poor prognosis."[147]

Long assessed the situation in Germany annually for years after the war and although tuberculosis rates for American troops in Germany were higher than those of Army personnel elsewhere, by 1948 they had returned to prewar levels in most of the American Zone except for Berlin, where high levels persisted.[148] Historian Albert Cowdrey has credited the American actions with preventing a number of postwar scourges: "No one can prove that a great typhus epidemic, mass deaths of prisoners of war, or widespread outbreaks of disease among the German population would have taken place without the efforts of Army doctors of the field forces and the military government." But, he continued, "conditions were ripe for such tragedies to occur, and Army medics brought both professional knowledge and military discipline to forestalling what might have been the last calamities of the war in Europe."[149] Thus, as usual, in public health the good news is no news at all.

In the United States the Army Medical Department also contended with increased tuberculosis rates, due not to an epidemic in the Army, but rather the systematic X-ray examination of all personnel as they separated from military service. These exams found about one in every 1,000 individuals had lung changes suggestive of tuberculosis, products of the cumulative effects of the stresses of war, the extended length of service for many troops, and/or exposure to tuberculosis overseas.[150] Having survived the war and preparing to return home, it must have been a terrible shock for these men and women to be detained or even disabled by a disease. A case in point is that of Lt. Col. Douglas Treat Davidson, Jr., a medical officer in the 101st Airborne Division who parachuted into Normandy on 6 June 1944 and received the Silver Star for courage in action for saving the lives of twenty wounded men. Injured during the Battle of the Bulge, Davidson recovered to celebrate the Allied victory. Upon his discharge examination, however, X-rays revealed tuberculosis and Davidson was hospitalized for eight months. Although he recovered enough to return to his medical practice, the war hero died eighteen years later from cancer and complications of tuberculosis.[151]

Catching people with tuberculosis before they returned home and could spread it to their loved ones was a key part of the Army Medical Department's strategy. One of Long's innovations was the careful storage and coordination of X-ray films, so that radiologists could compare individuals' induction films to their separation X-ray films and more easily detect any changes. The VA took over all X-ray films for filing and storage, and to assist in determining benefit claims for the veterans.[152] Long seized these pairs of X-rays (4 x 5 inch induction films and 14 x 17 inch separation films) as an opportunity to study the development of tuberculosis in a wartime army. The study, conducted with statistician Seymour Jablon and published in 1955, examined 6,000 randomly selected sets of X-rays and found that although educational background and civilian occupation did not impact the tuberculosis rate, medical personnel had above average rates, "which might well have been due to excessive exposure in the occupation itself," they wrote. Long and Jablon also concluded that both endogenous and exogenous sources caused the tuberculosis, that is, some soldiers developed active cases from their own latent infections and some were infected by others. They also noted that one-half of the men discharged for tuberculosis most likely had the disease when they entered the service, which underscored Long's recommendation that induction films be read by two radiologists to improve accuracy.[153]

The separation examinations discovered so many cases of tuberculosis that in January 1946 the Army designated Moore General Hospital in North Carolina, which at the time was repatriating many of its POW patients, as a center for patients with minimal tuberculosis or a good prognosis[154] (Figure 8-7). Acutely aware of the post-World War I experience, VA officials also sought to prepare for the onslaught of tuberculous veterans.[155] Maj. Gen. Paul R. Hawley, chief of medical services in the European theater, became chief medical director at the VA after the war. Given that the peak year for treating tuberculous veterans after World War I was 1922 when 44,951 patients had accounted for 43 percent of all hospitalized veterans, Hawley called for 15,000 additional tuberculosis beds by

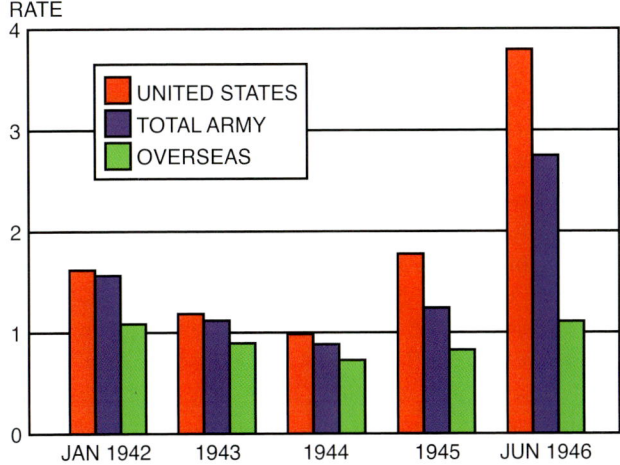

Figure 8-7. Chart showing the incidence of tuberculosis among U.S. Army troops in the United States and overseas, January 1942 to June 1946. In Esmond R. Long, "Tuberculosis," in John Boyd Coates, Robert S. Anderson, and W. Paul Havens, eds., *Internal Medicine in World War II, Medical Department, U.S. Army in World War II*, vol. 2, *Infectious Diseases* (Washington, DC: Office of the Surgeon General, Department of the Army; 1961), 336.

his predicted peak year of 1950.[156] The Federal Board of Hospitalization therefore oversaw the establishment of twenty-one VA hospitals for tuberculous veterans, enabling the government to avoid the overcrowding and public outcry of World War I. By 1950 the VA had reached Hawley's goal of 15,000 beds, and in 1954 was caring for almost 16,000 tuberculosis patients.[157]

But tuberculosis hospitals alone would not solve the problem. Patient behavior and morale threatened to undermine Army and VA control efforts. When Long inspected Moore Hospital in February 1946 he found poor morale among some patients who "resent their retention in the Army, at a time when they are feeling well and were about to be discharged."[158] But, he wrote to a colleague, the problem of poor morale "is a general one, not limited to tuberculosis. It arises in all diseases in which there is temporary complete disability for military service, but excellent prospect of full recovery within a few years."[159] Before the war, Fitzsimons' commander Col. Buck had complained that financial incentives encouraged veterans to leave the hospital before they were well. Receiving a monthly disability stipend, discharged tuberculosis patients could live in the Denver area and come to Fitzsimons for pneumothorax refills as outpatients. But, noted Buck, "they are not under constant supervision and cannot be trusted to observe the controlled life, including rest periods and proper food that is so essential to satisfactory progress in collapse therapy."[160] This problem persisted during the war. Col. Frederick Wright at Fitzsimons told an inspector that "the Army is discharging patients with open tuberculosis into the civil population."[161] Despite the

War Department's requirement that Army installations discharging men with tuberculosis advise the health departments of the men's home states, the Medical Department observed that "many stations failed to comply with this regulation." The Maryland Department of Health advised the Office of The Surgeon General that when it received a list of 123 names of veterans with tuberculosis, only fifty of them included information on their whereabouts.[162]

In June 1943 Louis Dublin, renowned statistician for the Metropolitan Life Insurance Company, went public with the problem when he told American Legion officers and a VA administrator that while private and state tuberculosis programs had been effective, "under the Veterans Administration it has been almost altogether a failure." Dublin noted that of more than 9,800 tuberculosis discharges in 1942 only 3 percent had left the VA with the disease "arrested," "apparently arrested," or "quiescent." The remaining cases were discharged from the hospital as "condition improved" (33 percent), "condition unimproved" (29 percent), "condition not stated" (16 percent), or deceased (19 percent).[163] In a series of articles published in 1943 and 1944 Dublin said the problem was that VA hospital patients were not subject to the same kind of discipline as in military institutions. Veteran patients "may come and go almost at will, irrespective of their condition and against medical advice. Six to eight admissions of the same patient are a frequent occurrence," he wrote. Forty percent of VA tuberculosis patients left against medical advice, and those who stayed were allowed a five-day furlough by law each month. Tuberculous veterans, he said, "have spread infection not only to their immediate families but to the larger circle of civilians with whom they have been in contact for longer or for shorter periods." Dublin also cited the "monetary incentive for discontinuing hospital treatment." Veterans discharged from the hospital received $70 to $100 per month, depending on the degree of disability, compared to only $8 to $20 per month as hospital patients, or the government paid $50 a month for a wife or other family member to care for a tuberculous veteran at home. Significantly, Dublin did not blame the VA. "The chief difficulty, in my judgment, has been the lack of appreciation on the part of Congress and of others interested in veterans' welfare, of certain fundamental conditions necessary for the effective treatment of tuberculosis." Therefore, he asserted, "the monetary incentives which have [wreaked] havoc with care of the men in tuberculosis hospitals should certainly be removed."[164] He called for isolating tuberculous veterans, canceling the five-day furloughs, improving case reporting to local authorities, hospitalizing veterans closer to home so that families could visit, and making hospital care more appealing.[165]

In response to such criticisms, the VA and the American Legion developed cooperative plans for follow up and treatment of tuberculous veterans once they left Army and VA hospitals.[166] The Wisconsin Anti-Tuberculosis Association publicized the problem in newspapers and magazines, established a speakers bureau, and issued a pamphlet educating the public on the dangers of discharging men before they were cured.[167] Such efforts were far from successful. Given the political sensitivity of holding veterans against their will, federal facilities would not institute stricter measures until the 1950s and 1960s when medical professionals and scientists, as well as veterans and their families, the general public, and elected officials more fully appreciated the nature and danger of tuberculosis transmission. The effect of all of these factors on tuberculosis rates in the United States was, thankfully, muted. Tuberculosis rates in the country did not increase during the 1940s, but wartime conditions did cause the rate of decrease to almost level off during the decade.[168]

But if World War II did not bring great improvements in the treatment and control of tuberculosis, it did transform American medicine in other ways. One scholar credits military medicine during the war for creating a postwar demand by Americans for a higher level of medical care than they were accustomed to.[169] World War II also dramatically increased federal government expenditures for basic biomedical research and accelerated the dominance of specialization in medical education and treatment. One reason for this increased support for and belief in medicine was that it was becoming more effective. Diseases transmitted by insects, especially mosquito-borne malaria in the Pacific theater and louse-borne typhus in the European theater, troubled all armies, but American employment of quinine derivatives and DDT in the Pacific, and sanitation, immunization, and DDT in Europe, dramatically reduced disease incidence.[170] Faster medical transport, blood plasma, and improved surgical techniques reduced death from battle wounds to below 5 percent. In addition to immunizing trainees against centuries-old plagues such as smallpox, typhoid, paratyphoid, tetanus, typhus, yellow fever, cholera, and plague, medical personnel now began to cure other bacterial infections. During the 1930s, researchers found that sulfa drugs were effective against streptococcus and other wound-infecting germs that killed millions of soldiers over the centuries, so in the 1940s soldiers carried individual first aid packets that contained sulfa powder and tablets. An injured man could sprinkle an open wound with the powder, cover it, and/or take the tablets even before he arrived at a first aid station.[171] Then came penicillin, effective against a broad spectrum of bacteria, from wound infections to sexually transmitted diseases. At first in short supply, the United States began mass-producing penicillin during the war and by late 1943 Gen. Hawley authorized penicillin for general hospitals in the European theater for life-threatening or persistent infections.[172] "The inoculating syringe and the insect repellent spray became secret weapons, providing our troops an important increased operating range," wrote George Darling, a member of the National Research Council's Division of Medical Sciences, when he later described World War II medicine. "The stories of penicillin, of blood plasma, of DDT and of the use of quinacrine (atabrine) in malaria, to name a few, are among the modern romances of medicine."[173]

The story of the discovery of a cure for tuberculosis is less romantic than that of penicillin or blood plasma. Neither sulfa drugs nor penicillin made a dent in tuberculosis, and there was no single "Aha!" moment in discovering a cure. Like everything else with tuberculosis, it was complicated and the development of an effective cure slogged on for a decade. But again, the Army Medical Department, with its specialized hospitals, expert tuberculosis physicians, nurses, and other personnel, and thousands of tuberculosis sufferers, was at the center of the action.

Notes

1. Marcus J. Smith, *The Harrowing of Hell: Dachau* (Albuquerque, NM: University of New Mexico Press, 1972), 6.
2. Biographical information on Long is drawn from Peter C. Nowell and Louis B. Delpino, "Esmond R. Long, June 16, 1890–November 11, 1979," *National Academy of Sciences, Biographical Memoirs* 56 (1987): 285–310.
3. John T. Greenwood and F. Clifton Berry Jr., *Medics at War: Military Medicine from Colonial Times to the 21st Century* (Annapolis, MD: Naval Institute Press, 2005), 113.
4. Only 26,309 soldiers died of their wounds of the 599,724 wounded in action, a 4.4 percent death rate. Frank A. Reister, U.S. Army Medical Department Historical Unit and U.S. Department of the Army, Office of The Surgeon General, *Medical Statistics in World War II, Medical Department, U.S. Army in World War II* (Washington, DC: U.S. Department of Defense, Department of the Army, Office of The Surgeon General, 1975 [hereafter cited as Reister, *Medical Statistics*]), 6–11.
5. During 1942–45, 28,395 of 2,967,246 admissions, according to Reister, *Medical Statistics*, 37–38. Also on military medicine during World War II, see the Medical Department series, especially Graham A. Cosmas and Albert E. Cowdrey, *The Medical Department: Medical Service in the European Theater of Operations,* World War II, 50th Anniversary commemorative ed., *U.S. Army in World War II* (Washington, DC: Center of Military History, 1992); Morris Fishbein, ed., *Doctors at War* (New York, NY: E. P. Dutton and Company, 1945); Albert E. Cowdrey, *Fighting for Life: American Military Medicine in World War II* (New York, NY: Free Press, 1994); and Mary Sarnecky, *A History of the Army Nurse Corps* (Philadelphia, PA: University of Pennsylvania Press, 1999).
6. Arthur S. McNalty, "Tuberculosis in Peace and War," *Tubercle* 23 (1942): 266.
7. Reister, *Medical Statistics*, 37.
8. On tuberculosis in wartime, see Matthew Smallman-Raynor and Andrew D. Cliff, "War and Disease: Some Perspectives on the Spatial and Temporal Occurrence of Tuberculosis in Wartime," in Matthew Gandy and Alimuddin Zumla, eds. *The Return of the White Plague: Global Poverty and the 'New' Tuberculosis* (London, UK: Verso, 2003).
9. Esmond R. Long, chap. 11, "Tuberculosis," in U.S. Army Medical Service, John Boyd Coates, Robert S. Anderson, and W. Paul Havens, eds., *Internal Medicine in World War II, Medical Department, U.S. Army in World War II*, vol. 2, *Infectious Diseases* (Washington, DC: Office of The Surgeon General, Department of the Army; 1961 [hereafter cited as Long, "Tuberculosis"]), 331–39.

10. *Annual Report of the Surgeon General,* 1941 (hereafter cited as *ARSG,* year), 2; and Clarence McKittrick Smith, *The Medical Department: Hospitalization and Evacuation, Zone of the Interior,* Kent Roberts Greenfield, ed. *U.S. Army in World War II* (Washington, DC: Office of the Chief of Military History, Department of the Army, 1956); and Leonard Rowntree, "Fit To Fight: The Medical Side of Selective Service," in Fishbein, ed., *Doctors at War,* 46–47.

11. Elias Huzar, *The Purse and the Sword: Control of Army by Congress through Military Appropriations, 1933–1950* (Ithaca, NY: Cornell University Press, 1950), 157–58.

12. C. S. Stephenson, Memorandum, Subcommittee on Tuberculosis, 24 July 1940, Record Group 52, Records of the Bureau of Medicine and Surgery [hereafter cited as RG 52], Entry 494, Box 6, National Archives and Records Administration [hereafter cited as NARA].

13. Long, "Tuberculosis," 331.

14. Benjamin Goldberg, "Presidential Address: War and Tuberculosis," *Diseases of the Chest* 7 (October 1941): 322–25. Louis Dublin said this figure was for 200,000 people, in "The Problem of the Tuberculous Veteran," *Diseases of the Chest* 10 (1944): 151.

15. Frank Walton Burge, "The Tuberculosis Problem in the Mobilization of Military and Naval Personnel," *Diseases of the Chest* 7 (1941): 20.

16. Robert S. Anderson and William B. Foster, U.S. Army Medical Service, U.S. Department of the Army, Office of The Surgeon General and U.S. Army Medical Service Historical Unit. *Physical Standards in World War II, Medical Department, U.S. Army in World War II.* (Washington, DC: Office of The Surgeon General, Department of the Army; 1967 [hereafter cited as Anderson and Foster, *Physical Standards*]), 31.

17. On X-ray technology see Ramsay Spillman, "The Value of Radiography in Detecting Tuberculosis in Recruits," *Journal of the American Medical Association* 115 (19 October 1940): 1371–79; Herman E. Hilleboe, "Opportunities in the Newer Methods of Tuberculosis Case Finding," *Public Health Reports* 58 (16 July 1943): 1094–1101; Alfred A. de Lorimier, "Army X-ray Examinations of the Chest," *Army Medical Department Bulletin* 61 (April 1942): 68–74; and Esmond R. Long and Seymour Jablon, *Tuberculosis in the Army of the United States in World War II: An Epidemiological Study with an Evaluation of X-ray Screening* (Washington, DC: GPO, 1955).

18. For example, C. M. Hendricks to Charles C. Hillman, 6 May 1941, RG 112, Entry 29, 1941–42, Box 241, NARA; and Cloyd M. Chapman to Charles Hillman, 28 September 1939, RG 112, Entry 29, 1938–40, Box 66, NARA.

19. Elias E. Cooley, "Routine Chest X-ray of Overseas Replacements," *Army Medical Department Bulletin* 38 (1937): 55–58.

20. W. Paul Havens, *Activities of Medical Consultants, Internal Medicine in World War II,* Leonard D. Heaton, ed., *Medical Department, U.S. Army in World War II,* vol. 1 (Washington, DC: Office of The Surgeon General, Department of the Army, 1961 [hereafter cited as Havens, *Medical Consultants*]), 403; and Charles C. Hillman, "The Tuberculosis Problem in the Army," *Diseases of the Chest* 9 (May–June 1943): 265–68.

21. Charles Hillman to F. S. Wright, 2 September 1941, RG 112, Entry 29, 1938–44, Box 205, NARA.

22. Mobilization Regulations 1–9, 15 March 1942, in Anderson and Foster, *Physical Standards,* 33.

Sources on tuberculosis screening during World War II include Long, "Tuberculosis"; Anderson and Foster, *Physical Standards,* 30–36, and an unpublished manuscript, Esmond R. Long, "Exclusion of Tuberculosis: Physical Standards for Induction and Appointment," RG 112, Entry 54-A, Box 453, NARA. See also Tamara M. Haygood and Jonathan E. Briggs. "World War II Military Led the Way in Screening Chest Radiography," *Military Medicine* 157 (1992): 113–16; and David C. Wheeler, "Physical Standards in Allied and Enemy Armies during World War II," *Military Medicine* (1965): 899–916.

23. Citing Spillman in Long, "Tuberculosis," 332.

24. Joseph R. Darnall and V. I. Cooper, *What Every Citizen Should Know About Wartime Medicine*, The Citizen Series (New York, NY: W. W. Norton, 1942), 161.

25. Thomas Parran, "Tuberculosis Control Program of the U.S. Public Health Service," *Journal of the American Medical Association* 121 (13 February 1943): 520–21; Thomas Parran, "The USPHS [U.S. Public Health Service] in War," in Fishbein, *Doctors at War*; Herman E. Hilleboe, "Tuberculosis Control in Action During Wartime," *Transactions of the National Tuberculosis Association* 38 and 39 (1942–43): 144–49; Herman E. Hilleboe and David M. Gould, "Tuberculous Control in Industry," *Diseases of the Chest* 11 (1945): 278–81.

The subcommittee debated whether the Public Health Service and induction boards should report the names of individuals found to have active tuberculosis to their local public health boards. Some members were concerned about stigmatizing individuals with apparently healed tuberculosis, but, Long observed, "There is no harm in telling a man the truth unless it be in relation to 'mental deficiency.' [The] apparently healed label shouldn't do any harm." "Notes on Conference of the Subcommittee on Tuberculosis of the National Research Council, 15 June 1942," RG 52, Entry 494, Box 6, NARA.

26. Coriss J. Williams, "The Tuberculous Registrant," *American Journal of Nursing* 41 (September 1942): 988.

See also "Problems of Personnel in Tuberculosis Sanatoriums," *Journal of the American Medical Association* 123 (11 September 1943): 97; Mapheus Smith, Lester T. Reynolds, and M. Ethel Hand, "Tuberculosis among Selective Service Registrants," *American Review of Tuberculosis* 60 (1949): 773–87; and Arden Freer, "Occurrence of Pulmonary Tuberculosis in Supposedly Screened Selectees," *Diseases of the Chest* 10 (May–June, 1944): 197–209.

27. Greenwood and Berry, *Medics at War*, 84. Men were not allowed in the Army Nurse Corps and women were not allowed in the Medical Corps until 1943, when Congress authorized commissions for women physicians and scientists to make up a shortfall in medical officers. Male corpsmen usually served nearer the front lines than nurses but women in the Women's Army Corps also served as dietitians, physical therapists, and scientists.

28. Frank Hines to Henry Stimson, 12 June 1942, RG 112, Entry 29, 1941–42, Box 93, NARA.

29. G. F. Aycock to Esmond Long, 6 May 1944, Esmond Long Papers, Box I, Military History Institute, Carlisle, PA.

30. Long, "Tuberculosis," 335–36.

31. Smith, Reynolds, and Hand, "Tuberculosis among Selective Service Registrants," 773; and Long, "Tuberculosis," 332.

32. Long and Jablon, *Tuberculosis in the Army*, 84; and E. R. Long et al, "Experiences with Dual Reading of Chest Photoroentgenograms," *U.S. Armed Forces Medical Journal* 7 (April 1956): 493–515.

33. This broke out annually to 24 in 1942; 4,643 in 1943; 3,533 in 1944; and 4,811 in 1945. See Long, "Tuberculosis," 331–39.

34. Marietta, "Tuberculosis in World War II," 268.

35. Greenwood and Berry, *Medics at War*, 92.

36. Greenwood and Berry, *Medics at War*, 103.

37. Long, "Tuberculosis," 357–64; and Alphonse E. Timpanelli, "Tuberculosis in the Southwest Pacific Theater," RG 112, Entry 54-A, Box 365, NARA.

38. Charles M. Wiltse, *The Medical Department: Medical Service in the Mediterranean and Minor Theaters*, U.S. Army in World War II, The Technical Services (Washington, DC: Office of the Chief of Military History, Department of the Army, 1965), 556.

39. Theodore L. Badger Papers, 1934–81, Finding Aid, Harvard University Library, available at: http://oasis.lib.harvard.edu/oasis/deliver/~med00001, accessed 24 August 2012.
40. Correspondence can be found in RG 112, Entry 31, Zone of the Interior, Box 1056, NARA.
41. Havens, "Medical Consultants," 403–4.
42. Theodore Badger, "Tuberculosis Survey, Interim Report #1," 28 June 1943, RG 112, Entry 31, Zone of the Interior, Box 1056, NARA.
43. Administrative Memorandum No. 22, 22 February 1944, Chief Surgeon, European Theater of Operations, in Havens, "Medical Consultants," 412; and Long, "Tuberculosis," 341.
44. Studies indicated that 25–50 percent of these cases would develop tuberculosis within five years. Long, "Tuberculosis," 370–72.
45. Circular Letter No. 100, Long, "Tuberculosis," 342; and Havens, "Medical Consultants," 431.
46. Daniel J. Feldman, "Tuberculosis in Military Service," unpublished paper," 1945, p. 1, Medical History Unit Collection, Professional Papers, Military History Institute, Carlisle, PA.
47. George T. McKean and Donald S. King, "Survey of Tuberculosis and 'Primary' Pleural Effusion for the Period of Activity of NATOUSA [North Atlantic Theater of Operations U.S. Army] and MTOUSA [Mediterranean Theater of Operations U.S. Army] to 1 April 1945," unpublished report, RG 112, Entry 31, Zone of the Interior, Box 1056, NARA.
48. McKean and King, "Survey of Tuberculosis," 20; and G. Thomas McKean and Donald S. King, "Tuberculosis in the Army in North Africa and Italy," *Bulletin of the U.S. Army Medical Department* 6 (October 1946): 452–55.
49. The 46th General Hospital was activated at the University of Oregon medical school in Portland in July 1942, and after a year of training at Fort Riley, Kansas, opened operations in Algeria in November 1943, specializing in skin diseases, sulfa-resistant gonorrhea, and tuberculosis. After eight months functioning as a hospital for the Mediterranean, the unit transferred to the European theater of operations and admitted its first patients at its facility in Besancon, France, September 1944. See 46th General Hospital, "Annual Report of Activities, 1944," 25 January 1945, RG 112, Entry 54-A, Box 419, NARA.
50. Samuel L. Diack, "A Report on Tuberculosis from the 46th General Hospital from November 1943 to August 1944," RG 112, Entry 54-A, Box 419, NARA.
51. Havens, "Medical Consultants," 443–44.
52. Theodore Badger to Esmond Long, 20 April 1944, RG 112, Entry 31, Zone of the Interior, Box 1056, NARA.
53. Esmond Long to Theodore Badger, 29 April 1944, RG 112, Entry 31, Zone of the Interior, Box 1056, NARA.
54. Havens, "Medical Consultants," 432. Others had made similar recommendations. See Esmond P. Long and C. M. Hendricks correspondence, April–August 1943, RG 112, Entry 29, 1943–44, Box 493, NARA.
55. Long, "Tuberculosis," 275.
56. Theodore L. Badger and Wesley S. Spink, "Sources of Tuberculous Infection among Nurses," *American Journal of Nursing* 36 (1936): 1100–4.
57. "Period Report, 46th General Hospital, 1 January 1945 to 30 June 1945," RG 112, Entry 54-A, Box 419, NARA; and Long, "Tuberculosis," 347.
58. Theodore Badger, "Tuberculosis in Nurses in the European Theater of Operations," 14 August 1944, RG 112, Entry 31, Zone of the Interior, Box 1056, NARA; Edna M. Cree, "Health of the Army Nurse Corps in the ETO [European Theater of Operations]," *American Journal of Nursing* 45 (November 1945): 915–16; and Long, "Tuberculosis," 342–43.

59. Greenwood and Berry, *Medics at War*, 98.

60. William H. Roper and James Waring, "Air Evacuation of Tuberculous Military Patients," *Annual Review of Tuberculosis* 61 (1944): 678–89; and "Air Transport of Tuberculous Patients," *Bulletin of the U.S. Army Medical Department* (April 1945): 8.

61. John Stephenson, "Fitzsimons Gives Victims of War New Hold on Life," *Rocky Mountain News*, 8 April 1943.

62. Hugh J. Morgan, "Inspection of Fitzsimons General Hospital," 13 April 1942, RG 112, Entry 31, 1941–42, Box 204, NARA; and "Fitzsimons Training Program is Speeded," *Denver Post*, 6 September 1940.

63. *Fitzsimons Annual Report*, 1940 [hereafter cited as *FZAR*, year], 1.

64. Long, "Tuberculosis," 383–85.

65. Jack Carberry, "Miracle Worked on Wounded Man at Fitzsimons," *Denver Post*, 31 March 1943. See also John Stephenson, "Fitzsimons Gives Victims of War New Hold on Life," *Rocky Mountain News*, 8 April 1943.

66. "Research Leaders Discuss Use of Penicillin,"*Stethoscope*, 1 October 1943.

67. Champ Lyons, "Penicillin Therapy of Surgical Infections in the U.S. Army," *Journal of the American Medical Association* 123 (1943): 1007–18. The War Department established Bushnell General Hospital with 1,500 beds near Brigham City, Utah, in 1942. It specialized in orthopedic, neuropsychiatric, and tropical diseases and was one of the first military hospitals to use penicillin. The War Department decommissioned the facility in 1946. See Utah History Encyclopedia Website, http://www.media.utah.edu/UHE/b/BUSHNELLHOSPITAL.html, accessed 30 October 2012.

68. *FZAR*, 1943, 50.

69. *FZAR*, 1943, 36.

70. Long, "Tuberculosis," 383.

71. *FZAR*, 1944, 53; Grover C. Penberthy, "A Visit to Fitzsimons General Hospital, Denver Colorado, December 6, 7, and 8, 1942," 1 January 1943, RG 112, Entry 31, 1943–44, Box 679, NARA; and John B. Grow, Omer M. Raines, and Ora L. Huddleston, "Reconditioning in Chest Surgery," *Journal of the American Medical Association* 126 (23 December 1944): 1059–60.

72. *FZAR*, 1946, 75.

73. Training Orders No. 3, "Training Directive," 15 August 1942, RG 112, FGH, HQ Memos, 1942, Box 1, NARA. See also Fitzsimons General Hospital, School for Medical Department Technicians, Annual Reports 1942–48, Box 7, NARA; and School for Medical Technicians newsletter, Fitzsimons General Hospital, 1943-44. *Soldiers in White*.

74. "Four Fitzsimons Schools to Begin Training Women," *Denver Post*, 19 October 1944.

75. See for example, "Miss America of 1943 Visits Fitz,"*Stethoscope*, 17 December 1943; "Gary Cooper Makes Two-Day Visit," *Stethoscope*, 14 August 1944; "Negro Choir at School Chapel," *Stethoscope*, 9 December 1944; and "Lamour Stars as Theater at Fitzsimons is Opened," *Rocky Mountain News*, 22 August 1943.

76. "Fitzsimons Operates Big-Scale War Garden," *Denver Post*, 3 September 1943.

77. "Fighting Soldier Leads Way in Bond Campaign with Record Purchase," *Stethoscope*, 4 February 1944.

78. *FZAR*, 1944, 44; and "Three Permanent Chaplains Now at Fitzsimons," *Denver Post*, 31 October 1942.

79. Long, "Tuberculosis," 381–83.

80. Bruns General Hospital Annual Report, 1944, RG 112, Entry 54-A, Box 63, NARA; and Esmond Long to C. C. Hillman, 21 October 1944, Esmond Long Papers, Box 1, Military History Institute, Carlisle, PA.

81. Hazel L. Rountree to Bruns General Hospital, 7 February 1946, RG 159, Record Group of the Inspector General (Army) [hereafter referred to as RG 159], General Correspondence, 1939–47, Box 1091, NARA.

82. Esmond Long to Surgeon General, "Visit at Bruns General Hospital," 11 February 1946, RG 112, Entry 31, 1945–46, Box 1426, NARA.

83. Stanhope Bayne-Jones, "Enemy Prisoners of War," in Leonard D. Heaton, editor, *Preventive Medicine in World War II*, vol. 9, *Special Fields* (Washington, DC: Office of The Surgeon General, 1969 [hereafter cited as Bayne-Jones, "Enemy Prisoners of War"]), 341–418. See also Arnold Krammer, "Japanese Prisoners of War in America," *Pacific Historical Review* 52 (1983): 67–91; and Matthias Reiss, "Bronzed Bodies behind Barbed Wire: Masculinity and the Treatment of German Prisoners of War in the United States during World War II," *Journal of Military History* 69 (2005): 475–504.

84. Bayne-Jones, "Enemy Prisoners of War," 412.

85. Verne R. Mason to Esmond Long, 14 September 1944, RG 407, 1940–45, Box 4150, NARA; and War Department Circular 347, 1944.

86. Prisoner of War Circular No. 11, 8 February 1944, Camp for Prisoners of War in Florence, Arizona.

87. Bayne-Jones, "Enemy Prisoners of War," 342–46; and U.S. War Department, "What's the Score on Our Prisoner of War Camps?" *Army Talk, Orientation Fact Sheet* 42 (21 October 1944); Long, "Tuberculosis," 393–94. On Glennan see Louis B. Laplace, "Pulmonary Tuberculosis at a Prisoner of War General Hospital: A Report on the Work of the Tuberculosis Section at Glennan General Hospital," Medical History Unit Collection, Professional Papers, Military History Institute, Carlisle, PA; Lewis B. Laplace, "Tuberculosis at a Prisoner of War Hospital," *Bulletin of the U.S. Army Medical Department* 8 (April 1947): 398–99; and inspection reports of Glennan General Hospital, RG 389, Records of the Office of the Provost Marshall [hereafter referred to as RG 389], Entry 461, Box 2661, NARA and RG 59, Entry 58, Box 27, NARA.

88. Fitzsimons General Hospital, Denver Colorado, 14 June 1944, RG 59, entry 461, Box 2661, NARA.

89. "3 Jap Captives in Hospital Try Hara-Kiri; Fail," *Chicago Daily News*, 12 August 1944.

90. Francis E. Howard to Special War Problems Division, 17 November 1944, RG 389, Entry 452-A, Box 1403, NARA. Other accounts of these events are found in RG 59, 1940–44, Box 2248, NARA.

91. Francis E. Howard to Special War Problems Division, 17 November 1944; see also RG 59, 1940–44, Box 2248, NARA; and "Prisoners Are Killed by Fitzsimons Guard," *Denver Post*, 30 October 1944.

92. Krammer, "Japanese Prisoners of War in America," 67–91. On military medicine during the war with Japan see Mary Ellen Condon-Rall, Albert E. Cowdrey, and Center of Military History, *The Medical Department: Medical Service in the War Against Japan* (Washington, DC: Center of Military History, GPO, 1998).

93. Reports found in RG 389, Entry 452-A, Boxes 1388 and 1403; and Entry 468, Boxes 1846 and 1848, NARA.

94. "Health of the Prisoners of War," *Bulletin of the U.S. Army Medical Department* (May 1945): 61–62.

95. Visit by Mr. Metraus on April 25, 1945, Bruns General Hospital, Santa Fe, New Mexico, RG 59, Entry 59, Box 23, NARA. On the provisions of the Geneva Convention, see Bayne-Jones, "Enemy Prisoners of War," 342–47.

96. Long, "Tuberculosis," 347. Bayne-Jones puts the figure at 325 patients, but I am using Long's figures.

97. Long, Circular No. 41 in, "Tuberculosis," 346.

98. "Period Report, 46th General Hospital, 1 January 1945 to 30 June 1945," 9, RG 112, Entry 54-A, Box 419, NARA.

99. "Annual Report of Activities, 1944," 46th General Hospital, 25 January 1945, RG 112, Entry 54-A, Box 419, NARA.

100. Theodore L. Badger, "Tuberculosis in the Russian RAMP [Recovered Army Military Personnel] at the 46th General Hospital," 30 March 1945, RG 112, Entry 31, Zone of the Interior, Box 1057, NARA.

101. Cosmas and Cowdrey, *Medical Service in the European Theater*, 487.

102. A. L. Cochrane, "Medical Experiences as a Prisoner of War in Germany," *Bulletin of the U.S. Army Medical Department* 7 (March 1947): 288; and A. L. Cochrane, "Tuberculosis among Prisoners of War in Germany," *British Medical Journal* 33 (10 November 1945): 656–58.

103. William H. Balzer, *World War II Questionnaire*, Military History Institute, Carlisle, PA.

104. Long, "Tuberculosis," 391–92. On recovered Allied military personnel see Long, "Tuberculosis," 346–49; and Bayne-Jones, "Activities of Medical Consultants," 444–52.

105. John R. Bumgarner, *Parade of the Dead: A U.S. Army Physician's Memoir of Imprisonment by the Japanese, 1942–1945* (Jefferson, NC: McFarland, 1995).

106. J. R. Bumgarner, "Phthisis: My Case History. Surviving a Fifteen Year Odyssey as POW and Patient," *North Carolina Medical Journal* 54, no. 6 (June 1993): 288–90.

107. Bumgarner, "Phthisis: My Case History," and Bumgarner, *Parade of the Dead*.

108. "Soldier Loses Three-Year Fight for Life; Survived March of Death, but Not Disease," *New York Times*, 4 August 1945.

109. Long, "Tuberculosis," 392.

110. Accidents such as automobile wrecks accounted for 44 percent of the deaths, followed by tuberculosis at 19 percent, with tuberculosis rates among prisoners of war of Japan higher than those of Germany. Bernard Milton Cohen and Maurice Z. Cooper, *A Follow-up Study of World War II Prisoners of War*, VA Medical Monograph (Washington, DC: GPO, 1954), 22–25, 38–39, and 46.

111. On liberation of the concentration camps see Robert H. Abzug, *Inside the Vicious Heart: Americans and the Liberation of Nazi Concentration Camps* (New York, NY: Oxford University Press, 1985); Sam Dann, *Dachau 29 April 1945: The Rainbow Liberation Memoirs* (Lubbock, TX: Texas Tech University Press, 1998); Flint Whitlock, *The Rock of Anzio: From Sicily to Dachau, a History of the 45th Division* (Boulder, CO: Westview Press, 1998); Ben Shephard, *After Daybreak: The Liberation of Bergen-Belsen, 1945* (New York, NY: Schocken Books, 2005); Howard A. Buechner, *Dachau: The Hour of the Avenger: An Eyewitness Account* (Metairie, LA: Thunderbird Press, 1986); Deborah A. Gomez, "The Exclusion of American Nurses from Imagery of Liberation," in *Virtual War: The Challenges to Communities*, Jones Irwin, ed. (Amsterdam: Rodopi Press, 2004); and Nerin E. Gun, *The Day of the Americans* (New York, NY: Fleet Publishing, 1966).

112. Marcus J. Smith, *The Harrowing of Hell: Dachau* (Albuquerque, NM: University of New Mexico Press, 1972), 80. For his work at Dachau Smith was nominated for a bronze star.

113. Smith, *Harrowing of Hell*, 81.

114. Smith, *Harrowing of Hell*, 88–89.

115. Smith, *Harrowing of Hell*, 93. The U.S. Holocaust Memorial Museum Web site, http://www.ushmm.org/, accessed 24 August 2012, and the Center for Holocaust and Genocide Studies, University of Minnesota Web site, http://www.chgs.umn.edu/about/, accessed 24 August 2012, provide overviews of the concentration camps.

116. David Schuman, Headquarters, 116th Evacuation Hospital, "Unit History through 30 June 1945," 27 August 1945, RG 112, HUMEDS [Historical Unit Medical Detachments], NARA. For an overview of these activities, see Long, "Tuberculosis," and the original manuscript for the chapter in RG 112, Entry 54-A, Box 453, NARA. In addition to Dachau, American medical personnel fought tuberculosis and typhus on a large scale at the Buchenwald and Mauthausen camps. On Buchenwald, see reports by Abner Zehm, "Historical Report, 45th Evacuation Hospital, January–June," and "In through the Gate, out through the Chimney," in RG 407, Records of the Office of the Adjutant General [hereafter cited as RG 407], Entry 427, Box 21500, NARA; Esmond R. Long, "Visit to Buchenwald Concentration Camp, Weimar, Germany," 3 May 1945, Esmond Long Papers, Box 2, Military History Institute, Carlisle, PA; "Buchenwald Concentration Camp, 1945," RG 112, HUMEDS, Box 36, NARA; David A. Hackett, *The Buchenwald Report* (Boulder, CO: Westview Press, 1995); and "Unit History," 120th Evacuation Hospital, Semimobile, 26 October 1945, RG 407, Entry 427, Box 21517, NARA. On Mauthausen, see "Organizational History, 131st Evacuation Hospital, Semimobile," 1945, RG 407, Entry 427, Box 2154, NARA; and "Period Report, Medical Department Activities, 131st U.S. Evacuation Hospital, Semimobile," 1945, RG 112, Entry 54-A, Box 409, NARA.

117. Aubrey L. Bradford, "Unit Medical History," 1 July 1945, RG 112, Entry 54-A, Box 408, NARA.

118. Dann, *Dachau, 29 April 1945*.

119. Elisabeth May Craig, "In the Wake of the War," excerpt *Portland Press Herald*, 8 May 1945, RG 112, HUMEDS, Box 86, NARA.

120. Craig, "In the Wake of the War."

121. Gun, *Day of the Americans*, 206.

122. Gun, *Day of the Americans*, 198–99.

123. Smith, *Harrowing of Hell*, 225.

124. Dann, *Dachau, 29 April 1945*, 32. On typhus in World War II see Chris J. D. Zarafonetis, "The Typhus Fevers," in *Medical Department of the U.S. Army in World War II, Infectious Diseases*, vol. 2, chapter 7, 143–202.

125. Dachau Concentration Camp Scrapbooks. Available at: http://www.scrapbookpages.com/DachauScrapbook/DachauLiberation/aftermath.html, accessed 24 August 2012.

126. Suge Fabregas, "Nursing Care in Typhus Fever," *American Journal of Nursing* 41 (May 1941): 558–60.

127. Schuman, "Unit History," 7.

128. Gun, *Day of the Americans*, 195.

129. Ben Shephard makes this point in *After Daybreak*, 78.

130. Robert Proctor, *Racial Hygiene: Medicine under the Nazis* (Cambridge, MA: Harvard University Press, 1988), 215.

131. Abner Zehm, "Buchenwald Concentration Camp, Historical Report, 45th Evacuation Hospital," 28 April 1945, RG 407, Entry 427, Box 21500, NARA.

132. Craig, "In the Wake of the War."

133. "Letter from Harold Porter to His Parents Describing Dachau Concentration Camp," 7 May 1945, Dachau Concentration Camp Scrapbooks. Available at http://www.scrapbookpages.com/DachauScrapbook/DachauLiberation/LiberationDay2.html, accessed 24 August 2012.

134. Dann, *Dachau, 29 April 1945*, 208.

135. Gun, *Day of the Americans*, 17–18.

136. Gun, *Day of the Americans*, 199.

137. Gun, *Day of the Americans*, 200.

138. Earl F. Ziemke, *The U.S. Army in the Occupation of Germany, 1944–1946* (Washington, DC: Center of Military History, United States Army, 1990).

139. A. D. Piatt, "A Radiographic Chest Survey of Patients from the Dachau Concentration Camp," *Radiology* 47 (September 1946): 234–48; and Long, "Tuberculosis," 350. On tuberculosis in postwar Europe, see Esmond Long, editorial, "Tuberculosis in Europe," *American Review of Tuberculosis* 57 (1948): 420–25; Marc Daniels, "Tuberculosis in Post-War Europe: An International Problem," *Tubercle* 28 (September 1947); and Johannes Holm, "Tuberculosis as a World Problem: Tuberculosis in Europe after the Second World War," *Transactions of the National Tuberculosis Association* 43 (1947): 315–29.

140. Long, "Tuberculosis," 353; and Esmond Long, "Tuberculosis Control in U.S. Zone of Germany," 9 October 1945, Esmond R. Long papers, Box 2, Military History Institute, Carlisle, PA.

141. Stan Sommers, "After Effects of Imprisonment," manuscript, 1980, Military History Institute, Carlisle, PA, citing an article by M. Dvorjetski, "Tuberculosis among Jewish Immigrants to Israel."

142. "Tuberculosis in Germany," *Bulletin of the U.S. Army Medical Department* 8 (July 1948): 564–66.

143. Marc Daniels, "Tuberculosis in Post-War Europe: An International Problem," *Tubercle* 28 (September 1947): 201–38. On tuberculosis in other countries during the war see also Frederick Heaf and Lloyd Rusby, "A Further Review of Tuberculosis in Wartime," *Tubercle* 23 (1942): 107–30; J.B. McDougall, "Tuberculosis and England during War," *Diseases of the Chest* 8–9 (1942–43): 228–35; J. B. Adamson, "Tuberculosis and World War II in the Canadian Army," *Diseases of the Chest* 11 (1945): 272; James A. Doull, "Tuberculosis Mortality in England and Certain Other Countries during the Present War," *American Journal of Public Health* 35 (July 1945): 783–87; Prof. Levitin, "The Fight against Tuberculosis: Current Problems in the USSR," *Tubercle* 26 (1945): 109–14; Umberto Carpi, "The Fight against Tuberculosis in Italy in the War," *Tubercle* 27 (May–June 1946): 60–62; "Tuberculosis in Europe," *American Journal of Nursing* 46 (July 1946): 480; Johannes Holm, "Tuberculosis as a World Problem: Tuberculosis in Europe after the Second World War," *Diseases of the Chest* 13 (1947) 315–29; and Miguel C. Anizares, "Tuberculosis as a World Problem: The Tuberculosis Problem in the Philippines," *Diseases of the Chest* 13 (1947): 352–58.

144. Edward P. Morgan, "Disease: Shadow over Europe," *Collier's* (23 March 1946): 14 and 73–77.

145. Long, "Tuberculosis Control in U.S. Zone of Germany."

146. Long, "Tuberculosis," 397–99.

147. Esmond R. Long, "Report of the Visit of Consultant on Tuberculosis to U.S. Zone Germany for Consultation on Tuberculosis Problems," 30 July–7 August 1947, RG 112, Entry 31, Zone of the Interior, Box 1057, NARA.

148. "Tuberculosis and Germany," *Bulletin of the U.S. Army Medical Department* 8 (July 1948): 564–66; Esmond R. Long, "Report of Visit of Consultant on Tuberculosis to U.S. Zone Germany for Consultation on Tuberculosis Problems, 13 July–20 July 1949," Esmond Long Papers, Box 2, Military History Institute, Carlisle, PA. These reports can also be found in RG 112, Entry 31, Zone of the Interior, Box 1057, NARA.

149. Cowdrey, *Fighting for Life*, 291.

150. "Discovery of Tuberculosis at Separation Centers," *Bulletin of the U.S. Army Medical Department* 5 (May): 489. See also Louis Schneider, "Separation Center Chest Survey," *Diseases of the Chest* 12 (1946): 147–52; and William Porter Swisher, "Tuberculosis and Discharged Soldiers," *American Review of Tuberculosis* 55 (1947): 481–87.

151. William H. Duncan, "Reflections on World War II" (unpublished paper), "William H. Duncan Papers," Item #04-310-002, Military History Institute, Carlisle, PA; 2004.

152. C. C. Hillman to E. R. Long, 24 September 1941, Esmond R. Long Papers, Manuscript Collection 362, National Library of Medicine.

153. Long and Jablon, *Tuberculosis in the Army*, 82–83.

154. "Specialized Center for Tuberculosis at Moore General Hospital," *Bulletin of the U.S. Army Medical Department* 5 (February 1946): 130.

155. See Roy A. Wolford, "The Tuberculosis Problem in the Veterans Administration," *Diseases of the Chest* (1943): 274–80; Louis I. Dublin, "Function of the Health Officer in the Control of Tuberculosis among Veterans," *American Journal of Public Health* 33 (December 1943): 1425–29; Roy A. Wolford, "The Care of the Tuberculous Veteran," *Diseases of the Chest* 11 (1945): 351–55; Roy A. Wolford, "The Tuberculous Veteran, Plans for his Future Care," *Diseases of the Chest* 13 (May–June 1947): 189–96; and Leo V. Schneider, "The Tuberculosis Control Program of the U.S. Veterans Administration," *Military Surgeon* 107 (August 1950): 97–102.

156. Paul R. Hawley, "The Tuberculosis Program of the Veterans' Administration," *American Review of Tuberculosis* 55 (1947) 1–7. On general hospitalization trends during and after the war, see Eli Ginzberg, "Federal Hospitalization," *Modern Hospital* 72 (April 1949): 61–64.

157. Administrator of Veterans Affairs, *Annual Report for Fiscal Year Ending June 30, 1954* (Washington, DC: GPO, 1955), 43.

158. Esmond Long, "Visit at Moore General Hospital," 19 February 1946, RG 112, Entry 31, 1945–46, Box 1432, NARA.

159. Esmond Long to H. W. Doan, 29 December 1947, Esmond Long Papers, Box 2, Military History Institute, Carlisle, PA.

160. C. D. Buck, "Revision of Policy on Tuberculous Soldier Patients," 19 February 1940, RG 112, Entry 29, 1938–40, Box 66, NARA.

161. Hugh J. Morgan, "Inspection of Fitzsimons General Hospital, Denver Colorado, April 8, 1942," RG 112, Entry 31, 1941–42, Box 204, NARA.

162. "Report to State Public Health Officers on Enlisted Men Discharged by Reason of Tuberculosis," 28 July 1945, and accompanying correspondence, Office of The Surgeon General, Office of History Files.

163. Louis I. Dublin, "Memorandum on the Care of Tuberculous Veterans," June 1943, and accompanying documents, RG 112, Entry 31, Box 1056, NARA.

164. Louis I. Dublin, "Function of the Health Officer in the Control of Tuberculosis among Veterans," *American Journal of Public Health* 33 (December 1943): 1425–29; Louis I. Dublin, "The Problem of the Tuberculous Veteran," *Diseases of the Chest* (1944): 151–54; also reprinted in *American Review of Tuberculosis* 50 (1944): 375–79.

165. Louis I. Dublin, "Memorandum on the Care of Tuberculous Veterans," June 1943, and accompanying documents, RG 112, Entry 31, Box 1056, NARA.

166. Bernard Milton Cohen and Maurice Z. Cooper, *A Follow-Up Study of World War II Prisoners of War, VA Medical Monograph* (Washington, DC: GPO, 1954)

167. Wisconsin Anti-tuberculosis Association, "Going Where?" n.d., drawn from Louis I. Dublin, "Informal Meeting of the Committee on Tuberculosis among Veterans, Chicago, Ill., May 11, 1944," RG 112, Entry 31, Box 1056, NARA.

168. Chart 1, "Tuberculosis Death Rates, United States, 1900–1957," *American Journal of Public Health* 48 (1958): 1440.

169. E. Ginzberg, "Everything I Know about Health Care I Learned in the Pentagon in World War II," *Academic Medicine* 66, no. 8 (1991): 439–42.

170. Cowdrey, *Fighting for Life*, passim; and Fishbein, ed. *Doctors at War*.

171. Cosmas and Cowdrey, *Medical Service in the European Theater*, 361; and Cowdrey, *Fighting for Life*, 175.

172. Cosmas and Cowdrey, *Medical Service in the European Theater*, 125–26.
173. George B. Darling, "How The National Research Council Streamlined Medical Research For War," in Fishbein, *Doctors at* War, 374.

Chapter Nine
Miracle Drugs?

On 23 November 1941, twenty-one-year-old Margaret E. "Midge" Wall and her good friend Iris Garrard swore their commitment to the Army Nurse Corps. They had graduated from Mount Sinai Hospital Nursing School that May, passed their licensing exams, and were working at the hospital. But now the young women were looking for something else, perhaps an adventure. As Wall later wrote, "On 6 November 1941, election day in Chicago, Iris and I were feeling very patriotic. We had just voted for the first time." They had the day off, and went down to the nurses' recruiting station to get information on the Army Nurse Corps. "By the end of the day," she said, "not only had we filled our applications for admission into the Army Nurse Corps, but we had our complete physical examination as well."[1]

Both from North Carolina, the young women had chosen nursing school in Chicago to see the world. Now, when offered assignments in either South Carolina or in Vancouver, Washington, "the latter struck our fancy. This would be a chance to go West, to travel." The night of their swearing-in they boarded a train for Vancouver and three days later were at the Vancouver Barracks Army camp. Wall remembered the American flag flying. "There was a beautiful green lawn, and this together with the neat rows of white buildings was a beautiful and peaceful site. Already we were in love with that place before we had actually driven through the gate." Wall was assigned to Ward No. 13, the contagious disease ward devoted to tuberculosis patients, in Barnes Hospital and immediately went to work. Most of her patients had been evacuated from Alaska. Some of them were Inuits, but most were American soldiers, "typical of the G. I. patients I have come to know so well and love." Many patients were very sick and confined to bed, so her duties involved feeding and bathing them, and assisting in performing and refilling pneumothoraces. Neither she nor the other nurses wore protective clothing or masks while caring for patients. On 7 December, a fellow nurse ran into her room with news of the Japanese bombing of Pearl Harbor. Listening to the radio, they realized that war was now upon them. "Yes, it was now here, and I had been in the Army only fifteen days." Wall would serve in the Army Nurse Corps for four-and-one-half years.

Wall asked for foreign duty but waited for two-and-one-half years for an overseas assignment. A diary she later wrote for *Stars & Stripes* about her life in the Army reveals that in addition to Ward No. 13, she worked in orthopedics and gastrointestinal wards during the years 1941 through 1943. Finally, in May 1943, she got her new assignment and after several months of training, boarded a ship out of San Francisco for the South Pacific theater. Her first post was the 27th Station Hospital in New Caledonia, where she contracted dengue fever, a serious disease transmitted by mosquitoes. But, more happily, she also met a "tall and handsome officer," Lieutenant (Lt.) John Gaule, an infantry officer with the Sixth Replacement Depot. The two became engaged and when they learned that her unit would be transferred out of New Caledonia, asked for permission to marry. (The War Department had lifted the prohibition on marriage for members of the Army Nurse Corps in 1943.) They wed on 3 January 1945 and after three months of married life, Midge, now Margaret Gaule, departed for the front lines and the Battle of Okinawa, one of the deadliest encounters of World War II. "I could hardly wait to get ashore and care for these wounded men of ours.... Now I finally had a chance to do the nursing I had wanted for so long to do," she later wrote. Assigned to the shock ward of the 74th Field Hospital on Buckner Bay, Okinawa, Gaule was able to give newly developed and life-saving whole blood and blood plasma units to severely wounded men. It was an experience that would stay with her for life. The War Department gave Gaule a commendation for her war service and discharged her on 25 March 1946 (Figure 9-1).

John and Margaret Gaule began their postwar life in John's hometown of Omaha, Nebraska, where he worked in the insurance business. By 1956, they had three sons. One Sunday evening in August of that year, returning from a trip to North Carolina to visit her family, Gaule was feeling tired and then had a "massive oral hemorrhage." Her husband rushed her to an Omaha hospital where several physicians examined her, including P. James Connor, M.D., just out of medical school.[2] Diagnosed with "chronic pulmonary tuberculosis, far advanced, active," Gaule entered the veterans' hospital in Omaha. When she wrote of her illness to Jean Greer, who had been the assistant chief nurse at Barnes Hospital, Greer responded, "I cannot tell you how shocked and sorry I was to receive the news that your letter brought yesterday.... Do not kid yourself—it is going to be a long and tedious battle." She knew, because she, too, had had tuberculosis, and had spent eighteen months in the hospital and more than eight years with a pneumothorax. She told Gaule that three other nurses from the Barnes tuberculosis ward—Cecilia Smith, Frances Van Hoomissen, and Gladys Larkin—had also developed tuberculosis. This meant that five of twenty-five nurses—20 percent—in tuberculosis Ward No. 13 at Barnes during the early war years developed active tuberculosis. Remembering that kiss under the mistletoe from a patient, Gaule later said, "I should have known there'd be a problem with Ward 13."[3]

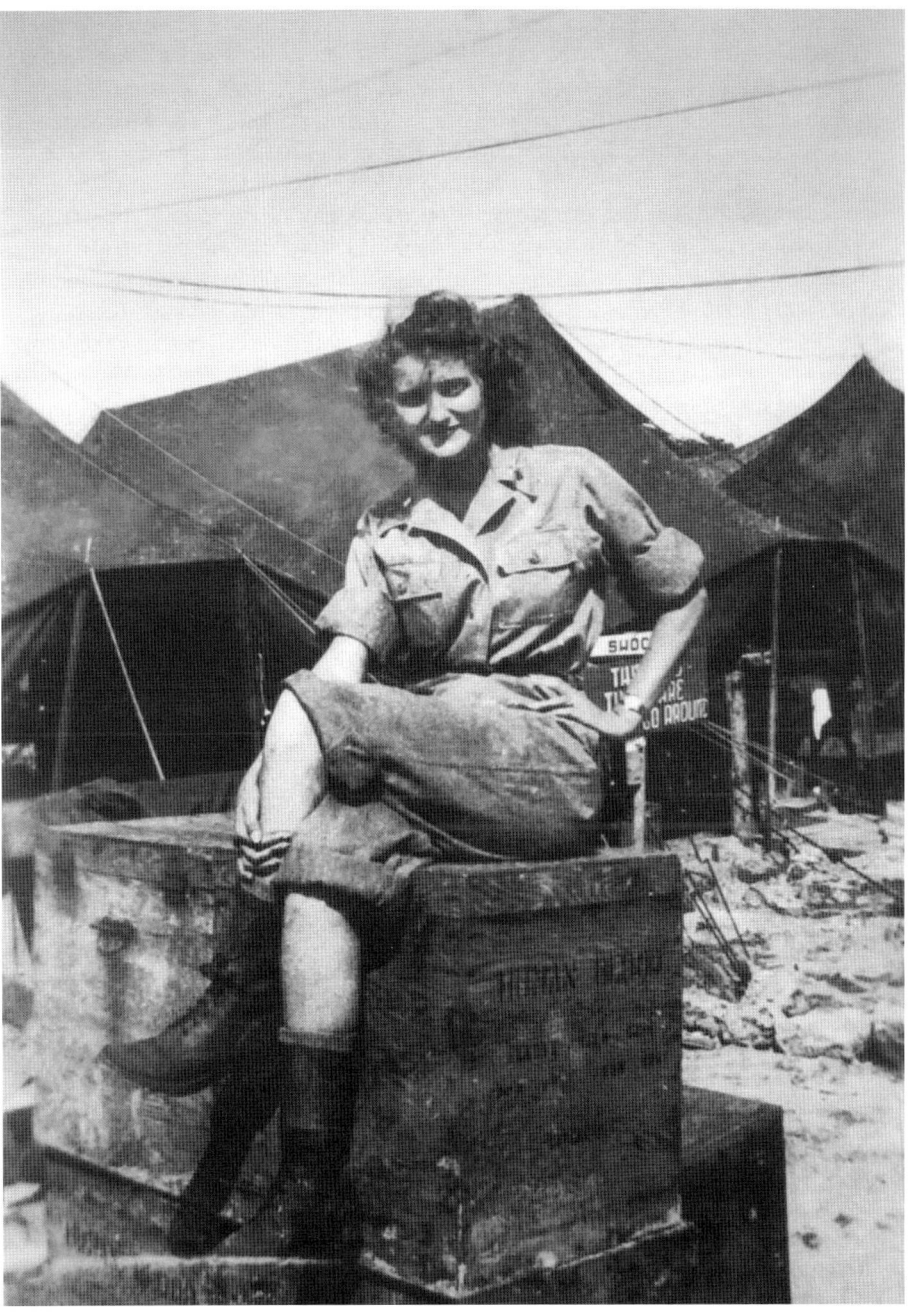

Figure 9-1. Margaret E. Gaule, nurse with the 74th Field Hospital on Buckner Bay, Okinawa, who participated in the Battle of Okinawa in 1945.
Photograph courtesy of the family of Margaret E. Gaule.

Although seriously ill, Gaule was fortunate to be in the first generation of tuberculosis patients during the era of effective treatment—but it was not a quick or miracle cure. Gaule spent eight months in the Omaha veterans' hospital on rest therapy and new antibiotic medications. Her physicians at the Veterans Administration (VA) considered surgery, but she and her husband got a second opinion at the Mayo Clinic, which recommended against it, so she refused surgical intervention.[4] Once she was discharged from the hospital, Gaule continued to take antibiotics for a year. Given the hardship, and the cost of care for her three young children while she was in the hospital, Gaule filed for veterans' compensation. In January 1958, however, the VA Board of Veterans' Appeals denied her claim because she had not developed active tuberculosis within three years of her termination of service in the Army Nurse Corps, and therefore fell outside of the presumptive period for benefits.[5] Unlike so many Army nurses over the years, Gaule was able to recover her health and had another baby boy. But her scarred lungs remained a lifelong reminder of the costs of being a tuberculosis nurse—and of the fact that the government had refused to recognize her sacrifice.

Airborne Transmission

While Gaule and other tuberculosis nurses were caring for patients without gloves or masks, the debate about airborne transmission and immunity continued in both military and civilian medical circles. In 1943 Army medical reserve officer Colonel (Col.) John Wakeman Turner reprised Bushnell's epidemiology of tuberculosis in *Military Surgeon*, lamenting the fact that many people "do not believe in the laws of tuberculous immunization," and that "such a state of mind is unfortunate and is not helpful in practical prophylaxis."[6] In 1948 a civilian physician similarly wrote, "It is estimated that about one half of the population of the United States is tuberculin positive.... Most doctors feel that a positive tuberculin indicates a greater resistance to a reinfection of the disease."[7] Others continued to worry, however, about high rates of tuberculosis among nurses. An *American Journal of Nursing* author said that tuberculosis should be considered an occupational disease for the nursing profession, but that "tuberculosis control among nurses is lagging far behind the control of silicosis in industry."[8]

Predictably, the issue of tuberculosis transmission transcended medical circles and entered the courts. In the 1940s some people began to make workers' compensation claims for contracting tuberculosis in the workplace and patients began to sue hospitals for developing tuberculosis while being treated for something else.[9] Two New York City physicians were frustrated that although "contagiousness is not a definite fixed characteristic of tuberculosis," in the courts "claims for compensation are granted daily by judges, referees and juries on the lay belief that tuberculosis is always a contagious disease."[10] In 1951 the journal *Chest* noted a study that found that only 247 of 4,539 general hospitals had "satisfactory programs" to prevent the transmission of tuberculosis in their institutions, and warned that "no hospital can afford to have contagious tuberculosis exist among its patients or personnel unless they are under rigid isolation technique."[11] Many hospitals had been compelled to compensate their employees and, *Chest* observed, "[C]ourts have granted awards to persons, who, as patients, were exposed to contagious cases of tuberculosis and later fell ill from this disease." This judicial involvement was regrettable, the editors believed, because when "rigid isolation technique was instituted...the fear of having tuberculosis patients in general hospitals because of contagion is unfounded."[12]

Several efforts, however, suggested the need for continued education and advocacy to encourage general adherence to the procedures. In 1955 the National Tuberculosis Association issued a fifty-page document on tuberculosis control procedures with rigorous contagious disease precautions, and the American College of Chest Physicians assembled a series of scientific papers on the issue for wide distribution. Some people called for more legal authority. Two physicians suggested that because some patients simply would not practice hygienic measures, "It appears that successful management can never be completely attained without the aid of a compulsory hospitalization law."[13] Others agreed that "tuberculosis is a serious communicable disease that should require isolation, enforceable by law."[14]

After the war, in addition to periodic tuberculin and X-ray examinations of its staff, Fitzsimons did gradually institute more stringent protective practices. In 1947, the hospital medical service reported that "a real effort has been made to establish good standard measures of aseptic technique."[15] Measures included special lectures, training on the wards, and the inevitable circulation of memoranda on the subject. The next year the construction of a "gown room" allowed medical personnel to scrub before and after entering the tuberculosis wards.[16] In 1949, Fitzsimons constructed a new administration building and a separate receiving ward for the tuberculosis section that provided additional isolation, and by 1950 nurses were attending a four-day orientation course on tuberculosis that included instruction on "protective technique, conducted by an especially trained Army nurse assigned permanently to the Chest Disease Section."[17] Out of step with these changes, a 1956 Army lesson plan on "The Fundamentals of Tuberculosis Nursing," by nurse Florence Bankhead, continued to emphasize the role of sputum rather than airborne infection in tuberculosis transmission. "Tuberculosis germs are carried from the mouths of people who have active tuberculosis to the mouths of well people," she wrote. "These germs are spread by kissing, coughing, spitting, sneezing, and also by putting things like pencils, pens, forks, spoons, or cups into one's mouth after they have first come into contact with germs from a person with active tuberculosis."[18]

Researchers continued to investigate tuberculosis transmission exploring routes such as skin punctures or abrasions, the alimentary tract, cigarettes and smoking, dust, and animal secretions.[19] Some scientists also began to uncover evidence of the power of tuberculosis bacteria to persist and travel in the air. In the 1930s, W. F. Wells, of the University of Pennsylvania's Department of Pathology, demonstrated that droplet nuclei could be suspended in the air for long periods of time. Citing this and other studies, Max B. Lurie, of the University of Pennsylvania and the Henry Phipps Institute in Philadelphia (Esmond Long's institution), stated in 1946 that "pulmonary tuberculosis is largely an airborne disease. It originates from the inhalation of invisible droplet nuclei or microscopic dust particles carrying tuberculosis bacilli."[20] In 1949 Esta McNett, a nurse and a consistent advocate of protective technique, urged the use of facemasks, stating the "modern medical opinion inclines strongly toward inhalation infection as the most important mechanism in the transmission of tuberculosis."[21] But the issue was still not settled.

In the mid-1950s Richard L. Riley, a student and colleague of W. F. Wells, theorized that tuberculosis bacteria could exist on these droplet nuclei and therefore travel far from a patient to be inhaled by other people.[22] To test this theory and to see if ultraviolet light could disinfect air containing tuberculosis bacilli, he installed two chambers with cages of guinea pigs in the air ducts above the rooms of patients with advanced tuberculosis in a Baltimore VA hospital. In one chamber, air from the patients' rooms was exposed to ultraviolet light before reaching the guinea pigs and in the other chamber it was not. After two years Riley found that none of the guinea pigs in the chamber using ultraviolet light had been infected with tuberculosis, but 71 of 156 guinea pigs in the other chamber had become infected. Besides proving the salutary effect of ultraviolet light, the latter finding also, even more strikingly, proved that tuberculosis bacteria could be airborne. After eliminating other sources of tuberculosis, that is, ensuring that the workers who cared for the animals had never been infected with tuberculosis and that the animals had not infected one another, Riley and his team asserted that their evidence "justifies the conclusion that all seventy-one guinea pigs were infected by aerial contamination produced by patients occupying a tuberculosis ward."[23]

In its 1959 article, "Aerial Dissemination of Pulmonary Tuberculosis: A Two-Year Study of Contagion in a Tuberculosis Ward," Riley's team was able "to demonstrate beyond question the fact of aerial dissemination and the probability of its predominant importance in the transmission of pulmonary tuberculosis." The air did not contain a large quantity of tuberculosis bacteria, but, team members argued, their work demonstrated that even a small number of bacilli could cause an infection. Given that epidemiological studies had shown that it took a tuberculin-negative nurse about a year to convert to positive, the Riley team could argue that "the amount of airborne tuberculosis in the vicinity of patients, though small, appears to be enough to account for the observed rate of infection, at least in nurses." Pulmonary tuberculosis, the team concluded, "is a classic example of air-borne contagion."[24] This theory was widely disseminated in a textbook by Riley and F. O'Grady, *Airborne Infection*, first published in 1961.[25] The National Tuberculosis Association awarded Riley its Trudeau Medal, given annually for the most meritorious contribution to increased understanding of the cause, prevention, and treatment of tuberculosis. The National Tuberculosis Association said that Riley's work "has shaped modern thinking about transmissibility, the uselessness of many traditional isolationist strictures, scientifically valid cautionary measures, and the place for air disinfection with ultraviolet radiation."[26]

This, finally, was the scientific proof needed to end the debate on transmission and protect tuberculosis workers, patients' families, and the public from infection. When the American Epidemiological Society reprinted the article as a classic in

1995, Dr. Michael B. Iseman, tuberculosis expert at the National Jewish Center for Immunology and Respiratory Medicine in Denver, wrote that "because of these findings, urgent steps have been taken to lessen the risks of institutional transmission of tuberculosis."[27] In a bittersweet irony, however, those precautions would become increasingly less urgent because researchers finally were able to devise a cure.

Antibiotics

The discovery of penicillin and its wonderful wartime success in curing a wide range of infections spurred increased research—indeed a race—to find additional antibiotic agents. In the spirit of this hunt, Rutgers University soil scientist Selman Waksman and his assistant Albert Schatz discovered in 1943 that streptomycin inhibited the growth of tuberculosis bacilli in the laboratory. There was little interest in their work, however, until 1945, when researchers at the Mayo Clinic showed streptomycin's effectiveness in treating patients with advanced cases of tuberculosis.[28] Then, as curiosity about the new drug surged, the National Research Council convened representatives of the Army, Navy, VA, and Public Health Service in mid-1946 to structure trials for streptomycin therapy and determine how to distribute the limited supply of the drug. The ubiquitous Esmond Long served as the acting chair and Fitzsimons became one of the leading institutions in the project. The process to develop an effective cure, however, took almost a decade during which time physicians continued to prescribe bed rest, lung collapse treatments, and surgery—in addition to antibiotics—to help their patients.

Military and VA hospitals were attractive research venues because of the often-large numbers of similar patients (young men) with the same disease or injury. Medical officers would identify patients whose condition and symptoms they believed would make them appropriate for new, experimental procedures or medicines, and then seek the patient's voluntary consent. (The power relationship between officers and enlisted men, physicians and patients, however, raises the question of the extent to which consent was indeed voluntary.[29]) The streptomycin trials also indicated that experimentation in military and veteran populations was becoming increasingly politically sensitive. Historian Harry Marks has described how streptomycin experiments on tuberculosis patients helped usher in a new era in scientific research using double-blind randomized drug testing that has become the standard today. The new procedures enabled scientists to compare results for patients receiving a new drug with results from a control group receiving placebos, and the randomized selection of subjects avoided biasing the test cohort and prevented physicians and patients from knowing which they were receiving.[30] Military and VA investigators were reluctant to use this protocol, however, due to concerns about fairness, physician control, and public relations.

Streptomycin seemed to be so promising, in fact, that the National Research Council committee decided against using placebos, believing the practice would not be fair to its patients. The committee instead agreed that the first cases on which to test the new drug should be those where the tuberculosis diagnosis was clear, and "moderately advanced in extent, with evidence of recent progression."[31] Long preferred to leave the choice of patient subjects to the research staff. He told Larry B. McAfee at Bruns Hospital, who participated in the trials, that medical officers at Fitzsimons were concerned about public relations because "[i]f the word gets around that some men have been selected for a 'Miracle Drug,' the press may seize the opportunity, and the Army may be accused of partiality." Therefore, he told McAfee "this office would rather leave the problem to your own judgment in this respect."[32] The VA representative on the committee was also reluctant to use a control group, and objected to the word "experiment," for the trials, preferring "investigation" or "observations" to avoid public censure.[33] The Public Health Service did not participate in the initial National Research Council studies due to lack of funding at the time, but rather conducted its own, smaller investigation and, in contrast to the Army, Navy, and VA researchers, did use control groups. Harry Marks argues that although "both studies testified favorably on behalf of streptomycin, it was the Public Health Service studies, properly randomized, that received credit for demonstrating the new drug's benefits in treating tuberculosis." Moreover, he concludes, the Public Health Service's work "served as an example of scientific progress in therapeutics."[34]

The first National Research Council trials began in June 1946, with groups of ten patients at a time receiving streptomycin, with a prescribed dosage of 1.8 grams per day for four months. Researchers were advised to watch for signs of toxicity. The National Research Council also appointed an outside review board to evaluate the results of the trials. In December researchers convened what would be the first of fourteen "Streptomycin Conferences," held from 1946 to 1955, to evaluate the results, coordinate the studies, and discuss clinical and laboratory issues.[35] At that meeting they found that streptomycin was effective in reversing the course of many cases of tuberculosis, and in particular was able to stop the progression of the usually lethal miliary and meninginal tuberculosis. Researchers also immediately recognized several limitations to streptomycin: (*a*) the drug reduced tuberculosis bacteria reproduction but did not kill them; (*b*) prolonged treatment allowed resistant bacteria to develop; (*c*) the drug could damage a cranial nerve responsible for hearing and balance; and (*d*) because the body did not absorb streptomycin well it needed to be administered by numerous, often painful injections.[36]

Patients' improvement was dramatic, nevertheless. Captains Stanley H. Hoffman and George A. Hyman at Fitzsimons reported on a "rather typical" patient whose progression showed the results of the combination of streptomycin and collapse therapy. The twenty-one-year-old white male arrived in April 1947 with "severe constitutional symptoms," including a cough, three-quarters cup of sputum a day, positive smear, and advanced tuberculosis with cavities in both the lungs. They collapsed his right lung and put him on streptomycin, two grams per day given in five injections, from 25 April to 25 August. The patient's temperature returned to normal after three weeks, his cough improved, and his sputum was negative by July. X-ray films in August "showed remarkable clearing with no definite evidence of cavitation visible," and the improvement continued even after the streptomycin injections were stopped.[37] Because of results such as these, institutions clamored to participate in the National Research Council trials. Torn between conducting careful, scientific studies on the effects of a possible miracle drug on a small number of patients, or making the drug available to a wide range of desperately ill patients, the Army, Navy, and VA researchers opted for the latter. By 1947 the oversight group had lost control over many of the protocols.

The treatment regime was rigorous at the start: large doses (up to two grams) of streptomycin divided into five or six injections daily, for three or four months, which could amount to 450 to 720 shots (this, before the advent of tiny, disposable needles). Many patients also underwent surgery in addition to the drug regime. Fitzsimons' researchers reported on twelve patients who each had from five to ten ribs removed in thoracoplasty, and then received streptomycin for four to eight months with a total dose ranging from 64 to 470 grams. All of the patients improved, losing their fever, gaining weight, and producing negative sputum tests. The fact that one of the twelve left the hospital against medical advice, though, and two others presented "severe disciplinary" problems is not surprising given the invasiveness of the surgery and multiple daily hypodermics.[38] Because some patients had trouble with their balance or hearing or even became deaf after several months of therapy, physicians at Fitzsimons confirmed that "streptomycin is definitely toxic to the great majority of patients." But so many patients responded well that "at present, it would seem folly to withhold the drug when indicated." They cautioned, however, that streptomycin should be used as a complement to and not a substitute for other types of treatment.[39]

Fitzsimons had a strong team guiding the introduction of antibiotic therapies during this time of transition. Col. James H. Forsee, chief of surgery from 1946 to 1953, and Col. Carl W. Tempel, chief of medical services from 1950 to 1955, led efforts to test various combinations of rest, antibiotics (which they called "chemotherapy"), and surgery to find the safest and most effective protocol for their patients. Forsee and Tempel followed similar career paths. Both graduated from medical school in St. Louis in 1929, Forsee from Washington University and Tempel from the St. Louis University Medical School, and then received their Army commissions immediately after graduation. Forsee's first Army assignment was at Fitzsimons General Hospital where he served until 1934, during which time he studied the tuberculin testing of staff and the question of tubercularization.[40] His subsequent assignments included service in Hawaii and at Walter Reed General Hospital. During World War II Forsee earned the Legion of Merit for his service as commander of the Second Auxiliary Surgical Group in Italy. After the war, he returned to Fitzsimons as chief of surgery, and wrote an extensive and widely read report on the front-line surgical treatment of the severely wounded.[41] After Fitzsimons, Forsee (Figure 9-2) served as a surgical consultant at Army posts in Asia and Walter Reed. Promoted to major general in 1962, he held the position of special assistant to the Surgeon General in Washington until his death in 1963 at the age of fifty-nine.

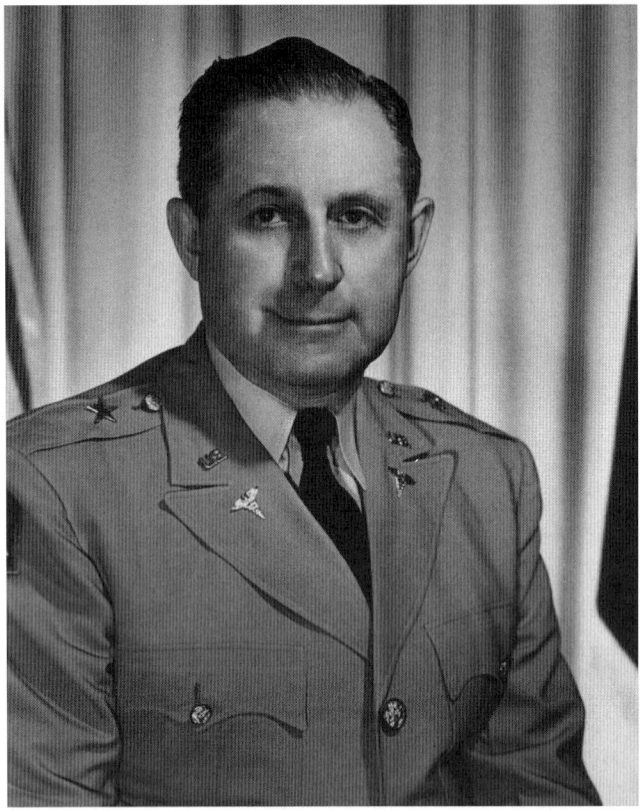

Figure 9-2. James H. Forsee, tuberculosis specialist at Fitzsimons General Hospital, in 1957. Photograph courtesy of the National Library of Medicine, Image #B012074

Carl Tempel's first assignment was at William Beaumont Army Hospital, after which he served at a number of Army hospitals, including Fitzsimons from 1937 to 1940. During the war he was assigned to Walter Reed and then commanded a general hospital in the Asia-Pacific Theater. After the war, he commanded the 42nd General Hospital in Tokyo, and returned to Fitzsimons in 1947, becoming chief of medical services in 1950. After another tour of duty in the Far East, Tempel (Figure 9-3) returned to Fitzsimons in 1960 as its nineteenth commander. Like Forsee, he attained the rank of major general. Tempel retired in 1962 and joined the administration of the Webb-Waring Institute for Medical Research at the University of Colorado Medical Center in Denver.[42] He died in 1979 and was buried at Fort Logan Cemetery in Denver.[43]

Forsee and Tempel were colleagues and friends at Fitzsimons. Their families lived next to each other on "Colonel's Row," and during their years of overlap in Denver they coauthored several articles on tuberculosis treatment, including "The

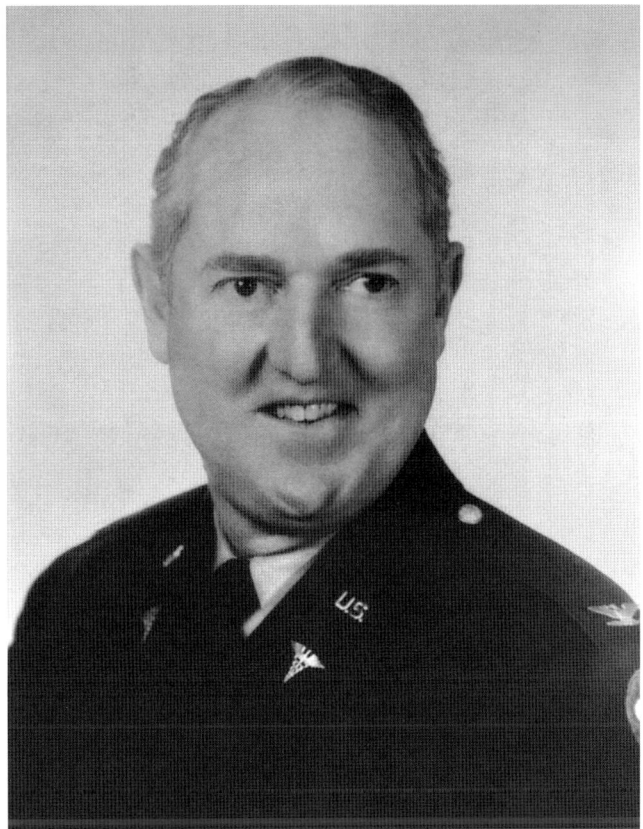

Figure 9-3. Carl W. Tempel, tuberculosis specialist at Fitzsimons General Hospital, in 1957. Photograph courtesy of the National Library of Medicine, Image #B024680.

Definitive Treatment of Pulmonary Tuberculosis," in *Military Surgeon*, 1950.[44] An example of their leadership includes Forsee's textbook, *The Surgery of Pulmonary Tuberculosis* (1954), based on his experience with the surgical treatment of patients at Fitzsimons. The Association of Military Surgeons of the United States Army also recognized Tempel with the Stitt Award in 1957 for his outstanding medical research with streptomycin.[45]

The challenge facing Forsee and Tempel in the late 1940s and early 1950s was to harness streptomycin's power against tuberculosis while minimizing the development of antibiotic resistance and the drug's toxicity to patients. They used all the tools at their disposal—bed rest, collapse therapy, surgery, and the new drugs. Forsee began to administer streptomycin prior to surgery, with the aim of "either improving the operability of the patient or for aiding in the conversion of an unsuitable operative risk in need of surgery to a reasonable surgical risk."[46] Fitzsimons' surgeons also tried resection or removal of diseased lung tissue followed by antibiotics with good results and found that reducing the streptomycin dosage reduced toxicity and bacterial resistance.[47] Tempel and his colleagues developed elaborate tables of treatment regimens according to the nature, location, and extent of the patient's infection. In 1947, for example, he prescribed seventeen possible treatment plans (Figure 9-4) combining bed rest, temporary or permanent lung collapse, surgical removal of lung tissue, and streptomycin injections.[48] Tempel also found that bacterial resistance to streptomycin increased with the length of time it was administered. Only 3.9 percent of patients treated for 60 days developed resistance, but fully one-third of patients did after 120 days of streptomycin.[49] Tempel concluded in 1949, therefore, that "streptomycin is only an adjunct to conventional methods of therapy,... chemotherapy will never replace surgical and other measures of therapy."[50]

Physicians soon had another weapon, however, because in 1949 Danish scientist Jorgen Lehman discovered the antibiotic properties of para-aminosalicylate (PAS). Daily doses of PAS given orally in combination with lower doses of streptomycin every other day effectively controlled tuberculosis and reduced the chances of side effects and bacterial resistance. Assessing the results at forty-two hospitals that treated 7,000 cases with streptomycin and PAS (2,000 of them at Fitzsimons), tuberculosis specialists at the 1949 Eighth Streptomycin Conference recommended against using streptomycin alone, due to the problems of toxicity and resistance and the availability of PAS.[51]

But the optimal treatment was not yet clear. The British journal *Tubercle* editorialized in 1950 that "for a long time clinicians have been feeling their way towards the best way of using the many therapeutic measures at their disposal in the treatment of pulmonary tuberculosis.... There is no settled technique of dosage or length of [the] course of treatment and no agreement as to which sorts of cases should or should not have them."[52] Perhaps in response to such pleas, Tempel, Forsee, and their colleagues published numerous articles outlining tuberculosis treatment, considering factors such as therapeutic effectiveness, lack of toxicity, bacterial resistance, ease of administration, patient acceptance, sustainability for prolonged use, and relative costs of various protocols.[53] As chemotherapy became more effective and less toxic, they also eased the bed rest requirements that were difficult for so many patients. Tempel began to prescribe bed rest only during the early months of hospitalization or in case of serious illness. Thereafter, patients on drug therapy had four hours out of bed daily for "self-care and limited educational and recreational pursuits on the ward." When patients' sputum was negative, chest X-rays were improved, and they had been free of symptoms for a period of six months, they could begin ambulatory outpatient care.[54]

Finally, in 1952, scientists at three different drug companies—Bayer, La-Roche, and Squib—identified a third drug, isoniazid, as effective against tuberculosis bacteria. Gerhard Domagk, a German scientist at Bayer who had won the 1939 Nobel Prize for developing a powerful sulfa drug, pioneered this work. Barred from leaving the country to accept his Nobel award, and despite Allied bombing raids and the Nazi harassment and seizure of his Jewish wife (who survived

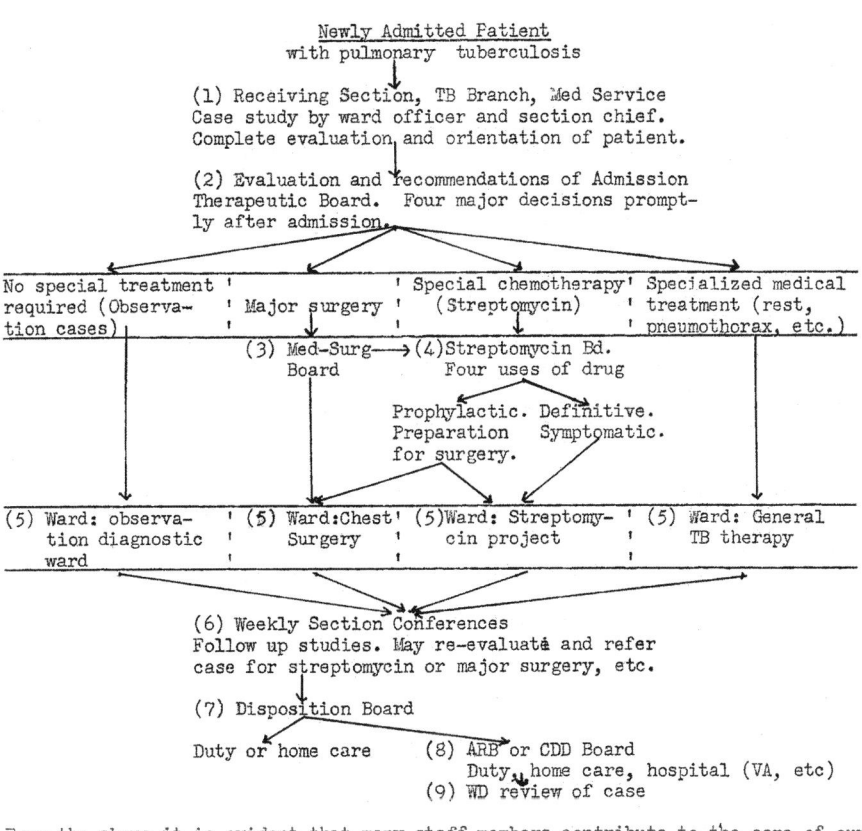

Figure 9-4. Table of treatment regimes for tuberculosis patients in "Annual Report of Fitzsimons General Hospital, Denver, Colorado, calendar year ending 31 December 1947," 76–77, FGH, Box 5, RG 112, National Archives and Records Administration, College Park, Maryland.

the war), Domagk continued his work on a tuberculosis cure. After the war, Allied scientists gained access to German research laboratories and discovered Domagk's work. Thus researchers at the three companies found isoniazid almost simultaneously.[55] At Fitzsimons, Tempel's team immediately tried isoniazid with streptomycin on sixty-one patients and found that they responded favorably.[56] In 1954 other researchers found that the three drugs together—streptomycin, PAS, and isoniazid—had greater therapeutic value and created fewer resistant strains than any previous combination.[57] Isoniazid therefore provided the final weapon that, in combination with PAS and/or streptomycin, safely and effectively cured tuberculosis. The treatment was not quick and easy—it involved taking two or three powerful drugs for several months, and sometimes even undergoing surgery—but for most individuals, it was a cure. Thus, as tuberculosis expert Michael Iseman explains, by 1954, "it was recognized that combining isoniazid, streptomycin, and PAS afforded nearly universal, lifetime cures of a scourge that had ravaged humankind like no other."[58]

Tuberculosis rates had already been steadily declining throughout the twentieth century in many countries, but with effective antibiotics the ability to save the lives of the very sick and to actually cure many tuberculosis cases marked a qualitative change in the fight against the disease and the status of tuberculosis medicine. The effect was—finally, thankfully—dramatic. In 1955, George J. Drolet and Anthony M. Lowell assessed "The First Seven Years of the Antimicrobial Era, 1947–1953," tracking the trajectory of tuberculosis death rates in the VA, Army, and Navy hospitals. They found that before streptomycin, the annual death rate for tuberculosis hospital patients was 20 percent to 23 percent; streptomycin reduced that to 17 percent, PAS and streptomycin brought it to about 10 percent, and the addition of isoniazid brought it down to 7.5 percent of VA and military tuberculosis patients, a two-thirds decrease in the death rate in less than a decade. The national trend was similar, with tuberculosis deaths in the United States falling 60 percent from 48,064 in 1947 to 19,393 in 1953. Other countries experienced declines ranging from a 38 percent drop in Mexico to an 83 percent reduction in Iceland. Drolet and Lowell believed that the shift from bed rest and collapse therapy to the "antimicrobial era" of chemotherapy and excisional surgery marked "the most rapid decline in tuberculosis mortality the world has ever seen."[59]

Others were equally elated. One writer said the trends vindicated Public Health Service epidemiologist Wade Hampton Frost's prediction that tuberculosis would one day be eradicated.[60] Louis Dublin, who had excoriated the VA's tuberculosis program for releasing infectious veterans, was ebullient. "The balance between the tubercle bacillus and man has finally given way in favor of man," he wrote. "We cannot say exactly when control will be complete, but there is every indication that it will be some time in the course of the next 20 years."[61] Most of the celebrants knew tuberculosis too well, however, to be sanguine. As the *American Journal of Public Health* observed in 1956, "While great gains against tuberculosis mortality have been achieved,...far more extensive measures are needed to eradicate infection from millions of adults who still harbor tubercle bacilli."[62] This would prove to be only too true.

Drug therapy did pose new problems. Because of the long duration of the treatment and antibiotics' side effects, some patients declined to complete the course of therapy. This enabled some bacteria to become resistant, and if the patient's tuberculosis resurged, made it more difficult to fight. By 1963, one study found that 8 percent of all new cases of tuberculosis in the country were resistant to streptomycin, PAS, or isoniazid.[63] Other issues emerged with regard to public health and tuberculosis that continue to be debated today. For example, if early cases of tuberculosis were the easiest to cure, Trudeau medalist James J. Waring at the University of Colorado Medical School asked, "just how minimal does tuberculosis have to be before one would not treat it with chemotherapy?"[64] Should public health officials treat people who had positive tuberculin tests but no other symptoms? Who should be in charge of tuberculosis treatment? Some believed that with effective chemotherapy and fewer patients, tuberculosis treatment could be returned to general practice medicine. But editors at the journal *Chest* countered that not all physicians and medical institutions understood the importance of educating patients about self-care and ensuring that they completed the full drug regimen. This, they cautioned, increased the chance of noncompliance, the development of bacterial resistance, and the spread of tuberculosis. They therefore advocated continuing to send tuberculosis patients to specialists who could provide comprehensive education and care.[65] Carl Tempel, in civilian life at the Webb-Waring Institute in Denver, cautioned in 1964 against "complacency in tuberculosis control," noting that one-quarter of the U.S. population was still infected with tuberculosis bacilli, and that many cases were not discovered until they were far advanced. He counseled continued vigilance and community education on tuberculosis to identify new cases and prevent strains from developing drug resistance.[66]

The new therapies did enable the Army to eliminate most tuberculosis from the ranks by screening out tuberculous recruits and then carefully overseeing the comprehensive application of the new treatments on any military patients. A study of VA and military patients successfully treated with chemotherapy from 1951 through 1954 reported that 86 percent returned to duty, work, or school. The researchers happily found that "working does not cause relapse, even when the work requires a high degree of physical exertion, even when pulmonary tuberculosis has been far advanced—if there has been definitive treatment of the disease."[67] By 1955 only 4.4 percent of veterans receiving disability payments had tuberculosis (91,000 of more than 2 million).[68]

This trend raised policy questions. After World War II, the U.S. Congress and the VA again struggled to define clear and equitable benefits for tuberculous veterans; the emergence of effective chemotherapy for the disease further complicated the issue. Postwar benefits provided disability compensation from 0 percent to 100 percent depending on the degree of a veteran's impairment. World War II tuberculosis veterans also had access to vocational rehabilitation and "G. I. Bill" education benefits and loans, and some of their survivors were eligible for Social Security benefits.[69] In the late 1940s, Congress authorized a three-year presumptive period for service-connected tuberculosis—the policy that denied Margaret Gaule's request for compensation. To the congressional mandate, the VA added additional coverage periods of six months for minimal tuberculosis, nine months for moderate tuberculosis, and twelve months for advanced tuberculosis. The government also continued to periodically revise the definition of service-connected tuberculosis as well as the level of disability and range of benefits to keep up with the evolving treatment regimes.[70]

A 1955 VA survey of civilian and military medical specialists' views on the validity of the disability rating system indicated the impact of antibiotics. One-fourth of the 153 respondents believed that tuberculosis benefits had become too liberal because diagnostic techniques and antibiotics often enabled the cure or arrest of the disease obviating the need for compensation.[71] One physician noted that "the arrested tuberculosis awards are in excess nowadays, with the new drugs and ambulatory therapy practiced and especially in those cases which have been operated on and for all practical purposes, cured."[72] The VA also became increasingly confident in its ability to treat tuberculosis. During one round of disability benefit adjustments in the 1970s, VA officials observed that "due to the impact of programs dealing with case-finding, diagnostic refinements, and improved chemotherapy, tuberculosis can now be quickly identified and up to 95% of new cases of tuberculosis can be quickly cured." They concluded that the relapse rate after effective treatment was so low as to be "virtually meaningless."[73]

Given such confidence and the fact that drug therapy shortened the bed rest requirements and hospital stays, hospitals across the country converted their tuberculosis wards to outpatient clinics, and sanatoriums slowly emptied; the last patient left Lake Saranac Sanatorium in New York in 1954. During the 1950s and 1960s tuberculosis institutions either had to adapt or close. Some, like the National Jewish Hospital in Denver, established programs for other respiratory diseases such as emphysema, cystic fibrosis, and asthma. In the early 1950s, the Army Medical Department's tuberculosis program at Fitzsimons reported a 55 percent reduction in occupied tuberculosis beds and an increasing number of outpatient visits; the hospital consequently took on new responsibilities.[74] In 1947 the Medical Department had designated Fitzsimons as an Army X-ray center for the treatment of malignant tumors, so that as tuberculosis rates fell and cancer rates increased, Fitzsimons' thoracic surgeons turned their skills to lung cancer and other diseases of the chest, and radiologists adapted their technology to therapeutic as well as diagnostic measures.[75] Fitzsimons also supported the postwar baby boom with a growing pediatrics program that cared for military dependents, and treated battle casualties from the Korean War in the 1950s, and Vietnam War in the 1960s and 1970s, specializing in chest wounds.[76] In 1955, the hospital found itself once again in the national spotlight, when, after a fishing trip in the Rocky Mountains, President Dwight D. Eisenhower suffered a heart attack and was rushed to Fitzsimons.[77] Seriously ill, the president stayed at the hospital in a special suite from 24 September to 11 November, and upon his departure commended the Fitzsimons staff for their medical care and extended his "very grateful thanks."[78]

With the end of the Cold War, however, and the contraction of Department of Defense facilities, Fitzsimons again faced the chopping block. Colorado's elected officials and Fitzsimons' partisans fought off several closure attempts, but in 1990 Congress passed the Defense Base Realignment and Closure Act that resulted in the closure of Fitzsimons in 1996 and the transfer of its healthcare responsibilities to the U.S. Army Medical Department Center and School at Fort Sam Houston, Texas. The Department of Defense then transferred the physical structures and land to what is now called the Fitzsimons Life Science District, which houses the University of Colorado Health Sciences Program and the Colorado Science and Technology Park for private enterprise. The District retained the Fitzsimons name for the campus but sought to "demilitarize" the post by converting the street names honoring military personnel to Denver city street names. Thus, names such as Bruns and Bushnell Avenues, Hutton and Halloran Circles, Moncrief Road, Quade Drive, Van Valzah Street, and Wright Loop are now gone.

But not all traces of the Army's "good tuberculosis men" have disappeared. If in the twenty-first century tuberculosis has become a minor, if not forgotten, presence at Fitzsimons, it remains nonetheless commemorated in the tall main hospital building that Lawrence Lewis dedicated in 1941. It is now called Building 500, but a new generation of medical personnel meets to discuss today's medical challenges in the Bushnell Auditorium and the Bruns Conference Room.

The Twenty-First Century

Despite the advent of antibiotic therapy, tuberculosis never submitted to significant control in those parts of the world lacking good housing, sanitation, nutrition, and robust medical and public health systems. In the 1980s, a new virus, human immunodeficiency virus/acquired immunodeficiency syndrome (HIV/AIDS), took hold in the country, lowering infected individuals' resistance, and thereby allowing myriad infections, including latent tuberculosis, to flourish. Tuberculosis therefore resurged in the United States, surprising a public health system that had lowered its guard and surveillance activities against the disease. Immigration from countries with high tuberculosis rates also contributed to American rate increases, as did persistent poverty, homelessness, and alcohol and drug abuse.[79] Fitzsimons felt the impact of HIV/AIDS with an average of 14 admissions a week, or 12 percent of inpatient admissions in 1986.[80] The hospital installed negative air pressure rooms, double air lock doors, and staff started using disposable gowns when treating infectious patients. Originally aimed at HIV/AIDS, these precautions soon became critical in the care of tuberculosis patients as well. Tuberculosis cases increased alarmingly in the nation, peaking in 1992 with 26,673 cases or 10.4 per 100,000 population. Rates thereafter declined annually, however, to 15,078, or 5.2 per 100,000 in 2001 and 10,528 cases or 3.4 per 100,000 people in 2011 in the United States.[81]

Tuberculosis never completely receded from Gaule's life. In 2004, eighty-four years of age and widowed, she reflected on her war experience, and resubmitted her request for veterans' benefits. This time the VA Board of Veterans' Appeals agreed to hear her appeal because "new and material evidence has been received to reopen the claim of service connection or residuals of pulmonary tuberculosis."[82] What was new? In the petition to the Board of Veterans' Appeals requesting a review of the case, Gaule's attorney William J. Lindsay Jr., stated that "evidence received subsequent to the January 1958 board determination raises a reasonable possibility of substantiating the claim of entitlement to service connection for pulmonary tuberculosis."[83] He attached a statement from Dr. P. James Connor, who, as a young physician had examined Gaule in Omaha in 1956 after her first lung hemorrhage. Connor, Lindsay explained, was "one of the few physicians in the United States who is still practicing who has had substantial experience with tuberculosis patients," and was also the Gaule's family physician.[84] Connor's letter stated that it was not unusual for active tuberculosis to turn up in people who had been exposed years before and cited his experience treating such patients between the 1940s and the 1960s. "Tuberculosis is an airborne disease and…Mrs. Gaule was exposed to it while in the service," he asserted, therefore "her chance of acquiring her tuberculosis was over 95% during her period of work as a nurse in the service of the United States government."[85] The appeals board concluded that "Dr. Connor's medical report clearly provides a potential nexus between pulmonary tuberculosis and military service which was not previously shown." Gaule's VA medical history also showed her scarred lungs, and that "substantial medical authority, including Internet research was submitted in support of the claim." It therefore agreed to reopen Gaule's application for service-connected benefits.[86]

On 15 February 2008, almost sixty-two years after she left the Army Nurse Corps, the VA granted Gaule's claim of disability noting "it is at least as likely as not that the pulmonary tuberculosis contracted in 1956 is related to your military service when you worked on Ward 13 at Barnes Hospital." The board assigned her a disability of "0%," however, because "medical evidence does not show that you have significantly disabling residuals to warrant a higher evaluation."[87] But in October 2009, after she was hospitalized with pulmonary hypertension, a condition that can be a result of tuberculosis, the VA recognized the connection and awarded Gaule $300 a month disability payments and $5,000 in retroactive compensation. The decision letter noted that "residuals of pulmonary tuberculosis, service connected, World War II, incurred static disability, 0% from 09/29/2003, 100% from 07/23/2009."[88] Gaule died on 20 February 2011 from complications following a stroke. She was ninety-one-years old.

The particulars of Gaule's case were no doubt central to the VA ruling, but the point here is that more than sixty years after World War II, the federal government was still negotiating policies concerning tuberculosis disability benefits. Today, although the Medical Department can exclude most tuberculosis from the Army, some troops will develop active disease while in service overseas or in the United States.[89] The Army Medical Department therefore continues to conduct tuberculosis surveillance in the ranks and to employ careful and rigorous protective measures when caring for confirmed or suspected tuberculosis patients.[90] This ancient, deadly disease, however, continues to elude understanding, and the search for improved diagnostics and treatments and an effective vaccine continues. According to the World Health Organization, tuberculosis ranks second behind HIV/AIDS as the most deadly single infectious agent for humans, and the combination of the two diseases is especially lethal: tuberculosis is the greatest single killer of people infected with HIV[91] (Figure 9-5). Equally troubling, tuberculosis bacteria continue to develop resistance to antibiotics, threatening decades of progress in disease control. Tuberculosis experts define multi-drug resistant tuberculosis (MDR-TB) bacteria

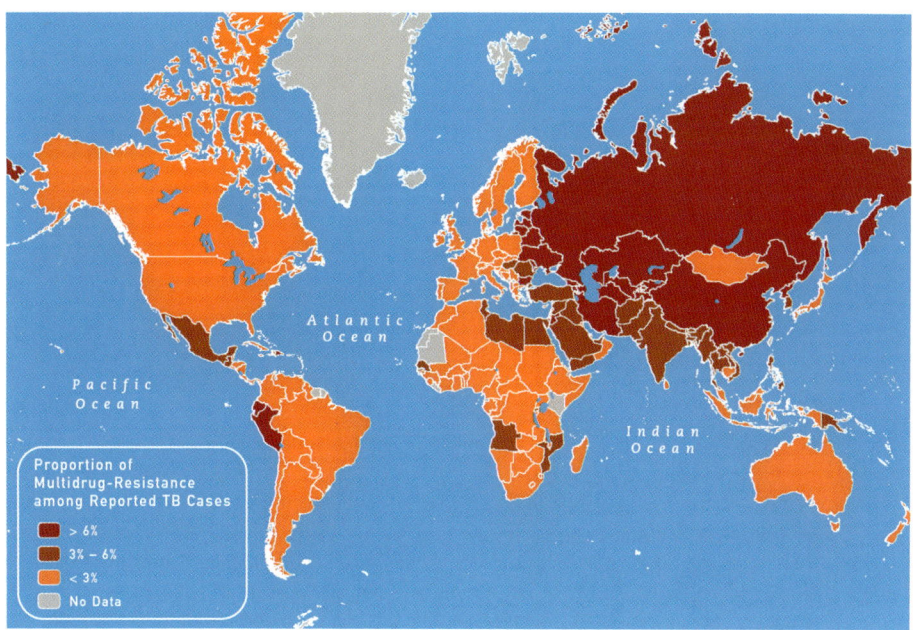

Figure 9-5. Map showing the infection rates of tuberculosis bacilli in the world population, from the Centers for Disease Control and Prevention Yellow Book, 2010. Available at http://wwwnc.cdc.gov/travel/images/map3-16-mdr-tb-large.png.

as those that do not respond to isoniazid and rifampicin, the two most powerful, first-line tuberculosis drugs, and extensively drug resistant tuberculosis (XDR-TB) bacteria as those resistant to isoniazid, rifampicin, and the most effective second-line drugs. Public health officials are now on guard for totally resistant strains that may have developed in patients in several countries in recent years.[92] The severity of these MDR and XDR tuberculosis infections has caused physicians to return to old methods of surgical excision and lung collapse to battle the disease, and to redouble research on *Mycobacterium tuberculosis*. In South Africa, for example, scientists have reproduced Richard Riley's studies on the airborne transmission of tuberculosis to better understand the transmissibility of XDR-TB.[93] As scientific knowledge of tuberculosis evolves, so will Army Medical Department tuberculosis policies and practice, continually redefining the disease experience as well as the hopes and fears of military and veteran patients and their families, doctors, and nurses who struggle with tuberculosis in the twenty-first century.

Notes

1. The following account is taken from Margaret Elizabeth Gaule, "The Diary of an Army Nurse by First Lieutenant Margaret Elizabeth Gaule," unpublished manuscript written in May 1945 on the island of Okinawa, in possession of the author.
2. P. James Connor to William J. Lindsay Jr., 31 July 2006, in possession of the author.
3. Author conversation with Gaule, 12 May 2006.
4. Margaret Gaule to Carol R. Byerly, 2007, in possession of the author.
5. Appeal of Margaret W. Gaule, Docket No. 05-25-216, Department of Veterans Affairs, 17 December 2007. The three-year presumption was approved by Congress in Public Law 573, 23 June 1950. See "The Veterans' Administration Disability Rating Schedule: Historical Development and Medical Appraisal," The President's Commission on Veterans' Pensions, Staff Report No. 8, Part B, 18 July 1956, House Committee Print No. 275, Committee on Veterans' Affairs, 84th Congress, 2nd sess.
6. John Wakeman Turner, "Colonel Bushnell's Epidemiology of Tuberculosis," *Military Surgeon* 92 (June 1943): 637.
7. Robert G. Lovell, *Taking the Cure: The Patient's Approach to Tuberculosis* (New York, NY: MacMillan, 1948), 60.
8. M. Pollak, "Don't Neglect Tuberculosis," *American Journal of Nursing* 44 (December 1944): 1133.
9. Leopold Brahdy, "Compensation for the Tuberculosis Nurse?" *American Journal of Nursing* 47 (June 1947): 381–82; and Theodore C. Waters and Mary Graham Mack, "Is Tuberculosis Compensable?" *American Journal of Nursing* 50 (December 1950): 776–79.
10. Edgar Mayer and Israel Rappaport, "Contagiousness of Tuberculosis: Its Relation to Compensation Claims," *Chest* 9 (1943): 500–9.
11. "Editorial," *Chest* 20 (1951): 564–67. The studies were: W. H. Oatway Jr., "Current Status of Routine Chest X-rays in General Hospitals in the United States," *Arizona Medicine* 6 (1949): 23; and W. H. Oatway Jr., "Aseptic Technic in the Care of Tuberculosis Patients," *American Journal of Nursing* 50 (March 1950): 164–66.
12. "Editorial," *Chest* 20 (1951): 564–67.
13. Dan Morse and R. H. Runde, "The Non-Cooperative Patient," *Diseases of the Chest* 18 (1950): 599–608.
14. James H. Sands et al., "Irregular Discharges of Tuberculous Patients: An Analysis of 273 Cases," *Chest* 28 (1955): 555.

15. *Fitzsimons Annual Report,* 1947 [hereafter cited as *FZAR*, year], 82.
16. *FZAR*, 1948, 83.
17. *FZAR*, 1950, 84; and *FZAR*, 1949, 88.
18. Florence A. Burkhead, "Lesson Plan: The Fundamentals of Tuberculosis Nursing," typescript, 1956, Military History Institute, Carlisle Barracks, PA.
19. For example, Esmond R. Long, "The Hazard of Acquiring Tuberculosis in the Laboratory," *American Journal of Public Health* 41 (July 1951): 782–87.
20. Max B. Lurie, "Control of Airborne Contagion of Tuberculosis," *American Journal of Nursing* 46 (1946): 809.
21. Esta H. McNett, "The Face Mask in Tuberculosis," *American Journal of Nursing* 49 (January 1949): 32–36.
22. For example, W. F. Wells, "Droplets and Droplet Nuclei," *American Journal of Hygiene* 20 (November 1934): 611–27.
23. R. L. Riley, C. C. Mills, W. Nyka, et al., "Aerial Dissemination of Pulmonary Tuberculosis: A Two-Year Study of Contagion in a Tuberculosis Ward," *American Journal of Hygiene* 70 (1959): 185–96. Reprinted as "Historical Paper," in *American Journal of Epidemiology* 142 (1995): 3–14.
24. Riley, Mills, Nyka, et al., "Aerial Dissemination of Pulmonary Tuberculosis,"196. Also, Richard L. Riley, W. Wells, C. Mills, et al., "Air Hygiene in Tuberculosis: Quantitative Studies of Infectivity and Control in a Pilot Ward," *American Review of Tuberculosis* 75 (1957): 420–30.
25. Richard L. Riley and F. O'Grady, *Airborne Infection: Transmission and Congress* (New York, NY: Macmillan, 1961).
26. L. Fred Ayvazian, "The Fifty-Five Trudeau Medalists (1926–1980): A Seventy-Fifth Anniversary Review," *American Review of Respiratory Disease* 121 (1980): 771. The Trudeau Medal is still given today, but for contributions for the "cause, prevention, and treatment of lung disease," and is awarded by the American Lung Association, the successor organization of the National Tuberculosis Association.
27. Michael D. Iseman, "Invited Commentary" on "Aerial Dissemination of Pulmonary Tuberculosis, " *American Journal of Epidemiology* 142 (1995): 2. See also Edward A. Nardell, "Catching Droplet Nuclei: Toward a Better Understanding of Tuberculosis Transmission," *American Journal of Respiratory and Critical Care Medicine* 169 (2004): 553–54.
28. H. C. Hinshaw and W. H. Feldman, "Streptomycin in Treatment of Clinical Tuberculosis: A Preliminary Report," *Proceedings of the Staff Meetings of the Mayo Clinic* 20 (5 September 5, 1945): 313–17; and H. Corwin Hinshaw, William H. Feldman, and Karl H. Pfuetze, "Treatment of Tuberculosis with Streptomycin: A Summary of Observations on 100 Cases," *Journal of the American Medical Association* 132 (30 November 1946): 778–82.
29. On human experimentation see W. H. Johnson, "Civil Rights of Military Personnel Regarding Medical Care and Experimental Procedures," *Science* 117 (1953): 212–15; Jordan Goodman, Anthony McElligott, and Lara Marks, "Making Human Bodies Useful: Historicizing Medical Experiments in the Twentieth Century," in *Useful Bodies: Humans in the Service of Medical Science in the Twentieth Century*, Jordan Goodman, Anthony McElligott, and Lara Marks, eds. (Baltimore, MD: Johns Hopkins University Press, 2003); Susan E. Lederer, *Subjected to Science: Human Experimentation on Americans before the Second World War* (Baltimore, MD: Johns Hopkins University Press, 1995); and Thomas G. Benedek, "The History of Gold Therapy for Tuberculosis," *Journal of the History of Medicine and Allied Sciences* 59 (2004): 50–89.

30. Harry M. Marks, *The Progress of Experiment: Science and Therapeutic Reform in the United States, 1900–1990* (Cambridge, UK: Cambridge University Press, 1997), 115.

31. Memorandum, "Streptomycin Conference," 18 June 1946, Esmond R. Long Papers, Manuscript Collection 362, National Library of Medicine; and Esmond Long to Surgeon General, "Visit at Fitzsimons General Hospital," 13 July 1946, Record Group 112, Records of the Surgeon General of the Army [hereafter cited as RG 112], Entry 31, 1945–56, Box 1428, National Archives and Records Administration [hereafter cited as NARA].

32. Esmond R. Long to Larry B. McAfee, 28 August 1945, Esmond R. Long Papers, Medical Historical Unit Collection, Personal Papers, Military History Institute, Carlisle Barracks, PA.

33. Marks, *The Progress of Experiment*, 116.

34. Marks, *The Progress of Experiment*, 127 and 115.

35. Chester S. Keefer et al, "Streptomycin in the Treatment of Infections: A Report of 1,000 Cases," *Journal of the American Medical Association* 132 (7 September 1946): 4–5; and Council on Pharmacy and Chemistry, "Effects of Streptomycin on Tuberculosis in Men," *Journal of the American Medical Association* 135 (8 November 1947): 634–43. Also, Virginia Cameron and Esmond R. Long, *Tuberculosis Medical Research: National Tuberculosis Association, 1904–1955* (New York, NY: National Tuberculosis Association, 1959), 92.

36. Selman A. Waksman, *The Conquest of Tuberculosis* (Berkeley, CA: University of California Press, 1964), chapter 9.

37. Stanley H. Hoffman and George A. Hyman, "The Combined Use of Streptomycin and Pneumoperioneum in the Treatment of Pulmonary Tuberculosis," *Diseases of the Chest* (March 1949): 354–65.

38. James H. Forsee, "Extrapleural Thoracoplasty Early in Caseo-pneumonic Tuberculosis," *Rocky Mountain Medical Journal* (June 1949): 452–59. A. E. Ellis' novel, *The Rack*, draws a chilling portrait of the impact on patients in this early stage of drug therapy. The protagonist, Paul, undergoes multiple surgeries, develops resistance to streptomycin, and is left to an excruciatingly drawn-out and painful death that gave the novel its title. A. E. Ellis, *The Rack* (London, UK: Penguin Books, 1958, 1961).

39. George W. Fishburn, Myron W. Fisher, and John D. Wallace, "Streptomycin in the Treatment of Tuberculosis," *Bulletin of the U.S. Army Medical Department* 7 (October 1947): 877–79.

40. "A Concise Biography of Major General James Hedges Forsee," May 1965, Biographical Background Files, RG 112, Box 16, NARA.

41. James H. Forsee, "Forward Surgery of the Severely Wounded," Office of The Surgeon General, Second Auxiliary Surgical Group Report to the Surgeon General (Washington, DC, Office of The Surgeon General, 1945); and Lyman A. Brewer III, "The Contributions of the Second Auxiliary Surgical Group to Military Surgery During World War II with Special Reference to Thoracic Surgery," *Annals of Surgery* 197 (March 1983): 318–26.

42. The Institute was initially established to honor Gerald Webb, George Bushnell's tuberculosis specialist in the American Expeditionary Forces during World War I, and James S. Waring, a Denver tuberculosis specialist who headed up some research programs at Fitzsimons during World War II. See Helen Clapsattle, *Dr. Webb of Colorado Springs* (Boulder, CO: Colorado Associated University Press, 1984), epilogue; and "Major General Carl W. Tempel, Medical Corps, U.S. Army," September 1960, Biographical Background Files, RG 112, Box 48, NARA.

43. Fort Logan National Cemetery Web site: http://www.interment.net/data/us/co/denver/logan/t/t02.htm, accessed 24 August 2012.

44. Carl W. Tempel and James H. Foresee, "The Definitive Treatment of Pulmonary Tuberculosis: General Therapeutic Principles as They Apply to Various Types of Chest Lesions," *Military Surgeon* 108 (1951): 375–83.

45. James H. Forsee, *The Surgery of Pulmonary Tuberculosis* (Philadelphia, PA: Lea and Febiger, 1954), which was translated into Japanese; "A Concise Biography of Major General James Hedges Forsee," May 1965, Biographical Background Files, RG 112, Box 16, NARA; author's conversation with James Hedges Forsee Jr., 12 March 2010; and "Major General Carl W. Tempel," September 1960, Biographical Background Files, RG 112, Box 48, NARA.

46. James H. Forsee, "Extrapleural Thoracoplasty Early in Caseo-pneumonic Tuberculosis." Barron Lerner writes that "The major role played by surgery in the 'conquest' of tuberculosis after World War II has been largely neglected." Barron H. Lerner, *Contagion and Confinement: Controlling Tuberculosis along Skid Row* (Baltimore, MD: Johns Hopkins University Press, 1998), 62.

47. Paul F. Ware, Hans-Karl Stauss, Robert J. Dillon, and Carl W. Tempel, "Present Status of Pulmonary Resection in the Treatment of Localized Necrotic Residuals of Pulmonary Tuberculosis," *American Review of Tuberculosis* 76 (1956): 175; Carl W. Tempel and William E. Dye, "Selecting the Streptomycin Regimen for Patients with Pulmonary Tuberculosis with Special Reference to Intermittent Dosage Schedule," *Diseases of the Chest* 16 (December 1949): 704–13; and Carl W. Tempel and John R. Durrance, "The Use of Streptomycin in Tuberculosis," *Bulletin of the U.S. Army Medical Department* 9 (April 1949): 312–15.

48. *FZAR*, 1947, 75–77.

49. Tempel and Dye, "Selecting the Streptomycin Regimen for Patients with Pulmonary Tuberculosis with Special Reference to the Intermittent Dosage Schedule."

50. Carl W. Tempel, "The Place of Streptomycin in the Treatment of Pulmonary Tuberculosis," *Bulletin of the U.S. Army Medical Department* 9 (January 1949): 25–34.

51. Annual Report, Fitzsimons General Hospital, Denver, Colorado, 1949, RG 90, Records of the Public Health Service, NARA Denver, folder 258; and Veterans Administration, "Minutes of the Eighth Streptomycin Conference," Fulton County Medical Society, Atlanta, GA, 10–13 November 1949, in Esmond R. Long Papers, National Library of Medicine.

52. "Streptomycin and PAS," *Tubercule* 73 (1950): 31.

53. Carl W. Tempel, James A. Wier, and Paul F. Ware, "The Classification and Treatment of Pulmonary Tuberculosis: Definitive Care Based on an Evaluation of Lung Pathology," monograph, Denver, CO: Fitzsimons Army Hospital, n.d., c. 1953; and Tempel and Forsee, "The Definitive Treatment of Pulmonary Tuberculosis." Other related articles can be found in Medical Historical Unit Collection, Professional Papers, Military History Institute, Carlisle, PA.

54. Tempel, Wier, and Ware, "Definitive Care," 12–13.

55. Michael D. Iseman, *A Clinician's Guide to Tuberculosis* (Philadelphia, PA: Lippincott Williams & Wilkins, 2000), 16–17.

56. Forrest W. Pitts et al., "Isoniazid and Streptomycin in the Treatment of Pulmonary Tuberculosis," *Journal of the American Medical Association* 152 (4 July 1953): 886–90.

57. See, for example, Albert R. Allen, Guy E. Marcy, and James K. Yu, "The Continuous and Concurrent Use of Streptomycin, Para-Aminosalicylic Acid, Isoniazid Plus Early Surgery in the Treatment of Tuberculosis," *Diseases of the Chest* 26 (July 1954): 41–43.

58. Iseman, *A Clinician's Guide to Tuberculosis,* 18; Michael D. Iseman, "Evolution of Drug-Resistant Tuberculosis: Tale of Two Species," *Proceedings of the National Academy*

of Sciences, U.S.A., (1994): 2428; Waksman, *The Conquest of Tuberculosis;* Frank Ryan, *The Forgotten Plague: How the Battle against Tuberculosis was Won—and Lost;* and Hubert Lechevalier, "The Search for Antibiotics at Rutgers University," in *The History of Antiobiotics: A Symposium*, ed. John Parascandola (Madison, WI: American Institute of the History of Pharmacy, 1980).

59. George J. Drolet and Anthony M. Lowell, "Whereto Tuberculosis; The First Seven Years of the Antimicrobial Era, 1947–1953," *American Review of Tuberculosis* 72 (October 1955): 442.

60. Floyd M. Feldmann, "How Much Control of Tuberculosis: 1937–1957–1977?" *American Journal of Public Health* 47 (October 1957): 1235–41.

61. Louis I. Dublin, "The Course of Tuberculosis Mortality and Morbidity in the United States," *American Journal of Public Health* 48 (November 1958): 1447–48.

62. Godias J. Drolet, "Whereat Tuberculosis?" *American Journal of Public Health* 46 (July 1956): 895–96.

63. Irving Willner, "Can Tuberculosis Be Eradicated?" *Chest* 43 (1963): 270.

64. James J. Waring, "The Achilles Heel of Tuberculosis Control," *Diseases of the Chest* 30 (1956): 438.

65. Editorial, "Care of Tuberculosis Patients in the 1970s. After the Sanitorium, Then What?" *Chest* 60 (October 1971): 309.

66. Carl W. Tempel, "Complacency in Tuberculosis Control," *Diseases of the Chest* 45 (1964): 223–24. See also Willner, "Can Tuberculosis Be Eradicated?" 270.

67. Morris W. Lambie and Kenneth A. Dening, "Employment and Clinical Follow-Up of 532 Tuberculosis Patients Discharged from 1951 to 1954," *Chest* 49 (1966): 37.

68. See "The Veterans' Administration Disability Rating Schedule: Historical Development and Medical Appraisal," The President's Commission on Veterans' Pensions, Staff Report No. 7, Part B, 18 July 1956, House Committee Print No. 275, Committee on Veterans' Affairs, 84th Congress, 2nd sess.

69. The President's Commission on Veterans' Pensions, "The Historical Development of Veterans' Benefits in the United States," Staff Report No. 1, 1956, House Committee Print No. 244, Committee on Veterans' Affairs, 84th Cong., 2nd sess.

70. The President's Commission on Veterans' Pensions, "The Historical Development of Veterans' Benefits in the United States."

71. Fourteen of the respondents were tuberculosis specialists, and included Esmond R. Long, Donald King of the North Africa tuberculosis program, and several medical officers from Fitzsimons Hospital. President's Commission on Veterans' Pensions, "The Veterans Administration Disability Rating Schedule," 262–66.

72. President's Commission on Veterans' Pensions, "The Veterans Administration Disability Rating Schedule," 202.

73. Veterans Administration, "Veterans Benefits, Rating Considerations Relative to Specific Diseases," *Federal Register* 43 (3 July 1978): 28824.

74. Fitzsimons Army Hospital, "Program Document FY 1957," RG 112, Records of US Army Hospitals, 1919–67, Fitzsimons General Hospital, Box 35, NARA.

75. FZAR, 1947, 192–94. Some of these changes are discussed in Cynthia A. Gurney, *Thirty-Three Years of Army Nursing: An Interview with Brigadier General Lillian Dunlap* (Washington, DC: United States Army Nurse Corps, 2001), 97–108.

76. FZAR, 1950, 106–7 and 155.

77. "Normally Quiet, Hospital Turns Into Busy Place," *Denver Post*, 25 September 1955, 3a.

78. Dwight D. Eisenhower, "Remarks on Leaving Denver, Colorado," 11 November 1955, The American Presidency Project, University of California at Santa Barbara, available at: http://www.presidency.ucsb.edu/ws/index.php?pid=10383&st=Denver&st1=, accessed 24 August 2012.

79. Randall Reves, "Epidemiology of Tuberculosis," in the "Denver TB Course," National Jewish Medical and Research Center, 26–29 April 2006, Denver, CO; Matthew Gandy and Alimuddin Zumla, eds., *The Return of the White Plague: Global Poverty and the 'New' Tuberculosis* (London, UK: Verso, 2003); and CDC Tuberculosis Surveillance Report, 2011, available at: http://www.cdc.gov/tb/statistics/reports/2011/pdf/report2011.pdf, accessed 6 November 2012.

80. *FZAR,* 1984, 22; *FZAR,* 1987, D-2; and *FZAR,* 1986, 20.

81. Centers for Disease Control and Prevention, *Reported Tuberculosis in the United States, 2011* (Atlanta, GA: U.S. Department of Health and Human Services, CDC, October 2012), 15.

82. Appeal of Margaret W. Gaule, Docket No. 05-25-216, Department of Veterans Affairs, 17 December 2007.

83. Appeal of Margaret W. Gaule, Docket No. 05-25-216.

84. Attachment to VA Form 9, Gaule, Margaret W., 07 870 022.

85. P. James Connor to William J. Lindsay, Jr., 24 January 2008, in possession of author.

86. In the Appeal of Margaret W. Gaule, C7 870 022, Board of Veterans' Appeals, Department of Veterans Affairs.

87. Department of Veterans Affairs, VA Regional Office, VA file number 07 807 022, Margaret W. Gaule, Rating Decision, 15 February 2008.

88. Department of Veterans Affairs, VA Regional Office, VA file number 07 870 022, Margaret W. Gaule, Decision on Appeal, 21 October 2009; author's phone conversation with Margaret W. Gaule, 3 March 2010; and conversation with Dennis Gaule, 29 November 2012. My thanks to Dennis Gaule, Margaret Gaule's son, for his assistance in documenting this decision.

89. One study identified 578 active cases of tuberculosis in the U.S. military from 1990 to 2006. J.D. Mancusco, S.K. Tobler, A.A. Eick, and L.W. Keep, "Active Tuberculosis and Recent Overseas Deployment in the U.S. Military," *American Journal of Preventive Medicine* 39 (August 2010): 157–63. See also Donald F. Thompson, Joel L. Swerdlow, and Cheryl A. Loeb, "The Bug Stops Here: Force Protection and Emerging Infectious Diseases," Center for Technology and National Security Policy, National Defense University, November 2005. Available at: http://www.ndu.edu/CTNSP/.../DTP%2021%20Bug%20 Stops%20Here.pdf, accessed 24 August 2012.

90. For the most recent Department of Defense policies regarding tuberculosis see the DoD Deployment Health Clinical Center Web site: http://www.pdhealth.mil/tuberculosis.asp#cg, accessed 24 August 2012. See also Jamie Mancuso, "Tuberculosis in the U.S. Military," presentation at Walter Reed Army Institute of Research, 15 September 2010, available online at: http://wrair-www.army.mil/Documents/TropMed/11-Mancuso-MTb-WRAIRTropMed.pdf, accessed 6 November 2012; James D. Mancuso, Steven K. Tobler, and Lisa W. Keep, "Pseudoepidemics of Tuberculin Skin Test Conversions in the U.S. Army after Recent Deployments," *American Journal of Respiratory and Critical Care Medicine* 177 (2008): 1285–89; and M. Renè Howell, "Screening for Mycobacterium Tuberculosis in the U.S. Military: Considerations for a Cost-Effectiveness Model," Johns Hopkins Medicine, Johns Hopkins University, n.d., available at: http://www.health.mil/dhb/afeb/meeting/021803meeting/TB%20Screening%20US%20Military%20Cost%20 Model.pdf, accessed 30 November 2012.

91. WHO tuberculosis fact sheet, available at: http://www.who.int/mediacentre/factsheets/fs104/en/, accessed 30 November 2012.

92. Gwen Huitt, "MDR/XDR-TB," Denver TB Course, 13 October 2012, available at: http://www.nationaljewish.org/pdf/Proed_TB_2012_Huitt_MDR_XDRTB.pdf, accessed 30 November 2012; and Centers for Disease Control and Prevention, Web site on Tuberculosis, available at http://www.cdc.gov/TB/default.htm, accessed 30 November 2012.

93. See for example, Russell R. Kempker, Sergo Vashakidze, Nelly Solominia, Nino Dzidzikashvili, and Henry M. Blumberg, "Surgical Treatment of Drug-Resistant Tuberculosis," *The Lancet Infectious Diseases* 12 (February 2012): 157–66; Edward A. Nardell, "Quantifying Transmission of MDR-TB: Riley Revisited," presentation at Department of Microbiology, Immunology, and Pathology, Colorado State University, 8 April 2008; and Lee B. Reichman and Janice Hopkins Tanne, *Timebomb: The Global Epidemic of Multi-Drug-Resistant Tuberculosis* (New York, NY: McGraw-Hill, 2002).

Selected Bibliography

PRIMARY SOURCES

National Archives and Records Administration, Washington, DC; College Park, MD; Denver, CO; and Fort Wayne, TX
    RG 15, Records of the Veterans Administration
    RG 51, Records of the Bureau of the Budget
    RG 52, Records of the Bureau of Medicine and Surgery
    RG 59, Records of the Department of State
    RG 90, Records of the Public Health Service
    RG 94, Records of the Adjutant General
    RG 112, Records of the Army Surgeon General
    RG 153, Records of the Judge Advocate General
    RG 159, Records of the Office of Inspector General
    RG 165, Records of the Office of the Chief of Staff
    RG 227, Records of the Office of Scientific Research and Development
    RG 247, Records of the Office of the Chief of Chaplains
    RG 338, Records of the U.S. Army Commands
    RG 389, Records of the Provost Marshall General
    RG 393, Records of the U.S. Army Continental Commands
    RG 407, Records of the Adjutant General

Government Reports
    Annual Reports of the Army Surgeon General
    Annual Reports of the Department of War
    Annual Reports of Fitzsimons Army Hospital
    Annual Reports of the Public Health Service
    Annual Reports of the Veterans Administration

Office of The Surgeon General. *The Medical Department in the World War*. Vols. 1–15. Washington, DC: U.S. Army, Office of The Surgeon General, 1921–29.

Select volumes from: Office of The Surgeon General. *Medical Department, U.S. Army in World War II*. Washington, DC: U.S. Army, Office of The Surgeon General, 1950–72.
> Anderson, Robert S., and William B. Foster, U.S. Army Medical Service, U.S. Department of the Army, Office of The Surgeon General, and U.S. Army Medical Service Historical Unit. *Physical Standards in World War II*, Washington, DC: Office of The Surgeon General, Department of the Army, 1967.
> Armfield, Blanche B., John Boyd Coates, Leonard D. Heaton, Charles Maurice Wiltse. U.S. Department of the Army, Office of The Surgeon General, and U.S. Army Medical Service Historical Unit. *Organization and Administration in World War II, Medical Department, United States Army in World War II*. Washington, DC: Office of The Surgeon General, Department of the Army, 1963.
> Coates, John Boyd, Frank B. Berry, Elizabeth M. McFetridge, Leonard D. Heaton, U.S. Department of the Army, Office of The Surgeon General, and U.S. Army Medical Service Historical Unit. *Thoracic Surgery*. 2 vols. *Medical Department, U.S. Army in World War II*. Washington, DC: Office of The Surgeon General, Department of the Army, 1963.
> Coates, John Boyd, and Ebbe Curtis Hoff, U.S. Army Medical Department Historical Unit, and U.S. Surgeon General's Office. *Preventive Medicine in World War II*. Washington, DC: Office of The Surgeon General, Department of the Army, 1955.
> Havens, Jr., W. Paul. U.S. Army Medical Department Historical Unit, and U.S. Department of the Army, Office of The Surgeon General, *Internal Medicine in World War II*, *Medical Department, U.S. Army in World War II,* vol. 2. Washington, DC: U.S. Department of Defense, Department of the Army, Office of The Surgeon General, 1963.
> Heaton, Leonard D., U.S. Department of the Army, Office of The Surgeon General, and U.S. Army Medical Service Historical Unit. *Activities of Surgical Consultants, Medical Department, U.S. Army in World War II*. Washington, DC: Office of The Surgeon General, Department of the Army, 1962.

Reister, Frank A. U.S. Army Medical Department Historical Unit and U.S. Department of the Army, Office of The Surgeon General. *Medical Statistics in World War II, Medical Department, U.S. Army in World War II*. Washington, DC: Office of The Surgeon General, U.S. Department of the Army, 1975

Smith, Clarence McKittrick. *The Medical Department: Hospitalization and Evacuation, Zone of Interior. U.S. Army in World War II*. Washington, DC: Office of the Chief of Military History, Department of the Army, 1956.

Military History Institute, Carlisle, PA

Bruns, Earl H. "The Tuberculosis Situation in the American Expeditionary Forces." Trier, Germany: Office of Civil Governor, American Area, Department of Sanitation and Public Health, 1919, unpublished manuscript.

Duncan, William H. "William H. Duncan Papers," 2004.

Johnson, Richard, " My Life in the US Army, 1899 to 1922," unpublished manuscript.

Medical Historical Unit Collection, Personal Papers.
    James Hedges Papers
    Esmond R. Long Papers
    Carl Willard Tempel Papers

Moncrief, William H., Papers, 1876–1973.

National Library of Medicine, Bethesda, MD

Bier, Robert A. "Fitzsimons General Hospital, Denver, Lecture notes, 1926–1927," typescript.

Association of Military Surgeons of the United States Biographical Sketch Collection, 1870–1940. Ms C142

Lectures on Tuberculosis, Fort Bayard, 1910–1913. Ms C12

Illustrations of Tuberculous Lesions. Fort Bayard, NM: U.S. Army General Hospital, 1908.

Papers of Esmond R. Long. Ms C362

U.S. Army Medical Department, 1942–45, Lectures, Talks, and Statements. Ms C26

Periodicals
    Biand-Foryu
    The Oteen
    Soldiers in White
    The Star Shell
    Stethoscope

Colorado Historical Society, Denver, CO
   Lawrence Lewis Papers, Scrapbooks, and Diaries

South Carolina Historical Association, Charleston, SC
   George S. Legare Papers, correspondence, 1907–08. In Legare Family Papers, Waring Family Papers

Tutt Library, Colorado College, Colorado Springs, CO
   Gerald Bertram Webb Papers

Periodicals
   American Journal of Nursing
   American Journal of Public Health
   American Medicine
   American Review of Tuberculosis/American Review of Pulmonary Diseases
   Annals of Medical History
   Archives of Internal Medicine
   Army and Navy Journal
   Boston Medical and Surgical Journal
   Bulletin of the United States Army Medical Department
   The British Journal of Tuberculosis
   British Medical Journal
   Denver Medical Times
   Denver Post
   Diseases of the Chest/Chest
   Journal of the American Medical Association
   Journal of Experimental Medicine
   Journal of Laboratory and Clinical Medicine
   Journal of the Outdoor Life
   Lancet
   Medical and Surgical Reporter
   Medical Record
   Military Surgeon/Military Medicine
   Modern Hospital
   New Mexico Medical Journal/Southwestern Medicine
   New York Medical Journal
   New York Times
   Public Health Reports
   Rocky Mountain Medical Journal/Colorado Medicine
   Rocky Mountain News

Transactions of the American Climatological Association
Transactions of the National Tuberculosis Association
Tubercle
U.S. Armed Forces Medical Journal
U.S. Navy Medical Bulletin
Western Medical Times

Published Documents

Ashburn, Percy M. *A History of the Medical Department of the U.S. Army*. Boston, MA and New York, NY: Houghton Mifflin, Co., 1929.

Aynes, Edith A. *From Nightingale to Eagle*. Englewood Cliffs, NJ: Prentice-Hall, Inc., 1973.

Bateman, Cephas C. "The Army Hospital at Fort Bayard: Fort Bayard, New Mexico." Lawrence, KS: Kansas Collection, University of Kansas Libraries, c. 1911.

Bumgarner, J. R. "Phthisis: My Case History. Surviving a Fifteen Year Odyssey As POW and Patient." *North Carolina Medical Journal* 54, no. 6 (June 1993): 288–90.

Bushnell, George. *The Diagnosis of Tuberculosis in the Military Service*. New York, NY: William Wood, 1917.

_____. "Record of completed cases of tuberculosis at the United States Army General Hospital, Fort Bayard, New Mexico." U.S. Army General Hospital (Fort Bayard, NM, 1908).

_____. *A Study in the Epidemiology of Tuberculosis with Especial Reference to Tuberculosis of the Tropics and of the Negro Race*. New York, NY: William Wood, 1922.

Carrington, Paul M.. *How Uncle Sam Fights the Great White Plague: Sanatorium of PHS and Marine Hospital Service at Fort Stanton, New Mexico*. Santa Fe, NM: n.p. 1907.

Crane, A. G. *Education for the Disabled in War and Industry. Army Hospital Schools: A Demonstration for the Education of Disabled in Industry*. Vol. 110. New York, NY: Teachers College, Columbia University, 1921.

Dublin, Louis I. *The Mortality from Tuberculosis: A Study of the Experience Among the Industrial Policyholders of the Metropolitan Life Insurance Company, 1911 to 1930, Monograph 2 in a Twenty-year Mortality Review*. New York, NY: Metropolitan Life Insurance Company, 1935.

Ellis, A. E. *The Rack*. London, UK: Penguin Books, 1958, 1961.

Fitzsimons Army Medical Center. *Manual on Management of Pulmonary Tuberculosis*. Denver, CO: 1953.

Fitzsimons General Hospital. *The Gift Book: Fitzsimons General Hospital, U.S.A.* Denver, CO: Wahlgreen Publishing, 1926.

Garrison, Fielding H. *An Introduction to the History of Medicine*. 4th ed. Philadelphia, PA: W. B. Saunders, 1929.

Hoppin, Laura Brackett. *History of the World War Reconstruction Aides*. Millbrook, NY: William Tyldsley, 1933.

Klebs, Arnold C., ed. *Tuberculosis: A Treatise by American Authors on its Etiology, Pathology, Frequency, Semeiology, Diagnosis, Prognosis, Prevention, and Treatment*. New York, NY: D. Appleton & Co., 1909.

Knopf, Adolphus S. *Tuberculosis as a Disease of the Masses and How to Combat It*. 5th ed. New York, NY: Fred P. Flori, 1908.

Long, Esmond R. "Tuberculosis in Modern Society." *Bulletin of the History of Medicine* 27 (1953): 302–16.

———. "Weak Lungs on the Santa Fe Trail." *Bulletin of the History of Medicine* 8 (1940): 1040–54.

Long, Esmond R., and Seymour Jablon. *Tuberculosis in the Army of the United States in World War II: An Epidemiological Study With an Evaluation of X-ray Screening*. Washington, DC: Government Printing Office, 1955.

MacDonald, Betty. *The Plague and I*. Philadelphia, PA: J. B. Lippincott, 1948.

Mann, Thomas. *The Magic Mountain*, 1924.

Myers, J. Arthur. *Tuberculosis: A Half Century of Study and Conquest*. St. Louis, MO: Warren H. Green, Inc., 1970.

The President's Commission on Veterans' Pensions. *The Historical Development of Veterans' Benefits in the United States*. Edited by Committee on Veterans' Affairs. U.S. Congress, 84th Cong., 2nd sess., House Committee Print No. 244 ed., *Report on Veterans' Benefits in the United States*. Washington, DC: Government Printing Office, 1956.

Riley, Richard L. and F. O'Grady. *Airborne Infection: Transmission and Control*. New York, NY: Macmillan, 1961.

Rixey, Presley Marion. *The Study of Tuberculosis in the United States Navy*. Carlisle, PA: Association of Military Surgeons, 1908.

Stewart, Donald. *Sanatorium*. New York, NY: Harper and Brothers Publishers, 1930.

Tempel, Carl Willard. *The Classification and Treatment of Pulmonary Tuberculosis: Definitive Care Based upon an Evaluation of Lung Pathology*. Denver, CO: Fitzsimons Army Hospital, 1953.

Tobey, James A. *A Manual of Tuberculosis Legislation*. New York, NY: National Tuberculosis Association, 1928.

———. *The Medical Department of the Army: Its History, Activities, and Organization*. Baltimore, MD: The Johns Hopkins University Press, 1927.

Waksman, Selman A. *The Conquest of Tuberculosis*. Berkeley, CA: University of California Press, 1964.

Webb, Gerald B. *Tuberculosis*. New York, NY: Paul B. Hoeber, 1936.

SECONDARY SOURCES

Abbot, Carl, Stephen J. Leonard, and Thomas J. Noel. *Colorado: A History of the Centennial State*. 4th ed. Boulder, CO: University of Colorado Press, 2005.

Abel, Emily K. *Suffering in the Land of Sunshine: A Los Angeles Illness Narrative*. New Brunswick, NJ: Rutgers University Press, 2006.

———. *Tuberculosis and the Politics of Exclusion: A History of Public Health and Migration to Los Angeles*. Edited by Rima D. Apple and Janet Golden, *Critical Issues in Health and Medicine*. New Brunswick, NJ: Rutgers University Press, 2007.

Abrams, Jeanne E. *Blazing the Tuberculosis Trail: The Religio-Ethnic Role of Four Sanatoria in Early Denver*. Denver, CO: Colorado Historical Society, 1991.

———. *Dr. Charles David Spivak: A Jewish Immigrant and the American Tuberculosis Movement*. Boulder, CO: University of Colorado Press, 2009.

Barr, Ronald J. *The Progressive Army: US Army Command and Administration, 1870–1914*. New York, NY: St. Martin's Press, 1998.

Bates, Barbara. "Quid Pro Quo in Chronic Illness: Tuberculosis in Pennsylvania, 1876–1926." In *Framing Disease: Studies in Cultural History*, edited by Charles E. Rosenberg and Janet Golden. New Brunswick, NJ: Rutgers University Press, 1992.

———. *Bargaining for Life: A Social History of Tuberculosis, 1876–1938*. Philadelphia, PA: University of Pennsylvania Press, 1992.

Bayne-Jones, Stanhope. *The Evolution of Preventive Medicine in the United States Army, 1607–1939*. Washington, DC: Office of The Surgeon General, 1968.

Budd, Richard M. *Serving Two Masters: The Development of American Military Chaplaincy, 1860–1920*. Lincoln, NE: University of Nebraska Press, 2002.

Byler, Charles A. *Civil-Military Relations on the Frontier and Beyond, 1865–1917*. Westport, CT: Praeger Security International, 2006.

Caldwell, Mark. *The Last Crusade: The War on Consumption*. New York, NY: Atheneum, 1988.

Charmaz, Kathy. *Good Days, Bad Days: The Self in Chronic Illness and Time*. New Brunswick, NJ: Rutgers Unversity Press, 1991.

Clapesattle, Helen. *Dr. Webb of Colorado Springs*. Boulder, CO: Colorado Associated University Press, 1984.

Coker, Richard. *From Chaos to Coercion: Detention and the Control of Tuberculosis*. New York, NY: St. Martin's Press, 2000.

Condrau, Flurin and Michael Worboys. *Tuberculosis Then and Now: Perspectives on the History of an Infectious Disease*. Montreal and Kingston: McGill-Queens University Press, 2010.

Connolly, Cynthia A. *Saving Sickly Children: The Tuberculosis Preventorium in American Life, 1908–1970*. New Brunswick, NJ: Rutgers University Press, 2008.

Cosmas, Graham A., Albert E. Cowdrey, and Center of Military History. *The Medical Department: Medical Service in the European Theater of Operations*. World War II, 50th anniversary commemorative ed, *U.S. Army in World War II*. Washington, DC: Center of Military History, 1992.

Courtwright, David. *Violent Land: Single Men and Social Disorder from the Frontier to the Inner City*. Cambridge, MA: Harvard University Press, 1996.

Cowdrey, Albert E. *Fighting for Life: American Military Medicine in World War II*. New York, NY: Free Press, 1994.

Cunningham, Andrew, and Perry Williams, eds. *The Laboratory Revolution in Medicine*. Cambridge, UK: Cambridge University Press, 1992.

D'Antonio, Patricia. *American Nursing: A History of Knowledge, Authority and the Meaning of Work*. Baltimore, MD: Johns Hopkins University Press, 2010.

Dillingham, Walter P. *Federal Aid to Veterans, 1917–1941*. Tallahassee, FL: University of Florida Press, 1952.

Dormandy, Thomas. *The White Death: A History of Tuberculosis*. New York, NY: New York University Press, 1999.

Dubos, René, and Jean Dubos. *The White Plague: Tuberculosis, Man, and Society*. New Brunswick, NJ: Rutgers University Press, 1952, 1987.

Duffy, John. *The Sanitarians: A History of American Public Health*. Champaign, IL: University of Illinois Press, 1990.

Eisner, Marc Allen. *From Warfare State to Welfare State: World War I, Compensatory State Building and the Limits of Modern Order*. University Park, PA: Pennsylvania State University Press, 2000.

Fairchild, Amy L., Ronald Bayer, and James Colgrove, with Daniel Wolfe. *Searching Eyes: Privacy, the State, and Disease Surveillance in America*. Berkeley, CA: University of California Press, 2007.

Feldberg, Georgina D. *Disease and Class: Tuberculosis and the Shaping of Modern North American Society*. New Brunswick, NJ: Rutgers University Press, 1995.

Fishbein, Morris, ed. *Doctors at War*. New York, NY: E. P. Dutton and Company, 1945.

Fitzsimons, Office of Public Affairs. *Fitzsimons Army Medical Center: The Life and History, 1918–1996*. Aurora, CO: Fitzsimons Army Medical Center, 1998.

Gamble, Vanessa Northington. *Germs Have No Color Line*. New York, NY: Garland Publishing, 1989.

Gandy, Matthew, and Alimuddin Zumla, eds. *The Return of the White Plague: Global Poverty and the 'New' Tuberculosis*. London, UK: Verso, 2003.

Geitner, Lawrence et al. *Ending Neglect: The Elimination of Tuberculosis in the United States*. Edited by Committee on the Elimination of Tuberculosis in the United States, Division of Health Promotion and Disease Prevention, Institute of Medicine. Washington, DC: National Academy Press, 2000.

Gerber, David A. *Disabled Veterans in History*. Ann Arbor, MI: University of Michigan Press, 2000.

Gillett, Mary C. *The Army Medical Department, 1865–1917*. Washington, DC: Center of Military History, 1995.

_____. *The Army Medical Department, 1917-1941*. Washington, DC: Center of Military History, 2009.

Ginn, Richard V. N. *The History of the U.S. Army Medical Service Corps*. Washington, DC: Office of The Surgeon General and Center of Military History, 1997.

Goode, Paul R. *The United States Soldiers' Home: A History of Its First Hundred Years*. Richmond, VA: [Publisher unknown], 1957.

Greenwood, John T., and F. Clifton Berry, Jr. *Medics at War: Military Medicine from Colonial Times to the 21st Century*. Annapolis, MD: Naval Institute Press, 2005.

Harrison, Mark. "Medicine and the Management of Modern Warfare." *History of Science* 34 (December 1996): 379–410.

Howell, Joel. *Technology in the Hospital: Transforming Patient Care in the Early Twentieth Century*. Baltimore, MD: Johns Hopkins University Press, 1995.

Huzar, Elias. *The Purse and the Sword: Control of Army by Congress Through Military Appropriations, 1933–1950*. Ithaca, NY: Cornell University Press, 1950.

Iseman, Michael D. *A Clinician's Guide to Tuberculosis*. Philadelphia, PA: Lippincott Williams & Wilkins, 2000.

Jones, Billy. *Health Seekers in the Southwest, 1817–1900*. Norman, OK: University of Oklahoma Press, 1967.

Karsten, Peter. *Soldiers and Society: The Effects of Military Service and War on American Life*. Abingdon, UK: Greenwood Press, 1978.

Kelly, Patrick J. *Creating a National Home: Building the Veterans' Welfare State, 1860–1900*. Cambridge, MA: Harvard University Press, 1997.

———. "Establishing a Federal Entitlement." In *The Civil War Veteran: A Historical Reader*, edited by Larry M. Logue and Michael Barton. New York, NY: New York University Press, 2007.

Kevles, Bettyann Holtzmann. *Naked to the Bone: Medical Imaging in the Twentieth Century*, *Sloan Technology Series*. New Brunswick, NJ: Rutgers University Press, 1997.

Killigrew, John W. *The Impact of the Great Depression on the Army*. Bloomington, IN: Indiana University Press, 1979.

Kleinman, Arthur. *The Illness Narratives: Suffering, Healing, and the Human Condition*. New York, NY: Basic Books, 1988.

Koistinen, Paul A. C. *Mobilizing for Modern War. The Political Economy of American Warfare, 1865–1919*. Lawrence, KS: University Press of Kansas, 1997.

Lee, Harriet S., and Myra L. McDaniel. *Army Medical Specialist Corps*. Washington, DC: Office of The Surgeon General, Department of the Army, 1968.

Lerner, Barron H. *Contagion and Confinement: Controlling Tuberculosis along Skid Row*. Baltimore, MD: Johns Hopkins University Press, 1998.

Linker, Beth O'Donnell. *War's Waste: Rehabilitation in World War I America*. Chicago, IL: University of Chjcago Press, 2011.

Longmore, Paul, and Lauri Umansky, eds. *The New Disability History: American Perspectives*. New York, NY and London, UK: New York University Press, 2001.

Marks, Harry M. *The Progress of Experiment: Science and Therapeutic Reform in the United States, 1900–1990*. Cambridge, UK: Cambridge University Press, 1997.

McQuien, Carolyn June. "Tuberculosis as Chronic Illness in the United States: Understanding, Treating, and Living with the Disease, 1884–1954." Ph.D. Dissertation, University of Texas at Austin, 1993.

Melosh, Barbara. *"The Physician's Hand": Work Culture and Conflict in American Nursing*. Philadelphia, PA: Temple University Press, 1982.

Molina, Natalia. *Fit to be Citizens? Public Health and Race in Los Angeles, 1879–1939*. Berkeley, CA: University of California Press, 2006.

Ortiz, Stephen R. *Veterans' Policies, Veterans' Politics*. Gainesville, FL: University of Florida Press, 2012.

Ott, Katherine. *Fevered Lives: Tuberculosis in American Culture Since 1870*. Cambridge, MA: Harvard University Press, 1996.

Phalen, James M. "Chiefs of the Medical Department, U.S. Army, 1775–1940." *Army Medical Bulletin* 52 (April 1940): 88–93.

Plante, Trevor K. "Genealogy Notes: The National Home for Disabled Volunteer Soldiers." *Prologue* 36, no. 1 (Spring 2004): 56–61.

Porter, Bruce D. *War and the Rise of the State: The Military Foundations of Modern Politics*. New York, NY: The Free Press, 1994.

Reiser, Stanley Joel., ed. *Medicine and the Reign of Technology*. Cambridge, UK: Cambridge University Press, 1978.

Reverby, Susan M. *Ordered to Care: The Dilemma of American Nursing: 1850–1945*. Cambridge, UK: Cambridge University Press, 1987.

Robbins, Jessica. "Class Struggles in Tubercular World: Nurses, Patients, and Physicians, 1903–1915." *Bulletin of the History of Medicine* 71, no. 3 (Fall 1997): 412–34.

Rogers, Frank B. "The Rise and Decline of Altitude Therapy of Tuberculosis." *Bulletin of the History of Medicine* 43 (1969): 1-16.

Rosenberg, Charles E. *The Care of Strangers: The Rise of America's Hospital System*. New York, NY: Basic Books, 1987.

———. ed. *Explaining Epidemics and Other Studies of the History of Medicine*. Cambridge, UK: Cambridge University Press, 1992.

Rosenkrantz, Barbara Gutman, ed. *From Consumption to Tuberculosis: A Documentary History*. New York, NY: Garland Publishing, 1994.

Rosner, David. *A Once Charitable Enterprise: Hospital and Health Care in Brooklyn and New York, 1885–1915*. Cambridge, UK: Cambridge University Press, 1982.

Rothman, Sheila. *Living in the Shadow of Death: Tuberculosis and the Social Experience of Illness in American History*. New York, NY: Basic Books, 1994.

Sarnecky, Mary T. *A History of the U.S. Army Nurse Corps*. Philadelphia, PA: University of Pennsylvania Press, 1999.

Shorter, Edward. *Doctors and Their Patients: A Social Study*. New Brunswick, NJ: Transaction Publishers, 1985, 1991.

Skocpol, Theda. *Protecting Soldiers and Mothers: The Political Origins of Social Policy in the United States*. Cambridge, MA: Belknap Press of Harvard University Press, 1992.

Stevens, Rosemary. *American Medicine and the Public Interest*. New Haven, CT: Yale University Press, 1971.

———. *In Sickness and in Wealth: American Hospitals in the Twentieth Century*. New York, NY: Basic Books, Inc., 1989.

Stover, Earl F. *Up From Handyman: The United States Army Chaplaincy, 1865–1920*. Vol. III. Washington, DC: Office of the Chief of Chaplains, Department of the Army, 1977.

Teller, Michael E. *The Tuberculosis Movement: A Public Health Campaign in the Progressive Era*. New York, NY: Greenwood Press, 1988.

Vogel, Morris J., and Charles E. Rosenberg. *The Therapeutic Revolution: Essays in the Social History of American Medicine*. Philadelphia, PA: University of Pennsylvania Press, 1979.

Weber, Gustavus A., and Laurence F. Schmeckebier. *The Veterans' Administration: Its History, Activities, and Organization*. Washington, DC: Brookings Institution, 1934.

Index

A

Abbot, Stephen, 51
Active tuberculosis, 176
Adams, Alva, 233, 246
Adjusted Compensation Act of 1924, 165
AEF. *See* American Expeditionary Forces
African Americans
    Buffalo Soldiers, 1–3, 13, 57, 128–130
    Fort Bayard patients, 56–57
    segregation of hospital wards, 128–130, 157
Agnes Memorial Sanatorium, 157
Alcohol therapy, 61
Alcoholism
    effect on tuberculosis rates, 8–10
    Fort Bayard issues, 66–67
Alexander, John, 183
AMA. *See* American Medical Association
American Association of Immunologists, 117
American College of Chest Physicians, 155, 319
American College of Surgeons, 159
American Epidemiological Society, 320–321
American Expeditionary Forces
    autopsy program, 119–120
    false positive tuberculosis tests, 115–116
    rejection rate due to tuberculosis, 115
    tuberculosis among soldiers, 115–121
    tuberculosis hospitals, 106, 117–118
American Federation of Labor, 261
American Legion, 169, 238, 302
American Medical Association, 18, 61, 106
American Nurses Association Relief Fund, 217
American Red Cross, 106, 129, 158, 290
American Sanatorium Association, 182
ANC. *See* Army Nurse Corps

Antibiotics, 321–333
Antituberculosis programs, 5, 158–59
Antituberculosis serum, 18
Appel, Maj. Daniel M.
    conference presentation on first two years of Fort Bayard tuberculosis hospital, 18
    court martial trial, 18–19, 21
    death of, 21
    establishment of hospital at Fort Bayard, 1, 12–13
    fraud and conspiracy charges, 18–19, 21
    hospital regimen, 14–15
    hospital staff management, 19–20
    leadership issues, 20–21
    life history, 12
    newspaper quotes, 19
    transfer to the Philippines, 21
Appel, Robert, 47
Army and Navy General Hospital, 11
Army Appropriation Bill, 254
Army Medical Department
    budget cuts during the Great Depression, 236–237
    budget shortages, 162–165
    disability discharges, 189–191
    tuberculosis hospitals, 106
    tuberculosis program, 107–115
    tuberculosis screening program, 109–112, 275–279
Army Nurse Corps, 52, 165, 207–216, 315
Army Nurse Reserve Corps, 165
Army of the Buffalo Soldiers, 1–3, 13, 57, 128–130
Army School of Nursing, 105, 237

Arrested tuberculosis, 176
Artificial pneumothorax, 180–182
Aspinall, Wayne N., 256
Associated Editors of Tuberculosis Publications, 158
Association of the Military Surgeons of the United States, 18
Auscultation chart, 60
Aycock, Lt. Col. George, 221, 278
Aynes, Maj. Edith A., 213

B

Babcock, Capt. Walter C., 72
Bacille Calmette-Guerin, 220
Badger, Col. Theodore, 280–282, 288–289
Baker, Newton, 135
Baker, Pvt. Charles F., 66
Ball, Laurence, 294
Balzer, William H., 290–291
Bankhead, Billy, 252
Bankhead, Florence, 319
Barney, Capt. Charles, 41, 51, 69, 91
Bartlett, Zilpha, 216
Base hospitals, 117–118
Bassett, Harold, 135
Bateman, Cephas, 42–43, 51, 55, 65, 67–68
Battle of Fredericksburg, 3
Battle of the Bulge, 283
Bayard, Brig. Gen. George D., 3
BCG, *See* Bacille Calmette-Guerin
Belanger, Helene, 212, 213, 222
Benefits. *See* Veterans benefits
Bier, Robert A., 175
Biggs, Hermann M., 5
Black, Robert L., 221
Black Regulars, 3
Blanton, Thomas L., 250
Blivins, Clara, 54
Bloombergh, Carl, 111
Bloombergh, Lt. H. D., 20
Bonus Act, 165
Booth, 1st Lt. Olin R., 55
Bradley, Harry C., 48
Branson, Mrs. Donald P., 48
Brewer, George, 114
Brooke, Col. Roger, 138, 253
Brown, Lawrason, 186, 188
Brown, Wilmot E., 56
Browning, Col. William S., 239
Bruns, Caroline, 39
Bruns, Col. Earl H.
    appointment as head of Fort Bayard, 105
    as chief of medical services at Fitzsimons General Hospital, 160, 164
    concern related to manageability of large hospitals, 159–162
    death of, 191
    evaluation of American Expeditionary Forces in Europe, 111
    health deterioration, 190
    medical duty at Fort Bayard, 49, 59, 61–62
    as rehabilitation advocate, 172–173
    tuberculosis illness, 39–40, 55, 160
    tuberculosis instruction for medical officers, 175–178, 180
    use of heliotherapy, 178–180
Bruns General Hospital, 285–286
Bubb, Capt. Charles B.B., 190
Buck, Col. Carroll S., 191, 239–240, 246–249
Buffalo Soldiers, 1–3, 13, 57, 128–130
Bullock, T.S., 14, 18
Bumgarner, John R., 291
Bureau of War Risk Insurance, 167–168
Burns, Joe, 250
Burro Mountain Copper Company, 122
Bushnell, Col. George Ensign
    appointment to Army Medical Department's tuberculosis section, 26–27
    approach to tuberculosis treatment, 40
    Army tuberculosis program, 107–115
    death of, 141
    establishment of the Office of Tuberculosis, 105
    grounds management at Fort Bayard, 43
    health deterioration, 138
    hospital construction management, 43–47
    hospital regimen, 27–28, 57–65
    leadership of hospital at Fort Bayard, 2, 24, 25–28, 42–43, 66–68
    life history, 26
    medical staff, 49–54
    patient discipline, 65–68
    provision of sanctuary for tuberculosis patients, 54–57
    recruiting of tuberculosis specialists, xi
    retirement of, 140–141
    screening soldiers for tuberculosis, 106
    treatment of Congressman George Legare's illness, 88—94
    tuberculosis illness, 26, 41–42
    tuberculosis immunity theory, 107–109, 120–121
    tuberculosis screening program, 109–112

C

Carrington, Paul M., 18, 50
Casper, Maj. Joseph, 183–184
CCC. *See* Civilian Conservation Corps
Chamberlain, Col. W.P., 190–191
Chamberlain, George E., 135
Chamberlain, J.L., 139
Chapin, Charles V., 218

Chatel Guyon, France
    Base Hospital No. 20, 118
Chemical weapons
    studies on effect of tuberculosis incidence, 119
Chenoweth, John, 262
Chest X-rays, 276–277, 279, 300
Circular No. 20, 109–110, 112, 117
Civilian Conservation Corps, 256–258
Clayton, Col. Jere B., 121–122, 125, 135
Clement, Thomas G., 137
Climatology, 5
Cochrane, Capt. A.L., 290
Collapse therapy, 180–182
Collins, Lt. Robert L., 20, 24, 28
Collins, Ross A., 249, 251–252
Comegys, Lt. Col. Edward
    death of, 25
    leadership issues, 22–24
    leadership of hospital at Fort Bayard, 1–2, 22–25
    malaria illness, 22
    retirement of, 24–25
    transfer to the Philippines, 24
Commission for the Prevention of Tuberculosis in France, 106
Committee on World War Veterans' Legislation, 169–170
Concentration camps, 292–298
Condé, Marlette, 209
Connor, P. James, 316, 332
Conroy, Pvt. Bernard, 56
Constantine, Joseph, 240
Cooley, Alford W., 47
Cooper, Lt. Col. Alexander, 182–183
Corbin, H.C., 25
Costigan, Edward, 246
Creed of the Disabled Soldier, 172
Culberson, C.A., 70
Cumming, Surg. Gen. Hugh S., 167
Cunningham, George, 57

D

Dachau concentration camp, 292–298
Daniel, Thomas, 224
Davidson, Lt. Col. Douglas Treat, 300
Davis, Charles E., 127
Defense Base Realignment and Closure Act, 330
Delano, Jane, 52
Deming, Dorothy, 222–223
Denison, Charles, 5
Denver, Colorado. *See also* Fitzsimons General Hospital
    General Hospital No. 21, 132–137, 139
    as urban community, 157–158
Denver Civic and Commercial Association, 132–133
Dern, George, 236, 254–256
Diack, Maj. Samuel L., 282
Diemer, F.E., 110
Dirks, Sedrick, 53–54
Disability benefits, 169–171
Disability discharges, 189–191
Disabled American Veterans, 169
Division of Internal Medicine, 105
Domagk, Gerhard, 326–327
Dormandy, Thomas, 188
Douglas, Louis W., 243–244
Drolet, George J., 328
Drum, Margaret, 14
Dublin, Louis, 302
Duffey, James, 67
Dunham, Kenneth, 170–171
Dunn, William LeRoy, 170–171
Dustbowl of 1933-39, 241
Dysentery
    effect on tuberculosis rates, 9–10

E

Economy Act, 238–239, 242, 245–246, 249
Edson, Carroll E., 57
EH. *See* Evacuation hospitals
Eisenhower, Dwight D., 330
Elliot, Walter, 51
Ellis, A.E., 181–182
European theater of war
    tuberculosis in, 283
Evacuation hospitals, 294
Evangelical Lutheran Sanitarium, 6, 157
Evanka, John, 135
Extensively drug resistant tuberculosis, 333

F

Farley, James A., 243
Federal Board for Vocational Education, 168
Federal Board of Hospitalization, 245, 248, 251–252, 254, 258, 301
Fike, Joseph, 55
Finney, Will, 57
Finsen, Niels Ryber, 177
Fishberg, Maurice, 109
Fisk, Samuel, 5
Fitzsimons, Lt. William, 139–140
Fitzsimons General Hospital
    antibiotic studies, 322–323
    the antituberculosis movement, 158–159
    approval of new construction, 255–256
    budget cuts during the Great Depression, 238–239
    budget shortages, 162–164
    closure of, 330–331
    Col. Buck as hospital commander, 191,

239–240, 246–249
    construction of new hospital, 258–263
    dedication of new hospital, 250–263
    description of, 159–162
    disability discharges, 189–191
    invasive tuberculosis therapies, 178–189
    nurses, 210–217, 221
    President Roosevelt's visit in 1936, 233–235
    rate of patient admissions, 155–156
    rehabilitation of patients, 172–174
    renaming of General Hospital No. 21, 139–140
    Rep. Lewis' efforts to keep hospital open, 241–246
    repair and renovation estimates, 239
    School for Medical Technicians, 285
    threats to close hospital during the Great Depression, 239–240, 249–255
    treatment of prisoners of war, 287–288
    treatment regimes table, 327
    tuberculosis protective practices, 319
    twenty-fifth anniversary, 225
    urban environment of, 157–158
    use during World War II, 283–286
Fitzsimons Life Science District, 331
Flick, Lawrence, 41, 65
Forbes, Col. Charles R., 168
Forsee, Col. James H., 220–221, 323–325
Fort Bayard, New Mexico
    African American patients, 56–57, 128–130
    alcohol abuse, 66–67
    building style, 44
    child patients, 48
    civilian laborers, 54
    civilian patients, 47–48
    classes of patients, 14
    closing of, 137–141
    criticisms of hospital during World War I, 121–126
    departure from, 69–73, 96–101
    desertion rate, 39
    establishment of, 2–3
    expansion to accommodate Navy patients, 21
    female patients, 48
    funding sources, 48–49
    grounds management, 43
    hospital construction, 43–47
    hospital personnel, 14, 43
    hospital regimen, 14–15, 27–28
    increase in number of hospitalized patients, 121–131
    leadership of, 1–2
    lifestyle of patients, 65–68, 94–96
    location of, 2–3
    map showing temporary structures during wartime emergency, 123
    medical officers, 49–51
    military personnel and beneficiaries as patients, 47
    morale issues, 66
    nurses, 52–53
    nurses' residence, 46
    patient discipline, 65–68
    patient education, 15–16
    patient statistics, 43
    physical plant, 43–47
    as sanctuary to tuberculosis patients, 54–57
    staff, 51–54
    transformation to tuberculosis hospital, 1, 4–6, 11–13
    treatment for tuberculosis patients, 57–65, 92–94
Fort Bayard National Cemetery, 56, 57, 72
Fort Stanton, New Mexico
    establishment of sanatorium, 11
    medical officers, 49–50
    patient survival rates, 65
France
    Base Hospitals, 117–118
    incidence of tuberculosis among soldiers, 105–106
Frost, Wade Hampton, 223–225

G

Garrard, Iris, 315
Gaule, Lt. John, 316
Gaule, Margaret E. Wall, 315–318, 331–332
General hospitals, 125–131
Gil, Pvt. Cornie, 130
Ginther, Stanley, 137
Glomsett, D.J., 120
Goldberg, Benjamin, 155, 276
Gonorrhea
    average hospital patient-days, 175
Goodrich, Annie, 124
Gorgas, Surg. Gen. William C., 26, 48, 105, 129
Gosling, Robert J., 185
Graham, Evarts C., 188–189
Granger, Edward W., 126
Great Depression
    Army Medical Department budget cuts, 236–238
    Rep. Lewis' efforts to keep Fitzsimons General Hospital open, 241–246
    threats to close Fitzsimons General Hospital, 239–240, 249–255
    War Department budget cuts, 235–236
Great Lakes Construction Company, 259
Green, Cleveland, 285
Greenlee, Maj. D.P., 284

Greer, Jean, 316
Gregg, William, 56
Gridley, Charles O., 242, 244, 250, 259
Grow, Col. John B., 284–285
Gun, Nerin, 295, 297
Gurley, Helen Kress, 48

H

Hagenmeister, Lt. Wolfgang, 287
Hall, Lt. Midge, 212–213
Hammer, Maj. William J., 126
Hammond, J.F., 111
Hardaway, Col. Robert M., 191
Harding, Warren G., 137
Harlow, William P., 133, 135
Hauch, Martha A., 205–207
Hause, William E., 135
Hawley, Maj. Gen. Paul R., 280, 282, 289, 300–301
Hayden, Carl, 114
Health benefits. *See* Veterans benefits
Heasley, Edward, 48
Heasley, Mrs. Edward C., 48
Heflebower, 1st Lt. Roy C., 50, 63
Heimbeck, Johannes, 217
Heliotherapy, 177–180
Henderson, First Lt. Albert B., 16–17
Henderson, Pvt. Albert, 20
Hendricks, C.M., 276
Henry Phipps Institute for the Study, Prevention and Treatment of Tuberculosis, 273
Herbst, Steward, 19
Hernandez, Lt. Pedro A., 55
Heroin, 61
Heyl, Col. Charles H., 24
Hill, Samuel, 71
Hill-Burton Act of 1946, 258
Hillman, Brig. Gen. Charles, 276–277
Hines, Gen. Frank T., 168, 171, 242, 244
Hines, John L., 141
HIV/AIDS, 331–332
Hoagland, Henry W., 167
Hoffman, Capt. Stanley H., 322
Holderness-Brunson treatment, 177
Holliday, John Henry, 4
Holmberg, Maj. Carl, 111, 128, 131
Holmes, Charles S., 242
Hoover, Herbert, 168
Hospital Corps, 52–54
Hospitals. *See* Tuberculosis hospitals
Howard, Col. Francis E., 287
Howe, Louis M., 244, 256
Hutton, Col. Paul C., 17, 68, 111, 126, 162–163, 191
Hyman, Capt. George A., 322

Hynes, Frank, 277

I

Influenza epidemic, 130–131
Invasive therapies, 174–189
Ireland, Surg. Gen. Merritte, 122, 126, 139, 164, 186, 208
Irons, Maj. James A., 20–21
Iseman, Michael, 321, 328
Isoniazid, 326–328, 333

J

Jablon, Seymour, 300
Jahr, Rhoda, 213
Jamme, Anna C., 124
Jewish Consumptives' Relief Society, 6, 157
Johnson, Capt. Thomas H., 51, 64, 66
Johnson, Col. Howard H., 136, 137
Johnson, Edwin C., 191, 233, 241
Johnson, Joseph, 101
Johnson, Pvt. Richard, 39–40, 52, 59–60, 68, 70
Johnston, L.C., 55
Jones, Lt. Edgar, 66
Jones, William, 57

K

Kane, Thomas L., 66
Kearns, Howard F., 137
Keating, Pvt. Walter P., 115
Kelley, Lt. Col. Dennis E., 288
King, Col. Donald S., 281
Kinney, Dita H., 20
Klebs, Arnold, 58
Knights of Columbus, 129–130
Knopf, Alfred, 131
Koch, Robert
    tuberculin discovery, 61
    tuberculosis bacilli identification, xvii, 5
Koerper, Capt. Conrad, 62, 111
Ku Klux Klan, 157

L

LaGuardia, Fiorella, 247
Larisey, H.L., 100
League of Nations, 132
Legare, George
    arrival at Fort Bayard, 85
    death of, 100–101
    letters to wife, 85–100
    life history, 87–88
    tuberculosis illness, 47, 85–101
Legare, Mary Frances Izlar, 85–100
Lehman, Jorgen, 326
Lerner, Barron, 223
Lever, Asbury, 101
Lewis, John L., 261

Lewis, Lawrence, 191, 233–235, 241–254, 260–262, 331
Lewis, W.F., 133
Limited Service Corps, 172
Lindsay, William J., Jr., 331–332
Lipow, Maj. E.G., 296
Locke, Frances Lafaye, 216
Logan, Walter B., 101
Long, Esmond R., 42, 121, 220, 224, 273–279, 297–301, 321–322
Long, Pvt. Edward, 17
Longworth, Nicholas, 52
Lovell, Robert, 219
Loving, Capt. R.S., 219
Lowell, Anthony M., 328
Lurie, Max B., 319–320
Lusk, Lt. Oscar, 70

M

MacArtan, Neill, 135
MacArthur, Gen. Douglas, 212, 236, 239–242, 244–245, 253, 256
Macon, John, 135
MacRae, R.D., 110
Magee, Maj. Gen. James C., 260, 261, 273
Malaria
  effect on tuberculosis rates, 9–10
Mann, Thomas, 182
Mariette, Ernst S., 219
Marshall, Gen. George C., 236, 289
Martin, John A., 233
Matson, Ralph C., 110
McAdoo, William, 166
McAfee, Brig. Gen. Larry B., 286
McAfee, Loy, 249
McCann, Matthew, R., 129
McCarty, Medora, 71
McCormack, John, 262
McCrae, Thomas, 111
McDill, Maj. John, 22
McGovern, Joseph, 67–68
McHale, Alberta M., 216
McIntyre, Marvin H., 233, 250–252
McKean, Capt. George T., 281
McKee, E.R., 135
McKinley, William, 26
McNalty, Arthur S., 274
McNett, Esta H., 216, 320
McQueen, Sgt. Homer, 61–64, 71–72, 98
MDR-TB. *See* Multi-drug resistant tuberculosis
Medical Administrative Corps, 236
Mediterranean theater of war
  tuberculosis in, 279–281, 283
Memford, Edgar W., 164
Metropolitan Life Insurance Company, 302

Miller, Pvt. Clarence, 54
Miller, Watson, 186
Minor, Charles L., 26, 57, 58–59, 127, 212
Moncrief, Col. William H., Sr., 162–164, 167, 189
Moore, R. Walton, 206
Moore General Hospital, 300–301
Morissette, William, 135
Morphine, 61
Multi-drug resistant tuberculosis, 332–333
Munson, Maj. Edmund
  efforts to control alcoholism rates, 9
  tuberculosis illness, 49
Munson, Maj. Edward L., 17
Murphy, Pvt. Peter, 12
Murray, Alexander, 48
Murry, Leslie, 109
Myers, J. Arthur, 217–218, 223, 224

N

National Association for the Study and Prevention of Tuberculosis, 5–6, 59
National Defense Act of 1940, 275
National Home for Disabled Voluntary Soldiers, 10, 67–68
National Jewish Hospital for Consumptives, 6, 65, 157, 330
National Research Council, 274, 276, 321–323
National Swedish Hospital, 157
National Tuberculosis Association, 120–121, 141, 158, 175, 217, 258, 319–320
Nazi concentration camps, 292–298
Neuman, James E., 291
New Deal programs, 255–261
New Mexico. *See* Fort Bayard, New Mexico
Nightingale, Florence, 6, 207, 210
North Africa theater of war
  tuberculosis in, 279–282
Noyes, Charles, 69
Nursing
  Army Nurse Corps, 52, 165, 207–216
  Army Nurse Reserve Corps, 165
  Army School of Nursing, 105
  nurses at Fort Bayard, New Mexico, 46, 52–53
  transmission of tuberculosis, 216–223
  tuberculosis nursing, 210–223

O

O'Brien, Reta M., 214
Office of The Surgeon General
  budget cuts during the Great Depression, 239, 249
  dissatisfaction with Comegys, 22
Office of Tuberculosis, 105

O'Grady, F., 320
Ohlinger, Loren, 24
O'Reilly, Surg. Gen. Robert M., 22, 24
Osler, William, 9, 108
Oteen, North Caroline
    General Hospital No. 19, 125, 138
Otis, Edward O., 108
Otisville, New York
    General Hospital No. 8, 125–127, 129–130
OTSG. *See* Office of The Surgeon General
Ozone treatment, 177

P

Palmer, George T., 109, 167
Panama Canal, 47–48
Para-aminosalicylate, 326–328
Parks, Roy, 134–135
Parks, Tilman B., 250
PAS. *See* Para-aminosalicylate
Patterson, Surg. Gen. Robert U., 190–191, 236–246, 249–255, 257
Peabody, Mrs. George, 135
Penicillin, 321
Pershing, John, 4
Petersen, Pvt. Charles, 54
Philippine Scouts, 9
Phrenectomy, 182–183
PHS. *See* Public Health Service
Piatt, A.D., 297
Plummer, Samantha C., 122, 124–125
Pneumothorax, artificial, 180–182
Poison gases
    studies on effect of tuberculosis incidence, 119
Pollock, William, 220–221
Portland, Oregon
    General Hospital No. 46, 289–290
Post Hospital, Fort Bayard, NM, 15
Pott's Disease, 179
Powers, E.F., 135
Powers, Lt. Robert, 13–14
POWs. *See* Prisoners of war
Presidio, 11, 70
Principles and Practice of Medicine, 9
Prisoners of war
    enemy POWs with tuberculosis, 286–288
    recovered American POWs, 290–292
Public Health and Marine Hospital Service, 11
Public Health Service, 49–50, 138, 167–168, 223, 258, 277
Public Works Administration, 255, 257, 259
Puffer, Ruth Rice, 224
PWA. *See* Public Works Administration

Q

Quade, Brig. Gen. Omar H., 263, 284

Quezon, Manuel, 212
Quiescent tuberculosis, 176

R

Racial segregation, 128–130, 157
Rafferty, Maj. Ogden, 71
Rankin, John, 171
Red Scare, 132
Reece, Carroll, 170
Rehabilitation benefits, 171–174
Rest therapy, 57–65
Reynolds, Col. Charles, 254–255, 258–259
Rifampicin, 333
Riley, Richard L., 320
Rixey, Surg. Gen. Presley M., 21, 47
Robbins, Hugh T., 66
Robbins, Walter, 61
Robert, H.R., 51
Robertson, H.E., 120
Rockefeller Foundation, 106
Rockhill, Lt. Col. Edward P., 122, 124, 128, 130
Rockwell, Robert F., 262
Rollier, Augusto, 177
Roosevelt, Eleanor, 258
Roosevelt, Franklin, 233–235, 238, 242, 245–249, 256–258, 273, 292
Roosevelt, Theodore, 6, 43
Root, Elihu, 21, 26–27
Ross, Leon, 57
Ross, Marion Ruth, 216
Ross, Steve, 296–297
Ross, William, 57
Rossiter, Surg. Gen. Percival S., 244–245
Rotzien, Mable Marie, 216
Roundtree, Hazel L., 286
Ruble, Minnie H., 20

S

Sanatoriums. *See also* Tuberculosis hospitals
    establishment of, 6, 11
Sanocrysin, 175
Sauerbruch, Ferdinand, 183
Savenay, France
    Base Hospital No. 8, 118
Schatz, Albert, 321
Scott, Capt. George, 50
Scott, Edyth M., 216
Scott, Maj. T.E., 219
Seibert, Florence B., 220
Sepkowitz, Kent, 206
Sexually transmitted diseases
    average hospital patient-days, 174–175
    effect on tuberculosis rates, 8–9
Sheehan, Mary, 213
Shepard, Maj. Charles A., 247
Shreiner, E.R., 136

Siler, Col. Joseph, 189
Sims, Demet C., 135
Skin tests, 220
Smith, Allen M., 126
Smith, Capt. Marcus J., 292–294, 296
Smith, Pvt. Horace, 57
Social Security, 258
Soldiers' Home, 9, 10, 47, 67–69, 166, 238
Sorensen, Helene, 212, 222
Spahlinger Cure, 175
Spanish-American War
    disease death rates, 10–11
Special Committee on World War Veterans Legislation, 169–170
Spit cups, 16
State homes, 10
Steele, Capt. Charles L., 16
Sternberg, Brig. Gen. George
    choice of Appel as commander of Fort Bayard tuberculosis hospital, 12
    efforts to control tuberculosis, 7–11
    report to Secretary of War concerning Fort Bayard tuberculosis hospital, 18
Stethoscope, 225
Stevens, Frederick C., 20
Steward, Luther F., 67
Stewart, Donald, 182
Steyskal, Julies, 52
Stimson, Col. Julia, 208–210, 214, 216, 238
Stimson, Henry, 48, 289
Stratton, Pvt. Virgil E., 284
Streptomycin, 321–328
Strohm, Col. J.G., 289
Sutherland, Halliday, 114
Swedish National Sanitarium for Consumptives, 6
Syphilis
    effect on tuberculosis rates, 9, 64

T

Taft, William H., 47, 85, 88, 92
Taylor, Ed T., 233
Tefft, Capt. W. H., 50, 111
Tempel, Col. Carl W., 323–327, 329
Thayer, William, 117
Thearle, Maj. William, 185–186, 188
Thomas, Pvt. Leslie, 66
Thomason, R.E., 250, 252
Thoracoplasty, 183–189
Thornton, Pvt. Clifford, 12
Townsend, Charles, 88, 101
Treaty of Guadalupe Hidalgo of 1848, 2
Treaty of Versailles, 132
Tropical diseases
    effect on tuberculosis rates, 9–10
Troutman, George W., 115

Trudeau, Edward, 41
Trudeau, Francis, 66
Trudeau Medal, 41
Tuberculin test, 61, 220
Tuberculin therapy, 60–61
Tuberculization theory, 223–224
Tuberculoallergy, 221
Tuberculosis
    antibiotic treatment, 321–333
    antituberculosis serum research, 18
    Army death and illness rates, 7
    chest sounds, 59–60
    classification of, 59
    climate therapy, 4–5
    complications of, 64
    death rates in U.S., xvii–xviii, 64–65
    diagnosis of, xxi, 58–61, 220
    disposition of patients, xxii–xxiii
    etiology, xix–xx
    extensively drug resistant tuberculosis, 333
    immunity theory, xx–xxi, 107–109, 120–121, 220–221, 224, 318
    incidence during World War I, 105, 278
    incidence during World War II, 273, 278, 301
    infection rates in the world population, 333
    invasive therapies for, 174–189
    multi-drug resistant tuberculosis, 332–333
    patient weight loss, 15
    rate of hospital care for veterans post-World War I, 156
    rest therapy, 57–65, 90–91, 177
    screening program, 106, 109–112, 275–279, 300
    transmission of, xx, 70, 318–321
    treatment of, xxi–xxii, 57–65, 92—94, 174–189, 321–333
    vaccine, 220
Tuberculosis hospitals. *See also* specific hospitals
    American Expeditionary Forces, 106
    difficulties during World War I, 125–128
    establishment of, 6
    increase in number of, 125
    racial segregation of wards, 128–130
Turner, Col. G. Soulard, 186–187
Turner, Col. John Wakeman, 318
Tyler, Pvt. Charles, 56–57, 70–71
Typhus, 296–297

U

U.S. Soldiers' Home, 9, 10, 47, 67–69, 166, 238
U.S. Typhus Commission, 296–297

V

Vaccines, 220

Valentine, Lt. Watts C., 10
van Hoff, Col. John R., 21
Van Horn, J.B., 51
Van Valzah, Maj. Shannon, 189, 247–248
Vancouver Barracks Army camp, 315
Vauclair, France
    Base Hospital No. 3, 117–118
Venereal disease
    effect on tuberculosis rates, 8–9, 64
Vestal, Capt. Solomon, 51, 71
Veterans Administration, 155, 238, 302, 329–330
Veterans benefits
    administration of, 166–168
    cuts during the Great Depression, 238
    disability, 169–171
    eligibility of, 168–169
    structuring, 165–166
    tuberculosis rehabilitation, 171–174
Veterans Bonus March of 1932, 165
Veteran's Bureau, 168
Veterans of Foreign Wars, 169
Veterans Rehabilitation Bureau, 167
Vocational Rehabilitation Act of 1918, 172
Vocational training, 172–174
von Pirquet, Clemens, 61

W

Wagner Act, 260
Waksman, Selman, 321
Walkup, Capt. Joseph O., 43, 50
Wall, Margaret E., 315–318, 331–332
Walter Reed Hospital, 11
War Mothers' Homes, 158
War Risk Insurance Act of 1917, 166–167, 171
Waring, Edward, 115
Waring, Ferdinanda Legare, 101
Waring, James, 41, 121, 188, 329
Watkins, Dena, 48
Watson, Corp. Howard O., 72
Waynesville, North Carolina
    General Hospital No. 19, 127–128, 129, 131
Webb, Gerald B., 41, 116–121, 129, 133, 188
Welles, Col. E.M., Jr., 138
Wells, W.F., 319
Wheaton, Clarence L., 111
Whipple Barracks, Arizona
    General Hospital No. 20, 128, 131
White, William Charles, 175
Whitney, Jessamine, 217, 221
Wilkie, Wendell, 261
Wilkins, Fred W., 19
Willing, Joseph, 135
Wilson, Charles, 135
Wilson, Theodore, 47
Wilson, Woodrow, 105, 132
Wisconsin Anti-Tuberculosis Association, 302
Women's Army Corps, 285
Wood, Leonard, 4
Works Progress Administration, 255, 257, 259
World War I
    Army tuberculosis program, 107–115
    autopsy program, 119–120
    closing of Fort Bayard, 137–141
    end of, 132
    false positive tuberculosis tests, 115–116
    incidence of tuberculosis among soldiers, 105, 278
    increase of hospitalized patients in the U.S., 121–131
    influenza epidemic, 130–131
    investigation of postwar hospital, 132–137
    screening soldiers for tuberculosis, 106
    soldier rejection rate due to tuberculosis, 115
    tuberculosis among soldiers, 115–121
World War II
    enemy prisoners of war with tuberculosis, 286–288
    incidence of tuberculosis among soldiers, 273, 278, 301
    Nazi concentration camp survivors, 292–298
    postwar disease, 298–303
    recovered American prisoners of war, 290–292
    refugees with tuberculosis, 288–292
    tuberculosis in the theaters of war, 279–283
    tuberculosis screening program, 275–279
    use of Fitzsimons General Hospital, 283–286
World War Veterans Act of 1924, 169
WPA. *See* Works Progress Administration
Wright, Col. Frederick, 261, 301

X

XDR-TB. *See* Extensively drug resistant tuberculosis

Y

YMCA, *See* Young Men's Christian Association
Young, Agnes, 54
Young Men's Christian Association, 129

Z

Zang, Adolph F., 243
Zehm, Abner, 296